Mind/Body Health
The Effect of Attitudes, Emotions and Relationships

FOURTH EDITION

Keith J. Karren

N. Lee Smith

Brent Q. Hafen

Kathryn J. Jenkins

Benjamin Cummings

San Francisco   Boston   New York
Cape Town   Hong Kong   London   Madrid   Mexico City
Montreal   Munich   Paris   Singapore   Sydney   Tokyo   Toronto

Acquisitions Editor: *Sandra Lindelof*
Assistant Editor: *Jacob Evans*
Managing Editor: *Deborah Cogan*
Production Supervisor: *Mary O'Connell*
Senior Marketing Manager: *Neena Bali*
Manufacturing Buyer: *Jeffrey Sargent*
Cover Designer: *Riezebos Holzbaur Design Group*
Text Designer: *Hespenheide Design*
Production Management and Composition: *Black Dot Group*
Copy Editor: *Black Dot Group*
Proofreader: *Black Dot Group*
Indexer: *Black Dot Group*
Text Printer: *Edwards Brothers Malloy*
Cover Printer: *Edwards Brothers Malloy*
Cover Art: *Brad Yeo Collection / Theispot*

Library of Congress Cataloging-in-Publication Data

Mind/body health : the effects of attitudes, emotions, and relationships / Keith J. Karren . . . [et al.]. —4th ed.
    p. ; cm.
  Includes index.
  ISBN-13: 978-0-321-59642-0
  ISBN-10: 0-321-59642-0
  1. Medicine, Psychosomatic. 2. Emotions—Health aspects. 3. Psychoneuroimmunology. 4. Mind and body. I. Karren, Keith J.
  [DNLM: 1. Psychosomatic Medicine. 2. Attitude to Health. 3. Emotions. 4. Personality. 5. Social Support. WM 90 M662 2010]
  RC49.M522 2010
  616.08—dc22

2009000260

Benjamin Cummings
is an imprint of

www.pearsonhighered.com

ISBN-10: 0-321-59642-0
ISBN-13: 978-0-321-59642-0
4 5 6 7 8 9 10—EBM—15 14 13 12

Contents

PART IV   SPIRITUALITY AND HEALTH

PART V   PERCEPTION AND HEALTH

Preface

The body is the shadow of the soul.

—Marsilio Ficino

Take your mind back 300 years to a simple, rough-hewn dinner table somewhere in colonial North America. Spread out across the table were the bounties of hunt and harvest—the succulent browned flesh of the pheasant, the savory goodness of carrot and parsnip, the robust sweetness of caramelized onions. Plump berries exploded from crusts glazed with milk and sugar, staining the folds of thick muslin used to carry the steaming dishes to the table.

Everywhere was evidence of the gardens, plotted in neat rows between the brick houses, shaded by the towering elms that lined the streets. Their harvest might have looked much like yours and mine—except that no one was eating tomatoes. Tomatoes were "poisonous." Everyone knew they were poisonous. After all, they were a member of the nightshade family, and members of the nightshade family were poisonous.

The fact that the French and Italians were eating plenty of tomatoes without any harmful effects did not encourage colonial Americans to try them. The very thought was an outrage: It simply did not make sense to eat poisonous food. And so America's tables, set by the warm yellow glow of lantern and lamp, peppered the colonies of New England without even a crimson hint of a ripened tomato. It took a rebel to turn the tide. Not until 1820, when Robert Gibbon Johnson ate a tomato on the steps of the courthouse in Salem, New Jersey, and survived, did the people of America slowly start to eat tomatoes. Centuries later, the tomato is prized not only for its flavor, but also for its versatility and nutritional value.

The history of the tomato in colonial America gave rise to what scientists call the tomato effect. It happens when something beneficial is ignored or rejected because it doesn't make sense in light of what we already "know." It gives us tacit permission to turn away from new ideas because they don't fit neatly into the framework we have already constructed with materials we have grown comfortable with. But consider this: We are tethered to that comfortable framework. Its comfort, at once secure and predictable, comes at a heavy price.

Today, the vestiges of colonial America survive only in the villages preserved as museums along the eastern seaboard. In those townships, curators work pits of clay into bricks with their bare feet and spin dense curls of wool into lengths of soft thread. They sit on needlepoint stools and stitch the tucked bodices of aprons by hand, or work the supple reeds that grow along the ditch into a basket for gathering the eggs. They drag thick-bristled brushes through the manes of chestnut horses and repair splintering carriage wheels. In those villages, you will see horehound candy and fresh-brewed ale. You will see cobbled walks and windows of thick-paned glass. You will see muskets and tin toys. But you will not see any tomatoes.

Not so in the rest of this nation—or the world. You've undoubtedly savored the rich pungency of a juicy tomato—either fresh from the garden, sliced and lightly sprinkled with salt, or cooked until thick and ladled over a steaming plate of firm spaghetti noodles. There's nothing poisonous there.

So we ask you to savor the evidence presented in this book. It may challenge notions you have held for a long time. It may ask you to step outside the comfortable framework you have constructed. It may seem to fly in the face of what you have "known" to be true. But, just like the warm tomato you pluck from the vine along the back fence on a languid late August afternoon, there's no poison here. Nothing here will hurt you. On the contrary, you may find information that will change your life, enhance your health, and help you live a richer, fuller existence.

What you find here comes from a new field of medicine that has shattered traditional ideas about sickness—and wellness. For hundreds of years, we have been mired in the paradigm that disease is all about organisms: bacteria and viruses and parasites invade our body, overpower our immunity, and make us sick. For hundreds of years, scientists focused on that premise. As a result, we made giant inroads in the war against communicable disease. Today, smallpox has been virtually wiped out. Polio is unknown in all but third world countries. The diseases that once killed people the world over in epidemic proportions are now controlled by simple antibiotics. We have waged war on the bacteria and viruses and parasites, and it's a war we are winning by increasing margins.

Even then, however, we had precious little information on the human immune system. We knew how to stimulate it with vaccinations and immunizations, how to make it recognize a previously encountered enemy and how to raise the armaments. But we did not know what made it strong. We could not explain why one of two children exposed to the influenza virus remained robust and healthy while the other huddled under layers of patchwork quilts, chattering with the chills of relentless fever.

Nor did we understand how to confront our nation's new killers: chronic maladies like heart disease and cancer that, for the most part, were not caused by microorganisms. These were caused instead by some inherent weakness in the complex physical structure. Just as we could not explain the child who scampered happily through the crackling autumn leaves while his brother lay weakened with the flu, we could not explain why one executive in the office suite had a heart attack—or why one member of the golf foursome was ravaged by cancer. Why not all the executives in all the offices along the winding corridor? And why not all—or none—of the golfers?

Researchers who clamored for the answers did a good job of identifying risk factors. You can probably name most of them. Cigarettes. Obesity. High blood pressure. Lack of exercise. A high-fat diet. Valid as they are, they paint only a small part of the picture. Why? Because they concern themselves with only a small part of the person: the body.

Look in the mirror. What you see is an intricate body composed of complex physical systems that work together to sustain life. What you don't see—but what you know is there, just as surely as if you could see it in the mirrored reflection—is a mind that is marked by eagerness and curiosity, emotions that can change in an instant, a spirit that yearns for meaning, and a personality that sets you apart from every other person on this earth. And thanks to the work of a growing army of researchers, we know that your mind, your emotions, your spirit, and your personality have a profound impact on your body—and are powerful determinants in who stays well and who gets sick.

What started out as a few radical pioneers has swelled into a respected body of scientists who are bringing us the information we need to live longer, healthier lives. You may recognize some of their names: Deepak Chopra, an endocrinologist who has synthesized ancient and modern medicine, physics, and philosophy, teaches that mental awareness results in physical chemistry—and that our reality is a result of our perception. His is a world of "infinite possibilities." Physician Larry Dossey argues that the emotional and mental currency of meaning actually enters the body and alters its cells. His provocative research on the power of prayer has led to large-scale studies that are influencing the direction of medicine. Medical psychologist Joan Borysenko demonstrates how the mind, body, and spirit are inseparably linked—and are at work in the intricacies of human immunity. These ideas at first seem surreal; even Dossey, who has pioneered many of them, admits that they are "stretching our conceptual paradigms to the breaking point."

With that stretch, however, comes discovery. With that stretch comes compelling research and irrefutable scientific evidence that proves that we are all the product of a mind, body, and spirit—and that all three play a critical role in health and wellness.

Some of the evidence is simple: The hormones that are pumped into your bloodstream when you're angry literally corrode the lining of your arteries. Could it be, then, that anger and hostility are as important in the development of heart disease as too many fat-laden meals? Some of the evidence seems to boggle the mind: Every emotion you experience literally creates a chain of molecules that subsequently attaches to immune system cells. Could it be, then, that attitudes of hope and optimism may physically boost immunity?

Scientific studies say so. Researchers who follow thousands of people for a dozen or more years draw inescapable conclusions about how the closeness of their community protects them from heart disease—even in the presence of hearty Italian cooking. Anecdotal evidence says so, too. Renowned researcher Henry Dreher remembers Michael Callen, an intelligent, gritty, compassionate man who lived for twelve years after being diagnosed with AIDS because he rejected its death sentence and concentrated instead on searching for meaning in his life. "I couldn't help but wonder if his personality had contributed to his unexpected survival," Dreher wrote. "The passage of time would only reinforce my suspicion that it had."

What started as a preposterous notion—that the brain and the immune system are interconnected—is now irrefutable fact. What started out as a "fringe" group of eccentric but courageous pioneers has swelled into a burgeoning army of researchers from the fields of medicine, psychology, immunology, endocrinology, and neurology. Because of their careful scientific work, spanning two decades, we know that the nervous, endocrine, and immune systems "talk" to each other in a language that consists of cell products—and that they take their direction from the mind. As Dreher writes, "We can no longer carve up our biological systems into separate work forces based on a false division of labor."

In the pages that follow, you'll read about their amazing discoveries. You'll learn what we know about how emotions and attitudes affect health. Drawing on landmark scientific studies by many distinguished scientists, many of whom are now at the forefront of medical research, we build a solid foundation of evidence that shows the undeniable connection between the mind and the body. You'll see how "negative" emotions such as worry, anxiety, depression, hostility, and anger, when nurtured, can increase susceptibility to disease. You'll discover how "positive" emotions such as optimism, humor, and a fighting spirit can protect your health and help to heal. In exploring the powerful connection between your mind and body, we discuss:

- How your body responds to the way you see yourself and your circumstances
- Why social support, friendship, and strong, stable relationships protect your health
- How different personalities are either prone to, or able to resist, disease
- The scientifically proven changes in your body chemistry, heart rate, and hormones that accompany various attitudes and emotions
- How attitudes and emotions actually affect your immunity from disease

We hope you will be able to see a little bit of yourself in these pages and will be able to make some affirmations about what you will do with the emotions you experience in the course of everyday living. Above all, what is written here may help you learn to appreciate the tremendous healing power of your mind and your heart, and may help you focus both on an appreciation of life itself. Perhaps former Saturday Review editor Norman Cousins said it best in these words:

> An appreciation of life can be a prime tonic for mind and body. Being able to respond to the majesty of the way nature fashions its art—the mysterious designs in the barks of trees, suggesting cave paintings or verdant meadows interrupted by silvery streams; the rich and luminous coloring of carp fish with blues and yellows and crimsons seemingly lit up from within; the bird of paradise flower, an explosion of colors ascending to a triumphant and jaunty crest of orange and purple; the skin of an apple, so thin it defies measurement but supremely protective of its precious substance; they say the climbing trunk of a tree will steer its growth around solid objects coming between itself and the sun; the curling white foam of an ocean wave advancing on the shore, and the way sand repairs and smoothes itself by the receding water; the purring of a kitten perched on your shoulder, or the head of a dog snuggling under your hand; the measured power of Beethoven's Emperor Concerto, the joyous quality of a Chopin nocturne, the serene and stately progression of a Bach fugue, the lyrical designs in a Mozart composition for clarinet and strings; the sound of delight in a young boy's voice on catching his first baseball; and, most of all, the expression in the face of someone who loves you—all these are but a small part of a list of wondrous satisfactions that come with the gift of awareness and that nourish even as they heal.

Acknowledgments

Our lives have collectively been blessed with many wonderful individuals who have made contributions to this fourth edition of *Mind/Body Health*. We were incredibly blessed to have the help of Rilla Leckie, our research assistant, and Hugo Rodier, M.D., our colleague who developed the original nutrition chapter.

A special thanks goes to our dear friend and colleague, Kathy Jenkins, whose writing and editing expertise has made this revision a success.

We also express much gratitude to Sandra Lindelof and Jacob Evans of Benjamin Cummings for positive prodding and requesting excellence. Though this was a challenging process, they kept us on track, helping us keep our goals in sight.

Lastly, we pay tribute to our dear, departed friend and colleague, Dr. Brent Hafen, whose foresight envisioned the importance of this book.

Finally, the many reviewers of this book gave us excellent direction and played an integral part of the revision. Many thanks Susan Rausch, University of Arkansas; Dickie Hill, Abilene Christian University; Holly E. Tatum, Ph.D., Randolph College; Joan Stehle Werner, University Of Wisconsin-Eau Claire; Kris Hammar, Diablo Valley College; Marilyn Dalton, Western Tech College; Susan Rausch, University of Arkansas-Fayetteville; Anna Tacon, Texas Tech University.

Psychoneuroimmunology: The Connection Between the Mind and the Body

Great men are they who see that spiritual force is stronger than any material force, that thoughts rule the world.

—Ralph Waldo Emerson

LEARNING OBJECTIVES

- Define *psychoneuroimmunology.*
- Understand the major historical milestones in the development of mind-body medicine.
- Define the role of and interplay between the brain and the immune system.
- Understand the role of emotions and immunity in major diseases, such as heart disease and cancer.
- Understand the criticisms of mind-body medicine.
- Understand the challenges for mind-body medicine as the century progresses.

In a pronouncement that at first surprised the medical community, if not the lay public, one practitioner proclaimed that an estimated 90 percent of all physical problems have emotional roots. He followed by saying that his estimate was, at best, conservative, but that should not have been an earth-shattering revelation: the link between the mind and the body is something that physicians have intuitively known and written about for centuries.[1]

A growing body of evidence now indicates that virtually every illness—from arthritis to migraine headaches, from the common cold to cancer—is influenced, for good or bad, by how we think and feel. Solid research is now confirming what many physicians have long observed: the state of the mind directly affects physical illness.[2]

There are compelling reasons to address the issue of disease beyond its personal effects. The global impact of physical illness is profound: unprecedented amounts of money are being spent on chronic diseases, such as cardiovascular disease, diabetes, and obesity, with staggering losses in productivity for the nation's economy. As part of the effort to focus on prevention, seemingly disparate lines of research have converged into the discipline of mind-body medicine, a science that examines the relationship between the mind, the emotions, and the body. Mind-body medicine is based on the premise that mental and emotional processes (the mind) can affect physiological function (the body), and a large body of evidence now supports this connection.[3]

A Definition

The scientific investigation of how the brain affects the body's immune cells and how the immune system can be affected by emotions and behavior is called psychoneuroimmunology, a term coined in 1975 by Robert Ader and Nicholas Cohen of New York's University of Rochester. The science of psychoneuroimmunology (PNI) focuses on the integrated information circuit between the mind, the brain, the nervous system, and the immune system and investigates the relationship between psychosocial factors (such as behavior), the central nervous system, the immune system, and disease.[4] What makes PNI different from earlier mind-body models is that it brings the immune system into the equation.

David L. Felten—who discovered a network of nerves leading to the cells of the immune system—underscores the importance of including the immune system in any examination of mind-body medicine. "The field of psychoneuroimmunology, as a scientific discipline—and I'm not talking about people who hang crystals from their rear-view mirrors, I'm talking about hard-core research—is showing that the nervous system and the immune system communicate with each other massively, extensively, and continuously," he says.[5]

As a science, PNI searches for exact mechanisms by which the mind, nervous system, body, and immune system interact.[6] It then provides a scientific framework for research into why disease develops and how the body heals, enjoying the endorsement of the National Institutes of Health and the support of prominent researchers.

Initial PNI research demonstrated convincingly that the brain communicates with the immune system, but research conducted over the ensuing fifteen years showed that the immune system also sends a flow of information to the brain, proving that the immune system is itself a messenger. This evidence, says Steven Maier, director of the Center for Neuroscience at the University of Colorado at Boulder, "says that things that go on in the body can have potent effects on the brain's activity."[7]

Today, PNI has moved beyond folklore, intuition, and speculation into solid scientific evidence. Researchers are proving that the way people think and feel influences the immune system. Immunologists, physiologists, psychiatrists, psychologists, and neurobiologists now work with psychoneuroimmunologists, who focus on the link between the mind, the brain, the nervous system, and the immune system. Candace Pert, visiting professor with the Center for Molecular and Behavioral Neuroscience at Rutgers University, points out that separate disciplines have made it difficult to make progress. As these disciplines come together under the PNI umbrella, she says, "I think we're moving toward a much more interdisciplinary way of looking at things."[8]

A Brief History

The concept of and controversy surrounding the effect of emotions and stress on health are not new; the relationship between physical and psychosocial well-being has existed throughout history and across cultures.[9] The influence of the mind over the body can be traced to the traditions of ancient civilizations, such as the Aztec and the Maya. The integration of the mind, body, and environmental factors has always been part of native Indian medicine throughout the Americas, and, despite having only mere glimpses, some African writings also show evidence of the mind-body connection. It has been widely taught and accepted in Hindu-related practices, Buddhism, shamanism, the Ayurvedic approach, and many others.[10]

More than 4,000 years ago, Chinese physicians noted that physical illness often followed episodes of frustration. Egyptian physicians of the same period prescribed good cheer and an optimistic attitude as ways to avoid poor health. Half a millennium before the birth of Christ, Hippocrates, considered the father of medicine, cautioned physicians that curing a patient required knowledge of the "whole of things," of mind as well as body. That philosophy persisted for hundreds of years. In one of the best-known examples, the Greek physician Galen observed during the second century AD that melancholic women were much more prone to breast cancer than women who were cheerful.

In 600 AD in India, a well-regarded compilation of texts called the Astangahradaya Sustrasthana demonstrated a strong relationship between mental state and disease. The texts counseled physicians to "reject" patients who were "violent, afflicted with great grief, or full of fear." Further, it gave a poor prognosis to patients who were afflicted by intensely negative emotions. The texts warned that emotions such as hatred, violence, grief, and ingratitude are stronger than the body's capability for healthy balance, and those patients who could not abandon their negative emotions create new diseases as fast as a physician can heal an old one.

In 1680, Transylvanian physician Papai Pariz Ferenc reiterated the teachings of Aristotle when he wrote, "When the parts of the body and its humors are not in harmony, then the mind is unbalanced and melancholy ensues, but on the other hand, a quiet and happy mind makes the whole body healthy."[11]

Studies published by Joseph Breuer and Sigmund Freud stated that numerous kinds of mental events have dramatic influence on the body, but this suggested relationship between mental state and disease was not left unchallenged.[12] In the seventeenth century, philosopher-scientist René Descartes advanced his theory of "dualism." He hypothesized that there were two separate substances in the world: matter, which behaved according to physical laws, and spirit, which was dimensionless and immaterial. The body was material, he claimed, and the mind was spiritual. His notion of a fundamental, unbridgeable chasm between the body and the spirit—between the brain and the mind—continued to dominate not only medical philosophy but religious philosophy as well, despite the beliefs of mavericks like Charles Darwin, who advanced the theory that somewhere in the distant development of the species, the nervous system and the immune system had been one and the same.[13]

Most subsequent researchers supported the theory of Descartes, rather than that of Darwin, and it gained momentum throughout the beginning of the twentieth century. Robert Koch, a German country doctor, found that germs cause anthrax in sheep—one of the most significant medical discoveries of the time. In crude experiments, he recovered the anthrax germs from dying sheep, injected them into healthy sheep, and then watched those healthy sheep sicken and die of anthrax.

Since anthrax germs caused only anthrax, and no other disease, Koch theorized that every disease had a simple, specific biological cause: germs. The most respected medical authority of the time, Rudolf Virchow, disagreed; he subscribed to the theory that germs undoubtedly play a role in disease but that many other factors also were involved—such as environment, heredity, nutrition, psychological state, preexisting health, and stress. Despite Virchow's arguments, Koch held stubbornly to his view, and so did most other practitioners of his day.

Attitudes started to change slowly when American physiologist Walter Cannon conducted a series of experiments early in the twentieth century proving that glands in the body respond to stress. His early experiments demonstrated the relationship between stress and the hypothalamus, pituitary, and adrenal glands, and Cannon established himself as a pioneer of the relationship between the body's response to stress and its physiological symptoms. Skepticism about the role of mood, cognitive events, and behavior in influencing the body remained, though, creating a situation in which both physicians and psychologists treated maladies as separate events.

Several decades later, the experiments of Austrian-born physician Hans Selye gave us what we now know as the "fight-or-flight response" to stress.[14] However, it was not until the 1960s that researchers began studying the immune system in earnest. The first time PNI was referred to as a science was in a 1964 paper by G. F. Solomon and R. H. Moos entitled "Emotions, Immunity, and Disease."[15]

The immune system proved to be so complex that researchers were overwhelmed with the task of identifying its parts and functions. The way in which science eventually unraveled the mysteries of the immune system helped define its role in mind-body interactions: initial studies of the immune system focused only on how the system responded to bacteria.[16] That led to discovery of antibody structure and antigen-antibody reactions—which eventually led through several other areas of study and resulted in the realization that the immune system is not autonomous and does not regulate itself. A number of researchers started publishing studies that indicated powerful links between physical disease and factors such as personality, stressful experiences, and mental states.

In 1977, researchers first showed that, when activated, the immune system released an actual product that caused a change in the firing rate of neurons at a specific location of the brain—the hypothalamus. That finding was intriguing, since the hypothalamus activates the brain's communication with the rest of the body.[17]

Not until the 1980s did immunologists finally start formally looking at the growing evidence that there might be anatomical links between the brain, the nervous system, and the immune system. This body of evidence split into three areas of research:

- The interaction between the nervous system, the immune system, and the neuroendrocine system.
- The psychosocial components that influence immunity and their effects on health and disease.
- The influence of immunity on psychological disorders and behavior.

Regarding the first branch of research, J. Edwin Blalock proposed a theory in 1985 that the immune and endocrine systems shared both mediators and receptors, allowing them to influence each other.[18] It is important to note that data from the last two branches of research are much more difficult to gather and interpret, leading to frequent controversy about research findings.

Today, the broad spectrum of scientists who devote their time to the study of the brain-immune system link have brought together the psychosocial (mental) and biomedical (physical) aspects of health under the single branch of medicine known as psychoneuroimmunology. This branch of medicine concentrates on how emotions work to either enhance or cripple immune response.

The Mind-Body Connection Today

What seemed to be missing from earlier efforts was a definitive link between the mind, the immune system, and the nervous system. Psychoneuroimmunology provides that link—and the work of psychologist Robert Ader, whose key experiments laid the foundation for the field of mind-body research, gave the following evidence for those connections:[19]

- The central nervous system is linked to both the bone marrow and the thymus (where immune system cells are produced) and to the spleen and lymph nodes (where such cells are stored).

- Scientists have found nerve endings in the tissues of the immune system. The lymphoid organs, such as the spleen, are thoroughly laced with nerve fibers.

- Changes in the brain and spinal cord affect how the immune system responds. That's not all: when researchers trigger an immune response in the body, there are changes in the way the brain and spinal cord function.

- Researchers have discovered that lymphocytes (important immune system cells) respond chemically to hormones and neurotransmitters and that they can actually produce hormones and neurotransmitters. Receptors for neuromodulators and neurohormones have been found on the T cells (or T lymphocytes).[20]

- Emotions trigger the release of hormones into the system—adrenaline (also known as epinephrine), noradrenaline (also known as norepinephrine), endorphins, glucocorticoids, prolactin, and growth hormones, among others.

- Cells that are actively involved in an immune response produce substances that send signals to the central nervous system.

- The body's immune response can be influenced by stress; stress and other psychosocial factors can make the body more susceptible to infectious diseases (such as the common cold), autoimmune diseases (such as arthritis), or cancer.

- The body's immune response can be "trained," modified by the same kind of classical conditioning used in psychological experiments to train dogs.

- Immune function can be influenced and changed by psychoactive drugs, including alcohol, marijuana, cocaine, heroin, and nicotine.

- The research into the relationship between the mind and the body has dramatic implications for treatment.

Simply stated, we no longer regard the immune system as an independent, closed, self-regulating system but understand instead that it works almost as a "sixth sense," informing the brain about events taking place not only inside but outside the body. We know, too, that two-way communication takes place, and that the neuroendocrine system is the link between the mind and the immune system.[21] We also know that hormones enable the endocrine system's two-way communication with the immune system.[22]

The impact of the mind-body connection goes far beyond isolated conditions and disorders; instead, it's a pervasive interaction that influences and is influenced by all other events, both psychological and physical. Well-documented examples of conditions in which psychoneuroimmunological interactions occur include: conditioning, the stress response, infections, tumor development, autoimmune diseases, therapeutic interventions, biofeedback mechanisms, the placebo effect, brain damage, neurological diseases, and virtually all classes of psychiatric disorders.[23]

What was once considered on the fringe of science is now a respected field of research attracting some of the nation's brightest minds. A number of medical schools have integrated PNI into their curricula, and a host of federal grants are underwriting more aggressive research. An increasing number of physicians are acknowledging that how a patient thinks and feels can be a powerful determinant of physical health. Widespread implementation of mind-body medicine based on PNI will depend on effective removal of the barriers that currently prevent its acceptance by both physicians and patients—including lack of appropriate knowledge and insight, a dramatic paradigm shift from the focus of most previous physician training, the tendency to see everything in a simple cause-and-effect relationship, and the willingness of patients to be treated in a more holistic way.[24]

PNI: The Major Components

The Brain

Five hundred years BCE, the Greeks knew the brain as a three-pound organ inside the head.[25] Through crude clinical observation over the ensuing years, beliefs about the brain and its function changed. In the Middle Ages, scientists regarded the brain as the seat of the soul. Today, our ability to measure and analyze the electrical activity of the brain and to obtain other visual recordings of brain activity (using technological advances such as positron emission tomography [PET] and magnetic resonance imagery [MRI]) has generated major advances in understanding its function.

What the Brain Is   The brain has a heart to supply it with blood, lungs to supply it with oxygen, intestines to supply it with nutrients, and kidneys and a liver to remove poisons from its environment. The most important part of our nervous system, the brain is the focal point of organization. For the body to survive, the nervous system (and particularly the brain) must be maintained; all other organs will sacrifice to keep the brain alive and functioning when the entire body is under severe stress.

By weight, 90 percent of the central nervous system is located inside the head in the form of the brain. A long extension of the brain, the spinal cord, descends down the back inside the spinal column. Nerves branch out to the sensory organs—the eyes, ears, nose and tongue—from the brain and the spinal cord. Nerves also branch out to the muscles, the skin, and all the organs of the body.

Brain functions are modulated by neuropeptides, body chemicals that act directly on the nervous system. At least seventy have been identified, including endorphins (which regulate pain relief and happiness), enkephalins (which regulate pain relief), glucocorticoids (which regulate mood, sexual behavior, sleep, and food intake), and adrenaline (which regulates fear).[26]

The neuropeptides play a major role in engineering communication between the brain, the immune system, and the endocrine system. They have also been shown to directly impact the function of certain kinds of cells, such as Langerhans cells (which produce insulin). Moreover, neuropeptides also influence cellular development and growth, immunity, recruitment of cytokines in the immune response, inflammation, and tissue repair.[27]

These neuropeptides alter behavior and mood, and they reside in various receptors. The receptors are proteins with three-dimensional folding patterns that provide a site where cells of all types receive most of their information about what surrounds them. In essence, a signaling molecule (called a ligand) fits into the receptor site and influences the behavior of the cells. These molecules, or ligands, can be free molecules (like hormones) or can be on the surface of other cells. When the molecules are located on the surface of other cells, the cells must come into actual contact in order for them to communicate.[28] The brain stem is rich with receptors—and we know that similar receptors are also found on the cells of the central nervous system and the immune system.

The neurotransmitters are responsible for the direct transfer of signals from one cell to another through the receptors. The neuropeptides set the "tone" by altering how effective the transfer of signals is.

What the Brain Does   The brain sends information to various parts of the body by masterminding nerve impulses that are carried throughout the body. It controls such voluntary processes as the direction, strength, and coordination of muscle movements; the processes involved in smelling, touching, and seeing; and other processes over which you have conscious control. The brain also controls many automatic, vital functions in the body, such as breathing, the rate of the heartbeat, digestion, bowel and bladder function, blood pressure, and release of hormones.

Finally, the brain is the cognitive center of the body where ideas are generated, memory is stored, and emotions are experienced. The emotions that so affect the body originate in the brain, then, and this process explains the brain's powerful influence over the body as well as its link to the emotions and the immune system.

Emotions Produced by the Brain   The emotions produced by the brain are, in a very real sense, a mixture of feelings and physical responses—and every time the brain manufactures an emotion throughout its loose network of lower brain structures and nerve pathways known as the limbic system, physical responses accompany those emotions.

A report published in *U.S. News and World Report* presents a vivid picture of what happens as feelings and physical responses are combined:

> Seeing a shadow flit across your path in a dimly lit parking lot will trigger a complex series of events. First, sensory receptors in the retina of your eye detect the shadow and instantly translate it into chemical signals that race to your brain. Different parts of the limbic system and higher brain centers debate the shadow's importance. What is it? Have we encountered something like this before? Is it dangerous? Meanwhile, signals sent by the hypothalamus to the pituitary gland trigger a flood of hormones alerting various parts of your body to the possibility of danger, and producing the response called "fight or flight": Rapid pulse, rising blood pressure, dilated pupils, and other physiological shifts that prepare you for action. Hormone signals are carried through the blood, a much slower route than nerve pathways. So even after the danger is past—when your brain decides that the shadow is a cat's, not a mugger's—it takes a few minutes for everything to return to normal.[29]

This description tracks what happens with fear, a relatively uncomplicated emotion. According to brain researchers, the pathways of more complicated sensations, such as sadness or joy, are much more difficult to trace, but they are just as responsible for physical effects in the body.

Chemicals Produced by the Brain

Endorphins. The natural, morphinelike chemicals called endorphins work as the brain's natural painkiller, sometimes exerting analgesic effects more powerful than those of narcotic drugs; they also produce a sense of calm, happiness, and well-being (responsible for the well-known "runner's high"). The hot spot for endorphin receptors is the part of the brain known as the amygdala, or pleasure center.

The role of endorphins is apparently much more complex than was originally thought. According to a report published in *Psychology Today,* endorphins play a role in "crying, laughing, thrills from music, acupuncture, placebos, stress, depression, chili peppers, compulsive gambling, aerobics, trauma, masochism, massage, labor and delivery, appetite, immunity, near-death experiences, and playing with pets."[30]

Scientists have also found that certain foods give people a "sensory hit" and stimulate the release of endorphins. The result is a "feel good all over" experience that causes us to relate pleasure with food. The main food that stimulates endorphin production is sugar.

Can there be a downside to all this ecstasy? Apparently so. In moderate amounts, endorphins can produce calm, inspire happiness, kill pain, and give us the thrill of anticipation over a warm-from-the-oven slice of spicy apple pie. However, when too many endorphins are released by the brain, the effect can be devastating to the immune system.

According to research conducted at the University of California–Los Angeles (UCLA), a flood of endorphins released in response to pain or stress can bind to the natural killer cells, immune system cells that search out and destroy tumor cells. When endorphins bind to the natural killer cells, they falter and become less effective in their role as the body's surveillance system; the immune system may not detect and subsequently destroy invaders.

Neuropeptides. Neuropeptides are intercellular messengers that are widely distributed throughout the nervous system, the gastrointestinal tract, and the pancreas.[31] One researcher compared the role of neuropeptides to a sophisticated conference call between the brain, the immune system, and the body's other organs and systems.[32] Pioneered by neuropharmacologist Candace Pert, neuropeptide research studies the hormones that govern communication between the brain and the body cells. "There's probably a peptide solution to every medical problem," she says.[33]

The Immune System

The immune system is a complex system consisting of about a trillion cells called lymphocytes (white blood cells) and about a hundred million trillion molecules called antibodies that patrol and guard the body against attackers, both from the outside and from within. Instead of operating within a biological vacuum, the immune system is very sensitive to a number of various influences.

A variety of factors influence immunity and the immune system, including genetics, gender, age, and personality traits. When something goes awry in the immune system, infection results; when the entire immune system is compromised, as in AIDS, victims eventually die from overwhelming infections.

The most basic requirement of the immune system is that it can distinguish between "nonself" and "self" cells and that it can then destroy the nonself invaders.[34] "Nonself" invaders, or antigens (cell-surface glycoproteins that the body recognizes as foreign), are unhealthy, dysfunctional, nonintegrated cells and tissues of the body, as well as foreign invading organisms such as bacteria and viruses. "Self" cells are the healthy, functional, integrated cells and tissues of the body. In destroying antigens, the immune system eliminates body cells and tissues that have mutated or been changed by disease or environmental factors.

Destruction of antigens is called natural or innate immunity. Acquired immunity occurs when the immune system is exposed to a certain type of antigen. The next time an individual encounters the same antigen, the immune system is primed to destroy it. The degree of immunity depends on the kind of antigen, its amount, and how it enters the body. Infants are born with relatively weak immune responses, but they do get natural immunity during the first few months of life from antibodies they receive from their mothers. Children who are nursed receive even more antibodies through breast milk. In addition to acquiring immunity naturally, it is possible to be immunized with a vaccine. Vaccines contain microorganisms that have been altered so they produce an immune response *without producing the full-blown disease.*

Organs of the Immune System   Spread throughout the body, the organs of the immune system are generally referred to as lymphoid organs because they regulate the growth, development, and deployment of lymphocytes, the key operatives of the immune system.[35] Lymphoid organs include the bone marrow, thymus, lymph nodes, and spleen, as well as the tonsils, appendix, and clumps of lymphoid tissue in the small intestine known as Peyer's patches.

Cells destined to become lymphocytes are produced in the bone marrow cells in the hollow shafts of the long bones. Some of these cells, known as stem cells, migrate to the thymus, a multilobed organ that lies high behind the breastbone. Stem cells that mature in the thymus are called T cells; they multiply and mature into cells capable of producing an immune response. Other lymphocytes that appear to mature either in the bone marrow itself or in lymphoid organs other than the thymus are called B cells.

Lymph nodes are small bean-shaped structures distributed throughout the body; they occur in strings in the neck, armpits, abdomen, and groin and bring together the various components needed to produce the body's immune response. Each lymph node contains a variety of specialized compartments. Some house T cells, others B cells. Still others are filled with another type of immunocompetent cell, macrophages (discussed in the next section). Lymph nodes also contain webbed areas that enmesh antigens.

Lymph nodes are linked by a network of lymphatic vessels similar to blood vessels; these carry lymph, a clear fluid that bathes all of the body's tissues and that contains a variety of cells, most of them lymphocytes. Like a system of small creeks and streams that empty into progressively larger rivers, the vessels of the lymphatic network merge into increasingly larger tributaries. At the base of the neck, the large lymphatic ducts empty into the bloodstream.

Lymph and the cells and particles it carries, including antigens that have entered the body, drain out of the body's tissues, seeping through the thin walls of the smallest lymph vessels. As the lymph passes through lymph nodes, antigens are filtered out and more lymphocytes are picked up. The lymphocytes, along with other assorted cells of the immune system, are carried to the bloodstream, which delivers them to tissues throughout the body. The lymphocytes patrol the entire body for foreign antigens, and then gradually drift back into the lymphatic system to begin the cycle all over again.

During their travels, circulating lymphocytes may spend several hours in the spleen, an organ in the abdomen that contains a high concentration of lymphocytes. Anyone whose spleen has been damaged by trauma or disease is very susceptible to infection.

The Immune System in Action   The immune system stores just a few cells specific to each potential invader; when any antigen appears, the immune system stimulates these few specifically matched cells, which then multiply into a full-scale army adequate for fighting the invader. Later, powerful suppressor mechanisms prevent the army of immune cells from proliferating wildly, similar to what happens in cancer.

Immune system cells include:

- B cells (lymphocytes, or white blood cells) secrete antibodies; each specific antibody exactly matches a specific invading antigen and inactivates it so it can't cause disease. The body is capable of making antibodies to millions of antigens.

- T cells (also lymphocytes) act as both messengers and destroyers in the fight against pathogens. Helper T cells activate B cells or other T cells; suppressor T cells turn them off, shutting down the immune response when it is no longer needed. T cells ravage healthy cells from another person's body, which is why organ transplant recipients need medication to prevent rejection. Scientists believe there are as many as 100 million different varieties of T cells and another 100 million antibodies.

- Natural killer cells attack and destroy other cells and begin working without being stimulated by a specific antigen. Most normal cells resist natural killer cell activity, but tumor cells as well as normal cells infected with a virus are susceptible. Natural killer cells are key elements in immune surveillance against cancer, hunting down cells that develop abnormal changes.

- Another twenty or so proteins circulate in the blood in inactive form and make up the immune system's complement system. These substances are triggered by antibodies that lock onto antigens, and they rapidly kill bacteria and other pathogens by puncturing their cell membranes. The result is inflammation with its accompanying redness, warmth, and swelling.

But when it comes to the interaction between the immune system, the emotions, and the brain, possibly the most important immune system cells are the macrophages and their companion monocytes—first on the scene of any infection, they act as scavengers to engulf and digest invading microorganisms. Monocytes circulate in the blood, whereas macrophages are seeded through body tissues in a variety of ways.

Macrophages actually initiate the immune response by "presenting" antigens to T cells in a way that allows the immune system to recognize them. Macrophages and monocytes also secrete an amazing array of powerful chemical substances called monokines that help direct and regulate the immune response.

Macrophages also create protein molecules called proinflammatory cytokines—interferon gamma, the various types of interleukin, and tumor necrosis factor alpha—that have specialized roles in fighting viruses, tumor cells, and other threats. These cytokines amplify the body's inflammatory response, assist in wound healing, and activate specific immune responses.[36] However, the real fascination for PNI researchers is the fact that, once the immune system is mobilized, these cytokines dispatch messages to the central nervous system and the brain (as well as other non–immune system cells[37]), alerting them to the existing injury or infection. What happens next is key to the interaction between the brain and the immune system: the brain produces its own cytokines, signaling the central nervous and immune systems to initiate the cascade of responses—including the release of powerful brain chemicals—that let us know we're sick.[38] The result is a sophisticated two-way communication between the brain and the immune system that allows the mind (and its emotions) to impact immunity. (Interestingly, researchers have found that these proinflammatory cytokines are also released during depression, mania, and bipolar disease and that cytokines produced by the brain are a factor in psychological illnesses.[39])

This bidirectional flow of data between the brain and the immune system provides powerful evidence that emotions actually cause illness instead of the reverse. Depression is a perfect example: for years, researchers maintained that being sick is depressing—and so, naturally, the depression was an expected side effect of disease. Cytokine research demonstrating the sensitivity of the immune system to signals from the brain instead has convinced scientists that emotions like depression can actually cause disease.

When proinflammatory cytokines are released in response to infection, inflammation, or any kind of injury to the body's tissues, the cytokines influence the central nervous system and behavior to create what is called "sickness behavior." Sickness behavior is a combination of physiological and behavioral changes that develop in response to the infection, inflammation, or injury—and it can include any combination of fever, fatigue, pain, sleepiness, decreased ability to concentrate, reduced food and water intake, sleep disorders, changes in coping ability, and loss of pleasure, appetite, and sexual drive. It can also cause lack of interest in social interaction and feelings of depression, hopelessness, irritability, anxiety, worthlessness, and guilt.[40] The implications of recognizing the impact of proin-flammatory cytokines on sickness behavior are profound: clearly the development of behavioral problems, such as depression, can readily result from a physical illness.

In most cases, the immune response overcomes the infection and heals the wound or injury. As the crisis passes, the release of cytokines tapers off and eventually stops. But the cytokines are like a two-edged sword.[41] If the immune response is impacted, the proinflam-matory cytokines are chronically produced, and inflammatory diseases—such as Crohn's disease, lupus, diabetes, and rheumatoid arthritis—can result. Chronic activation of cytokines can also result in chronic symptoms of sickness, which can also lead to mood and cognition disorders. And if the immune response is insufficient, the release of cytokines can spiral out of control and can flood areas of the body other than the one that is injured or threatened. Uncontrolled and widespread release of cytokines can injure tissues, cause shock, reduce blood supply to the organs, result in blood clotting, and even cause death.[42]

Malfunctions of the Immune System   Unfortunately, a number of factors can cause breakdown or failure of the immune system. One is aging. The thymus shrinks; by age twenty it has lost approximately 75 percent of its size and function, and it is virtually gone by age sixty, a process that significantly changes the number and activity of T cells. Aging also upsets the ratio of helper to suppressor cells, turning off the immune response. Still another effect of aging is the production of antibodies by B cells. Overproduction of antibodies for any reason causes an allergic overreaction to substances that are usually harmless; in the extreme, the result is asthma or anaphylactic shock.

A similar malfunction of the immune system is autoimmune disease, in which the immune system reacts to normal body cells as though it were allergic to them. Simply stated, the body attacks and destroys its own tissues and organs. Examples include rheumatoid arthritis and systemic lupus erythematosus.

The immune system can also be suppressed by cancer and can be damaged by the drugs and radiation used to treat cancer. While these treatments kill the rapidly growing cancer cells in the body, they can also destroy normal cells, especially those of the immune system.

Cells of the immune system themselves may become cancerous, resulting in diseases such as lymphoma or leukemia. The immune system may also be damaged or even destroyed by viral infections (such as AIDS) or congenital diseases; these immune system failures are called immunodeficiency diseases. In these cases, the body is overwhelmed by infections and cancers because it can't destroy invading organisms.

The Brain-Immune System Connection

As mentioned, the key connection between the brain and the immune system are the cytokines, protein molecules that carry messages. Discovery of these cytokines is proba-bly the most compelling and exciting area of PNI research. For years, scientists *suspected* that the brain and the immune system were talking to each other, but none knew how it was being accomplished.

Scientists knew of some possibilities. We knew that the brain communicates with cells through the nerves that innervate the glands and organs. For example, the thymus gland plays an essential role in the maturation of immune system cells, and researchers have discovered extensive networks of nerve endings laced throughout the thymus gland.[43] Rich supplies of nerves also serve the spleen, bone marrow, and lymph nodes, which provided researchers with evidence of a link between the brain and the immune system.

There are other connections, too. The surface of the lymphocytes contains receptors for a variety of central nervous system chemical messengers, such as catecholamines, prostaglandins, serotonin, endorphins, sex hormones, thyroid hormone, and growth hormone.[44] National Institute of Mental Health researchers discovered that "certain white blood cells were equipped with the molecular equivalent of antennas tuned specifically to receive messages from the brain."[45]

Because of these receptors on the lymphocytes, physical and psychological stress alter the immune system. Stress has been shown to affect the T cells, B cells, natural killer cells, and lymphocytes. One of the most frequently implicated ways in which stress alters immunity, however, is by suppression of the natural killer cells, which could have important implications on cancer prognosis and the progression of HIV infection.[46]

Stress also causes the hypothalamus of the brain to release several powerful neurohormones, including catecholamines, corticosteroids, and endorphins that bind with the receptors on the lymphocytes and alter immune function. Corticosteroids, in fact, have been found to have such a powerful influence in suppressing the immune system that they are widely used to treat allergic conditions (such as asthma and hay fever) and autoimmune disorders (such as rheumatoid arthritis and rejection of transplanted organs).

While those factors certainly play a part in communication between the brain and the immune system, the key players are clearly the cytokines. Because the cytokines are produced by both the brain and the immune system, there is bidirectional communication between the two. If the brain interprets a threat (as in fear), it produces cytokines that alert the immune system and the rest of the body's systems to get ready to meet the threat. If the immune system interprets a threat (such as from invading bacteria), it produces cytokines that alert the brain and the rest of the body's systems to get ready to meet that threat. In both cases, the system on the other end produces its own cytokines that then respond.

The Immune System and Emotion

The second principle behind mind-body medicine is that the peptides carry not only information about the nervous system and the body's physical functions, but also information about the emotions. Information about the emotions is carried throughout the body, potentially impacting every body system. Decades of research demonstrate that strong negative emotions are associated with significant health problems.

One of the reasons why strong negative emotions may be linked to illness is that negative emotional response—whether it be stress, anger, or sadness—may disrupt the immune system. When you experience strong emotions, your body responds much like it would in the classic "fight-or-flight" response model. Endocrine system activity sends hormones coursing through the bloodstream, which in turn send messages to the brain. The brain manufactures cytokines that send messages to the immune system. As the chemical response gradually builds, your body reaches its physical threshold and ability to deal with the stress of negative emotion. In a state of exhaustion, your body becomes more susceptible to illness.

To say that emotions cause disease is far too simplistic. More accurately, emotions are only one important factor in the body's ability to resist any of the variety of things that can cause illness or disease. Normal homeostasis—the optimal balance of hormones, immunity, and nervous system functioning— protects us from the many threats to health we encounter daily. Disrupted emotional responses are one factor that lead to disrupted homeostasis. Physiological processes are then disrupted. Interestingly, the same part of the midbrain that keeps physiology balanced also controls emotional response, allowing responses to be appropriate.

There is another physiological reason why emotions can impact health. Different parts of the brain are associated not only with specific emotions, but also with specific hormone patterns. The experience ("release") of certain hormones, then, is associated with different emotional responses, and those hormones affect health.[47] As one example, we know that emotionally induced shifts in hormones can lead to chronic disease, such as high blood pressure. When a person is aggressive and anxious, too much noradrenaline and adrenaline are secreted, even at rest. The arteries thicken, and the excess hormones cause blood vessel muscles to constrict. The gradual rise in blood pressure can then result in hypertension, stroke, or heart failure.[48]

Feeling emotions is only one factor in the subsequent development of disease. Many researchers believe that the inability to express emotions is an even greater cause of disease. Studies have confirmed that the failure to perceive and express emotions can lead to various disease states.[49]

In a battery of tests conducted by Leonard Derogatis, it was found that breast cancer patients who showed little emotion were the ones who died early on. The "survivors" were the ones who felt and openly expressed a lot of anger, fear, depression, and guilt.[50] The process of suppressing emotion somehow contributed to the tenacity of the disease.

Infectious diseases—such as infectious hepatitis or gonorrhea—are caused by identifiable microorganisms such as bacteria or viruses, but emotions can determine in part how susceptible we are to these infectious agents and whether they will actually make us sick.

An excellent example is the herpes simplex virus, which causes fever blisters and cold sores. Most adults harbor this virus in a quiescent state at all times. It often resides around the nostrils and the mouth but remains dormant and does not cause sores. Sometimes, in response to lowered resistance, it flares up, especially when the person is ill with something else (such as the common cold). Many times, it flares up in response to emotional upset. In fact, mental stress is the most common precipitant of herpes skin lesions.

A number of studies have demonstrated the power of emotions in bringing on an attack of herpes virus infection. In one, students who had a high prevalence of cold sores throughout college found that their cold sores occurred less frequently after graduation, when stress levels were lower.[51]

The Role of Religion and Spirituality

Throughout recorded history, most religions have included healing practices; all early human civilizations dealt with physical illness in spiritual or religious terms, including the Mesopotamian, Egyptian, Indian, Chinese, Greek, and Roman civilizations.[52] These healing methods often used supernatural kinds of treatment, such as incantations, prayers, or religious pilgrimages. Until the last several decades, no one considered that the healing associated with spiritual or religious beliefs could actually be tied to natural mechanisms, such as psychosocial and behavioral factors.

We now know that spiritual and religious factors do have substantial impact on the factors that increase health and immunity. Religion and spirituality help people cope with stress; in one survey, 78 percent of Americans of all ages—and nearly 90 percent of older adults—said religion provided comfort and support.[53] Almost half of the medical patients in another survey indicated that religion was the most important factor in enabling them to cope with serious illness; the other half said it helps to a moderate or large degree.[54] Religion and spirituality have also been shown to contribute to positive emotions—such as life satisfaction, happiness, well-being, optimism, and hope—which have been shown to help protect the immune system. People who are involved in religious practice also consistently report stronger social support—a finding that holds true even for those who participate only in private religious practices, such as prayer.[55] Those who attend religious services have a significantly higher number of in-person contacts, non-kin ties, telephone calls, and instrumental support, all of which benefit health. In the last decade, twelve of thirteen studies have demonstrated a significant relationship between greater religious involvement, better physical health, and longer survival.[56]

There are several other reasons why religious and spiritual practice *can* enhance physical health and improve immune function:[57]

- Health behaviors. Religious involvement has been associated with a lower incidence of many high-risk behaviors such as cigarette smoking, alcoholism, drug use, risky sexual activity, drinking while driving, and failure to use seat belts. While these certainly explain some of the association between religious activity and health, researchers caution that they should not minimize the importance of religion itself.

- Health care practices. Often because of the increased social support (which is a protective factor in itself), people involved in religious practice are more likely to have their medical illnesses diagnosed sooner, monitored more regularly, and treated more effectively. People who are active in religious faith also tend to be more compliant with medical treatment.

- Stress buffering. Spiritual faith and religious involvement tend to produce a more hopeful and optimistic worldview, which helps people cope with both short-term and chronic stress. Religious people tend to turn to their faith for help in dealing with stressful situations (including serious illness and death) instead of to practices that could harm them, such as alcohol, cigarettes, or drugs.

The Emotion-Immunity Connection in Heart Disease, Cancer, and Other Conditions

Heart Disease

Solid research shows that psychological factors can be substantial risk factors for both coronary artery disease and myocardial infarction.[58] Psychological risk factors have been classified into three categories, depending on their duration:

- Acute triggers, like acute stress or outbursts of anger. Outbursts of anger can cut off oxygen to the heart, resulting in myocardial infarction; acute anger has been shown to double the risk of heart attack. In advanced stages of cardiovascular disease, angry outbursts can cause the rupture of arterial plaque, resulting in stroke or heart attack.

- Factors that last from several weeks to several years, including exhaustion and depression.

- Chronic factors, including negative personality traits (such as hostility) and low socioeconomic status.

Angina (chest pain that occurs when the heart muscle is temporarily deprived of oxygen) can be caused by physical exertion but is also aggravated by emotional stress. "Excessive stress can trigger an angina attack," points out James L. Levenson, assistant professor of psychiatry at the Medical College of Virginia. "In some forms of stress the adrenal glands secrete epinephrine—the hormone associated with the 'fight-or-flight' response. This, in turn, increases heart rate and blood pressure and hence the workload on the heart. . . . Some patients may be more vulnerable to artery spasms at these times."

According to comprehensive research, the most common feature of sudden cardiac death is "marked emotional perturbation," a flood of strong emotion. The most provocative emotional circumstances that lead to sudden death include the death of, or threat of injury to, a loved one; the early grief period following any loss; and the threat of personal injury.

Extreme emotional stress in people with otherwise structurally normal hearts can lead to primary arrhythmias (disturbance in heart rhythm that causes it to beat unusually fast or slow). In people who have coronary artery disease, the effects of emotional stress are even more severe and can result in angina, silent ischemia, or fatal arrhythmias.

Cancer

For years, researchers studying the mind-body connection thought that depression—characterized by sadness, submissiveness, and a tendency to suppress or repress feelings—raised the risk of developing cancer. We now know that isn't true. Several large-scale studies involving thousands of people as well as the pooled results of many other studies have found no evidence suggesting that personality or mood has any influence in either preventing or initiating the onset of cancer.[59]

While psychological factors almost certainly do not *cause* cancer, researchers are still considering whether they may impact the progression or recurrence of cancer. Some studies show that psychological factors do seem to have an impact on the progression of already-established cancers.[60] However, the findings have been inconsistent, and anecdotal claims about the mind's influence over cancer have further muddied the waters.[61] Various studies have shown that cancer patients who are isolated, unmarried, feeling hopeless, or going through a financial crisis were more likely to die than those who did not have these kinds of stresses in their lives. Other studies, however, show that stress in the year prior to cancer diagnosis or in the five years following it does not affect the rate of recurrence of cancer. And an analysis of fifty-eight studies found that attributes such as a fighting spirit, denial, fatalism, helplessness, or hopelessness had no effect on either cancer survival or recurrence—just the opposite of what researchers had earlier believed.[62]

We do know that exposure to the hormones and chemicals resulting from chronic stress impacts the immune system and makes it less able to respond to threats. We know that a loss of immunity could possibly promote the growth of tumors. We know that stress affects the activity of natural killer cells, which are the body's surveillance system against tumors. What we *don't* know is how those factors impact the onset, development, or recurrence of cancer.

Scientists are continuing their research of the possible connections, just as they are continuing research into any of the many things that may contribute to cancer. Psychoneuroimmunology research in this area is particularly difficult for a number of reasons. For one, by the time cancer is diagnosed, it has had months, if not years, to adjust to the internal workings of its host. How far back do researchers look, and is it even possible to isolate a time when the onset of cancer occurred? For another, causes and effects are sometimes very difficult to distinguish; for example, a cancer patient who is depressed may be depressed because he has cancer and may not have cancer because he is depressed. People with the most serious disease are likely to be more depressed, anxious, or distressed—but may die sooner because the disease was more serious, not because they were depressed, anxious, or distressed. And the symptoms of a number of psychological problems (sadness, loss of appetite, fatigue, and insomnia, among them) can also be caused by chemotherapy, radiation treatment, or the cancer itself. Even looking at people who have outlived their prognosis isn't a sound approach: these people may simply be statistical anomalies.

Physicians at Harvard University caution that the possible effects of the mind, mood, or personality on cancer should not be exaggerated to cancer patients. "If people are led to think they can be cured by cultivating the right feelings, they may also blame themselves if they do not recover quickly," say researchers.[63] Possibly the greatest role of treating patients with behavioral and psychological regimens is not to prolong their lives, but to improve the quality of life while they fight their disease.

Diabetes

The link between emotions and diabetes was made as early as the seventeenth century, when British physician Thomas Willis noted that diabetes first appeared in many cases among patients who had experienced significant life stresses. Nearly 200 years later, Claude Bernard, considered the father of modern physiology, found that he could produce diabetes in a normal animal by making a lesion in or close to the hypothalamus.

That finding helps explain why there could be a link between stress, anxiety, and diabetes, which may be linked to an upset in the central nervous system.

Chronic Pain

Research has shown that the pain center of the brain—the anterior cingulate cortex (ACC)—is directly influenced by emotions. As a result, emotional pain can cause literal physical pain. In a study by UCLA scientist Naomi I. Eisenberger published in *Science*, research shows that a rejected lover's broken heart may cause as much distress in the pain center of the brain as an actual physical injury. In commenting on the study, Bowling Green State University psychologist Jaak Panksepp wrote, "Throughout history, poets have written about the pain of a broken heart. It seems that such poetic insights into the human condition are now supported by neurophysiological findings."[64]

While patients with chronic pain overuse the health care system and drive up health care costs, they rarely get significant relief from their symptoms when given traditional medical treatment. Convincing evidence shows that mind-body medicine is much more effective in the treatment of chronic pain.

In one important study,[65] more than 100 patients with various types of chronic pain symptoms received mind-body treatment. At the end of the first ten weeks, the patients still had pain but reported less anxiety, depression, and hostility. As treatment continued, the pain began to decrease, and the other symptoms continued to improve as well. By the end of a year, the patients were visiting the clinic 36 percent less often; visits continued to decline during the second year of treatment. The savings from medical care were significant during the first year, and doubled during the second year. What are the implications? Using mind-body therapies to treat victims of chronic pain could result in improvement for the patients and cost savings for the health care system.

Based on current studies, researchers estimate that as much as 95 percent of all back pain—some of the most stubborn chronic pain—is triggered by the psyche, not by physical abnormalities or by heavy lifting. According to New York psychiatrist Hans Draus, back muscles tense up in response to emotional stress. If the muscles remain tensed too long, they start to hurt. In people whose backs hurt the most, the best predictor of pain is a psychological problem, such as depression.[66] Tense muscles are more prone to injury—so those who are emotionally upset and whose back muscles are tense are more likely to injure their backs with even minor exertion.

The Mind and Longevity

Can the way that we think and feel directly impact longevity? One interesting study that looked at the factors that influence longevity was conducted in an area of southern Sweden comprised of one major city, eight smaller towns, and a number of small communities and rural districts.[67] For each person in the study, researchers did the following:

- Conducted a medical examination that included, among other things, taking blood tests, taking blood pressure measurements, obtaining a medical history, and asking questions about smoking habits, alcohol consumption, and diet.

- Conducted a psychological assessment that included, among other things, tests for memory, learning retention, reaction time, behavior, and personality rating.

- Gathered sociological data that included, among other things, marital status, type of housing, socioeconomic status, satisfaction with professional life, education, social network, feelings of loneliness, and formal/informal social support.

- Interviewed each person about quality of life, both during their entire preceding life span and at the time the interviews were conducted.

Researchers found that genetics definitely played a role in whether the people in the study reached the age of 100. There were also several medical factors that played a key role; the two most important were body composition and blood pressure. The incidence of severe disease was also low. Most in the study had never smoked. However, researchers also identified a number of factors indicating that the mind plays a powerful role in longevity.

According to the study, the centenarians were more responsible, capable, relaxed, easygoing, and emotionally stable and were less prone to anxiety than the population in general. Social characteristics seemed to be especially important. Most had grown up in stable homes; their parents had been extremely long lived. (While the mean age of death for their fathers was 71.6 years and for their mothers was 74.3 years, the average age for survival from birth at that time in Sweden was only 40 years for men and 44 years for women.) Marriage played an important role; only 2 percent of the centenarians had been divorced, and only 19 percent had never married. Only 9 percent said they often felt lonely. They felt their quality of life—both at present and over their lifetimes—had been good.

Other studies show that the impact of the mind on longevity probably has to do with the relationship between the mind and the immune system. Generally, old age is associated with decline in immunity. The thymus gland stops influencing the growth and development of white blood cells at around the age of sixty. The T cells become less responsive with age and decline in numbers during the three years before death. While the B cells do not decline in number, they lose the ability to function with age. Similarly, most studies indicate that the body produces fewer natural killer cells as it ages.[68]

Research has shown that impairment of the immune system is probably not characteristic of aging per se because a considerable percentage of the elderly maintain robust and healthy immunity. Instead, these changes may be due in part to the fact that the events of old age (such as retirement, loss of an active role in society, and bereavement) are likely to cause a high level of stress, and we know that stress impacts the immune system.[69]

Depression and bereavement, common during old age, have also been shown to impair immunity. Research shows that the more depressed a person is during bereavement, the greater the impairment of the immune system. Thirty-five studies found that depression was related to significant alterations in immunity, including reduced white blood cells and lowered natural killer cell activity—both of which affect the ability to fight off disease. The effect of depression may be partly related to stress (since depression can either cause stress or result from stress) and partly related to the way depressed people tend to behave: the depressed tend to sleep less, eat a less balanced diet, get less exercise, drink more alcohol, and smoke. The immune effects of depression have been found to be even greater among the elderly or those who are hospitalized.[70]

Other stressful events associated with aging include:

- Increased economic stress, including a reduction in income that often accompanies retirement.
- Progressive loneliness (caused by death of a spouse, move or death of friends, and/or being forsaken by children).
- Isolation (caused by institutionalization).
- Poor or declining physical health caused by age-dependent diseases.
- Loss of mobility.
- Physical disability.
- A perception of uselessness.

Those who adapt—who learn to cope with these changes—tend to suffer far fewer health effects than those who do not, further indicating that stress instead of aging may be the major culprit in reduced immunity with aging. Those who are unable to adapt suffer impaired immunity as they age; the result is an especially high frequency of autoimmune and infectious diseases.

Criticisms of the Mind-Body Approach

The field of PNI and the resulting application of mind-body medicine has come a long way in the last decade; and, as chemical messengers in the body have been identified and analyzed, mainstream science has become much more accepting of what was once largely debunked as folklore. But there are still critics and detractors who take a skeptical look at claims of solid connection between the brain, the immune system, and the endocrine system.

Some critics accurately point out that just as the immune system itself is extremely complex, so are the studies that attempt to unravel its functioning. According to one work on PNI, the complexity of research includes "biobehavioral involvements, endocrine measure, immune indicators, and health outcomes. When one also takes into account the heterogeneity of study designs, the problem of drawing broadly based conclusions and generalizing results appears overwhelming."[71] Researchers, say the authors, need to be aware of potential limitations, subtle biases, "holes" in the data (areas where few studies have investigated potential relationships), and the temptation to make generalizations—especially when combining the findings of several different studies.

According to Robert Ader, what we observe in the research "is not nature itself, but nature exposed to our method of questioning."[72] As Ader points out, the training of scientists, the formulation of hypotheses, the implementation of research, and even the funding of that research takes place within a system limited by the way we have divided biomedical researchers and by our own intellectual limitations. Those divisions and limitations may keep us from the most stunning discoveries of all.

Other criticisms of PNI and mind-body medicine include:[73]

- The general tendency to isolate mind-body health from sociopolitical, economic, and environmental health—which of necessity disregards factors like poverty, limited access to health care, and risky environmental factors.

- The relative neglect of some important areas of health, such as smoking addiction.

- The danger that mind-body approaches could supplant advanced drugs and higher-technology treatment plans for chronic illness, which makes mind-body medicine a "competing" approach instead of a complementary one.

- The cost in terms of training and time commitment to bring practitioners up to speed with mind-body approaches at a time when medical clinics are being forced to cut budgets in the face of managed care cutoffs.

Psychoneuroimmunology (PNI) Resources

As PNI continues to attract research efforts, a number of organizations are furthering the development of PNI as a science. Some of these organizations include:

1. The PNI Research Society, an international organization for researchers in a number of scientific and medical disciplines—including psychology, neurosciences, immunology, pharmacology, psychiatry, behavioral medicine, infectious diseases, endocrinology, and rheumatology—who are interested in interactions between the nervous system and the immune system, as well as the relationship between behavior and health.

2. The UCLA Cousins Center, which brings together research expertise in the behavioral sciences, neuroscience, and immunology to understand the interplay of psychological and biological factors in disease and how the resiliency of the human body can be aided by positive behaviors, attitudes, and emotions.

3. The Association for the Advancement of Applied Psychoneuroimmunology, whose purpose is to serve as a resource for information and education concerning the field of PNI; it aims to apply PNI in the areas of management of chronic illness and disability and to inspire more general immuno-supportive lifestyle changes as they relate to individual self-responsibility for wellness.

4. *Advances in Mind/Body Medicine,* a publication of the Fetzer Institute, whose major functions are to support research, education, and service programs exploring the integral relationships among body, mind, and spirit.

5. Association for Applied Psychophysiology and Biofeedback (http://www.aapb.org/), a nonprofit organization largely composed of clinicians, researchers, and educators in biofeedback and related mind-body therapies.

6. Center for Mind-Body Medicine, a nonprofit organization aimed at transforming medicine into a more compassionate, open-minded, and effective model of health

care and health education, addressing the mental, emotional, social, spiritual, and physical dimensions of health and illness.

7. Institute of Noetic Sciences (IONS), which studies the mind and its diverse ways of knowing in a truly interdisciplinary fashion; IONS is a research and education foundation that produces several publications, organizes educational events, and provides grants for scholarly research.

8. International Society for the Study of Subtle Energies and Energy Medicine, an interdisciplinary organization for the study of the basic sciences and medical and therapeutic applications of subtle energies.

9. Mind/Body Medical Institute and Mind/Body Medical Clinic, a nonprofit scientific and educational organization dedicated to promoting the relaxation response and belief systems. The institute conducts basic and clinical research and offers training to health care professionals and others.

10. National Institute for the Clinical Application of Behavioral Medicine, which establishes practitioner-oriented conferences and seminars for health care providers, specifically on the interface between health and psychology.

11. Society of Behavioral Medicine, a multidisciplinary, nonprofit organization that provides a scientific forum for behavioral and biomedical researchers and clinicians to study the interactions of behavior, physiological, and biochemical states.

An example of treatment centers that focus on PNI include, but are not limited to:

1. The Life Sciences Institute of Mind-Body Health, Topeka, Kansas, founded by health professionals who pioneered applications of biofeedback to mental and physical problems such as stress-related disorders, addictive disorders, attention deficit disorder, depression, anxiety, immune deficiencies, and urinary incontinence. The institute also offers support in accessing particular states of consciousness associated with concentration or creativity.

2. Mind/Body Medicine, Harvard Vanguard Medical Associates, Boston, Massachusetts, a center that treats patients with chronic or recurrent illnesses and physical and/or emotional problems that are stress-sensitive and helps patients become aware of their unique stress response patterns and learn skills for making healthy changes.

3. The Mind-Body Wellness Center, Meadville, Pennsylvania, which focuses on treating the whole person with an open-minded approach that focuses on each individual in a caring, comprehensive and coordinated manner. The center offers treatment and courses in many mind-body therapies.

4. St. Elizabeth's Medical Center, Boston, Massachusetts, which teaches participants in an eight-week program to incorporate meditation and yoga into their lives for the purpose of relieving stress and its effect on the mind and body.

Major PNI web resources include:

1. Alternative Health News Online: Mind/Body Control.
   http://www.altmedicine.com/altmind.htm: Provides links to sites offering information on an overview of mind-body healing and discussions on various

mind-body techniques, such as music therapy, art therapy, yoga, hypnosis, biofeedback, and guided imagery.

2. Cygnus: Books on Mind-Body Medicine.
   http://www.cygnus-books.co.uk/ and http://www.mind-body.com/: A brief list of mind-body books, with a description of the book and links to books on related topics.

3. Health World Online.
   http://www.healthy.net/: Choose links to general mind-body topics such as medicine, health, exercise. Also has comprehensive links to specific mind-body therapies, such as bodywork, guided imagery, etc.

4. OnHealth: Mind/Body Medicine.
   http://onhealth.com/alternative/resource/althealth/item,15041.asp. Brief descriptions on mind-body medicine therapies, including biofeedback, guided imagery, hypnosis, meditation, yoga, and more. Also offers an overview of mind-body medicine and tips on choosing a practitioner.

5. Yahoo! Health: Mind-Body Medicine.
   http://sg.yahoo.com/health/alternative_medicine/mind_body_medicine/. Provides several links on mind-body medicine, with definitions, related resources, biofeedback, meditation, hypnosis, PNI, and more.

The Challenge for the Twenty-First Century

A unique challenge—and unique opportunity—faces the field of medicine as we continue through the twenty-first century. Consumer confidence in traditional medicine is waning. In an article directed at primary care physicians, the medical director of a family clinic wrote:

> In spite of impressive advances in immunology, imaging, and therapeutics, many patients are increasingly dissatisfied with their medical care. The side effects and inadequacies of many drugs and procedures have been discussed at length in the lay press, and many Americans have begun to look beyond conventional medicine for health care. Not surprisingly, most people seeking out unconventional therapies are those with chronic diseases. Although the treatment of many acute and infectious illnesses has improved, it has become clearer that the biomedical health care model is not equally effective for all types and stages of illness. Many physicians have noticed that patients experiencing emotional stress often complain of chronic physical symptoms that respond poorly to medications. This phenomenon has led to a growing scientific movement charged with exploring the mind's capacity to affect the body.[74]

Clearly, there are some limitations in both behavioral and traditional medical treatments. For example, a person with meningitis needs intravenous antibiotics; a person with appendicitis requires immediate surgery. Behavioral treatment would be inappropriate in situations like these. On the other hand, for vast numbers of patients who suffer with stress-related complaints, traditional medicine falls short, and behavioral techniques can offer tremendous benefits. And for chronic and degenerative diseases that have not responded well to traditional treatment, including some cancers, AIDS, osteoarthritis, collagen vascular diseases, chronic fatigue, and chronic pain, a combination of traditional and behavioral treatments may provide the answer. Some believe that mind-body therapies are best used in conjunction with appropriate standard medical therapies and may be most effective for stress-related illnesses.[75] As physicians were instructed in the professional journal *Primary Care,* "Mind-body therapies have been used successfully for many varied medical conditions. . . . The potential uses are vast, but research has not yet unequivocally defined which medical conditions are most improved by mind-body therapies."[76]

When it comes to exploring the mind's capacity to affect the body, we have learned a great deal, but there is still far to go. The body of knowledge we have so far is exciting, full of promise for the prospect of a whole new horizon on how we look at and treat disease—and, most important, burgeoning with possibilities of how we might prevent it. But, to paraphrase Stanford University psychologist David Spiegel, who wrote in the *Journal of the National Cancer Institute,* we have entered the twenty-first century with twentieth-century science and technology and a nineteenth-century understanding of what it tells us about mind-body relationships.

To address the organizational barriers that have kept researchers from effectively communicating about the scope and results of their efforts, the National Institutes of Health is implementing several initiatives that will facilitate interdisciplinary research—and that will ultimately lead to the development of new hybrid disciplines that can give us a greater understanding of PNI.[77] As we learn more about how the brain, the immune system, and the endocrine system work together to influence disease, we may need to redefine the nature of some diseases—and seriously reassess how we treat those diseases.

More than three decades ago, physicians were challenged to embrace a model of health and illness that recognized psychological and social variables as important contributors to health and disease. The ensuing thirty years of important scientific work have altered the specific applications, but not the general implications, of that challenge.

WHAT DID YOU LEARN?

1. How would you define *psychoneuroimmunology*?
2. Do the mind, the immune system, and the nervous system constantly communicate with each other? Is there any scientific proof for this?
3. What are the major components of psychoneuroimmunology?
4. What have we learned about the emotion-immunity connection in heart disease, cancer, and other health conditions?
5. What are the major criticisms of the mind-body approach?

ENDNOTES

1. M. Viljoen, A. Panzer, J.L. Roos, and W. Bodemer, "Psycho-neuroimmunology: From Philosophy, Intuition, and Folklore to a Recognized Science," *South African Journal of Science* 99 (July/August 2003): 332.

2. Joel S. Lazar, "Mind-Body Medicine in Primary Care: Implications of Applications," *Primary Care* 23, no. 1 (March 1996): 169.
3. Delia Rossetto Chiaramonte, "Mind-Body Therapies for Primary Care Physicians," *Primary Care* 24, no. 4 (December 1997): 788.
4. Karl Goodkin and Adriaan P. Vissar, eds., *Psychoneuroimmunology: Stress, Mental Disorders, and Health* (Washington, DC: American Psychiatric Press, Inc., 2000), 1.
5. Franklin Hoke, "Alternative and Conventional Biomedical Research: A Creative Synergy," *The Scientist* 8, no. 5 (March 7, 1994): 1.
6. Michael R. Irwin, "Human Psychoneuroimmunology: 20 Years of Discovery," *Brain, Behavior, and Immunity* 22 (2008): 129–139.
7. Tori DeAngelis, "A Bright Future for PNI," *Monitor on Psychology*, 33, no. 6 (June 2002).
8. Hoke, "Alternative and Conventional Biomedical Research."
9. Historical data are summarized from "Emotions and the Body," *Executive Health Report* 11, no. 10 (July 1985): 1–4; and Gina Maranto, "The Mind Within the Brain," *Discover* (May 1984): 34–43.
10. Viljoen et al., "Psycho-neuroimmunology."
11. Ibid.
12. Ibid.
13. Ibid.
14. "Mind Within the Brain."
15. G. F. Solomon and R. H. Moos, "Emotions, Immunity, and Disease: A Speculative Theoretical Integration," *Archives of General Psychiatry* 11 (1864): 657–74.
16. Viljoen et al., "Psycho-neuroimmunology."
17. H. Besedovsky, E. Sorkin, D. Felix, and H. Haas, "Hypothalamic Changes During the Immune Process," *European Journal of Immunology* 7 (1977): 323–325, in Virginia M. Sanders and Annemieke Kavelaars, "Adrenergic Regulation of Immunity," pp. 63–78 in Robert Ader, ed., *Psychoneuroimmunology*, 4th ed., vol. 1 (New York: Elsevier, Inc., 2007), 63–78.
18. J. E. Blalock, D. Harbour-McMenamin, and E. M. Smith, "Peptide Hormones Shared by the Neuroendocrine and Immunologic Systems," *Journal of Immunology* 135 (1985): 858s–861s.
19. Daniel Goleman and Joel Gurin, eds., Mind/Body Medicine: *How to Use Your Mind for Better Health* (New York: Consumer Reports Books, 1993), 58–59.
20. J. C. Fidelibus, "An Overview of Neuroimmunomodulation and a Possible Correlation with Musculoskeletal System Function," *Journal of Manipulative and Physiological Therapeutics* 12, no. 4 (1989): 289–92.
21. Viljoen et al., "Psycho-neuroimmunology."
22. Robert H. McCusker, Kelemen Strle, Suzanne R. Broussard, Robert Dantzer, Rose-Marie Bluthe, and Keith W. Kelley, "Crosstalk Between Insulin-like Growth Factors and Pro-Inflammatory Cytokines," pp. 171–188 in Robert Ader, ed., *Psychoneuroimmunology*, 4th ed., vol. 1 (New York: Elsevier, Inc., 2007), 171.
23. Viljoen et al., "Psycho-neuroimmunology."
24. Ibid.
25. Donald B. Calne, *The Brain* (Bethesda, MD: National Institutes of Health, NIH Publication #79-1813), 7–10.
26. G. Miketta, TRIAS ed., *Netzwerk Mensch*, 1st ed. (Stuttgart: Georg Thieme Verlag, 1991).
27. Hanneke P. M. Van Der Kleij and John Bienenstock, "Significance of Sensory Neuropeptides and the Immune Response," pp. 97–130 in Robert Ader, ed., *Psychoneuroimmunology*, 4th ed., vol. 1 (New York: Elsevier, Inc., 2007), 98.

28. Phil Evans, Frank Hucklebridge, and Angela Clow, *Mind, Immunity, and Health: The Science of PNI* (London: Free Association Books, 2000), 15.

29. Erica Goode, "Accounting for Emotions," *U.S. News and World Report*, (June 27, 1988): 53.

30. Marvin R. Brown and Laurel A. Fisher, "Brain Peptides and Intercellular Messengers," *Journal of the American Medical Association* 251 (10): 1310–14.

31. Joan Goldberg, "Peptide Power," *American Health* (June 1990): 35–41.

32. Ibid.

33. John L. Stump, "Threads of Psychoneuroimmunology in Sport," *The Sport Journal* 6, no. 1 (Winter 2003):36–41.

34. Signe Hammer, "The Mind as Healer," *Science Digest* (April 1984): 49.

35. National Institute of Allergy and Infectious Diseases, *Understanding the Immune System* (Bethesda, MD: National Institutes of Health, NIH Publication #85-529), 2–10.

36. Christopher J. Czura, Mauricio Rosas-Ballina, and Kevin J. Tracey, "Cholinergic Regulation of Inflammation," pp. 85–96 in Robert Ader, ed, *Psychoneuroimmunology*, 4th ed., vol. 1 (New York: Elsevier, Inc., 2007), 85.

37. Robert Danzer, "Immune System Effects on Neural and Endocrine Processes and Behavior," pp. 267–270 in Robert Ader, ed., *Psychoneuroimmunology*, 4th ed., vol. 1 (New York: Elsevier, Inc., 2007), 267.

38. DeAngelis, "Bright Future for PNI."

39. Robert Danzer, "Expression and Action of Cytokines in the Brain: Mechanisms and Pathophysiological Implications," pp. 271–280 in Robert Ader, ed., *Psychoneuroimmunology*, 4th ed., volume 1 (New York: Elsevier, Inc., 2007), 271.

40. Viljoien et al., "Psycho-neuroimmunology."

41. Dantzer, "Expression and Action of Cytokines," 277.

42. Robert Dantzer, Rose-Marie Bluthe, Mathalie Castanon, Keith W. Kelley, Jan-Pieter Konsman, Sophie Laye, Jacques Lestage, and Patricia Parnet, "Cytokines, Sickness Behavior, and Depression," pp. 281–309 in Robert Ader, ed., *Psychoneuroimmunology*, 4th ed., vol. 1 (New York: Elsevier, Inc., 2007), 282.

43. Dossey, *Meaning and Medicine* (New York: Bantam, 1991),105–6.

44. Stephen S. Hall, "A Molecular Code Links Emotions, Mind, and Health," *Smithsonian* (June 1989), 231–239.

45. Shannon Brownlee, "The Body at War," *U.S. News and World Report* (July 2, 1990), 48–54.

46. Goodkin and Vissar, Psychoneuroimmunology, 13.

47. Helen Carter, Christine McKenna, Roderick MacLeod, and Robyn Green, "Health Professionals' Responses to Multiple Sclerosis and Motor Neurone Disease," *Palliative Medicine* 12, no. 5 (1998): 393.

48. James P. Henry, "The Arousal of Emotions: Hormones, Behavior, and Health," *Advances* 6 (2):59–62; and James P. Henry, "Neuroendocrine Patterns of Response," in R. Plutchik, ed., *Biological Foundations of Emotions* (New York: Academic Press, 1986), 37–60.

49. J. P. Henry and P. M. Stephens, *Stress, Health, and the Social Environment: A Sociobiologic Approach to Medicine* (New York: Springer, 1977)

50. Bernie Siegel, *Love, Medicine, and Miracles* (New York: Harper & Row, 1986), 98.

51. *General Dentistry* (November/December 2003).

52. H. G. Koenig, M. McCullough, and D. B. Larson, *Handbook of Religion and Health* (New York: Oxford University Press, 2001).

53. Princeton Religion Research Center, 1982, 120.

54. H. G. Koenig, "Religious Beliefs and Practices of Hospitalized Medically Ill Older Adults," *International Journal of Geriatric Psychiatry* 13: 213–24.

55. Harold G. Koenig and Harvey Jay Cohen, *The Link Between Religion and Health: Psychoneuroimmunology and the Faith Factor* (New York: Oxford University Press, 2002).
56. Ibid.
57. Ibid.
58. Willem J. Kop, "The Integration of Cardiovascular Behavioral Medicine and Psychoneuroimmunology: New Developments Based on Converging Research Fields," *Brain, Behavior, and Immunity* 17 (2003): 233–7.
59. "Cancer and the Mind," *Harvard Mental Health Letter 20*, no. 1 (July 2003).
60. Anil K. Sood, Susan K. Lutgendorf, and Steven W. Cole, "Neuroendocrine Regulation of Cancer Progression: I. Biological Mechanisms and Clinical Relevance," pp. 233–250 in Robert Ader, ed., *Psychoneuroimmunology*, 4th ed., vol. 1 (New York: Elsevier, Inc., 2007), 233.
61. Alastair J. Cunningham, "Do Some People Overcome Cancer By Mental Change? Commentary on Katz/Epstein," Advances, 21, no. 3–4 (Fall/Winter 2003), 17.
62. "Cancer and the Mind."
63. Ibid.
64. Naomi I. Eisenberger, Matthew D. Lieberman, and Kipling D. Williams "Does Rejection Hurt? An fMRI Study of Social Exclusion"Science 10 October 2003, Vol. 302. no. 5643, pp. 290 - 292; and Jaak Panksepp "NEUROSCIENCE: Feeling the Pain of Social Loss" *Science* 10 October 2003:Vol. 302. no. 5643, pp. 237 - 239
65. Chiaramonte, "Mind-Body Therapies for Primary Care Physicians."
66. Christie Aschwanden, "A Cure for the Back Blues," *Health* 15, no. 2 (March 2001): 158.
67. S. M. Samuelsson, B. Bauer Alfredson, B. Hagberg, G. Samuelsson, B. Nordbeck, A. Brun, L. Gustafson, and J. Risberg, "The Swedish Centenarian Study: A Multidisciplinary Study of Five Consecutive Cohorts at the Age of 100," *International Journal of Aging and Human Development* 45 (3; 1997): 223–53.
68. Taylor et al.
69. Luisa Guidi, Augusto Tricerri, Daniela Frasca, Marcello Vangeli, Andrea R. Errani, and Carlo Bartoloni, "Psychoneuroimmunology and Aging," *Gerontology* 44 (1998): 250.
70. Ibid.
71. Goodkin and Vissar, *Psychoneuroimmunology*, 10.
72. Robert Ader, ed., *Psychoneuroimmunology*, 4th ed., vol. 1 (New York: Elsevier, Inc., 2007), xv.
73. Henry Dreher, "A Challenge to the Mind-Body Health Movement," *Advances in Mind-Body Medicine* 17, no. 2 (Spring 2001): 147.
74. Chiaramonte, "Mind-Body Therapies for Primary Care Physicians," 787.
75. Ibid., 790.
76. Ibid., 791.
77. Ader, *Psychoneuroimmunology*, xv.

2

The Impact of Stress on Health

The only difference between a diamond and a lump of coal is that the diamond had a little more pressure put on it.

—Anonymous

LEARNING OBJECTIVES

- Define the health effects and costs of stress.
- Differentiate between healthy and unhealthy stress.
- Identify the physiological effects of stress on specific body systems.
- Clarify the key elements of job stress.
- Understand how to handle stress.

No one is free of stress. According to figures from New York's American Institute of Stress published in *Time* magazine, 90 percent of all American adults experience high stress levels one or two times a week; a fourth of all American adults are subject to crushing levels of stress nearly every day. A survey of American women revealed that 57 percent felt excessively distressed much or most of the time.

So is stress good or bad? Philosophers, spiritual guides, physiologists, and now physicians and health educators have been exploring the remarkable ramifications of that question for millennia. Medically speaking, however, stress is a fairly new concept. Only in the last sixty years or so have researchers been able to pinpoint some of the effects of stress on human illness—and only in the last few years have scientists understood how the complex network of communications within the body interacts in response to stress.

Much of what we know about stress today originated with pioneer researcher Hans Selye. Early in the twentieth century, physicians believed that each disease was caused by a distinct and separate agent. But Selye, then a medical student in Prague, was puzzled by something he observed in the hospital: patients with a wide variety of illnesses shared a number of symptoms (particularly fatigue, joint pains, and weight loss). If distinct organisms caused each disease, Selye wondered, how could patients with so many different diseases all have the same symptoms?[1]

Unable to solve the mystery, Selye moved on, largely forgetting the puzzling patients in the hospital. Ten years later, a totally unrelated experiment with rats focused Selye's mind sharply back on those hospital patients. Selye set out to test a chemical extract that he believed contained a new ovarian hormone. The experiment required that the laboratory rats be injected at frequent intervals with the extract; a control group of rats was injected at the same frequency but with ordinary saline. After days of being jabbed with the needle, the rats that were receiving the chemical extract started developing an unexpected set of symptoms: enlarged and overactive adrenal glands, withered thymuses (a sign of a deteriorating immune system), and gastric ulcers. Surprisingly, the same set of symptoms developed in the rats that were injected with only the saline solution.

Selye thought back to the hospital where he had worked ten years earlier. What occurred to him then became the cornerstone of stress research: He realized that both the patients and the rats were reacting to stress, and he believed that, no matter what causes distress (whether it's a terminal illness, an overdrawn checking account, or a fight with a spouse), the body's reaction is the same. Selye called that reaction "the stress response," and it has become well documented during the ensuing decades of medical research.

We know that stress causes illness—and for decades the focus of stress research centered on the immune system. We now know that the effects of stress and their ability to cause illness and disease extend far beyond the tissues of the immune system, and that stress alters the function of other systems that are not part of the immune system.[2]

Definitions of Stress

Practitioners gathered at the 1949 Conference on Life and Stress and Heart Disease provided some of the first formal recognition that stress could precipitate chronic disease. Here, stress was given one of its earliest formal definitions: "A force which induces distress or strain upon both the emotional and physical makeup."[3] Scientifically speaking, stress is "any challenge to homeostasis" (the body's internal sense of balance). Stress occurs whenever there is change and whenever we are forced to adapt to that change. It is actually a constellation of events that start when a stressor precipitates a reaction in the brain, which then activates responses throughout the body.[4]

Our understanding of stress has come a long way in the last four or five decades. Early stress researchers categorized all stress as negative or bad; today, we understand that stress is anything in the environment that causes the need to adapt and that a "stressful" situation can be either happy (like the birth of a baby) or sad (like the death of a loved one).

We also understand that stress isn't limited to what goes on in our thoughts. A physical wound or invasion by a virus elicits a physical stress response. This response, called allostasis, is elicited whenever we don't already have an easy, automatic way of handling the stress—particularly if it's threatening—and is designed to bring the whole person back to a state of equilibrium (homeostasis).[5] Mental stress is a biological and biochemical process that begins in the brain and spreads through the nervous system, causing the release of hormones from the endocrine system and eventually exerting an effect on the immune system. Communication among these three systems (the nervous system, the endocrine system, and the immune system) maintains all bodily functions in a balanced, controlled way, the condition known as homeostasis. These three systems are totally integrated subsystems of what Dr. Richard Chapman (at the Pain Research Center of the University of Utah) calls an overall "supersystem."[6] Any disturbance in one kicks off a response in the others. The result is a complex domino effect in the body, eventually involving an entire series of body systems and a whole range of powerful hormones.

In fact, some researchers look at stress itself as a system: the "stress system" involves the brain, the hormone receptors, and the hormones. When the system is functioning normally, you experience homeostasis as well as normal physical and mental health. The opposite occurs when the system is not functioning normally. Many systems are generally involved. For example, when stress causes an increase in blood pressure, the impact isn't limited to the cardiovascular system: it also affects the brain, the eyes, and the kidneys, to name a few.[7]

Back to the original question: Is stress good or bad? Part of the answer depends on how you deal with the stress. If stress is relentless and uncontrolled, it can cause misery and disease. If you deal with it well, stress can be stimulating and can raise you to new heights. It also depends on the way you think about it, which in turn impacts how you deal with it. Finally, stress can be tempered by your coping ability and by other moderating factors.[8] For example, fascinating new research shows that, depending on how your body handles a neurotransmitter called serotonin, you may be born with a genetic propensity to be either more resilient or vulnerable to stress.[9] It's not all genetic, though: your learned styles of coping with stress play a major role in determining how much impact your genetics have.

A good example of how stressful situations can be altered by perception and outlook was witnessed by Colorado cardiovascular researcher Dr. Robert Eliot while he was traveling in the Middle East.[10] In downtown Riyadh, Saudi Arabia, Eliot saw two Arabs, both driving Mercedes, crash into each other. The two men, uninjured, jumped out of their cars and began hugging and laughing instead of yelling at each other. Curious about their odd exchange, Eliot asked his interpreter what the two men were saying. The interpreter explained that the two men were thanking Allah for the chance to meet this way.

Perception is crucial. When it comes to stress, says Margaret Kemeny, director of the Health Psychology and Behavioral Neuroscience program at the University of California at San Francisco, "The body is responding to what's going on in the brain, not to what's going on in the environment."[11] American Institute of Stress President Paul J. Rosch likens stress to a ride on a roller coaster. "There are those at the front of the car, hands over head, clapping, who can't wait to get on again," he points out, "and those at the back cringing, wondering how they got into this and how soon it's going to be over." Or, to put it another way, one roller-coaster passenger "has his back stiffened, his knuckles are white, his eyes shut, jaws clenched, just waiting for it to be over. The wide-eyed thrillseeker relishes every plunge, can't wait to do it again."[12] These two very different responses illustrate that stress is not always "out there" being done to us as much as it is "in here," determined by the ways we have learned to think about the stressor.

Distress and Eustress

Differences in perception cause some stress to be good stress (eustress) rather than bad stress (distress). An example is career stress: whether it's good or bad seems to depend not so much on how busy you are, but on what drives your hard work: love of it, curiosity about it, and satisfaction in it (eustress)—or fear of failure or anxiety over trying to prove yourself (distress).

While distress may cause disease, eustress can actually improve health. Eustress promotes productivity and facilitates our efforts; distress leads to a loss of productivity.[13] Eustress is exhilarating: you're under control but excited, like riding a canoe in a swiftly flowing stream. Some of the happiest moments of life occur when you're under some stress but respond with a sense of highly effective "flow." The opposite happens with distress: out of control, you feel like a victim in a runaway train.[14] The key to good health is learning how to turn bad stress (distress) into good stress (eustress).

Distress has been shown to affect almost all body systems, resulting in cardiovascular disease, neuromuscular disorders (including headache and chronic back pain), respiratory and allergic disorders, immunological disorders, gastrointestinal disturbances (including peptic ulcer disease, irritable bowel syndrome, nausea, vomiting, and diarrhea), skin diseases, dental problems, and a host of other disorders. Since most diseases are caused by a variety of different factors instead of a single cause, distress usually does not cause illness by itself, but it clearly reduces adaptability to other causes of illness. Various studies have demonstrated a strong link between distress and the onset of disease. In fact, the most effective preventive medicine may well lie in creating stress resilience. The best strategy, in addition to simplifying your life is to change your attitude toward the things you can't prevent. That's the process of turning distress toward eustress.

Types of Stress

There are three basic types of stress: physical, psychological, and psychosocial.

- Physical stress involves stressors in the environment—such as environmental pollution, constant noise, an inadequate supply of oxygen, injury, infectious agents, or excess exertion.

- Psychological stress stems from the way we react toward anything that is threatening, whether the threat is real or imagined.

- Psychosocial stress involves stressors from interpersonal relationships and conflicts with people around us. It can also occur when there is isolation as a result of inadequate social interactions.[15]

The Stress Response

When the body becomes stressed, regardless of the source of the stress, it undergoes the stress response: usually, it's the fight-or-flight response used by primitive people as they faced the various threats in their environment. When facing one of their enemies—a saber-toothed tiger, let's say—their bodies reacted in a very specific way that prepared them to either fight the tiger or run for their lives.

Unfortunately, our bodies still react the same way to threats—real or imagined—even though, for today's stressors, fighting or fleeing are both usually inappropriate. As Boston University psychiatrist Peter Knapp pointed out, "When you get a Wall Street broker using the responses a cave man used to fight the elements, you've got a problem."[16]

Each phase of the stress response carried with it benefits for the primitive man or woman who faced physical dangers, and those same benefits have become hazards for the modern man or woman who faces today's social stresses. Let's look at a dozen phases of the stress response and examine why yesterday's benefits are today's drawbacks.[17]

1. The adrenal glands start pumping out a group of hormones such as cortisol and catecholamines (the body's chemical messengers of stress). In the right quantities, these are essential for life, but in excessive amounts they can impair the immune system and reduce healing,[18] making it difficult to fight off even a minor cold. Too much cortisol over a prolonged time causes lymph glands to shrivel, bones to become brittle, and blood pressure to rise; it can even cause blood sugars to spike into diabetic ranges.

2. The thyroid gland pumps out thyroid hormones, which accelerate metabolism and enable fuels to burn faster to give energy for fight or flight. It does the same thing to us today as it did for the primitive people; but, because we're not engaged in life-or-death battles, it produces a different set of symptoms: insomnia, shaky nerves, heat intolerance, and exhaustion. This is why some people lose weight under stress.

3. The hypothalamus releases endorphins, powerful natural painkillers that enabled primitive people to fight or flee even when injured. However, chronic, relentless stress depletes endorphins and can in turn aggravate headaches, backaches, and even arthritis pain. Located in the part of the brain that connects thinking to peripheral body processes, the hypothalamus also releases the brain's key chemical initiator of the stress response, corticotropin-releasing hormone (CRH). Injected into the midbrain, CRH causes anxiety and up-regulates the nervous system to overrespond to stimuli. People who continue to obsess about past trauma or perceived abuse continue to secrete high amounts of CRH, and they continue to scan for danger and overrespond to stimuli. This overresponsiveness triggers many common medical disorders.[19]

4. Sex hormones (female progesterone and male testosterone) are reduced. That served an important function in primitive times: the decreased libido and fertility came in handy during times of drought, overcrowding, and decreased food supply by giving the community fewer mouths to feed, and by redirecting attention from amorous adventures to the threat at hand. Sadly, the same thing happens to you under stress: You may lose your sex drive, become infertile, or suffer from sexual dysfunction (such as premature ejaculation or failure to reach orgasm). Women under acute stress may have an early menstrual period; unrelenting, chronic stress may cause irregular periods or a complete lack of periods (amenorrhea).

5. Coordination of the digestive tract shuts down. In primitive people, all blood was diverted to the muscles, rendering them capable of extraordinary feats of power; the mouth went dry, too. The same things happen today. Eating while under stress can result in stomach bloating, nausea, abdominal discomfort or cramping, and even constipation or diarrhea. The dry mouth problems persist, too. Ask any public speaker whose mouth is so dry that he or she can't speak. Dry mouth is such an acute symptom of stress, in fact, that in China it's used as a lie detector test.

6. Release of sugar (glucose) into the bloodstream is followed by a boost in insulin to metabolize it, something that provided primitive people with "fuel for the sprint" or a burst of short-lived energy. That same scenario today can cause either high or low blood sugars. Continuously high insulin levels can cause weight gain and lead to elevated blood pressure and lipids (cholesterol). This insulin resistance (induced by stress hormones) can lead to the "metabolic syndrome" that puts you at high risk for cardiovascular disease.

7. Cholesterol is released into the bloodstream, mostly from the liver; it took over where blood sugar left off in supplying sustained energy to the muscles. But today's man or woman under chronic stress doesn't generally need more cholesterol to sustain energy, so the cholesterol is deposited in the blood vessels. The result is well documented by our nation's rate of heart disease fatalities.

8. The heart begins racing, a physiological response that pumps more blood to the muscles and lungs, carrying more fuel and oxygen to the muscles—something primitive people needed when under duress. Blood flow to the muscles of the arms and legs increases 300 to 400 percent when a person is stressed. The result today is high blood pressure; left unchecked, it can lead to stroke, heart attack, or kidney problems.

9. Breathing rate increases, providing greater air supply. While usually helpful, the increased demand on the lungs can be problematic for people with lung disease, such as asthma. Unfortunately, anxious breathing is usually shallow and high in the chest, which is not very efficient. Try breathing in a shallow way, rapidly and at near full lung expansion; quite soon, you are likely to start feeling anxious and stressed. When breathing is anxious, the mind becomes anxious. Now see what happens to your mind when you breathe slowly and more deeply with your diaphragm (relaxed breathing); in most cases, your mind will rapidly become calm. Note that just as the body's stress responses follow the mind's direction, your mind's responses also follow what is happening with your body.

10. The blood thickens and coagulates more readily. If wounded (a stressor), thickening of the blood enabled primitive people to stop bleeding. However, when the blood turns thick under chronic stress today, the result can be heart attack, stroke, or embolus (blood clot).

11. The skin "crawls," blanches, and sweats. This heightened the sense of touch, provided a cooling mechanism for overheated muscles, and diverted blood away from wounds. Today, it decreases the resistance of skin to electricity (the principle behind most lie detector tests).

12. All five senses become acute. In primitive people, pupils dilated to enhance night vision, overall mental performance was sharpened, the senses of hearing and touch were improved, and the entire body was brought to peak function. The same thing happens today; but, without the burst of physical energy that brings an end to a sporadic stressful situation, we are more likely to suffer from chronic stress. Thus, the senses are constantly on red alert, sometimes resulting in pain from stimuli that shouldn't cause such pain, such as a headache getting worse in response to light, sound, or smells.

Prolonged stimulation of the twelve phases of the stress response leads to what Robert S. Eliot calls the vigilance reaction.[20] According to Eliot, while the vigilance reaction may have once protected us from external dangers or scarcity, today it wreaks havoc on our bodies. Hypervigilance can cause the nervous system to overrespond to various normal stimuli, leading to such common diseases as irritable bowel syndrome, palpitations, migraine, chronic pain, anxiety disorders, and even medically unexplained neurological symptoms such as dizziness, numbness, or tingling.

That's not all: when stress becomes chronic, the effectiveness of the neurohormones is reduced. As stress continues, the stress hormones themselves can cause inflammation. When the body fails to adapt and resolve the inflammation, the risk of cardiovascular disease and metabolic syndrome is increased. The same process has been shown to play a role in the development of a variety of other disorders, including Parkinson's and Alzheimer's diseases, multiple sclerosis, pain, and AIDS-associated dementia.[21]

While the stress response outlined above is the best-known and best-accepted in the scientific community, maverick researchers are proposing that there may be other ways in which people respond to stress. Research by a team at the University of California San Francisco, headed up by psychoneuroimmunology researcher Margaret Kemeny, recognizes the fight-or-flight response to stress but maintains there is also a second reaction to stress—a withdrawal reaction in which the person pulls back to conserve energy.[22] Shelley E. Taylor, a psychoneuroimmunology researcher at UCLA, proposes that women may respond to stress with what she calls a "tend-and-befriend" reaction, in which they engage in nurturing activities that protect themselves and their children. Taylor believes that the pituitary hormone oxytocin—which provides a calming effect and is strongly linked to maternal behavior—may foster the tend-and-befriend reaction to stress.[23]

Costs and Outcomes of Stress

Distress is costly. While no one can put a precise price tag on the various health costs of stress, figures from a variety of sources give us a fairly good idea of its devastating impact. The American Institute of Stress estimates that more than 75 percent of all visits to health care providers result from stress-related disorders. The American Academy of Family Physicians estimates that two-thirds of all office visits to family doctors are prompted by stress-related symptoms.

According to a 2006 study by HR.com, a website devoted to human resources issues, stress costs U.S. businesses more than $300 billion annually—a number that has doubled in just more than ten years. Stress accounts for 40 percent of employee turnover.

In a 2004 American Psychological Association poll, one in four people said they have taken a "mental health day" due to work-related stress. In fact, half of the 550 million working days lost each year in the United States from absenteeism are stress-related. That might not be the worst of it; *presenteeism*, lost productivity from stress while on the job, appears to cost even more than the absenteeism.[24]

There's something else you can't put a price tag on: left unchecked, unremitting distress can also shorten your life. In one study of more than 600 people over twelve years, the existence of distress at the beginning of the study was a good predictor of who would die during the ensuing twelve years. Even when researchers tried to "juggle" the results by controlling for factors such as smoking, cholesterol levels, obesity, or high blood pressure, or by excluding people with chronic heart disease, the figures remained the same.[25]

A similar study in Sweden found that men who were under stress were more likely to die prematurely than those who weren't under stress. However, the researchers also found that certain kinds of stress had more pronounced effects than others. For example, those who felt insecure at work had a 2.4-fold increased risk of dying. Those who had been divorced or separated from their wives or who were in serious financial trouble during the year before the evaluation had triple the risk of dying. Those who had been sued had 7.7 times the risk of dying prematurely than those who had not. Overall, say the researchers, suffering three or more stressful life events more than tripled the risk of dying for the men involved in the study.[26]

The good news is that situational stress doesn't have to knock you out. Research shows that some people manage to be resilient to stress, exhibiting what scientists call "hardiness" (an ability to resist the ill effects of stress). Research has also clarified things that help you cope better with stressors. To figure out where you stand, it's important to know the factors that lead to distress, the physiological reactions of the body when under stress, and the way that mental stress can compromise the immune and other body systems, and thus lead to illness.

Factors Leading to Distress

Stress arises both from external events and from the way you think about them. During the early 1950s, University of Washington psychiatrist Thomas Holmes noted that patients had come down with tuberculosis after a cluster of disruptive events, such as a death in the family, a new job, or a difficult marriage. Based partly on that observation and partly on his extensive research, Holmes pronounced that the single common denominator for stress is "significant change in the life pattern of an individual." Holmes emphasized that stress did not cause the tuberculosis—tuberculosis bacteria had to be present—but that stress somehow weakened the body or made it more vulnerable to the disease.[27] Any major change—even a good one—is a stressor, disruptive of old automatic responses.

Branching out in his research, Holmes began to search for specific links between disease and what he called life events, those things in life that call for the greatest adjustment. He found that the more life events a person was subjected to within a brief period of time, the more likely he or she was to become ill. Holmes developed a social-readjustment rating scale along with his colleague Richard Rahe; commonly known as the Holmes-Rahe scale, it assigns a numerical score to the almost four dozen stressors, or life changes, that are known to increase the risk of disease. Subsequent research by hosts of independent scientists has verified the accuracy of the Holmes-Rahe scale.

The Holmes-Rahe Scale

Listed below are the items in the Holmes-Rahe scale, along with their numerical scores. Note that not all the items on the scale are "bad" things. Only a few of us would consider things like marriage, an outstanding personal achievement, a vacation, or Christmas to be negatives. If seen as a production that needs to be perfect (but usually isn't), even these potentially happy events can be distressful. You begin to see how it is not so much the event itself that is good or bad, but rather your thinking and expectations about the event.

The key word is change. Each item on the Holmes-Rahe scale describes something that requires you to change your routine, to adapt. The thing that requires change or adaptation can be positive or negative—you largely determine whether your reaction is positive or negative.

So where do you stack up? Scan the list of life changes, pinpoint the ones you have experienced within the last year, and add up the numerical scores to get a total. The score for each represents the relative impact of that item compared to the others.

100 Death of spouse

73 Divorce

65 Marital separation

63 Jail term

63 Death of close family member

53 Personal injury or illness

50 Marriage

47 Fired at work

45 Marital reconciliation

45 Retirement

44 Change in health of family member

40 Pregnancy

39 Sexual difficulties

39 Gain of new family member

39 Business readjustment

38 Change in financial status

37 Death of close friend

36 Change to different line of work

35 Change in number of arguments with spouse

31 Mortgage or loan over $10,000

30 Foreclosure of mortgage or loan

29 Change in responsibilities at work

29 Son or daughter leaving home

29 Trouble with in-laws

28 Outstanding personal achievement

26 Spouse begins or quits work

25 Change in living conditions

24 Change in personal habits

23 Trouble with boss

20 Change in work hours or conditions

20 Change in residence

19 Change in recreation

19 Change in number or type of church activities

18 Change in number or type of social activities

17 Mortgage or loan under $10,000

16 Change in sleeping habits

15 Change in number of family get-togethers

15 Change in eating habits

13 Vacation

12 Christmas

11 Minor violations of the law

According to Holmes and Rahe, if you score between 150 and 199 in one year, you have a 37 percent chance of getting sick during the following year. If you score between 200 and 299, your chances of getting sick jump to 51 percent; if you score over 300, you have a 79 percent chance of getting sick during the following year. All of these odds are altered considerably, however, as you become more stress resilient. In fact, if you are hardy, you might even embrace and enjoy change.

The mind is extremely powerful. Research has shown that merely thinking about one of the stressors on the list can evoke emotions so strong that they can induce the stress response. Isolating one of the items on the list, Holmes said that "a person often catches cold when a mother-in-law comes to visit. Patients mentioned mothers-in-law so often that we came to consider them a common cause of disease in the United States."[28]

Major Life Events and Cancer

Without an adaptive attitude or perception, major life events can weaken the system enough to bring on serious illness or disease. Yale oncologist and surgeon Bernie S. Siegel attributes some of the cancers of his patients to traumatic loss or crisis in their lives. One study of children with leukemia showed that 31 of the 33 children in the study had experienced a traumatic loss or move within the two years prior to their diagnosis. A separate study at Albert Einstein College of Medicine found that children with cancer had twice as many recent crises as similar, cancer-free children. Even career reversals may play a role, says Siegel: "The defeats of Napoleon Bonaparte, Ulysses S. Grant, William Howard Taft, and Hubert Humphrey have often been implicated in their fatal cancers."[29] This is not to say that stress causes cancer, but it may play a role in one's resistance to the usual causes.

Still another study involved more than 3,000 women who came to the Heidelberg University Gynecological Clinic for breast examination. The women who were not diagnosed with cancer were compared to those who did have cancer as diagnosed through various tests. Researchers determined that three life events had significant relationships to the development of cancer. One was the death of the mother before the woman was sixteen. The second was divorce, separation, or widowhood at any time during the woman's life. And the third was at least one traumatic event during World War II that caused considerable disturbance (researchers noted events like air raids, the death of close relatives, becoming a refugee, transfer of population, encampment, being buried alive, or injury to relatives as among the most disturbing).[30]

A study of 8,000 cancer patients with various types of tumors concluded, ". . . in most of the cases, the cancer appeared during a period of severe and intense life stress often involving loss, separation, and other bereavements."[31] To sort out genetic factors from those attributable to stress, W. H. Green at the University of Rochester studied pairs of identical twins in which one had developed leukemia and found that one twin in each pair usually developed leukemia shortly after a major psychological upheaval, while the stress-free twin did not (despite identical genetics.)

Hassles

Another factor involved in stress is what researchers call hassles. Charles Bukowski aptly illustrates the theory in an excerpt from his poem:

> . . . It's not the large things that
> send a man to the
> madhouse . . . no, it's the
> continuing series of
> small tragedies
> that send a man to the madhouse . . .
> not the death of his love but a shoelace that snaps
> with no time left. . . .[32]

Research into stress shows that commonly it's not the major events, but often the minor hassles, that accumulate and cause problems—things like running out of gas on the way to work, having unexpected company drop in, or getting delayed at a busy intersection. Various studies show that hassles are strongly related to episodes of illness, even when there are no major life events to consider.

As an example, psychiatrist and behavioral scientist Ian Wickramasekera points out that men "who experience such important life changes as divorce or the death of a wife may then be exposed to a wave of minor hassles (paying bills, dressing children, cooking, or doing the laundry) as they encounter new responsibilities (moving from father and husband, for example, to father and housekeeper)." A person in this kind of situation often develops back pain, headaches, stomach distress, or chest pain. "Sometimes it is not the mountain in front of you," he says, "but the grain of sand in your shoe that brings you to your knees."[33]

Attitudes Toward Stress

Your attitudes, perceptions, and the way you look at stressful events in life appear to be even more important than the events themselves, and realizing this can help you resist the ill effects of stress. A perfect example of resilience to stress was uncovered by University of Michigan researcher Louis Ferman. He found a "hard-luck victim" who had been laid off three times: first in 1962 when the Studebaker Corporation folded, next in the 1970s by a truck manufacturer that went out of business, and finally during cutbacks at a Chrysler plant. Ferman said that by all accounts, "He should have been a basket case, but he was one of the best-adjusted fellows I've run into." Asked his secret, the man replied, "I've got a loving wife and go to church every Sunday."[34] The specifics of creating healthy attitudes toward stress will be taken up later in this chapter in the discussion of stress resilience.

Age-Related Stressors

Prenatal   People are susceptible to different stressors at different stages of their lives. The impact of stress begins before we are even born: a variety of studies have shown that chronic stress during pregnancy contributes to preterm labor,[35] and stress experienced by a pregnant woman has definite physiological effects on her unborn baby. In one study of more than 500 rural women, those who experienced increasing stress levels between the second and third trimester had a significantly higher rate of complications, including neonatal death, neonatal illness, and low birth weight. These findings held true even when the researchers figured in all the standard risk factors.[36] One group of researchers found that babies born to stressed mothers cried more, slept less, were more irritable, and did not eat or have bowel movements with normal frequency.[37]

There is some evidence that the neurochemical abnormalities of major stress, depression, or anxiety disorders may influence the fetal brain development in ways that affect personality and behavior long after delivery. Speculation has been raised about whether the depression seen in children of depressed mothers is all genetic or could be influenced by programming in the uterus of the developing brain by the mother's neuro-hormones. This raises some very practical dilemmas for the physician and mother if, while pregnant, she were to get moderately depressed or have panic disorder. If these problems cannot be controlled without medication, is the risk to the baby greater if the mother goes untreated or takes medication that may or may not be safe during pregnancy? With the more recent data documenting risks to the baby when the mother has mental stress disorders, more physicians are opting to treat with medication when it's really needed. The improved results at and after birth tend to support that decision, and even long-term effects on the baby are beginning to encourage treatment of the mother's depression or anxiety.

Children and Adolescents The most tremendous stress an infant faces, of course, is its own birth.[38] Other infant stress is related to the syndrome known as "failure to thrive" (a child simply does not grow, despite there being no known biological problem). Researchers also believe that, while some amount of stress is healthy for an adult, infants do not benefit from any stress at all.[39] The first year of life is, in some very important ways, critical to the global worldview a person later carries. "Is the world a safe and nurturing place, or it is hostile and dangerous? Can I express my needs and feelings safely and will they be honored, or am I likely to get zapped if I do so?" Things as simple as how a cry is responded to can establish longstanding attitudes and expectations in the baby and can later affect the person's ability to express feelings and needs or can influence the person's propensity to look at the world in a hostile, competitive way.

Much mental programming occurs in these early years, even if there is no conscious memory of whence it arose. Either abuse or neglect early in life has been shown to activate the gene for the brain neuropeptide corticotropin-releasing factor (CRF). The resulting long-term increases in this brain hormone cause significant anxiety and up-regulate the nervous system to overrespond to stimuli. This chronically overresponsive nervous system can be responsible for much of the increased pain, bowel symptoms, and anxiety experienced by such individuals, even later in life.[40]

School-aged children are understandably stressed by many of the same things that stress preschoolers—divorce of parents, serious illness that requires hospitalization, and witnessing violence. When school enters the picture, so does a whole new host of stressors. According to researchers, the most common stressors of school-aged children include anxiety about going to school, bullies, changing schools, conflicts with the teacher, forced competitiveness, difficulty with classmates, fads, dares with classmates, failing exams or getting failing grades, failing to make an athletic team, having to give oral reports in front of the class, learning disorders, being unable to complete homework assignments, lack of parental interest in achievements, parental pressure to achieve, dealing with the reputation of older siblings (bad or good), worrying about taking tests, and even special recognition (for making the honor roll, winning a debate match, and so on). A significant amount of stress stems from peer teasing—about, for example, being overweight, being of a different race, wearing glasses, having red hair, or wearing dental braces.[41]

Characteristically, school-aged children react to stress in a number of behavioral ways. They may regress (start wetting the bed or sucking their thumbs, for example), have problems getting along with classmates, lose motivation or concentration, become irritable, or withdraw from social contacts. These can also be signs of clinical depression in children. According to researchers, however, there are a number of physical signs and symptoms as well: school-aged kids under stress may suffer headaches, stomachaches, poor appetite, asthma or excess allergies, and sleeplessness.[42]

Parental reaction to the stress-induced illness can also be important. If illness becomes a safe haven because much nurturing and attention are given, it can become an unconsciously automatic response ("illness behavior") when safety and nurturing are needed. It may be kinder in the long run to make it a not-so-pleasant time, perhaps with bed rest, isolation, and not much that's fun to do—administered with kindness, of course. This is a tricky call because serious organic disease may heal faster with loving support.

Typical stressors in adolescence include the major transitions of moving from dependent childhood to independent adulthood, yet not being fully equipped for such independence.[43] Parents are wise to understand that this is a time when the need for independence and acceptance is foremost. A teenager knows he or she must become his or her own person, autonomous and "okay." The problem, often, is that a teen lacks the experience to make wise decisions, and parents may undermine the very empowering of their children by offering what they call "constructive criticism" in ways that imply they are not capable or acceptable and that they need to depend on the parent to make the right decision for them. The best parental balance seems to be to (1) creatively teach natural consequences of choice (and be sure those consequences "naturally" occur), then (2) encourage empowering independence, with (3) expressions of love and encouragement no matter which choices the teen makes.

Adults   College students are generally stressed by academic pressure, course overload, career decisions, self-doubt, changing roles in the family, and the pressures associated with developing intimate relationships. Young and middle-aged adults often suffer from family and career stressors and often financial problems.

The elderly face the unique stresses associated with adjusting to retirement, failing health, deteriorating sight and hearing, the loss of friends and family members, and the stress of facing their own deaths.[44] A major source of distress for those who are aging is Western society's notion that one's worth as a person depends on productivity and on looking young. This same heavy emphasis on productivity causes great stress for workers.

Factors that Influence How We Cope with Stress

A number of important factors enable some people to cope better with stress than others. For example, genetic susceptibility to distress may be indicated by parents or grandparents who die before the age of sixty-five.[45] The Wisconsin Primate Laboratory, studying mother monkeys for their stress resilience to separation from their family, found that the animals could be bred in stress-resistant and stress-vulnerable strains.[46] This might be similar to the genetic inheritance for depression and for alcoholism. For example, a person may inherit the tendency to produce too much of an enzyme (monoamine oxidase, or MAO) that removes brain neurotransmitters (such as serotonin and dopamine) involved in maintaining control and pleasurable mood.

If these neurotransmitters are removed too rapidly by MAO, a person tends to be shy, "on guard," more antisocial, and more prone to seeing the negatives in life—and, as a result, more distressed. If the MAO is low, on the other hand, the neurotransmitters increase, and a person is more likely to be a risk-taker who fails to see dangers. Other genes for some of these neurotransmitters have similar effects. Combinations of these vulnerability-inducing genes contribute to how well we deal with stress. If stress vulnerability runs in your family, it becomes doubly important to give attention to the methods of creating resilience (discussed later in this chapter and in Chapter 22).

Factors that increase the ability of children to cope with stress include gender (girls are generally more resilient under stress, though researchers are not sure why), high intelligence, easygoing temperament, a strong internal locus of control, the availability of adults who exhibit warmth and structure, and families with a high socioeconomic status.[47] Attitudes and learned ways of thinking about situations are also major factors in the ability to cope with stress. Other factors include a good sense of humor, a well-balanced and nutritious diet, realistic goal setting, plenty of sleep, thorough job preparation, financial security, stability at home, an understanding of stress, and use of relaxation skills.[48]

Meditators are particularly at an advantage when it comes to coping with stress. Other documented protective factors include high self-esteem, learning to be flexible and innovative in solutions, close personal relationships, having success/mastery experiences, self-discipline (including good control of time), and positive expectancy (hope). How to implement these factors will be discussed throughout this book.

The Physiological Reactions to Stress

When something sets off the complicated series of physiological responses in the body, the resulting "stress response" involves a series of more than 1,400 known physiochemical reactions. Some of the most common physical signs and symptoms of stress include headache, backache, insomnia, tightness in the neck and shoulders, indigestion, loss of appetite or excessive eating, and a pounding heartbeat.

The aches and pains we feel in response to stress can be the result of a complex physical reaction. For example, levels of the neurotransmitters serotonin and noradrenaline—which not only regulate mood, but help to modulate pain—drop during chronic distress.[49] When levels in the central nervous system fall too low, pain is up-regulated—that is, a small pain stimulus is perceived as a much greater stimulus. Chronic stress can result in chronic pain. Thus, antidepressant medications or behavioral interventions that increase a sense of control and raise these central neurotransmitters can be very helpful in reducing chronic pain.[50]

In 1936, stress pioneer Hans Selye called the stress response pattern the general adaptation syndrome[51]; it involves three major stages of the body's reaction to stress:

1. **Alarm reaction.** In the first stage, the alarm reaction, the body immediately responds to stress; neurotransmitters are released in response to an *external* stressor, and various physiological changes occur that enable the body to combat stress (the fight-or-flight reactions discussed earlier). If the stress is brief, the body's response is limited to that of the alarm reaction. When the stress ends, so does the reaction. In this case, the body tends to bounce back and recover quickly. The stress response system seems designed to facilitate this adaptive acute response.

2. **Resistance.** In stage two, resistance, physiological changes enable the body to adapt to prolonged stress. The body actually works overtime to bring immune response and resistance up to par. During this second stage, the body's immunocompetence is

actually stronger than normal, an attempt by the body to keep itself in fighting form. At this stage of increased immune response, a person may get disorders of excess immunity, such as increased allergies or autoimmune diseases (in which the immune system attacks the body's own tissues). This is when the immune system memory of how to respond is established.

3. **Exhaustion.** If the stressor doesn't relent, the body eventually loses the ability to keep up with the demands, and it enters the third stage, exhaustion (and dysregulation). Simply stated, the body has its limits. They're different in every person; but, when the body reaches its limit, protective immune function breaks down, sometimes with mixtures of too much antibody immunity (causing allergies) and, at the same time, too little cellular immunity (causing susceptibility to infection). This results in some of the diseases of adaptation, the diseases we know as stress-related disorders.[52]

Interestingly, the immune system usually goes through the same three stages in response to an *internal* stressor (such as a wound or bacteria): (1) an alarm (communicated by cytokines) when a wound occurs; (2) inflammatory resistance (and antibody memory of how to respond next time); and (3) dysregulation (such as autoimmunity) or exhaustion (such as system-wide infection) if the stressor is uncontrolled. When stress occurs, the resulting cascade of molecules and hormones actually keep the three key systems in communication:

- The nervous system releases *neurotransmitters*, which communicate with and significantly affect the immune and endocrine systems.

- The immune system releases *cytokines*, which communicate with and significantly impact the nervous and endocrine systems.

- The endocrine system releases *hormones*, which communicate with and effect significant changes in the nervous system and immune systems.

For example, in response to the physical stress of infection, the immune system releases proinflammatory cytokines (like interleukin-1), which cause mental depression; that's why you get all the symptoms of depression when you get the flu. The nervous system releases neurotransmitters in response to mental stress that can trigger allergic reactions in the immune system, which is why you may get hives when stressed. In fact, researchers have shown that the mechanisms in allergies and the changes of the immune system in response to stress have many things in common.[53]

The hyperaroused nervous system appears to trigger a more prolonged hyperaroused immune system. Conversely, an exhausted nervous system (such as occurs with clinical depression) is associated with depressed cellular immunity, and thus worsened susceptibility to infections.[54]

The bottom line of all this is that stress on one system (such as mental stress) creates significant alarm reactions in the other systems that in turn impact physical disease.[55] And, in a real sense, while the person represents the physiological supersystem within himself or herself, the person is also a subpart of a much larger biopsychosocial supersystem that impacts the stress he or she feels (and imparts to other nearby people).

Note that there is significant difference between the acute and chronic stress responses. Acute stress is defined as stress that lasts anywhere from a few minutes to a few hours; chronic stress is defined as stress that lasts for several hours a day for an extended period, usually months or years.[56] Studies of stress must always take this difference into account. It's much easier to test the effects of short-term, acute stress than to test the effects of chronic stress, which has many more unknown variables. Again, much more chronic physical disease is associated with the chronic stress response than with acute responses.

How long you can endure without breaking down and becoming exhausted is highly individualized. The same factors that help you cope with stress help determine how susceptible you are to developing chronic stress and its illnesses. A particularly important factor is the way we think about the stress. Different modes of thinking produce significantly different responses. For example, the comment, "You're looking good!" could be received by an older person as a compliment, as patronization, or as an implication that the person looks good for such an old person. Or a cynical person may ask in response to the compliment, "What do they want out of me?" In each case, the stress response would be very different. Stanford University biologist Robert Sapolsky emphasizes that it's not the stressor that's important, but the perception of it: "The exact same external event can happen to two different people, and, depending on the psychological baggage of the individual experiencing it, the outcome will be different, the disease will be different."[57]

There is apparently even a difference between the way men and women respond to stress. New research shows that though women complain more about the symptoms of stress, such as headaches and backaches, they actually suffer fewer long-term stress-related problems, such as cardiovascular disease. Researchers aren't sure why, but they think the key may lie in female hormones. In one study, women asked to perform stressful tasks registered higher blood pressure and higher heart rates after menopause than before.[58] Other reasons may well involve a woman's greater propensity to express feelings and seek support.

While the stress response is complex, you can more easily understand some of the profound effects of stress by understanding how it affects major body systems.

Stress and the Brain

The brain is usually the first body system to recognize an external stressor. It reacts with split-second timing to release neurotransmitters that instruct the rest of the body how to adjust to the stressor. The brain continues to stimulate the "stress reaction" for as long as 72 hours after a traumatic incident.

The brain is not always a good discriminator of stressors. It reacts the same whether the stress is physical (you are almost hit by a car that comes careening around the corner when you step off the curb), emotional (your boss calls you in for another of his "talks"), or even immune-mediated (your body is confronted by a threatening infection). If the brain overresponds to an emotional stressor, it may well overrespond to a pain or gut stressor or even an immune stressor, resulting in allergy. What that reaction entails, basically, is the release of a cascade of hormones and brain chemicals that course through the bloodstream, instructing other organs—such as the pituitary, the thyroid, and the adrenals—to release their respective hormones. Just as the brain is the organ that turns on the stress response, it is also the organ that finally turns it off.

Unfortunately, all this hormonal brain activity takes its toll. Elevated levels of stress hormones kill off significant numbers of vitally important brain cells. According to Sapolsky, the stress hormones, the glucocorticoids, help us adapt when we are confronted by danger; but, when chronically high, "...these all-important glucocorticoids also trigger a curious cascading death of the very brain cells that those hormones are meant to protect."[59] This can result, for example, in reduced memory and impaired thinking. University of Kentucky researchers under the direction of Philip Landfield exposed rats to prolonged stress—five days a week for six months. After only three weeks, the rats showed reduced electrical activity in the hippocampus (the crucial memory area of the brain that is most affected by Alzheimer's disease). When examined in autopsies at the end of six months, the rats that were exposed to stress had lost twice as many brain cells—50 percent of all their brain cells—as same-age rats that had been spared the stress.[60]

In separate studies at Stanford University[61] and at the Rockefeller University Laboratory of Neuroendocrinology, researchers found that the stress hormone cortisol makes the cells of the hippocampus smaller. In addition, it results in fewer nerve branches throughout the hippocampus. The stress does not necessarily need to be prolonged in order to have a significant effect: Excessive cortisol changes the nerve cells and branches of the hippocampus in as brief a time as three weeks. This shrinking of thinking and memory cells occurs in part as a result of cortisol suppressing the nerve growth factors that keep neurons healthy and which stimulate the formation of new nerve tracts created for new memory.[62]

Stress and the Endocrine System

The function of the endocrine system, with its network of glands, is to secrete hormones. When the body is under stress, two main hormone groups, the catecholamines and the corticosteroids, are galvanized to combat it. The catecholamines—adrenaline (or epinephrine) and noradrenaline (or norepinephrine)—cause the heart to beat faster, the blood vessels to constrict, the muscles to tense up, the respiratory system to work more rapidly, the blood to thicken and clot in case of injury, more energy to be released, and the brain to be more alert.

When catecholamine levels are too high, as in chronic stress, the effects can range from minor problems (such as tics and muscle tremors) to more serious, potentially long-range problems, such as diabetes, heart attack, and stroke. In the blood vessels, for example, norepinephrine can cause damage to the vessel lining that allows cholesterol into the wall and can stimulate clotting, both of which can lead to the thickening (plaque) that causes cardiovascular disease.

The other major hormone group secreted in response to stress is the corticosteroids, including cortisone and cortisol. Too much cortisol can suppress immunity, cause insulin resistance (leading to weight gain and diabetes), increase blood pressure, and cause progressive nerve loss in the hippocampus and other thinking parts of the brain.

The changes that occur in the hippocampus as a result of excessive cortisol mimic the loss of cells that results from aging. Studies done at New York University Medical Center point out that aged people are less able to regulate their stress response, and, as a result, levels of cortisol produced during stress don't return to normal for long periods of time. Under these stressed conditions the aged can suffer rapid shrinking of brain cells. The New York researchers concluded that stress can actually play a role in the development and progression of Alzheimer's disease.[63]

Apparently, stress can also interfere with the hormones that influence fertility and can result in infertility. Perhaps the most serious complication of chronic high cortisone levels is suppression of the immune system. High cortisol levels can cause shrinkage of the spleen and thymus, which are vital for the production of white blood cells. Known as powerful immunosuppressants, each of the corticosteroids, especially cortisol, "breaks down lymphoid tissues in the thymus and lymph nodes, reduces the level of T helper white blood cells and increases T suppressors, and inhibits the production of natural killer cells. Cortisol also reduces virus-fighting interferon."[64] Nevertheless, cortisol is not the whole story in stress-induced immunosuppression, since mental distress will suppress immunity even when the adrenal gland (the source of cortisol) has been removed.

According to research investigating the link between stress hormones and the immune system, a wide range of diseases is associated with elevated cortisol levels, including cancer, hypertension, ulcers, heart attack, diabetes, stroke, Parkinson's disease, multiple sclerosis, myasthenia gravis, and a variety of infections. Researchers believe that elevated cortisol levels associated with stress may contribute to depression and psychoses of the aged; "elevated cortisol levels are even reported to be a useful predictor of suicide."[65]

Stress and the Gastrointestinal System

How the gastrointestinal system reacts to the challenges of stress depends in large part on personality traits. A study that called on men to solve arithmetic problems and anagrams while under stress showed that some had an increase in gastric acid while others actually had a decrease. The difference, say the researchers, was due to personality traits—in other words, the way people coped with stress.[66] Those who produce too much acid may be at risk for stress-induced ulcers of the stomach or upper small intestine.

One study showed that the important factor seems to be *perceived* stress. More than 4,500 people took part in the National Health and Nutrition Examination Survey Epidemiologic Follow-Up Study. At the beginning of the study, participants did not have peptic ulcer disease; during the thirteen years of the study, researchers followed the participants to see who developed it. Interestingly, during that time, those who perceived themselves as stressed were 1.8 times more likely to develop ulcers than those who did not perceive themselves to be stressed, regardless of how many stressors actually existed.[67]

A far more common effect of stress on the gastrointestinal tract is that of "functional bowel disorders," such as irritable bowel syndrome, nonulcer dyspepsia, and esophageal spasm. These are the most common disorders diagnosed in gastroenterology clinics, and they are highly associated with central nervous system disorders (more than 80 percent of patients also have clinical depression or anxiety disorders).[68] This association of depression and anxiety with functional bowel problems makes sense because their cause really resides not so much in the bowel as in the central nervous system and that part of the peripheral nervous system that innervates the intestines. Abnormalities of the same neurotransmitters involved with stress and depression are the primary culprits in causing the bowel to overrespond to normal bowel stimuli, such as eating food (causing excessive spasm, pain, and bowel movement abnormalities).[69] These same neurotransmitter abnormalities cause the nervous system to overrespond to stress stimuli in an anxiety disorder.

Stress and the Cardiovascular System

As early as 1628, physician William Harvey maintained that ". . . every affection of the mind that is attended either with pain or pleasure, hope or fear, is the cause of an agitation whose influence extends to the heart."[70] Today, stress is recognized as a major contributor to heart disease. In his book *From Stress to Strength*, cardiologist Robert S. Eliot describes exactly how stress causes coronary artery disease:

- First, stress causes the blood pressure to spike. The increased pressure of the blood pounding through the vessels pummels and weakens the delicate, protective inner lining of the arteries.

- When the lining is damaged, the body starts its first attempt at repair: fats are deposited in the arteries. The result? Blood vessels are narrowed, blood circulation is slowed, and the likelihood of clotting becomes high.

- The body continues its arsenal of healing: Platelets are mobilized to the damaged arteries. Clots start to form. More fatty material is deposited, and the arteries finally become rigid and inflexible. All of this leads to heart attacks and strokes.[71]

Researchers have noted that in parts of the world where stress is uncommon, so is heart disease.[72] And stress can be life-threatening to a person who already has coronary heart disease: the resulting increased heart rate and blood pressure are a deadly combination to someone whose arteries are already narrowed by disease. The result is coronary occlusion, damaged heart tissue, and, sometimes, cardiac arrest.[73]

Effects on the Heart and Blood Pressure   Increases in heart rate and blood pressure caused by stress contribute to the increased load on the heart. Stress-induced high blood pressure is even greater among men whose arteries are already clogged by the fatty deposits of atherosclerosis.[74] According to North Carolina A&T researcher Andrew Goliszek:

> The stress of factory noise, for example, has been closely linked to high blood pressure in factory workers exposed to prolonged, daily noise; flood victims experiencing devastating property and financial loss have developed permanent high blood pressure during their recovery periods; and executives in their early thirties, who were chronically angry and hostile but who suppressed their anger and hostility because they couldn't express themselves, developed high blood pressure before they reached their fifties. Even school children are susceptible to high blood pressure when placed in stressful situations.[75]

Added to this scenario is the problem with some people whom researchers have dubbed "hot reactors," people whose blood pressure seems normal at rest but shoots up to dangerously high levels during stress.[76] Again, this relates to a sensitive nervous system overresponding to stimuli. Eliot estimates that as many as one in five people exhibits undetected daily blood pressure changes that place him or her at high risk for stroke or sudden cardiac death. Eliot has identified ten possible complications of hot reacting: permanent high blood pressure, damaged blood vessel linings, atherosclerosis, accelerated blood clotting, ruptured heart muscle fibers, heart rhythm disturbances, kidney and heart failure, heart attack, stroke, and sudden death.[77]

People who reduce stress enjoy the benefit of lower blood pressure. Research by psychologists at Harvard University followed residents of eight Massachusetts nursing homes for three years. Researchers randomly selected some of the patients in each nursing home and taught each to meditate as a way of reducing stress. At the end of three years, the survival rate among the people who meditated was 100 percent: not a single one of the patients who meditated had died, and most had significant drops in systolic blood pressure. Among the patients who did not meditate, survival rate was only 62.6 percent.[78]

Serum Cholesterol   Stress can also elevate levels of serum cholesterol. In one of the first studies showing a link, researchers followed forty accountants who, because of their work, were forced to meet stressful deadlines at specific times of year. The researchers found that the most strenuous work periods coincided with the highest levels of cholesterol, even though the diets and activity levels of the accountants remained unchanged.[79] During the tax preparation period from January 1 to April 15, the cholesterol levels of the accountants rose as much as 100 points over their normal levels.[80]

A number of studies duplicate these findings. One group of researchers measured serum cholesterol levels of medical students a few hours before final examinations and again 48 hours later. In all but one student, the serum cholesterol value was an average of 20 percent higher in the stress period before the exam.[81] A similar study showed that the highest cholesterol levels among military pilots in training occurred during examination periods. Similarly, studies among college students showed an increase of 11 to 17 percent in cholesterol levels during testing periods.

Almost any kind of stress can cause significantly increased quantities of cholesterol to be released into the bloodstream. A number of studies show that shift work is extremely stressful, particularly for those on the night shift. One study found that night labor was associated with significantly elevated cholesterol levels.[82]

Spasm in Damaged Blood Vessels   Traditional risk factors fail to account for half the cases of clinical coronary artery disease worldwide,[83] yet more than a half million deaths in the United States every year are attributed to arteriosclerosis. Stress delivers a double whammy to people who already have coronary artery disease: stress causes vessels already choked by plaque to narrow even more, boosting the chance for heart attack. In studies at Harvard Medical School, researchers put subjects under stress to determine the multiplied effect of stress on already damaged arteries. While under stress, the damaged arteries constricted 24 percent more and blood flow declined by 27 percent in the damaged vessels, though it didn't decline in the smooth vessels.[84] This coronary spasm is increased even more if the person has clinical depression (see Chapter 6).

In one study, researchers monitored patients hospitalized in London who were being evaluated for possible coronary bypass surgery. The researchers carefully studied heart function but also measured the levels of stress hormones in the urine and asked patients themselves to record their feelings at various times during the day. The findings showed that the higher the levels of stress hormones in the urine, the more frequent the episodes of silent ischemia.[85]

Cardiovascular Disease Events   Research has shown a strong link between stress and sudden cardiac death. In one study, researchers examined a hundred cases of sudden cardiac death drawn from a coroner's records. The researchers found that almost two-thirds of the victims were under moderate to severe stress on the final day of life, and more than one in five were experiencing acute stress during the last 30 minutes of life. The coroners' reports revealed stressors such as receipt of divorce papers, a fight over a game, an automobile accident, and an attack by dogs as some examples.[86] The sudden deaths were probably due to an irregular heart rhythm caused by catecholamines and increased heart demand as a result of stress.

A growing body of research has shown that, among heart disease patients, mental stress is as dangerous to the heart as physical stress.[87] Mental stress testing of coronary patients shows the same kind of coronary ischemia abnormalities as exercise stress testing.[88]

While early research on cardiovascular disease centered on diet and exercise, it has taken a dramatic swing toward the examination of stress as a leading factor. Maryland psychologist David Krantz summarizes heart disease as "some interaction of mind, body, and behavior. Your coronary risk probably depends on how your mind interprets situations, how your body reacts, and how often your behavior leads you into stressful situations."[89] This connection between stress and cardiovascular disease will be discussed in more detail in Chapters 3 and 4.

Stress and the Immune System

As research continues into the link between stress and the immune system, as discussed in Chapter 1, fascinating medical outcomes of that effect continue. One study of family infections showed that stress was four times as likely to precede an infection as to follow it. Throughout the year of the study, only about one-fifth of the low-stress families had any infection, whereas half of the high-stress families did. Does stress cause infection? Researchers don't think so. They are convinced, however, that stress compromises the immune system enough for infection to take hold.[90] One way in which that happens could involve the phenomenon known as acquired immunity: once the body is exposed to a certain virus, the immune system sets up a defense for that particular virus; the next time the body is exposed to that agent, it mounts an immune defense that kills the virus, preventing illness. That's the principle upon which vaccines are founded. Through a variety of effects, stress can delay and sometimes even prevent acquired immunity, leaving you susceptible to another bout of the cold or flu you just got over.[91]

How stress impacts immunity depends on a number of factors. Certainly psychological resilience—which stems from things like optimism, a sense of control, social support, early life experiences, and coping mechanisms—has a significant effect. So does physical resilience, which depends on things like genetics, nutrition, environment, and sleep. Researchers have learned that other factors also affect how much immunity is impacted by stress; these include the duration, intensity, and timing of the stress as well as whether and how intensely the systems of communication within the body are activated (including the neurotransmitters, cytokines, and hormones).[92]

Other research also shows that different ways of coping with stress seem to modify the impact of stress on immunity. Early research showed that the ability to control and predict stress decreased the physical consequence of that stress; in well-known experiments, laboratory rats that could predict or control a series of shocks were able to avoid the ill effects of stress suffered by the rats that could not predict or control the shocks.[93] That is, getting a mental sense of control seems to induce better immunological control. Different styles of coping with stress appear to affect the way stress impacts the immune system.[94]

Because of the impact of stress on the immune system, scientists have come up with a veritable shopping list of conditions caused or aggravated by stress: coronary heart disease, arteriosclerosis, atherosclerosis, high blood pressure, coronary thrombosis, stroke, angina pectoris, respiratory ailments, ulcers, irritable bowel syndrome, ulcerative colitis, gastritis, pancreatitis, diabetes, hyperthyroidism, migraine headache, myasthenia gravis, epileptic attacks, chronic backache, kidney disease, chronic tuberculosis, allergies, rheumatoid arthritis, systemic lupus erythematosus, impotence, infertility, psoriasis, eczema, cold sores, shingles, hives, asthma, Raynaud's disease, multiple sclerosis, cancer, and an entire spectrum of endocrine and autoimmune problems, to name just a few.

Physicians caution, however, that "few of these diseases are caused or triggered solely by stress." Other factors must also be considered.[95] While enough bacteria in the right place can cause disease in almost anyone, some people exposed to the usual causes of disease get sick and some do not. The difference usually resides in that person's "host resistance" to illness. Immunity is part of that resistance. Several mental factors also have proven to be important in host resistance, such as loving support and mature coping styles. (See the chapters on social support and disease-resistant personality, such as Chapter 8.) On the other hand, some mental factors undermine resistance, such as hostility, fear, or depression (also discussed in later chapters). Other positive mental factors optimize both immune and mental responses. Researchers have recently learned that, while stress generally suppresses the immune system, there are certain situations in which acute—not chronic—stress might actually enhance immunity.[96]

Self-Perceptions of Stress

Obviously, distress can be very detrimental. And, just as obviously, no one can live without some stress. Are we all, then, destined to become victims of stress? Fortunately not.

The researchers who have pinpointed the effects of stress also know that changing the way a person perceives stress and the way he or she copes with it can keep it from making him or her sick. Attitudes, beliefs, and perceptions can help keep humans well. Ample evidence, cited throughout this book, shows how factors like optimism, faith, hope, and a good explanatory style can help overcome the devastating effects of stress. All of these can be actively cultivated.

Epidemiologist Leonard Sagan remarked that "whether altered conditions are viewed as threatening or challenging, and whether the consequences contribute to personal growth or apathy and despair, is the result of the interaction of two factors: the magnitude and quality of the external stressor and the capacity of the individual to cope."[97]

How to Protect Yourself from Stress

Since everyone is confronted with stress, are there ways we can protect ourselves from the adverse effects of stress? Absolutely! One of the first ways, says Baylor College of Medicine psychologist Michael Cox, is to face the stress head on. Recognize it, and get ready to deal with it. "Avoiding and denying that stress exists won't make it go away," he says. "Look at different ways you can change the situation to lessen the stress, make your decision, and face the stress head on. Action is the fastest way to reduce the level of stress."[98] Be prepared for the worst possible scenario, but then leave it behind and work for the best outcome.

Sometimes, for health, a philosophical checkup can be even more useful than a medical one. What is life all about for you? Does life have more to do with proving yourself competitively by generating production numbers, or does it have more to do with discovering and experiencing the sources of joy? Or perhaps learning how to give and receive love? Or becoming wise? If joy or love or wisdom seems key to you, are all the busy things being done enhancing that, or are some getting in the way of it (your joy)? Is your style of responding to life's stressors what you like and admire? Or would you like to temper or modify it somewhat? What kind of style do you admire in people of great wisdom or goodness? Some methods for changing to your desired style will be explored in Chapter 22.

Following are some ideas from cardiologist Robert S. Eliot and others as to how you can reduce the effects of stress:

- Develop what Eliot calls a game plan for your personal aspirations, both short-term and long-term ones. Take a personal inventory, and reestablish important priorities. You need to balance your talents and goals, similar to the way in which you'd balance your financial portfolio. Work to get things back into balance, and figure out where your long-term goals may be losing out to short-term pressures, Eliot says.

- Do something nice for yourself every day. Take the time to read something you love, soak in a warm bath, take a brisk walk, or call an old friend.

- Commune with nature.

- Develop a system of time management that will help you plan your day without becoming a stressor itself. When you're scheduling your time, remember to leave time for play, time for hobbies and friends, and time for simple relaxation. If you have to, schedule in time for breaks.

- Just as you need to develop a game plan for your personal aspirations, Eliot advises developing a game plan for your career or work. Especially important in today's economy is the ability to adapt, continually assess where you are, look ahead, and anticipate and prepare for change.

- If you commute to work, make sure you plan enough time to arrive without feeling stressed. If you can, turn your commute into something pleasant: ride the bus instead of driving, and take the chance to catch up on some favorite books or magazines. If you have to drive, try out some entertaining tapes or music instead of the usual radio fare.

- Once at work, try the following strategies: Pair up with people you like. Instead of letting the telephone control you, control the telephone; have someone take messages, and block out several periods during the day in which to return calls. Delegate as much work as you can. Do what you can to reduce environmental stresses at work (noise, temperature extremes, and so on). At least once a day, concentrate on doing at least one task—no matter how small—that brings you satisfaction.

- Save a little money each month. Take frequent nonbusiness weekends away from home, preferably with someone you love and care about.

- Get married if you're not. Marriage, particularly if carefully nurtured, has been shown to protect against illness.

- Be realistic in your expectations of your children. According to Eliot, it's crucial to accept who they are and let children express their own ideas. Eliot also advocates giving children at least one adult they can look up to and letting them stay closer to home until they have the skills and resources to make it on their own in an increasingly complex world.

- Take a look at your neighborhood. What's going on? Do as much as you can to create a calm, controlled, quiet, comfortable neighborhood and home.

- Pay attention to your physical health. Have regular checkups, and take care of health problems promptly. If you notice unusual symptoms, have a doctor check them out as soon as possible. Above all, believe that you are well.

- Get plenty of sleep. British researchers concluded that flexibility, spontaneity, and originality of thought can be seriously undermined by as little as one sleepless night.

- Eat a balanced diet; avoid tobacco, caffeine, and excess alcohol. During periods of particular stress, go for a small, high-protein meal featuring something like chicken breast, turkey breast, nuts, tuna, or Swiss cheese.

- Get plenty of exercise.

- Stay socially connected. According to Eliot, "Friends are not just nice, they are a necessity." If you have problems, talk them out with a trusted friend; if you're facing something difficult, rehearse it with a friend first. Share your feelings often.

- Develop at least one confidant, someone with whom you can share your deepest thoughts and feelings. Write your thoughts down on a regular basis. Keeping a journal is good, but so is jotting your thoughts on scraps of paper. *In particular, write down daily two or three things that happened that day for which you are grateful; this can be exceptionally helpful.*

- Find and trust in a higher power; develop a sense of spiritual support. Attend your church or synagogue on a regular basis, affiliate with the religious community there, and practice forgiveness on a daily basis. Fill your life with faith; let go of guilt and shame.

- Get a pet! Research has shown that pets reduce stress, lower blood pressure, and provide a type of social support that enhances health.

- Learn to laugh at yourself, and fill your life with humor.

- When things get tough, take a warm bath or shower, or sip a cup of warm herbal tea. Above all, stay flexible. There may be more ways to cope with any situation than are apparent at first.[99]

Job Stress and Health

In today's fast-paced society, it's important to look at another common source of stress: the job. The stress connected with certain kinds of jobs can, indeed, hurt your health—and if stress on the job gets too intense, it can kill you. On the other hand, good and satisfying work can greatly enhance health, well beyond not working at all. So what makes the difference?

High-powered executives who cope with the stress of running corporations, humoring clients, balancing budgets, and solving personnel problems are not those most likely in danger. They're under stress, but research indicates that the people most likely to be negatively affected by job stress are the ones who have little control or decision-making power: assembly line workers, factory workers, or computer operators who are constantly scrutinized by supervisors. Another high-risk group is middle management, who are often given tasks from above with which they may disagree but have the burden of getting those who they manage to carry the task out—again feeling a lack of control both from above and below. Jobs that seem without meaning and purpose, or without recognition for work well done, can also lead to health problems.

Estimates are that job stress costs American industry more than $300 billion a year from absenteeism, illness (resulting in health insurance payouts and workers' compensation claims), employee turnover, and even theft and sabotage. That can add up to more than the company's profits.[100] In an attempt to dull the effects of job stress, a staggering number of employees are turning to drugs and alcohol on the job—a trend that is draining the honesty, energy, and reliability of American workers. Mental depression has been shown to be the major source of on-the-job loss of productivity,[101] yet curiously, employers (fearful of insurance premium increases) have been the largest barrier to getting full insurance coverage for treating such mental disorders and to changing job characteristics to minimize the risk of depression.

To sum it up, says New York Medical College psychiatrist Paul J. Rosch, who heads the American Institute of Stress, "Work stress may be America's number-one health problem."[102]

Job Burnout

A surprising number of people today, particularly in helping professions in larger companies, are experiencing burnout. For example, in a survey of the physicians in California's Sacramento Medical Society, 40 percent said they felt some symptoms of depression, and a third were planning to leave their practices within three years.[103]

Burnout often results from feeling a loss of personal control and a loss of meaning in the work. This phenomenon often follows excessive demands, expectations of

Table 2.1   Comparison of Characteristics of Stress and Burnout

Stress	Burnout
Characterized by overengagement	Characterized by disengagement
Emotions are overreactive	Emotions are blunted
Produces urgency and hyperactivity	Produces helplessness and hopelessness
Loss of energy	Loss of motivation, ideals, and hope
Leads to anxiety disorders	Leads to detachment and depression
Primary damage is physical	Primary damage is emotional
May kill you prematurely	May make life seem not worth living

ever-increasing productivity, and management scrutiny. Long work hours combined with lack of recreation and sleep frequently also trigger burnout.

Burnout is really different from stress. Stress is usually obvious and characterized by *too much*, and is often associated with anxiety. On the other hand, burnout can sneak up on you and is often characterized by *too little*—too little meaning, too little hope, too little interest. Table 2.1 illustrates the differences between stress and burnout.[104]

Burnout is much more difficult to solve, but it starts with stress, so identifying and addressing it in the stress stage is important because much can be done there. The loss of meaning is a major source of burnout (even in healing professions, which have great inherent meaning), as are overwork (often driven by "productivity" concerns), loss of sleep, and lack of recreation. Table 2.2 illustrates the results of an interesting study of this phenomenon that involved the measurement of attitudes of medical interns at the beginning and end of their grueling internship year (invariably with excessive workloads and sleep deprivation).[105]

These young physicians came out of school with significantly better moods, energy, and empathy (and less anger) than the general population; but, by the end of a hard job year, many of these benefits had been trained out of them.

Table 2.2   A Survey of Medical Interns

	Normal Population	Beginning of the year	9–12 Months later
Profile of Mood States			
Anxiety	13.5	10.8	10.4
Depression	14.1	5.1	10.7
Anger/Hostility	9.6	3.8	10.5
Fatigue	10.6	4.7	10.4
Interpersonal Reactivity Index			
Empathic Concern	10.6	22	20.7
Personal Distress	10.9	8.8	10.7

Why are we working so hard that we burn out? Consider how we calculate one's "worth"—generally it's by productivity, as measured by money, competition, or hours worked. Those of old age in the United States may be seen as not of much value because they are less "productive" in the quantifiable sense. But here's the paradox: the current demand to generate ever-increasing numbers, greater productivity, and better products than anyone else is driving workers and managers toward exhaustion. The incessant demand by employers for higher productivity actually causes less productivity because it leads to stress-related illness and burnout.[106]

Health Effects of Job Stress

Work is the source of a great deal of "ordinary" stress. In one British study, researchers for the National Survey of Health and Development questioned more than 1,400 26-year-old men. Those who were under stress were asked to pinpoint the source of their stress. Surprisingly, only 8 percent of the men reported stress at home or in some other arena of their personal lives. A staggering 38 percent reported work as the source of severe stress in their lives, and almost half of those said they were physically ill as well.[107]

In a series of studies done at Cornell University Medical College, researchers evaluated a total of 260 men who worked at various jobs in New York City. Men who worked in high-stress jobs—those characterized by plenty of pressure but little power to make decisions—were more than three times as likely to have high blood pressure as the men who worked in low-stress jobs.[108] This was further confirmed in a second three-year follow-up study.[109]

Stress has also been shown to increase both cortisol levels and blood pressure among working men and women. In one study, people with the highest levels of over-commitment at work were found to have cortisol levels that were an average of 22 percent higher than those of workers with the lowest levels of overcommitment.[110]

Apparently, the boss—and the boss's style—have a lot to do with mediating the effects of a stressful situation on the job. Researchers studied nearly 200 AT&T employees during a tumultuous period; those with supportive bosses suffered only half the illness of those with unsupportive bosses. Those with unsupportive bosses, in fact, suffered two times the illness, obesity, sexual problems, and depression that their colleagues with supportive bosses did.[111]

Both too little or too much work has ill effects. Unemployment can be devastating to health. One of the most conclusive studies was conducted in Scotland and reported in the *British Heart Journal*,[112] which found that the strongest predictor of coronary heart disease among the men in the study was found to be unemployment. On the other hand, excessive work is also a problem. Workaholism is a compulsive disorder, described by one writer as being "as ravaging and insidious as alcoholism or eating disorders."[113] Another called it "the only lifeboat guaranteed to sink." Diane Fassel, author of *Working Ourselves to Death*, calls it "a killer stalking our society."[114]

Studies show that job stress can even continue to affect people after they retire. One Swedish study followed more than 600 men who had retired. The Swedish researchers found that those who had job stress while working had nearly twice the relative mortality risk after retirement. Researchers also found that if job stress during work had been coupled with weak social support, the risk of early death jumped by more than 400 percent.[115]

Job Stress and Metabolic Syndrome

One of the most dangerous effects of job stress is metabolic syndrome—a syndrome characterized by a group of metabolic risk factors in one person. Those risk factors include:[116]

- Abdominal obesity (excessive fat tissue in and around the abdomen)
- Blood fat problems (such as high triglycerides, low high-density-lipoprotein [HDL] cholesterol, and high low-density-lipoprotein [LDL] cholesterol) that contribute to the buildup of plaque in the artery walls
- Elevated blood pressure
- Insulin resistance or glucose intolerance (which means the body can't properly use insulin or blood sugar)
- Factors in the blood that contribute to clotting (such as high fibrinogen)
- Proinflammatory state (such as elevated C-reactive protein in the blood)

People with the metabolic syndrome are at increased risk of not only coronary heart disease and other diseases related to plaque buildups (such as stroke and peripheral vascular disease), but also type 2 diabetes. It's estimated that more than 50 million Americans have metabolic syndrome.

Important new research shows that job stress is a particular risk factor for metabolic syndrome. The authors of the study defined metabolic syndrome by the presence of at least three of the factors listed above, and they defined job stress in situations in which people had a high number of job demands but little control. On an average, the people in the study were followed for fourteen years, which allowed for a meaningful collection of data.

The degree of job stress over time significantly increased the risk of the metabolic syndrome. Those people with lower grades of employment suffered disproportionately from the effects of stress as a risk factor for the metabolic syndrome, and men were more susceptible to the effects of stress than women.[117]

Job Characteristics Help Determine Job Stress

Just as some stress is critical to life, some stress is essential on the job. It's what keeps us motivated, inspired, and productive—as long as it's kept to a healthy level and a person has some sense of control as to how to deal with it well. In their book *Healthy Work*, authors Robert Karasek of the University of Southern California and Dr. Tores Theorell of Sweden's National Institute for Psychosocial Factors and Health say that the following are characteristics of healthy jobs:[118]

- **Skill discretion.** Your job allows you to make maximum use of your skills and provides the opportunity for you to increase or broaden your skills.
- **Autonomy.** Your job allows you some sense of control. You don't feel as though you are a child being disciplined. You get to participate in long-term planning, and your employer allows flexible hours.

- **Control.** You control the machines at your workplace, not the other way around.

- **Psychological demands.** You have some say over the magnitude of the demands placed on you, and the routine demands you are faced with are mixed with new, unpredictable challenges that help keep the job exciting.

- **Social relations.** You're encouraged to collaborate with your coworkers. There's a sense of teamwork and support.

- **Social rights.** When problems arise, democratic procedures are used to solve them. If you have some kind of a grievance, you know there's an accepted way for you to solve it.

- **Meaningfulness.** Your job has some meaning for you. You know what you're producing, and who it's for. You have ready access to feedback from your customers (the people you work for all day).

- **Integration of family and community life with work.** The people on the job share the responsibilities of running the business, so there's time—and energy—left over for activities other than work.

How Much Stress Is Enough?

Every job is going to include some stress.[119] It might be thunderous noise and wilting heat from the blast furnace of a steel plant, or it might be the inescapable deadlines of reporting for a newspaper. It might be the monotonous repetition of working on an assembly line or the crushing stress of running a multimillion-dollar corporation. No one would want a job that is totally devoid of stress. Somewhat stressful challenges make life (not to mention a job) interesting. But what are the signs that enough is enough, when you've inched over the line toward stress that is debilitating?

Basketball great Bill Russell of the Boston Celtics described the rush that can come from the right level of job stress when he told how the pressures of a professional game begin to percolate: "It usually began when three or four of the ten guys on the floor would heat up," he explained. "The feeling would spread to other guys, and we'd all levitate. . . . The game would be in the white heat of competition, and yet somehow I wouldn't feel competitive. . . . I'd be putting out the maximum effort . . . and yet I never felt the pain. My premonitions would be consistently correct. . . . There have been many times in my career when I felt moved or joyful, but these were moments when I had chills pulsing up and down my spine."[120]

A healthy level of job stress is one that provides a sense of cohesion, intense satisfaction, great challenge, supreme accomplishment, and personal control. Mihaly Csikszentmihaly, in some classic studies on human happiness, called these peak experiences "flow."[121]

When there's enough stress to stimulate challenge, satisfaction, and control, you'll feel certain emotions, and you'll find that your job performance meets certain standards. An optimum level of stress is characterized by high energy, mental alertness, high motivation, calmness under pressure, thorough analysis of problems, improved memory and recall, sharp perception, and an overall optimistic outlook.[122]

The signs of too little or too much stress on the job are much the same. Whether absence of job stress has created a monotonous environment devoid of challenge and excitement, or you're in over your head at a job you can't perform to anyone's liking, the signs generally include boredom, apathy, a high accident rate, frequent grievances, absenteeism, a negative outlook toward the employer, widespread fatigue, insomnia, changes in appetite, increased errors, indecisiveness, and increased use of tobacco, drugs, or alcohol.[123]

In summary, keys to healthy work involve creating some sense of personal control, establishing a sense of support, finding intrinsic meaning and purpose in one's work, and hoping to create even better things to come. Stress with an internal sense of control and being able to respond well makes life good.

Keys for Handling Job Stress

The same researchers who found that job stress is a killer have also identified a buffer: social support on the job. It might be a boss who treats you with respect. It might be a great feeling of camaraderie with coworkers. It might be regular feedback from customers who appreciate the job you're doing. It might be professional networking with others. Or it might be membership in a labor or professional union. In fact, say researchers Karasek and Theorell, social support on the job "may be one of the most important factors in improving health and well-being in the work environment."[124] As in all other facets of life, the people around us can be the key to good health and long life (see Chapter 9).

In addition to increasing your social support on the job, try the following measures to alleviate job-related stress:

- Take a hard look at the meetings you have to attend. Start by avoiding unnecessary meetings. Could you accomplish the same thing by memo or a few phone calls? When you do find yourself scheduled for a meeting, go in with a clear objective, then stick to the task.

- Set your priorities every morning. Make sure you accomplish at least one thing every day that has high value for you. We all have more items on our "to do" lists than there is time to do them. If one is stuck on the thought, "I have to do it all," frustration results. Usually doing the low-priority items that are right in front of you results in failing on the more subtle high priorities (such as great relationships, for example) for which one needs to consciously block out time. Remember, with "too many things to do," it's really okay not to do it all—and, in fact, saying "no" to low-priority items allows you to complete more high priority projects. The resultant sense of control over your life is highly health promoting.

- Fridays tend to be "down days," so save the last hour or so on Friday for house-keeping tasks, such as straightening your desk, sorting your mail, returning phone calls, or listing your tasks for Monday. Then save something you really like to do for Monday morning, to get your week started off on a pleasant note.

- Take frequent breaks. You know you need a break when you find yourself day-dreaming, you start procrastinating, you have a mental block, or you're feeling tense. Remember that you should take more frequent breaks if you are doing work that requires a lot of concentration. And people who take regular vacations are much less prone to burnout.

- Find meaning and purpose in work.

Rachel Naomi Remen, a physician deeply concerned about the phenomenon of burnout and loss of meaning in the workplace, has found some simple techniques that can be very useful in rediscovering the purpose and meaning you once felt toward your work: she suggests taking ten minutes at the end of the day to journal the answers to the following three questions:[125]

- "What surprised me today?"
- "What moved or touched me today?"
- "What inspired me today?"

Look for the stories. After some time, instead of seeing the answers six or more hours later, you will start to see them as they happen and find meaning in the moments.

Such techniques allow you to recapture the purposes for which you chose your work. For life to be satisfying, your work needs to have intrinsic value— a quality that you look forward to—rather than just the extrinsic rewards. It has been said that happiness consists of meaningful, good work to do and someone to love.

Ultimately, since much of life's stress can only be modified but not eliminated, the real key is turning distress into eustress, the principles of which will be discussed in the chapter on disease resilience (Chapter 8) and in Chapters 21 and 22.

WHAT DID YOU LEARN?

1. What is the difference between distress and eustress?
2. What is the difference between stress and burnout?
3. Describe how three body systems are affected by distress.
4. What is *flow*?
5. From the list of methods in "How to protect yourself," choose four that would be most helpful for you, and start to implement them.

ENDNOTES

1. Susan Jenks, "Further Clues to CAD-Stress Link," *Medical World News* (June 13, 1988): 108.
2. Bruce Rabin, "Stress: A System of the Whole," pp. 709–718 in Robert Ader, ed., *Psychoneuroimmunology*, 4th ed., vol. 2 (New York: Elsevier, Inc., 2007), 709.
3. Jenks, "Further Clues to CAD-Stress Link."

4. Firdaus S. Dhabhar and Bruce S. McEwen, "Bi-directional Effects of Stress on Immune Function: Possible Explanations for Salubrious as Well as Harmful Effects," in Robert Ader, ed., *Psychoneuroimmunology*, 4th ed., vol. 2 (New York: Elsevier, Inc., 2007), 723–50.

5. B. S. McEwen, Allostasis and Allostatic Load: Implications for Neuropsychopharmacology. *Neuropsychopharmacology* 22 (2000):108–24

6. R. C. Chapman, R. P. Tuckett, and C. W. Song, "Pain and Stress in a Systems Perspective: Reciprocal Neural, Endocrine and Immune Interactions," *Journal of Pain* 9 (2008):122–45.

7. Rabin, "Stress," 718.

8. Dharma Singh Khalsa, "Stress-Related Illness," *Postgraduate Medicine* 78, no. 6 (1985): 217–21.

9. Avshalom Caspi, et al., "Influence of Life Stress on Depression: Moderation by a Polymorphism in the 5-HTT," *Gene Science* 301, no. 5631 (18 July 2003): 386–389.

10. Jenks, "Further Clues to CAD-Stress Link."

11. Tori DeAngelis, "A Bright Future for PNI," *Monitor on Psychology,* 33, no. 6 (June 2002). Accessed at http://www.apa.org/monitor/jun02/brightfuture.html

12. Paul Rosch, "Good Stress: Why You Need It to Stay Young," *Prevention* (April 1986): 29.

13. Mihaly Csikszentmihaly. *Flow: The Psychology of Optimal Experience* (Harper Perennial, 1991).

14. Emrika Padus, *Positive Living and Health: The Complete Guide to Brain/Body Healing and Mental Empowerment* (Emmaus, PA: Rodale Press, 1990).

15. Mary F. Asterita, *The Physiology of Stress* (New York: Human Sciences Press, 1985), 4–5.

16. Claudia Wallis, "Stress: Can We Cope?" *Time* (June 6, 1983): 48–54.

17. Peter G. Hanson, *The Joy of Stress* (Kansas City, MO: Andrews, McMeel, and Parker, 1986).

18. Lawrence E. Lamb, "Your Vital Adrenal Steroids (Corticosteroids)," *The Health Letter* 34, no. 4 (1989): 1–8. Also, Charles B. Nemeroff, "The Persistent Neurobiological Consequences of Early Life Trauma: Implications for the Pathophysiology of Mood and Anxiety Disorders," American Psychosomatic Society 59th Annual Scientific Meeting March 10, 2001, Monterey CA

19. K. E. Habib P. W. Gold, and G. P. Chrousos. "Neuroendocrinology of Stress," *Endocrinology Metabolism Clinics of North America* 30 (2001): 695–728.

20. Robert S. Eliot, *From Stress to Strength* (New York: Bantam Books, 1994), 24.

21. National Institutes of Health, "Functional Links Between the Immune System, Brain Function, and Behavior."

22. Tori DeAngelis, "A Bright Future for PNI."

23. Ibid.

24. M. Boles, B. Pelletier, and W. Lynch. "The Relationship Between Health Risks and Work Productivity," *Journal of Occupational and Environmental Medicine* 46, no. 7 (July 2004): 737–45. Also W. N. Burton et al. "The Association of Medical Conditions and Presenteeism," *Journal of Occupational and Environmental Medicine* 46, no. 6 Suppl. (June 2004) S38–45.

25. P. D. Somervell, B. H. Kaplan, and G. Heiss, "Psychologic Distress as a Predictor of Mortality," *American Journal of Epidemiology* 130, no. 5 (1989): 1013–23.

26. A. Rosengren, K. Orth-Gomér, H. Wedel, and L. Wilhelmsen, "Stressful Life Events, Social Support, and Mortality in Men Born in 1933. *British Medical Journal* 307(6912) (1993): 1102–1105.

27. Hanson, *The Joy of Stress.*

28. Wallis, "Stress: Can We Cope?," 48–54.

29. Bernie S. Siegel, *Love, Medicine, and Miracles* (New York: Harper and Row Publishers, 1986).

30. Horst Scherg and Maria Blohmke, "Associations Between Selected Life Events and Cancer," *Behavioral Medicine* (Fall 1988): 119–24.

31. H. J. F. Baltrush, reported at the Third International Symposium on Detection and Prevention of Cancer, (New York, April 16–May 1, 1976).

32. Ibid.

33. Ian Wickramasekera, "Risk Factors Leading to Chronic Stress-Related Symptoms," *Advances* 4, no.1 (1987): 21.

34. Wallis, "Stress: Can We Cope?," 48–54.

35. Haim Omer and George S. Everly, Jr., "Psychological Factors in Preterm Labor: Critical Review and Theoretical Synthesis," *Advances* 7, no. 1 (1990): 11–3, adapted from *American Journal of Psychiatry* 145, no. 72 (1988): 1507–13.

36. Harold A. Williamson, Jr., Michael LeFevre, and Melvin Hector, Jr., "Association Between Life Stress and Serious Perinatal Complications," *The Journal of Family Practice,* 29, no. 5 (1989): 489–96.

37. Lynne C. Huffman and Rebecca del Carmen, "Prenatal Stress," in L. Eugene Arnold, ed., *Childhood Stress* (New York: John Wiley and Sons, Inc., 1990), 144–72.

38. Marie L. Lobo, "Stress in Infancy," in L. Eugene Arnold, ed., *Childhood Stress* (New York: John Wiley and Sons, Inc., 1990), 173–92.

39. Ibid.

40. Charles B. Nemeroff, "The Persistent Neurobiological Consequences of Early Life Trauma: Implications for the Pathophysiology of Mood and Anxiety Disorders." American Psychosomatic Society 59th Annual Scientific Meeting March 10, 2001, Monterey CA

41. Susan Jones Sears and Joanne Milburn, "School-Age Stress," in L. Eugene Arnold, ed., *Childhood Stress* (New York: John Wiley and Sons, Inc., 1990), p. 42.

42. Ibid.

43. Robert L. Hendren, "Stress in Adolescence," in L. Eugene Arnold, ed., *Childhood Stress* (New York: John Wiley and Sons, Inc., 1990), 247–66.

44. Age-related stressors summarized from Jerrold S. Greenberg, *Comprehensive Stress Management,* 3rd ed. (Dubuque, IA: Wm. C. Brown Publishers, 1990), 299–393.

45. Hanson, *The Joy of Stress.*

46. G. P. Sackett, "Genotype Determines Social Isolation Rearing Effects on Monkeys," *Developmental Psychology* 17 (1981): 313–8.

47. Ann S. Masten, "Stress, Coping, and Children's Health," *Pediatric Annals* 14, no. 8 (1985): 546.

48. Hanson, *The Joy of Stress.*

49. Stephen M. Stahl, "Does Depression Hurt?" *Journal of Clinical Psychiatry* 63 (2002): 273–4. Also Stephen M. Stahl, "The Psychopharmacology of Painful Physical Symptoms in Depression," *Journal of Clinical Psychiatry* 63, no. 5 (2002): 382–3.

50. H. J. McQuay et al. "Sytematic Review of Outpatient Services for Chronic Pain Control," *Health Technological Assessment* 1 (1997): i–iv, 1–135; C. Redillas and S. Solomon, "Prophylactic Pharmacological Treatment of Chronic Daily Headache," *Headache* 40 (2000): 83–102; A. G. Lipman, "Analgesic for Neuropathic and Sympathetically Maintained Pain." *Clinics in Geriatric Medicine* 12 (1996): 501–15.

51. Andrew G. Goliszek, *Breaking the Stress Habit* (Winston-Salem, NC: Carolina Press, 1987).

52. Ibid.

53. Gailen D. Marshall and Sitesh R. Roy, "Stress and Allergic Diseases," pp. 799–818 in Robert Ader, ed., *Psychoneuroimmunology,* 4th ed., vol. 2 (New York: Elsevier, Inc., 2007), 815.

54. S. Cohen, D. A. Tyrell, and A. P. Smith, "Psychological Stress and Susceptibility to the Common Cold," *New England Journal of Medicine* 325 (1991): 606–12. Also see J. B. Imboden, A. Cantor and L. E. Cluff "Convalescence from Influenza, A study of the Psychological and Clinical Determinants." *Archives of Internal Medicine* 108 (1961): 393–9.

55. R. C. Chapman, R. P. Tuckett, and C. W. Song, "Pain and Stress in a Systems Perspective: Reciprocal Neural, Endocrine and Immune Interactions," *Journal of Pain* 9 (2008):122–45.

56. Dhabhar and McEwen, "Bi-directional Effects of Stress," 723.

57. Bruce S. McEwen, "Hormones and the Nervous System," *Advances* 7, no. 1 (1990): 50–4.

58. Kelly Costigan, "What Is a Woman's Most Stressful Occupation?" *Complete Woman* (April 1988): 32–3.

59. Jerry Lazar, "New Proof That Stress Ages the Brain," *Longevity* 2, no. 3 (1988): 25.

60. "Workplace Warning: Stress May Speed Brain Aging," *New Sense Bulletin* 16, no. 11 (1991): 1.

61. Bruce S. McEwen, "Hormones and the Nervous System."

62. Maletic V. et al. "Neurobiology of Depression: An Integrated View of New Findings," *Clinical Practice* 61, no. 12 (2007): 2030–40. Also R. S. Duman et al. *Archives of General Psychiatry* 54 (1997): 595–606; and P. S. Ericson *Acta Neurologica Scandinavia* 110 (2004): 275–80

63. Bruce S. McEwen, "Hormones and the Nervous System."

64. Michael A. Weiner, *Maximum Immunity* (Boston: Houghton Mifflin Company, 1986).

65. Ibid.

66. G. Holtmann, R. Kriebel, and M. V. Singer, "Mental Stress and Gastric Acid Secretion: Do Personality Traits Influence the Response?" *Editor's Citation Abstract* 35, no. 8 (1990): 998–1007.

67. R. F. Anda et al., "Self-Perceived Stress and the Risk of Peptic Ulcer Disease: A Longitudinal Study of U. S. Adults," *Archives of Internal Medicine* 152 (1992): 829–33.

68. R. B. Lydiard, et al. "Prevalence of Psychiatric Disorders in Patients with Irritable Bowel Syndrom." *Psychosomatics* 34 (1993): 229–34. Also E. A. Walker, P. P. Roy-Byrne, and W. J. Katon. Irritable Bowel Syndrome and Psychiatric Illness. *American Journal of Psychiatry* 147 (1990): 565–72.

69. Gershon, *Alimentary Pharmacology and Therapeutics* 13, suppl. 2 (1999): 15–30. Also Humphrey et al., *Alimentary Pharmacology and Therapeutics* 13, suppl. (1999): 31–38; and Bearcroft et al., *Gut* 42 (1998): 42–6.

70. Andrew G. Goliszek, *Breaking the Stress Habit* (Winston-Salem, NC: Carolina Press, 1987).

71. Eliot, *From Stress to Strength*, 30–1.

72. Goliszek, *Breaking the Stress Habit.*

73. "Stress Can Make You Sick," *Consumer Reports Health Letter* 2, no. 1 (1990): 1, 3.

74. "Can Stress Clog Arteries?" *Consumer Reports on Health* (December 1993): 133.

75. Goliszek, *Breaking the Stress Habit.*

76. Susan Jenks, "Further Clues to CAD-Stress Link."

77. Robert S. Eliot and Dennis L. Breo, "Are You a Hot Reactor? Is It Worth Dying For?" *Executive Health* 20, no. 10 (1984): 18.

78. Stephen Brewer, "Anti-Old-Age Stress," *Longevity* (June 1990): 82.

79. Larry A. Tucker, Galen E. Cole, and Glenn M. Friedman, "Stress and Serum Cholesterol: A Study of 7,000 Adult Males," *Health Values* 2, no. 3 (1987): 34–9.

80. Eliot, *Stress to Strength*, 40.

81. S. Bloch, C. J. Brackenridge. Psychological, performance and biochemical factors in medical students under examination stress. *Journal of Psychosomatic Research* 16(1) (1972): 25–33. Also see J. Dreyfuss, J. W. Czaczkes. Blood Cholesterol and Uric Acid of Healthy Medical Students Under the Stress of an Examination. *Archives of Internal Medicine* 103(5) (1959): 708–11.

82. Tucker, Cole, and Friedman, "Stress and Serum Cholesterol," 34–9.

83. John E. Sutherland, "The Link Between Stress and Illness," *Postgraduate Medicine* 89, no. 1 (1991): 162.

84. K. A. Fackelmann, "Stress Puts Squeeze on Clogged Vessels," *Science News* (November 16, 1991): 309.

85. Marjory Roberts, "Stress and the Silent Heart Attack," *Psychology Today* (August 1987): 7.

86. Peter Riech, "How Much Does Stress Contribute to Cardiovascular Disease?" *Journal of Cardiovascular Medicine* (July: 1983): 825–31.

87. C. Noel Bairey et al., "Mental Stress as an Acute Trigger of Left Ventricular Dysfunction and Blood Pressure Elevation in Coronary Patients," *American Journal of Cardiology* 66 (1991): 28G.

88. C. K. Kim, et al. "Detection and Reproducibility of Mental Stress-Induced Myocardial Ischemia with Tc-99m Sestamibi SPECT in Normal and Coronary Artery Disease Populations." *Journal of Nuclear Cardiology* 10(1) (2003): 56–62.

89. Cited in John Tierney, "Stress, Success, and Samoa," *Hippocrates* (May/June 1987): 84.

90. Steven Locke and Douglas Colligan, *The Healer Within: The New Medicine of Mind and Body* (New York: E. P. Dutton, 1986), 127–8.

91. Michael T. Bailey, David A. Padgett, and John F. Sheridan, "Stress-Induced Modulation of Innate Resistance and Adaptive Immunity to Influenza Viral Infection," pp. 1097–1105 in Robert Ader, ed., *Psychoneuroimmunology*, 4th ed., vol. 2 (New York: Elsevier, Inc., 2007), 1097.

92. Dhabhar and McEwen, "Bi-directional Effects of Stress," 748.

93. P. Mormède, R. Dantzer, and B. Michaud, "Influence of Stressor Predictability and Behavioral Control on Lymphocyte Reactivity, Antibody Responses and Neuroendocrine Activation in Rats," *Physiological Behavior* 43 (1988): 577–83.

94. Robert Dantzer, "Stress and Immunity: What Have We Learned from Psychoneuroimmunology?" *ACTA Physiologica Scandinavia* 161(1997): 640.

95. S. I. McMillen, *None of These Diseases*, rev. ed. (Old Tappan, NJ: Fleming H. Revell Company, 1984).

96. M. Viljoen, A. Panzer, J. L. Roos, and W. Bodemer, "Psychoneuroimmunology: From Philosophy, Intuition, and Folklore to a Recognized Science," *South African Journal of Science* 99 (July/August 2003): 332–37.

97. Leonard A. Sagan, *The Health of Nations* (New York: Basic Books, 1987).

98. "Learn to Manage the Stress in Your Life," *Healthline* (September 1993).

99. Eliot, *Stress to Strength*, 107–44.

100. Walt Schafer, *Stress Management for Wellness* (New York: Holt, Rinehart & Winston, Inc., 1987), 310.

101. W. N. Burton et al., "The Association of Medical Conditions and Presenteeism," *Journal of Occupational and Environmental Medicine* 46 (June2004): S38–45.

102. Paul J. Rosch, "The Health Effects of Job Stress." *Business and Health* - Vol. 1(No. 6):5-8 - May 1984; also see Paul J. Rosch, "Stress and Cardiovascular Disease." *Comprehensive Therapy* 1983: 9(10): 6–13.

103. R. N. Remen, "Burnout in Health Professionals." *Internal Medicine News* (January 15, 2002), 5.

104. R. Crowtcher, "Stress and Burnout in Ministry." Accessed online (2008) at http://www.churchlink.com.au/churchlink/forum/r_croucher/stress_burnout.html; also at http://www.helpguide.org/mental/burnout_signs_symptoms.htm

105. L. M. Bellini, Baime, J. A. Shea. Variation of Mood and Empathy During Internship, *Journal of the American Medical Association* 287 (2002): 3143–6.

106. M. Boles, B. Pelletier, and W. Lynch, "The Relationship Between Health Risks and Work Productivity," *Journal of Occupational and Environmental Medicine* 46, no. 7 (July 2004): 737–45.

107. Cooper and Payne; Schafer; Matteson and Ivancevich; and Arthur P. Brief, Randall S. Schuler, and Mary Van Sell, *Managing Job Stress* (Boston: Little, Brown, 1980), 13–4. Also J. V. Johnson, E. M. Hall, T. Theorell, "Combined Effects of Job Strain and Social Isolation on Cardiovascular Disease Morbidity and Mortality in a Random Sample of the Swedish Male Working Population," *Scandinavian Journal of Work, Environment & Health*. 15, no. 4 (Aug 1989): 271–9.

108. J. V. Johnson, E. M. Hall, and T. Theorell, "Combined Effects of Job Strain and Social Isolation." Also P. A. Landsbergis et al.,"Association Between Ambulatory Blood Pressure and Alternative Formulations of Job Strain," *Scandinavian Journal of Work, Environment & Health* 20, no. 5 (Oct 1994): 349–63.

109. P. L. Schnall, et al., "A Longitudinal Study of Job Strain and Ambulatory Blood Pressure: Results from a Three-Year Follow-up," *Psychosomatic Medicine* 60, no. 6 (Nov 1998): 697–706.

110. A. Steptoe et al., "Effort-reward Imbalance, Overcommitment, and Measures of Cortisol and Blood Pressure Over the Working Day," *Psychosomatic Medicine* 66 (2004):323–9.

111. "Good Boss, Good Health," *Your Personal Best* (September 1990): 3.

112. I. K. Crombie, M. B. Kenicer, W. C. S. Smith, and H. D. Tunstall-Pedoe, "Unemployment, Socioenvironmental Factors, and Coronary Heart Disease in Scotland," *British Heart Journal* 61, no. 2 (1989): 172–7.

113. Bryan E. Robinson, "Are You a Work Addict?" *East/West* (August 1990): 50.

114. Diane Fassel, "Work- and Rushaholics: Spotting a Lethal Disease," *Longevity* (September 1990): 78.

115. Anders Falk, Bertil S. Hanson, Sven-Olof Isacsson, and Per-Olof Ostergren, "Job Strain and Mortality in Elderly Men: Social Network, Support, and Influence as Buffers," *American Journal of Public Health* 82, no. 8 (1992): 1136–8.

116. The American Heart Association, May 31, 2008, http://www.americanheart.org/presenter.jhtml?identifier=4756.

117. T. Chandola, E. Brunner, and M. Marmot, "The Ominous Consequences of Stress at Work," *British Medical Journal* 332 (2006): 521–5.

118. R. Karasek and T. Theorell, *Healthy Work* (New York: Basic Books, 1990), Chapters 1–4.

119. Cooper and Payne; Schafer; Matteson and Ivancevich; and Brief, Schuler, and Van Sell, *Managing Job Stress.*

120. University of California. *Healthy Lives: A New View of Stress.* (Health Letters Associates, Fernandine Beach, FL)

121. Mihaly Csikszentmihaly. *Flow: The Psychology of Optimal Experience* (Harper Perennial, 1991).

122. Rosalind Forbes, *Corporate Stress* (Garden City: Doubleday, 1979), 43.

123. Ibid., 44.

124. Karasek and Theorell, *Healthy Work*, 138, (see Figure 4-5 a–b).

125. Remen, *Internal Medicine News, 5.*

The Disease-Prone Personality

The tragedy of life is what dies inside a man while he lives.
—Albert Schweitzer

LEARNING OBJECTIVES

- Define the concept of personality.
- Understand the relationship between personality and disease.
- Explain the existing controversy around disease-prone personalities.
- Identify the "toxic core" of personality traits.
- Explain the research around a cancer-prone personality.
- Identify personality patterns that have been linked to specific diseases.

Psychologist and clinical professor of community medicine at the University of California Howard S. Friedman wrote, "I have never seen a death certificate marked 'Death due to unhealthy personality.' But maybe pathologists and coroners should be instructed to take into account the latest scientific findings on the role of personality in health."[1]

Definitions and Foundation

Personality is the whole of your personal characteristics, the group of behavioral and emotional tendencies that distinguish you from everybody else.[2] It is the way your habits, attitudes, and traits combine to make the person that is uniquely you. Because of your personality, you act in a similar and generally consistent way from one day to the next. Personality depends partly on the unique set of genes you inherited from your parents, but it is also shaped powerfully by the family you grow up in, the environment that surrounds you, and the culture and subcultures that influence you.[3]

The theory that personality affects health is, as world-renowned psychologist Hans J. Eysenck put it, a theory "based on centuries of observations made by keen-eyed physicians."[4] The notion that a certain personality type leads to heart disease dates back more than 2,000 years to Hippocrates.

Early studies piqued the interest of scientists, but most of them involved people who were already ill. Had the personality traits contributed to the illness, or had the illness caused the personality traits? What science needed was a study involving healthy people—a study that would characterize participants' personality traits, monitor them for a number of years, note which ones got ill, and determine whether there was any correlation between personality traits and the tendency to develop certain diseases.

Yugoslav psychologist Ronald Grossarth-Maticek took on the challenge. He started by identifying large random samples of subjects. He recorded each person's current physical health, smoking and drinking habits, and other health behaviors. Then he devised several ways to measure personality. At the end, Grossarth-Maticek categorized people into one of six categories, one of which was prone to develop cancer and one to develop heart disease.[5]

He followed each group closely for at least ten years, some for thirteen years. The results were remarkable. He was able to predict death from cancer with six times greater accuracy than it was possible to predict it based on cigarette smoking.

Among the groups he said were prone to develop cancer (those with inhibited, self-centered expression and a helpless, victimized personality style), almost half did die from cancer, but fewer than one in ten died from heart disease. Among those he predicted to be prone to heart disease (those with a hostile, aggressive personality style and barriers to self-centered expression), more than a third did die of heart disease, but only one in five died from cancer. Among the groups he predicted to be prone to good health, there were relatively few deaths.[6] Though there have been criticisms of and issues with his methodology,[7] to his credit, Grossarth-Maticek's ideas "in the early 1960s agree almost perfectly with the most recent results of American and British research in this field."[8]

Grossarth-Maticek then set out to determine whether the outcome of disease could be affected by changing some personality traits. In one study, he identified people with disease-prone personalities. Then he split that group randomly in half: Half received counseling that included modeling, suggestion, relaxation, visualization, desensitization, and other standard behavioral techniques used to modify personality. The other half received no counseling at all. The group that received counseling had lower death rates from both cancer and heart disease. He later repeated the studies with Eysenck.[9] Together, they found they could reduce by half the death rates from cancer and heart disease with as few as six hours of group therapy.

Grossarth-Maticek's work is the subject of considerable controversy. One report on his work maintains that his claims have "raised eyebrows, skeptical inquiries, and even some charges of scientific fraud."[10] Others charge that his work was riddled with technical and statistical problems that can cast doubt on the data.[11] In defense of the work, however, one editor opined,

> Many great scientific discoveries, of course, have had uncertain and spotty histories. Physicist Niels Bohr won a Nobel Prize for his model of the atom, which turned out to be inaccurate but inspired the research that got it right. Gregor Mendel made serious mistakes in his genetics experiments, but his research led to our modern understanding of human genetics and biology. And despite the criticism, no one, since Grossarth-Maticek began publishing his findings in 1980, has been able to knock down his numbers.[12]

Even though critical reviews since that time have challenged Grossarth-Maticek's numbers,[13] University of South Florida psychologist Charles Spielberger says that therapies aimed at changing personality traits may have some validity after all. "Even if the benefits of these therapies were reduced by one-half, or two-thirds, one could not reasonably allow the information to be suppressed," Spielberger says. "In the five or ten years needed to replicate these findings, thousands of men and women will die from cancer and heart attacks." As Spielberger points out, preventive psychotherapy isn't going to hurt anyone, and if it helps some, "more power to it."[14]

Regardless of the controversies surrounding Grossarth-Maticek's findings, say the experts, they endow us with hope and encourage further research to pinpoint what influence personality may have on health.

We don't know everything about the link between personality and health, but we do know a great deal about how personality influences health and which personality traits seem particularly connected to certain diseases. A warning is in order, however. First and foremost, we need to be cautious about overemphasizing personality or behavior patterns without looking at the myriad of other factors that likely affect the disease process. To do so causes inaccurate study results that could cause more harm than good.

There's more. With all of our research into the impact of personality on disease, we must carefully avoid blaming any person for his or her illness. Any person can get almost any illness. Personality styles or mental stress do not cause disease so much as they act as a risk factor that, when combined with other risk factors, increases vulnerability.

If you breathe high levels of cigarette smoke or certain other pollutants, there is a good chance that you will develop lung cancer. If you are a woman whose mother, aunts, and sisters developed breast cancer, there is a good chance that you will develop breast cancer. In cases like these, your emotional responses may not play a significant role in preventing the cancer. Disease is influenced not only by psychological factors, but also by the genes we are born with and the environment in which we live. In fact, most instances of disease are caused by a convergence of factors. As many well-known cases demonstrate, it is a sad fact of life that some people contract cancer and die of it at a young age, regardless of personality or heroic struggle.[15]

Even when people accept blame for an illness, it may be a mistake to assume that they "brought it on" themselves. Such a viewpoint may lead to inhumanity and a lack of compassion for people who need it most.

Why, then, is it important to study the links that we know exist between personality and disease? Because there is a great deal you can do to protect and preserve your own health. It won't work all of the time for all of the people in all circumstances, but many can probably help themselves stay healthy—and a fair share of those who become ill can help themselves recover.

Disease and Personality: Exploring the Connection

Most people, whether they know it or not, associate certain personality types with particular illnesses. Workaholics have heart attacks. Worriers get ulcers. People who get too uptight have asthma attacks. In reality, can they be so neatly categorized?

Not yet, but researchers have made tremendous strides in demonstrating that personality does have an impact on health. They have found that the way we look at things, as determined by our personality, may actually contribute to illness (or help keep us well).

A variety of studies dating back more than four decades has exposed the "tip of the iceberg" as far as personality and health connections are concerned. In 1948, a group of medical students at Johns Hopkins University described what they saw in ten Rorschach inkblots. What they saw tells a great deal about their outlook and the substantial differences in their personalities. Some saw the inkblot as a young couple kissing, two people shaking hands, or two dancers; others saw in the same pattern two dogs snarling at each other or two cannibals boiling Macbeth in a kettle.[16]

More than three decades later, psychologist Pirkko L. Graves and her colleagues combined the responses of those medical students with the responses of other groups of students (some of whom had been tested as recently as 1964). Graves rated the students according to an eleven-point scale, and then categorized them according to their general personality and personal interaction style.

No one was surprised to learn that the distant, withdrawn students who had a generally "negative" approach to interactions were much more likely to develop a severe mental disorder in the three decades following the first study. What was a surprise was that those students were also much more likely to have developed cancer—especially cancers of the stomach, pancreas, rectum, large intestine, and lymph nodes, as well as Hodgkin's disease, leukemia, and multiple myeloma.[17]

Recent analysis looked at the notion that prominent people are more prone to develop Parkinson's disease—and explored the possibility that the traits that lead people to rise to positions of authority might be the same personality traits that increase the risk of Parkinson's disease.[18] In a study that focused on Wilhelm von Humboldt and Adolf Hitler, research showed that those traits—ambition, perfectionism, rigidity, and repressed emotions—appear to boost the risk not only of Parkinson's disease, but also of general infection.

Other research[19] shows that certain personality traits are strongly associated with how people perceive their own health. After studying a large sample of adults between ages 25 and 74, researchers determined the existence of a solid relationship between personality traits and the way people perceive their health. Regardless of whether the people were healthy or ill, several traits were consistently associated with a perception of good health—including openness to experiences, extraversion, and conscientiousness. Similarly, several traits were consistently associated with a perception of poor health, including neuroticism. The association remained significant even after adjusting for factors like age, gender, race, marital status, and education.

The most recent research indicates that the most likely link between personality and disease depends on the way people deal with stress.

Differing Views on Personality and Disease

Generic View   Additional studies have also shown a link between personality and health. In an analysis of 101 studies conducted between 1945 and 1984, researchers concluded that there are "strong links" between personality and health.[20] While not ready to attach a single personality trait to a single disease, they did conclude that there was a strong connection between certain personality traits and "all diseases except ulcers," the most damaging personality traits being depression, anxiety, anger, and hostility.[21] "Personality may function as diet does: Imbalances can predispose one to all sorts of diseases."[22]

One viewpoint, then, holds that certain personality traits (or, in essence, a certain personality type) increase susceptibility to disease in general. Researchers who support this point of view believe that there may be a generic "disease-prone personality" but not individual "disease personalities" (such as cancer personality or ulcer personality, for example).

Disease-Prone Personality View   Other researchers disagree, saying that certain "personalities" or personality traits can be specifically linked to certain diseases. Most prominent in research has been the "coronary-prone personality," the hard-driving and competitive type A personality who is also hostile, angry, and suspicious. Also prominent in current research is the "cancer-prone personality," characterized by people who demonstrate little emotion, are ambivalent toward self and others, and were not close to their parents.

Disease Cluster View   A third group of researchers believes that a specific personality may make a person susceptible to a "cluster" of conditions, not just to a specific disease. Based on extensive research, Caroline Bedell Thomas and her coworkers at the Johns Hopkins School of Medicine believe that people can be categorized into three broad personality types—alphas, betas, and gammas—which can determine whether they are more prone to become ill or stay healthy.[23]

Alphas. Alphas are slow and solid, wary in new situations, gradually adaptable, and undemanding. Only about one-fourth of the alphas became seriously ill in the thirty years of Thomas's study.

Betas. Betas are cool and clever, quick to respond to new situations, articulate, and understanding. Only about one-fourth of the betas became seriously ill within thirty years. This group was most prone to be healthiest.

Gammas. The group with the greatest health problems were the gammas. They are either too careful or devil-may-care; often brilliant, but also moody and confused in new situations; and either too demanding or not demanding enough. In one of Thomas's studies, 77 percent of the gammas developed cancer, mental illness, high blood pressure, or heart disease or committed suicide. In another study, half of all the sick students were in the gamma group.

The Personality Cluster View   A similar viewpoint focuses on personality clusters. Rather than grouping people by personality traits, some researchers have identified what they call clusters or cluster groups—groups that have similar specific personality types. Researchers then identify diseases that seem most closely related to that cluster type. One group of researchers at Georgia State University identified five clusters of illnesses and determined which patterns of personality were strongly associated with each cluster.[24]

The Controversy

Most researchers now accept the notion of an "immune-prone personality," one whose hardiness enables him or her to tolerate the ravages of stress without becoming ill. There is not such widespread acceptance of the notion that certain personality traits are linked to illness so much as there is an acceptance of a tendency for those traits to be linked to an ability to remain healthy.

Contemporary research on personality and health has been surrounded by controversy for many reasons.[25] First, many physicians are simply not trained to think that way. They want a simple or tangible reason for a disorder so they can "fix it." Second, many physicians still think of the mind and the body as two separate entities that do not affect each other. Third, many physicians (and patients) are skeptical about unusual approaches, including the notion that personality affects health. Finally, the notion that personality affects health is simply not as financially rewarding for a practitioner. Our medical delivery system pays far more for mechanical procedures than for knowledgeable patient teaching and "healing." A surgeon who removes a diseased gallbladder makes hundreds of dollars for an hour's work; not so for a doctor who spends an hour talking to a depressed patient troubled by headaches.

The controversy was fueled a few years ago in response to the report of a study by Barrie R. Cassileth and her colleagues at the University of Pennsylvania. Her research team declared that neither positive attitudes nor feelings of depression or hopelessness had any effect on the survival rates of more than 350 people with advanced cancer. Cassileth's study was printed in the *New England Journal of Medicine*, which prompted pathologist and senior deputy editor of the journal, Marcia Angell, to editorialize, "Our belief in disease as a direct reflection of mental state is largely folklore."[26]

In her editorial, Angell criticized the medical community and the media for giving too much credit to personality and emotions as factors in physical health. "We are told," she wrote, that "type A people are vulnerable to heart attacks, repressed people (especially those who have suffered losses) are at risk of cancer, worry causes peptic ulcers, and so on."[27] Further, Angell said that studies relating personality to health were flawed in their design, analysis, or interpretation and that it was dangerous for patients to believe their emotional attitude can save them from serious illness because it could cause patients to forego necessary medical control in favor of some "method of mind control."[28]

Angell's editorial was incendiary. The journal was flooded with letters from physicians and former cancer patients disputing the editorial's claims. The 60,000-member American Psychological Association issued a statement attacking Angell's piece as "inaccurate and unfortunate."[29] In the years that have followed, the debate has continued.

Shortly after the editorial appeared, the journal *MD* conducted a poll of its physician readers, asking, "Does emotional state affect disease?"[30] The doctors could hardly have been more unequivocal in their answers: Of the 126 who responded, 124 said yes; only 2 said no. Some of the physicians who responded did not believe that emotions or personality "cause" illness, but almost all conceded that personality has a profound effect on the outcome of an illness.

Explaining the Differences in People

Regardless of where you stand on the controversy over personality and health, there's one clear fact: We all respond differently to the stresses and problems that confront us in life. Whether it's a bad day or a chronic emotional crisis, some of us sail through valiantly and others of us get sick. Even among those who get sick, there are differences; some suffer from insomnia, others from crippling headaches, and still others from indigestion.

We know that stress can cause physical illness. What we have not known until recently is why it has such a different effect on different people. Researchers think that part of the answer is personality.

The process begins when the brain directs various glands in the body to secrete hormones, which circulate through the bloodstream giving "orders" to various tissues and organs. They may direct the blood vessels to constrict, for example, or instruct the body to metabolize sugar. Once the specific task has been completed, a feedback system signals the brain, and the hormone level subsides. Everyone has the same network, the same sets of hormonal switches and cycles. They control how we respond in all kinds of situations, including stressful ones.

If everyone has the same general physiological makeup, why do we react so differently? Personality may play a key role—as do diet, accidents, early childhood experiences, and our genetic makeup. These factors create what researchers call weak links, which determine where stress is apt to strike a given person.[31] Psychoanalyst Herbert J. Freudenberger points out that these weak links, part of our personality, are for the most part "learned and reinforced behaviors."[32] It explains why one person under stress gets a backache while another gets an ulcer. In essence, it's another explanation of how personality can affect health.

Regardless of the illness involved, researchers reporting their findings in the *British Journal of Medical Psychology* pointed out perhaps one of the most telling traits of a disease-prone personality. Researchers at the University of Helsinki studied almost 200 people with various diseases and found an amazing difference: Unlike their normal counterparts, those with disease-prone personalities felt more emotionally stable when they were ill. More than anything else, that finding may help us distinguish those who, as Friedman wrote, may suffer "death due to unhealthy personality."[33]

Type A Personality: The Coronary Artery Disease–Prone Personality?

One of the most active areas of health research sought to identify and explain the relationships between personality and heart disease. At every stage of heart disease, state of mind appeared to play a role.[34]

In a summary of research printed in *Psychology Today,* a writer editorialized,

> By treating the heart as an unfeeling pump, surgeons have been able to create pacemakers and work their way up to the ultimate in high-tech medicine: the artificial heart. But even as Barney Clark and other courageous patients were testing the electronic pumps, scientists were using chemistry, psychology, and hard data to discover that trouble in the heart may come in part from sickness of the soul.[35]

That sickness of the soul has evolved over the past three decades from a notion called the "type A personality" to a broader-based concept that some call the "type A behavior pattern." Two bits of good news have emerged from the most recent research: First, because the behavior pattern consists of a set of habits, it can be changed. Second, some of the more desirable parts of the type A behavior pattern (such as increased productivity) apparently do not contribute to heart disease; one can safely retain some of those positive characteristics and change the harmful parts.

Personality traits that increase your risk for coronary artery disease are not inherent flaws. They are patterns of behavior that have been shown to potentially boost the risk of heart disease. For ease of discussion throughout this chapter, we will refer to this collection of personality traits by the name most researchers have used: the type A personality.

Definitions of the Type A Personality

Type A behavior "refers to the behaviors of an individual who reacts to the environment with characteristic gestures, facial expressions, fast pace of activities, and the perception of daily events and stresses as challenges, all leading to an aggressive, time-urgent, impatient, and more hostile style of living."[36] Those with type A behavior are characterized as more driven, energetic, ambitious, and impatient than those without this behavior.[37]

Cardiologist Ray Rosenman and his colleague Meyer Friedman originated the theory of type A personality more than three decades ago. They defined the type A personality as "an action-emotion complex that can be observed in any person who is aggressively involved in a chronic, incessant struggle to achieve more and more in less and less time, and if required to do so, against the opposing efforts of other things or other persons."[38]

That struggle against time and other people, Friedman contended, is what causes physical damage. As one researcher put it, type A personalities "are not only more hostile, competitive, and impatient" but are also guided by the central view that they "are indeed responsible for everything, control everything, and are not only the captains of their own ship but the crew and cargo as well."[39]

The opposite type of the type A behavior pattern is the type B behavior pattern: A person who is less driven, is more relaxed, and takes life at an easier, less hectic pace. Some researchers think that a number of different traits actually compose the type B behavior pattern.[40]

The first description of the type A personality, though it was not given that name, occurred at the turn of the twentieth century when American physician Sir William Osler attributed heart disease to "the high pressure at which men live and the habit of working the machine to its maximum capacity."[41] Other researchers followed; in the 1930s, the Menningers noted that coronary artery disease patients often exhibited a "strongly aggressive personality." A decade later, one psychosomatic medicine pioneer described a "coronary personality," whose pattern consisted of the hard-driving, goal-directed behavior he often saw among coronary heart disease patients.[42]

The most significant and far-reaching work on coronary personality came in the mid-1950s from cardiologists Meyer Friedman and Ray Rosenman. It began as somewhat of an accident: An upholsterer who came to their office to repair some furniture pointed out that the fabric was worn only on the very edge of the couches and chairs. It was a sign, he mused, that the patients were literally "on edge." Armed with evidence that their patients were consistently perched on the edge of their seats, Friedman and Rosenman launched the landmark series of studies that led to identification of the type A behavior pattern,[43] a pattern they initially dubbed "the hurry sickness."

Why the name "type A?" This time the advice came from a scientist, not an upholsterer. Friedman and Rosenman began applying for federal funding to conduct their studies, requesting funds to research a "coronary-prone personality." Their repeated requests were denied, apparently because the scientists who were reviewing the funding applications did not believe that personality could increase the risk of heart disease. Finally, a scientist at the National Institutes of Health advised the pair to come up with a more generic name for their research project. Friedman and Rosenman came up with the harmless label "type A behavior"; they called the opposite personality simply "type B." With the new name, funding was approved.[44]

Friedman and Rosenman made two bold proclamations:

1. There are literal biochemical reasons why behavior can increase the risk for coronary heart disease.

2. Certain behavior patterns can be used as a tool for predicting who will get heart disease—not just as a detail to be confirmed at a postmortem exam.

In 1960, the two began the Western Collaborative Group Study, involving more than three thousand men in their forties and fifties who did not show any signs of existing coronary heart disease. At the end of the eight-year study, Friedman and Rosenman said that those who had been classified as type A at the beginning of the study were more than twice as likely to get heart disease as those who had been classified as type B.[45]

The Western Collaborative Group Study established type A behavior as an independent risk factor for heart disease.[46] Type A behavior was added to the list of heart disease risks and was accepted as such for nearly two decades. In 1981, in fact, the National Heart, Lung, and Blood Institute concluded that type A behavior was an independent risk factor of cardiovascular disease.

A second larger study then cast doubt on the relationship between Type A personality and coronary heart disease. A decade-long study, the Multiple Risk Factor Intervention Trial (MRFIT), was conducted by the National Heart, Lung, and Blood Institute at a cost of more than $100 million. Researchers studied more than 12,000 men who did not yet have signs of heart disease but who did have specific factors that placed them at high risk for a heart attack.

Researchers found no relationship between type A behavior and any kind of coronary heart disease event. Of ten subsequent studies conducted during the late 1970s and early 1980s, eight also failed to confirm the type A hypothesis.[47]

More study results surfaced in 1988: Those in the Western Collaborative Group Study who had suffered heart attacks during the eight and a half years of the study were followed for a total of 22 years. The researchers learned that if the men survived the first 24 hours after a heart attack, the type A men actually had a significantly better long-term survival rate. In fact, they died at only about half the rate of the type Bs who had heart attacks. [48]

Advocates of the theory began what pioneer researcher Redford Williams calls the "second generation" of type A research. They hypothesized that type A is more of a risk factor for those under age 50 years and that it varies as a risk factor depending on the level of cholesterol in the blood.

In the meantime, a growing number of scientists found that some components of type A behavior were relatively harmless, while others formed what researchers called the "toxic core" of the personality type. Researchers believed that the positive components of type A behavior could increase the chances of survival after a heart attack, but the negative ones—the so-called "toxic core"—could significantly increase the risk of suffering a heart attack in the first place.

Later research indicated that depression might also play a factor—but not in the way scientists originally thought. In a study[49] involving 100 healthy young adults—half of whom were clinically depressed—researchers found that depression led to weight gain. (Interestingly, there was no evidence that the weight gain caused the depression.) The accumulation of adipose tissue caused the release of chemicals that in turn activated an inflammatory response that caused coronary heart disease.

Later research[50] also indicated that various personality traits might exert greater impact at different stages of cardiovascular disease. According to the research, hostility appears to have the most significant impact in the early stages of the disease. During the transition from stable to unstable disease, the most significant factors appeared to be depression and exhaustion (common in the type A behavior pattern). During acute episodes, the most significant factors seemed to be mental stress and anger.

The "Toxic Core" of Type A Behavior

With three decades worth of research pointing to different conclusions, what's the current thinking on the type A personality? Simply, studies have discounted the relationship of type A personality to heart disease.[51] The hurry-sickness attributes of the type A personality are probably the best known, but they are also the least detrimental to health. The set of traits that creates major health risks for people of all personality types (not just the type A personality) is a "toxic core" consisting of hostility, anger, cynicism, suspiciousness, and excessive self-involvement. Recent research at Duke University shows that hostility, anger, and depression are the most harmful traits and that they increase the risk of high blood pressure and coronary heart disease, as well as diabetes, in men.[52] Remember that these personality traits have been found to increase the risk of heart disease across the board, not just in people who have been labeled with a specific "personality."

Free-Floating Hostility   Free-floating hostility is a permanent, deep-seated anger that hovers quietly until some trivial incident causes it to rupture to the surface in a burst of hostility; it is the tendency to experience anger, irritability, and resentment in response to even common events and to react with antagonism and disagreeableness.[53]

Detailed research shows that there may actually be two separate components to free-floating hostility:[54]

- Expressive hostility, characterized by frequent expressions of anger and annoyance, the tendency to argue in a loud voice, and the potential for physical aggression when provoked.

- Neurotic hostility, characterized by chronic anger, low trust, and hostility that is not openly expressed. By itself, neurotic hostility has not been shown to increase the risk of heart disease; but, in combination with expressive hostility, it is a potent factor in heart disease.

Researchers Margaret Chesney, Nanette Frautschi, and Ray H. Rosenman believe that type A persons often have an "enhanced potential for hostility."[55] This potential can be created by either genetic or learned factors. Because the enhanced potential is chronic, or ever present, even minor irritations or upsets can trigger a hostile rage. People who have free-floating hostility react with seething anger and dwell on the objects of their contempt. They become irritated and explosive and find it difficult not to become physically abusive. Sometimes the anger that accompanies free-floating hostility is displaced: a woman who gets angry and hostile in a traffic jam may lash out at a child in the back seat, for example.

Important and still-controversial studies have made a startling conclusion about the hostility factor: apparently you can have many of the characteristics typically associated with the type A personality—such as competitive drive, an aggressive personality, and impatience—without running the risks of a heart attack, as long as you are not hostile.

Renowned experts, such as Duke University's Redford Williams, point to hostility as one of the most crucial elements in heart disease. "We have strong evidence that hostility alone damages the heart," Williams emphasizes. In one study, hostility was shown to increase the risk of heart disease by a staggering seven times. "The kind of person at risk is someone who generally feels that other people are not to be trusted," Williams adds, "that they'll lie and cheat if they can get away with it."[56]

In a report published in *Psychology Today*, the kind of personality Williams describes as being at highest risk is "deeply suspicious. They feel that they must remain constantly on guard against others, whom they believe are dishonest, antisocial, and immoral." The Duke University team of researchers claims that this kind of hostility predicts not only blockages in the coronary arteries, as measured by X-ray studies of patients suffering chest pains,[57] but also death from heart disease and other causes.[58]

Psychologist Timothy Smith of the University of Utah reported to the 2004 Society of Behavioral Medicine meeting that couples with no history of heart disease developed the early signs of disease if they were hostile and domineering in their interactions—even those over things as basic as household chores, in-laws, money, and children. Smith's research showed that those who were hostile began developing calcium deposits in their coronary arteries—an early sign of arterial damage. The more hostile and strained their relationship, Smith says, "the more severe this silent atherosclerosis tended to be."[59]

Part of the reason why hostile people run a greater risk of heart disease is that they more frequently trigger the cascade of potentially damaging hormones that are released as part of the fight-or-flight response. As Williams puts it, "Trusting hearts may live longer because for them the biologic cost of situations that anger or irritate is lower."[60]

Another reason why hostility may be correlated so strongly with heart disease is that people who are hostile tend to drive others away, and social support, social networking, and social integration have been repeatedly proven to be strong protectors of health.

Anger   Another dangerous trait sometimes seen in the type A behavior pattern is anger, defined by researchers as "an emotional state incorporating feelings ranging from irritation and aggravation to rage and fury."[61] (Anger is often confused with hostility, which is an habitual way of evaluating people or events in a negative, cynical, paranoid way.) Researchers believe that the powerful combination of hostility and unexpressed anger carries the greatest risk of heart disease.

The particular combination is deadly, say researchers, and it appears to have a much greater impact on health than any single factor. "It isn't the impatience, the ambition, or the work drive," says Redford Williams. "It's the anger: It sends your blood pressure skyrocketing. It provokes the body to create unhealthy chemicals. For hostile people, anger is poison."[62]

Some say that the greatest risks are from unexpressed anger, or "anger-in," a specific way of reacting to the people or situations that make a person angry. People who harbor unexpressed anger are not able to express their angry feelings, even when those feelings are appropriate or justified. Others disagree; in some studies, those who did best were the ones who "blew up" on a regular basis. It appears that the presence of ongoing anger may be more important than how it is expressed.

Cynicism   Cynicism, anger, and hostility are closely related emotions: As Redford Williams describes it, cynical mistrust of others is the driving force behind hostility. It almost starts a chain reaction, he explains:

> Expecting that others will mistreat us, we are on the lookout for their bad behavior, and we can usually find it. This generates the frequent anger to which the hostile person is prone, and that anger, combined with a lack of empathy for others—a natural consequence of the poor opinion we hold of others in general—leads us to express our hostility overtly, in the form of aggressive acts towards others.[63]

When cynicism is paired with hostility, the effects can be devastating to health. In one experiment, Duke University Medical Center researchers asked a group of college students (some of whom were hostile and some of whom were not) to solve a difficult series of scrambled word puzzles. Physiological responses, such as blood pressure, were measured during the experiment.

At the end of the first part of the experiment, researchers found that there was no difference between the two groups as they were doing the puzzles. Then they added another factor designed to separate students who were also cynical: researchers stood over the students while they were doing the puzzles and made snide remarks like "Stop mumbling; I can't understand what you are saying" and "Remember, you're getting paid to do this."

Once the element of harassment was added, the students who were cynical showed sharp differences in physiological responses. They had higher blood pressure, higher blood flow, and more anger while they were doing the puzzles and being harassed, and their blood pressure remained high for fifteen minutes after they did the puzzle. Researchers attribute the changes in the cynical students to the fact that hostile people "view other people's actions and motives very cynically. They thought the researchers were 'out to get them,' felt threatened, and reacted, while low hostiles did not perceive the researchers' actions as a personal attack."[64]

Suspiciousness   Suspiciousness is a trait closely allied to cynicism. In a study at Duke University's Center for the Study of Aging and Human Development, researchers noted that "people who are suspicious are constantly on guard, and there's evidence to suggest that this may raise levels of potentially harmful stress-induced hormones in the blood."[65] In the same study, those who scored high on a test of suspiciousness were significantly more likely to become ill and die during the fifteen years the study was conducted. The greater risk for illness and death due to suspiciousness held up even after researchers took into account other risk factors, such as age, sex, physician rating of functional health, smoking, cholesterol, and alcohol intake.[66]

In a separate study, Friedman and Rosenman studied 1,990 middle-aged men who had not yet developed coronary heart disease. Each man was given the Minnesota Multiphasic Personality Inventory, as well as a questionnaire that evaluated sixteen personality factors. The study subjects were then monitored for five years to determine which ones became ill or died. Those most likely to develop coronary heart disease were the men who showed higher levels of suspiciousness.[67]

Excessive Self-Involvement   One of the most interesting theories about behavioral traits and their potential link to heart disease points to a personality trait that researchers think is a killer: excessive self-involvement. A person whose language is excessively peppered with references to I, me, mine, and other self-references seems to be at the greatest risk of all for coronary heart disease.

Self-involvement seems to be such an important factor because people who are self-involved tend to be "hot reactors"; they have extreme cardiovascular reactions when subjected to stress, including precipitous increases in blood pressure and health-harming chemical changes.[68] Excessive self-involvement may be what actually causes the hostility and anger that have been so strongly linked to heart disease. The facts are that self-involvement may be related to, and often accompanied by, other dangerous type A traits such as hostility.

Effects of Coronary-Prone Behavior

Coronary-prone behavior causes health problems because it literally wreaks havoc on the body. In his book *Super Immunity*, psychologist Paul Pearsall gives a vivid description:

> The supersystem sizzles with neurochemical changes, we roast in our hormonal stew, and, as if by some universal wisdom, the body can be stopped in its tracks by adopting an "enough is enough" strategy. We overload, our heads start pounding for attention, our hearts get attacked for our lack of intimacy, and our vessels cause the doctor's mercury gauge to warn us that things are getting too high. Even our bowels can get irritated with us and show their displeasure in their own unique language. Somewhere in our bodies, through our overuse and abuse of our supersystems, something is burning out.[69]

The behavioral traits that are linked to heart disease are essentially an exaggerated stress response, and the body begins pumping out hormones needed to fight or flee. It's the classic fight-or-flight reaction we all have in response to stress, whether mental or physical (see Chapter 2). The hostile person lives in a chronic state of what Redford Williams calls vigilant observation.[70] The body is on constant alert. It never relaxes. The result is increased circulation and levels of blood cholesterol, blood triglycerides, and blood sugar.

The physical effects begin in the hypothalamus, a complex portion of the brain that lies at its base, directly over the pituitary gland. The hypothalamus sends out signals to various parts of the body in response to emotion. The anger and hostility are processed by the hypothalamus as it would process an intense physical struggle. As a result, the system is bathed with excessive catecholamines, adrenaline (epinephrine), testosterone, estrogen, thyroxine, and insulin. Other effects include:

- An increase in adrenaline-like hormones (norepinephrine) that cause microvascular drainage in blood vessel walls, allowing cholesterol in the blood to seep into the wall and eventually creating atherosclerotic plaques.[71]

- An increase in coronary artery spasm further narrows the vessels supplying oxygen to the heart muscle.

- An increase in blood pressure increases the heart's workload and oxygen requirement. The increase in norepinephrine, which constricts the blood vessels, results in high blood pressure.[72]

- Blood platelets become more "sticky," part of the process that leads to atherosclerosis and clotting to complete the obstruction of the narrowed arteries, a definite risk factor for coronary heart disease.[73]

- All of the above phenomena lead to oxygen imbalance in the heart and may result in myocardial infarction (heart attack).

Unfortunately, the anger, hostility, and struggle are chronic, so the body is always pumped full of excess hormones. Even during supposedly "low-voltage" periods of the day, type A individuals expose their bodies to "high-voltage" chemicals that can damage and even eventually destroy it. Some of the most profound effects of chronic overload of stress hormones are increased levels of cholesterol and fat, blood platelet changes, alterations in the heart and arteries, excess insulin secretion, magnesium deficiency, and defective immune system function.

Type D Personality

We know that stress, chronic anger or hostility, and social isolation can contribute to the development of heart disease. Those traits have been grouped into a behavior pattern—the "type D (distressed) personality,"[74] characterized by the tendency to experience negative emotions, to suppress those emotions, and to avoid social contact—that has also been linked to heart disease. The most recent research indicates that type D personality traits are at least as important as other, more conventional coronary heart disease risk factors.[75]

The hallmark of the type D personality is worried pessimism—once these people develop a high degree of emotional distress, they consciously suppress their feelings. Pressure builds up, and the system breaks down.[76] This constellation of traits has also been shown to increase the circulating levels of cytokine tumor necrosis factor (which in turn increases the risk of death from chronic heart failure).[77]

Here's what happens as a result: Stress hormones—especially the heart-harming cortisol—are so poorly regulated that the heart beats faster, blood pressure rises, extra sugar is released into the bloodstream, platelets get stickier, and inflammation increases. All of these factors combine to damage the blood vessels, break up atherosclerotic plaques on the walls of the vessels, and encourage the formation of clots.[78]

The negative traits that are part of the "type D personality" include depressed mood, anxiety, anger, and hostile feelings.[79] Apparently the constellation of negative emotions has a much greater impact on the development of heart disease when it is combined with what is referred to as "social inhibition," or the inability to easily make contact with others, talk to strangers, express opinions to others, make "small talk" (even with close acquaintances), carry on an easy conversation, impact others, take charge in group situations, or feel at ease in a group. Researchers have labeled the combination of negative emotions and social inhibition as Type D Scale–16 (DS16). Those who score high on both social inhibition and negative feelings are said to have a "distressed" personality (thus the name *type D*). Scientists found that the presence of either negative emotions or social inhibition without the other did not necessarily increase the risk of heart disease but that the combination can be deadly.[80]

The problem isn't the occasional experiencing of these negative emotions, but the tendency to experience these negative emotions across time and a variety of situations[81] and the tendency to suppress negative emotions.[82] Researchers have also found that people diagnosed with affective disorders are also significantly more likely to develop both fatal and nonfatal coronary artery disease.[83]

A large body of scientists found that certain negative emotions—such as anger,[84] anxiety,[85] depression,[86] worry,[87] and hopelessness[88]—all increased the risk of coronary artery disease. Heart bypass patients who are depressed at the time of their surgery are more than twice as likely to die during the next five years when compared to people whose conditions are the same but who are not depressed.[89] Other factors, including social isolation, have also been shown to impact the heart—and the emotional stress of being alone causes heart attack survivors to die at twice the rate of those who live with others. "They're heartbroken in more ways than one," says Dr. Herbert Benson, president of Boston's Mind/Body Medical Institute.[90]

Long-range research conducted over a period of ten years involving almost 300 men and women between the ages of 30 and 80 found that type D personality:[91]

- increases the risk of cardiac death, especially among patients with established coronary heart disease.[92]

- causes increased risk of subsequent heart attack among myocardial infarction patients.

- increases the risk of death by four times among coronary artery disease patients.

Research also shows that close relationships help to ease the emotions related to type D personality.[93] In one study reported in September 2004 by psychologist Timothy Smith of the University of Utah, simply looking at a picture of someone you love helps reduce the stress response, thereby reducing heart rate and blood pressure. Massachusetts cardiologist Harvey Zarren found that heart patients' abnormal heart rhythms stabilized and high blood pressure fell to normal when he rode in an ambulance with them and asked them to describe what they loved most in life. Unlike his colleagues, Zarren never had a patient progress to cardiac arrest while in the ambulance.

The Controversy

Researchers are waiting to see if the type D personality as a coronary risk factor has more staying power than its predecessor, the type A personality. However, the entire notion of coronary-prone personality is a controversial one, possibly because behavior is much more difficult to pinpoint as a risk factor than are other, more specific risk factors that can be measured in a laboratory (such as high blood pressure or elevated cholesterol). "Behavior comes from the soft, fuzzy science of psychology, rather than from the hard, precise, biomedical sciences," psychologist Ethel Roskies points out, a fact that may make it difficult for medical researchers to accept the coronary-prone personality. Medical personnel may have even more difficulty with the concept, she adds, "if behavioral modification, rather than conventional medical and surgical techniques, is seen as the treatment of choice for this new type of risk factor."[94]

Type C Personality: The Cancer-Prone Personality

At one time, researchers considered the possibility of a cancer-prone personality, a set of traits that might predispose a person to the development of cancer. There were a number of problems leading to controversy from the time the research started. For one, the exact effect of personality on cancer is difficult to assess: During the course of a study, people can be exposed unwittingly to carcinogens that may play a role. There can also be a vast difference in a number of factors between the time of prognosis and the time of diagnosis, and we know that most cancers have lurked in the system for months or even years before they are diagnosed, leading to confusion about which factors were actually part of the cause, if any. Despite these problems, some researchers and physicians did believe that there could be a link between personality and cancer, and a number of studies were conducted.

The notion of a possible cancer-prone personality has historical roots. The second-century physician Galen noted that "melancholic" women had a greater tendency toward breast cancer than their more "sanguine" counterparts. Medical writers in the eighteenth century described in detail the personality traits and experiences they observed were shared by cancer patients. Eminent British physician Sir James Paget noted in 1870, "The cases are so frequent in which deep anxiety, deferred hope, and disappointment are quickly followed by the growth or increase of cancer that we can hardly doubt that mental depression is a weighty addition to the other influences that favor the development of the cancerous constitution."[95]

Researchers became keenly interested in the possibility of a cancer-prone personality during the 1950s, when psychologist Eugene Blumberg began noticing a "trademark" personality among cancer patients in a Long Beach veterans' hospital. He wrote, "We were impressed by the polite, apologetic, almost painful acquiescence of the patients with rapidly progressing disease as contrasted with the more expressive and sometimes bizarre personalities of those who responded brilliantly to therapy with remissions and long survival."[96] He observed that the patients with the fastest-growing tumors were the ones who were "consistently serious, overcooperative, overly nice, overly anxious, painfully sensitive, passive, and apologetic"[97]—and had been all their lives.

At about the same time, physicians at San Francisco's Malignant Melanoma Clinic were noticing a "disturbing pattern" in the personalities of patients with melanoma (a particularly virulent form of skin cancer). The patients were "nice"—too nice. In fact, they were passive about everything, including their cancer. Doctors didn't think it was coincidence, so they asked University of California School of Medicine psychologist Lydia Temoshok to talk to the patients and determine whether a personality pattern emerged.

After talking to 150 of the clinic's melanoma patients, Temoshok noted a distinct pattern. The cancer patients were indeed very, very nice. They never seemed to express any negative emotion—not fear, sadness, anger, denial, or any of the other emotions common to a patient struggling with a terminal disease. The patients couldn't express negative emotion, assert themselves, acknowledge or attend to physical pain, or admit their own needs. In fact, say the researchers, these patients "were the rock of stability for their families. Even in the face of cancer, they maintained this composure. When one of them was diagnosed, she might say, 'I'm doing fine. But I'm really worried about my husband. He takes things so hard,'" explained Temoshok.[98] The hallmark of the pattern as she defined it was nonexpression of emotion.

Temoshok described what she called the type C personality, people who are overwhelmed by emotions they have not been able to express or resolve. Temoshok maintained that the type C individual was at high risk for cancer, and she and others did subsequent research that seemed to point in that direction. Subsequent analysis of her own and other studies convinced Temoshok that while behavior patterns might not cause cancer, they might affect the outcome of the disease; other research seemed to show that personality and behavior traits correlated with how aggressively cancer progresses.[99]

Throughout, Temoshok emphasized that "people did not bring cancer on themselves. No one can be blamed for mind-body factors in cancer, because no one intentionally develops the cancer-prone behavior pattern. . . . When brought about with compassion and self-care, awareness of type C behavior offers the person opportunities for growth and empowerment, not self-blame."[100]

About the same time Blumberg was puzzling over his "nice" cancer patients in the veterans' hospital, psychologist Lawrence LeShan was fascinated by a striking similarity in the life histories of cancer patients he interviewed, and he noticed three specific "life events" common to the cancer patients: a "bleak" childhood, strong emotional commitment as a young adult, and then loss of the emotional investment.[101]

Researchers looked at a variety of personality traits that might have been connected in some way to the development or progression of cancer. One of the primary factors they examined was stress. While stress may play some sort of role in the progression of the disease, researchers don't believe that stress alone causes cancer. Initial research indicated that many (but certainly not all) cancer patients characteristically react to stress, loss, or change with a feeling of helplessness, hopelessness, or an overwhelming inability to cope, leading researchers to wonder whether a person's response to stress might be a factor. If stress can be implicated at all, it is more likely a function of the impact of stress on immunity (see Chapter 2).

Interesting research conducted at Tel Aviv University indicates that stress may play a role in the recurrence of cancer—and that stress reduction and management might be a powerful way to help prevent cancer from recurring.[102] The study, led by Shamgar Ben-Eliyahu, scientifically demonstrated that stress impairs immune system functioning before, during, and after cancer surgery—especially at the critical point where a tumor is being removed.

According to the research, stress hormones are released before and during surgery, and those hormones weaken the immune system. "There is a short window of opportunity, about a week after surgery, when the immune system needs to be functioning maximally in order to kill the tiny remaining bits of tumor tissue that are scattered around the body," explains Ben-Eliyahu. A weak immune system is one of the major factors leading to cancer metastases.[103]

Research has shown that stimulating the immune system for a week or two before surgery and then blocking stress hormones during and following surgery might increase the long-term survival rates from postoperative cancer by 200 to 300 percent.[104]

Other personality factors, such as helplessness and hopelessness, appeared to play a possible role in who is able to survive cancer. "It is well-known, if quietly admitted, that the best medicine may be to no avail when given to someone who has already given up the struggle for life," stated one researcher. "Even if there is no strong relationship between the origins of cancer and some personality type, the evidence does suggest that the way in which a person responds to the threat may have a lot to do with surviving the physical insult of cancer."[105]

While there does not seem to be a personality "type" that causes or encourages the development of cancer, mind-body techniques have been shown to help in cancer treatment; even if they have not resulted in a cure, they have improved the quality of life for cancer patients. At Boston's Dana-Farber Cancer Institute, an ancient Chinese movement and meditation technique—qigong—has been used to reduce pain and anxiety among cancer patients. Tens of thousands of cancer patients are now using mind-body techniques to help them cope with pain, depression, and anxiety and to help them sleep better; these techniques include yoga, talk therapy, visualization, tai chi, music therapy, relaxation techniques, and prayers, among others.

Of the nation's 26 major cancer centers, 14 now offer complementary medicine programs that include mind-body techniques, bringing together oncologists and alternative practitioners. The Society for Integrative Oncology, founded by Dr. Barrie Cassileth, chief of integrative medicine at New York's Sloan-Kettering Cancer Center, held its first international conference in late 2004.

Lorenzo Cohen, head of integrative medicine at Houston's M. D. Anderson Cancer Center, says that mind-body techniques will soon become as much a part of standard cancer care as chemotherapy or radiation. "In the not-so-distant future," he says, "oncologists will send patients to learn tai chi or yoga the way cardiac specialists now send patients to stress-management courses after they've had a heart attack."[106]

The Rheumatoid Arthritis–Prone Personality

Of all the forms of arthritis, rheumatoid arthritis is the most crippling and most devastating. As an autoimmune disease, it is characterized by the immune system turning against the body and attacking the collagen in the joints' connective tissue. Because it isn't associated with wear and tear, rheumatoid arthritis attacks people of all ages, including children.

The disease has long been considered to have a powerful psychological component. Some researchers are so convinced of the arthritis-personality connection that they have described rheumatoid arthritis as the "expression of a personality conflict."[107]

Identical Twin Study

Study of the link between personality and rheumatoid arthritis began in earnest in the early 1960s, when a team of researchers from the University of Rochester studied eight pairs of identical twins—one of whom had rheumatoid arthritis while the other did not. Because only one twin in each set had the disease, researchers knew that genetics was not the sole determining factor.

Researchers interviewed each of the twins—all women—in great detail to determine not only personality traits, but also life events that may have led to the diagnosis of rheumatoid arthritis. They found some strikingly similar patterns among the women afflicted with arthritis. In each pair of twins, the one with arthritis seemed to put herself under a great deal of stress; in fact, these women actually seemed to seek out stress. The disease seemed to manifest itself only after each woman had decided to dedicate her energies to a particularly stressful or distasteful situation.[108] For example, one woman took a job she really didn't want so she could impress her in-laws. Another gave up personal pursuits to spend her life caring for her psychotic stepfather.

Other striking similarities emerged. The healthy twins felt free to express criticism and to argue but described their marriages as happy ones. The arthritic twins spoke ill of their husbands and apparently put up with considerable abuse in their marriages, yet they never argued with their husbands.[109] In summing up that peculiar dichotomy, one researcher remarked that people with rheumatoid arthritis "will endure stressful situations longer than their siblings. The arthritic patients' inability to express anger may make some situations more stressful to them than these same situations would be to other people."[110]

The healthy women described themselves as people who liked people. They said they were easy to get acquainted with, were active, were constantly busy, were productive workers, and enjoyed life in general. The self-image of the arthritic twins was just the opposite. They described themselves as moody and easily upset. They claimed they were nervous, tense, worried, depressed, and high-strung. While the healthy sisters enjoyed life, the arthritic ones said that they were struggling.

The results of the identical twin study are consistent with what other researchers have found. One researcher who examined more than 5,000 rheumatoid arthritis patients found "that in a high percentage of cases the patients suffered from worry, work pressures, marital disharmony, and concerns about relatives immediately prior to the onset of disease."[111] Others characterize rheumatoid arthritis patients as people who appear to be calm, composed, and optimistic and who rarely, if ever, express anger. Some believe these patients don't even feel anger. On the rare occasions when these patients express anger or rage, they feel overcome with remorse and guilt and feel a strong need to punish themselves. Research has established that people with rheumatoid arthritis are more likely to suffer from emotional disturbance and that they tend to suffer from perfectionism, chronic anxiety, depression, hostility, and introversion.[112]

The Solomon and Moos Study

Stanford University School of Medicine psychiatrist George Solomon and his colleague Rudolf Moos asked to examine each patient who came into the San Francisco General Hospital emergency room complaining of a tender, inflamed, or "hot" joint. Emergency room personnel administered laboratory tests to each patient—a simple blood test indicates the presence of an antibody in the blood. While patients were waiting for the results of the test, Solomon and Moos asked them to participate in a psychodrama.

Solomon and Moos knew that rheumatoid arthritis patients were characteristically unassertive and inhibited. So they constructed a psychodrama that would put that trait to its most severe test: They asked patients to return an item (an iron for women, a shaver for men) to someone playing a hostile department store clerk. The role required great assertiveness, and the researchers watched carefully as each suspected—but yet undiagnosed—patient play-acted.

Based on how each patient interacted with the "hostile clerk," Solomon made his own diagnosis, predicting which patients would eventually be proven to have rheumatoid arthritis and which would not. He was able to predict with 100 percent accuracy exactly which patients had rheumatoid arthritis simply by watching how they asserted themselves in an unpleasant situation.

Following their initial experiment, Moos compiled everything he could find on the link between personality and arthritis, and he became familiar with the case studies of more than 5,000 people with rheumatoid arthritis. Based on his exhaustive studies, he concluded that there was a distinct psychology involved in the rheumatoid arthritis process.[113]

The Immune System Factor

Since rheumatoid arthritis is an immune disorder, researchers have looked at how the personality affects the immune system among arthritis sufferers.[114]

In both animals and humans, emotional distress has significant effects on both immune dysfunction and the inflammatory response characteristic of arthritis.[115] Rheumatoid arthritis patients have been shown to have an imbalance in the white blood cells (lymphocytes) that regulate much of the immune response. In their blood and joint fluid, rheumatoid patients have a disturbed "immunoregulatory ratio" of helper

T lymphocytes (which enhance the immune response) to suppressor T lymphocytes (which decrease the response).[116]

Other neurochemicals that modulate immune function and inflammation are endorphins, the body's natural painkillers.[117] These are well-known to be affected by mental state; for example, happy excitement turns them on, depression turns them off. Less well-known is the fact that endorphins are deficient in both the blood and the brain in many arthritis patients.[118] Endorphins not only reduce pain perception in the brain but also block the release in tissues of inflammation-producing neurochemicals, such as substance P and prostaglandins. Substance P has also been thought to be a mechanism by which the nervous system might be involved in rheumatoid arthritis.[119]

Two of the traits common to arthritis victims, chronic anxiety and repressed hostility, have been shown in repeated studies to compromise the immune system. In one study, researchers carefully studied 33 women who suffered from rheumatoid arthritis. They looked at the number of daily "hassles" each went through, the major challenges they faced, and the amount of psychological distress each one had. They then measured the immune function of each woman. As expected, the researchers found major effects on the immune system, and those effects were stronger among the women who suffered greater psychological distress, major challenges, and minor hassles.[120]

Based on several decades of research into the connection between personality and rheumatoid arthritis, one researcher constructed what he believes to be an accurate picture of the arthritis patient's personality.[121] He maintains that individuals with rheumatoid arthritis are likely to be dependent and feel inadequate, but they deny their dependency by overcompensating with an outward façade of independence, self-assurance, and self-control. They are aware of strong, unexpressed feelings of anger, but they are severely blocked in their ability to express anger or other emotions. They tend to court others' favor, but they avoid closeness in interpersonal relationships. They tend to become overactive—a way of dealing defensively with their tensions—and they overreact to even the slightest criticism or rejection. The single most powerful precipitating factor in rheumatoid arthritis "was the loss of, or separation from, important key figures upon whom these patients depended for support."[122]

The Ulcer-Prone Personality

Physicians have long acknowledged that the physiology behind development of gastric ulcers is simple: The ulcer sufferer secretes too much gastric acid. That acid eats away at the lining of the stomach, causing erosion; in severe cases, the ulcer becomes perforated, eating a hole through the wall of the stomach. Most ulcers are caused by infection with a bacterium (*Helicobacter pylori*) that interacts with the acid. Whether mental stress in a susceptible person increases the likelihood of persistent *Helicobacter* infection, as it does with other infections, has not yet been studied.

Use of tobacco, alcohol, caffeine (especially coffee), and aspirin have all been shown to increase gastric acid production. Cigarette smoking is a double-edged sword, since it also delays healing. Certain emotions can also increase acid; the most powerful seem to be frustration, hostility, and resentment. Some people experience an increase in gastric acid when they see, smell, taste, or chew food—or even think about it.

Anti-inflammatory medications like aspirin (which are more commonly used by stressed patients) can compound the problem by breaking down the mucous barrier that protects the stomach and intestinal lining from the acid.

Pioneering Research

Recent research has indicated the presence of an "ulcer personality." Much like the cancer personality or arthritis personality, the ulcer personality may actually cause ulcers, or it may affect the overall severity of the ulcers.

One of the first recorded observations of the emotional link to ulcers occurred in the mid-nineteenth century:[123] Dr. William Beaumont had a patient whose abdominal wall had an opening clear into his stomach. That opening afforded the perfect window through which to view the rate of stomach secretion—and Beaumont noticed that the secretion of stomach juices changed when the man became emotionally stressed.

Pioneering research on the ulcer-personality link has been conducted by Dr. Charles Richardson and Dr. Mark Feldman, professors of internal medicine at the University of Texas Health Science Center in Dallas.[124] They found that ulcer patients seem to have the same number of stressful situations as people who don't have ulcers, but they perceive the situations as being far more negative than do other people. When faced with a job change or relocation, for example, ulcer patients perceived disaster and upset instead of adventure or a positive change. In addition, ulcer patients seemed much more likely than others to be neurotic—preoccupied with their own aches and pain and too concerned about their bodily functions. They expected the worst and felt threatened by a wide variety of situations, even situations that did not pose much of a real risk.

Characteristic Traits

The ulcer personality is characterized by excessive dependency on others and a tendency to rely on other people in ways that are not healthy. Even though such people are very dependent, they enjoy far less social support than most healthy people do. Many ulcer patients express the feeling that they have few friends or relatives on whom they could depend in times of crisis. They tend to suffer from excessive worry, annoyance, and fear of common situations or circumstances. And, unfortunately, ulcer patients seem to have more times of crisis than others, possibly because the ulcer personality is also marked by deep pessimism or the tendency to always expect the worst. Finally, ulcer patients who have been given psychological tests show a fairly consistent quality: while other people are able to bend with stress, an ulcer patient tends to break. This tendency leads to higher rates of emotional distress, anxiety, and depression among those with ulcers. The situation is aggravated by doing other things to damage the lining of the stomach, such as drinking too much coffee or alcohol.

However, researchers are quick to point out the bright side of ulcer personality research: with help and determination, ulcer patients can learn to change the way they look at things; and, with a change in personality traits, the tendency toward ulcers can diminish considerably.

An Asthma-Prone Personality?

Research shows that several factors may be at work in the personality traits of an asthmatic. Initially, many asthma episodes are caused by bronchial infection or an allergic reaction; air passages narrow, the victim can't get enough air, and that feeling is profoundly distressful. Any attending emotional reaction just makes the asthma worse. Asthma is usually maintained by an inflammatory process in the airways that may have some of the same underlying mechanisms involving the central nervous system as those for rheumatoid arthritis. It is not uncommon to see the airway disease of anxious or depressed asthmatics improve significantly when those mental conditions are treated appropriately.

It is now believed that some people later develop an almost Pavlovian response to whatever triggers their asthma. Simply thinking, "I feel a cold coming on; it's going to cause an asthma attack" or "The pollen count is going to be high today" can be enough to trigger a full-fledged asthma attack without an actual physical insult.

There's also a vicious cycle among asthmatics, especially childhood asthmatics, that is very difficult to break. An asthma episode tends to engender sympathy, attention, and compassion and to keep the child home from school. If that's what asthmatic persons need in their life—more sympathy, attention, and compassion—attacks may become more frequent. Although the biology of the attack is very real, it is precipitated by emotional need.

A few traits seem more common among those with asthma. Many are anxious and feel powerless. Even though they are angry and hostile, they feel weak and out of control of their lives. Finally, many feel ready to strike out at those around them.

Reducing Your Risks

Is it possible to overcome a disease-prone personality? Some researchers think it is. Any approach toward improving health should be balanced and should take into account all the factors that we know contribute to disease. In his landmark book, *Self-Healing Personality: Why Some People Achieve Health and Others Succumb to Illness*, Howard S. Friedman cautions that no single diet, fitness regime, or self-improvement program can promise health. Why? Every individual has a unique combination of genetics, behavioral habits, and emotional responses that work together to contribute to wellness or illness.

In an address before the National Institute for the Clinical Application of Behavioral Medicine, Henry Dreher suggested the following ideas for change:[125]

- Develop an awareness of your own needs. You can start on a small scale; maybe you need a few minutes alone when you get home from work before you plunge into family life, for example.

- Discover what Dreher calls an "inner guide"—essentially, an awareness of your innermost thoughts and feelings. If you're used to suppressing emotion or ignoring your needs, it can take some real concentration.

- Reframe your ideas about your feelings. If you're troubled by the thought that you are angry toward an abusive parent, stop feeling guilty for your anger. Find appropriate ways to express your anger, work through it, and then build on what is left, even eventually forgiving your abuser.

- Learn the skills of emotional expression. Everyone occasionally feels angry, hostile, disappointed, depressed, or resentful. The key is to acknowledge your emotion, express it appropriately, and then move on.

- Take charge of your medical care; find a physician who will take the time to talk to you, who will explore options, and who will answer questions. Find out all you can, and make your own decisions.

- Get as much social support as you can. A broad network of family and friends is ideal, but you should cultivate at least a few close friends in whom you can confide.

- Work through your feelings of hopelessness. Getting information is the first step; next, figure out what your challenges might be, and then work out a game plan for each. As soon as you realize that you have viable options, you'll find that you feel in charge instead of hopeless.

- Cultivate a fighting spirit; be willing to face challenges head-on and to fight to the finish.

To stress components that are more positive and productive, Dr. Meyer Friedman uses the following drills to help people change the negative components of personality into more health-protective characteristics:[126]

- Smile at yourself in the mirror for a minute or two.

- Don't interfere with someone who is doing a job more slowly than you would do the same job.

- Eliminate two phrases from your vocabulary at work: "How much?" and "How many?"

- Take regular breaks from work; try daydreaming, meditating, or even playing with your pet.

Other effective practices to modify health-harming personality traits and behaviors can include the following suggestions involving practicing mindfulness; that is, do one thing at a time, being completely present with full attention. Give yourself with caring creativity to whatever is chosen to be done in the present moment.[127]

- While waiting in lines, practice the enjoyment that comes with socializing or doing relaxation exercises.

- Smile at the competitive antics of yourself or others.

- Drive around the block when you try to beat someone out in traffic.

- Read books that have nothing to do with your vocation.

- Take restful breaks during the day, perhaps using relaxation exercises.

- Eat slowly and mindfully.

- Ask, "What did I do well today, and what's worth remembering?"

- Practice conditioning a relaxation response after exercise and other arousal.[128]

In making the transition, it's more important to envision what you want (valued personality traits) than to try not to be hostile. (The brain doesn't do well with "not" commands because it needs to picture clearly the desired outcome before change can occur.) As you try to envision the effective traits, work toward these habits:

- Have less time urgency: Give more attention to the central task at hand. Be less eager to move on to something else. Be on time but without frenzy or rage. Be patient. Contemplate, especially beauty and metaphor. Tend to see the whole more than the parts. Value and enjoy the things you've already done (or you're doing now) as much as the things you will do in the future.

- Relinquish control: Delegate. Be tolerant of, or even enjoy, differences. Inspire creative involvement with others.

- Value yourself: Appreciate yourself for what you are as much as for what you do. Accept and value yourself as you are. Understand that self-identity is far more than numbers. Feel valued and of worth, regardless of your achievements. Work hard, but don't let failure collapse your self-esteem. Learn to love growth and the process of getting better through mistakes. Compete with yourself, not with others.

- Get rid of free-floating hostility: Don't find fault with others to bolster your own ego. Accept with equanimity the trivial errors of subordinates. Enjoy empowering and lifting others. Don't feel tense or induce tension in others. Be self-confident enough to be objective, to see through another's eyes. Be capable of both feeling and expressing affection; enjoy intimate relationships.

The behavior change methods that develop these characteristics are beginning to be proven some of medicine's most valuable preventive approaches!

WHAT DID YOU LEARN?

1. Is there such a thing as a disease-prone personality? Any proof for or against its existence?
2. What significant finding did Ronald Grossarth-Maticek make?
3. What is the connection between disease and personality?
4. What are the major conflicts of the theory of disease-prone personality?
5. What is the research to support a heart disease–prone personality?

ENDNOTES

1. Howard S. Friedman, *The Self-Healing Personality* (New York: Henry Holt and Company, 1991), 1.
2. Clive Wood, "Type-Casting: Is Disease Linked with Personality?" *Nursing Times,* 84, no. 48 (1988): 26.
3. Friedman, *The Self-Healing Personality,* 22.

4. Hans J. Eysenck, "Personality, Stress, and Cancer: Prediction and Prophylaxis," *British Journal of Medical Psychology* 61 (1988): 1, 57–75.

5. S. Yousfi, G. Matthews, M. Amelang, and C. Schmidt-Rathjens, "Personality and Disease: Correlations of Multiple Trait Scores with Various Illnesses," *Journal of Health Psychology* 9, no. 5 (2004): 627–47.

6. R. Grossarth-Maticek, D. T. Kanazir, P. Schmidt, and H. Vetter, "Psychosomatic Factors in the Process of Carcinogenesis: Theoretical Models and Empirical Results," *Psychotherapy and Psychosomatics* 38 (1982): 284–302. Also R. Grossarth-Maticek, D. T. Kanazir, P. Schmidt, and H. Vetter, "Psychosomatic Factors in the Process of Carcinogenesis: Preliminary Results in the Yugoslavian Prospective Study," *Psychotherapy and Psychosomatics* 40 (1983): 191–210.

7. S. Yousfi et al., "Personality and Disease."

8. Eysenck, "Personality, Stress, and Cancer," 30.

9. Ibid.

10. Joshua Fischman, "Fighting Cancer and Heart Disease: The Character of Controversy," *Psychology Today* (December 1988): 27.

11. S. Yousfi et al., "Personality and Disease."

12. Fischman, "Fighting Cancer and Heart Disease."

13. "Nineteen Critical Commentaries," *Psychological Inquiry: An International Journal of Peer Commentary and Review* 2, no. 3, 1990.

14. Fischman, "Fighting Cancer and Heart Disease."

15. Friedman, *The Self-Healing Personality*, 94–6.

16. Bruce Bower, "The Character of Cancer," *Science News* 131 (1987): 120.

17. Ibid.

18. R. Horowski, L. Horowski, S. M. Caine, and D. B. Caine, "From Wilhelm von Humboldt to Hitler: Are Prominent People More Prone to Parkinson's Disease?" *SBU Therapeutics* 6, no. 4 (2000): 205–14.

19. R. Goodwin and G. Engstrom, "Personality and the Perception of Health in the General Population," *Psychological Medicine* 32, no. 2 (2002): 325–32.

20. Judy Berlfein, "An Ill Nature," *Psychology Today,* n.d., 16.

21. Ibid.

22. Ibid.

23. Joann Rodgers, "Longevity Predictors: The Personality Link," *Omni* (February 1989): 25.

24. Douglas J. Stanwyck and Carol A. Anson, "Is Personality Related to Illness? Cluster Profiles of Aggregated Data," *Advances* 3, no. 2: 4–15, 1998.

25. Friedman, *The Self-Healing Personality*, 15.

26. Marcia Angell, "Disease as a Reflection of the Psyche," *New England Journal of Medicine* 312 (1985): 1570–2.

27. Ibid.

28. Ibid.

29. Ibid.

30. June Zimmerman, "Does Emotional State Affect Disease?" *MD* (April 1986): 30, 41.

31. Joel Davis, "Anxiety Aches," *Self* (January 1985): 100.

32. Steven Locke and Douglas Colligan, *The Healer Within: The New Medicine of Mind and Body* (New York: E. P. Dutton, 1986), 140.

33. L. Kelti Kangas-Jarvinen, " 'Psychosomatic Personality': A Personality Constellation or an Illness-Related Reaction?" *British Journal of Medical Psychology* 62, no. 4: 325–31, 1989–1990.

34. Anne Underwood, "For a Happy Heart," *Newsweek* (September 27, 2004): 54.

35. T. George Harris, "Heart and Soul," *Psychology Today,* n.d.

36. Ray Rosenman, "Do You Have Type 'A' Behavior?" *Health and Fitness* 87 S12–3, p. 3.

37. "Personality Types A, B, and C and Disease," St. Louis Psychologist and Counseling Information and Referral, http://psychtreatment.com, Updated March 19, 2006.

38. Ethel Roskies, *Stress Management for the Healthy Type A* (New York: Guilford Press, 1987), 8.

39. Paul Pearsall, *Super Immunity* (New York: McGraw-Hill, 1987), 38–39.

40. "Personality Types A, B, and C and Disease," 2006.

41. Redford Williams, "The Trusting Heart," *New Age Journal* (May/June 1989): 19.

42. Roskies, *Stress Management,* 6.

43. Roskies, *Stress Management,* 8.

44. Williams, "The Trusting Heart," 22.

45. Ibid., 25–6.

46. Ibid., 27.

47. Ibid., 37.

48. R. B. Williams, T. L. Haney, J. A. Blumenthal, and Y. Kong, "Type A Behavior, Hostility, and Coronary Atherosclerosis," *Psychosomatic Medicine* 42(6): 539–549, 1980.

49. G. E. Miller et al., "Pathways Linking Depression, Adiposity, and Inflammatory Markers in Healthy Young Adults," *Brain, Behavior, and Immunity* 17, no. 4: 276–85, 2003.

50. Willem J. Kop, "The Integration of Cardiovascular Behavioral Medicine and Psychoneuroimmunology: New Developments Based on Converging Research Fields," *Brain, Behavior, and Immunity* 17 (2003): 233–7.

51. Michael Craig Miller, "What Is Type D Personality?" *Harvard Medical Health Letter* (November 2005): 8.

52. "Brain Behavior Immunity Research Featured in the New York Times," *Brain Behavior and Research* (August 2007). http://www.pnirs.org/news/brain-behavior-immunity-research-featured-in-the-new-york-times.html Updated August 17, 2007.

53. Gary Felsten, "Five-Factor Analysis of Buss-Durkee Hostility Inventory, Neurotic Hostility and Expressive Hostility Factors: Implications for Health Psychology," *Journal of Personality Assessment* 67, no. 1: 179, 1996.

54. B. J. Bushman, H. M. Cooper, and K. M. Lemke, "Meta-Analysis of Factor Analyses: An Illustration Using the Buss-Durkee Hostility Inventory," *Personality and Social Psychology Bulletin* 17: 344–9, June 1991.

55. Ibid., p. 346.

56. Ibid., p. 348.

57. R. B. Williams et al., "Type A Behavior, Hostility, and Coronary Atherosclerosis," *Psychosomatic Medicine* 42 (1980): 539–49.

58. R. B. Shekelle, M. Gale, A. Ostfeld, and D. Paul, "Hostility, Risk of Coronary Artery Disease and Mortality," *Psychosomatic Medicine* 45 (1983): 109–14; and J. C. Barefoot, W. G. Dahlstrom, and R. B. Williams, "Hostility, CHD Incidence, and Total Mortality: A 25-Year Follow-Up Study of 255 Physicians," *Psychosomatic Medicine* 45 (1983): 59–63.

59. Underwood, "For a Happy Heart," 55.

60. Chris Raymond, "Distrust, Rage May Be 'Toxic Core' That Puts 'Type A' Person at Risk," *Journal of the American Medical Association* 261, no. 16: 813, 1990.

61. Roskies, *Stress Management,* 17.

62. Earl Ubell, "The Deadly Emotions," *Parade* (February 11, 1990): 46.

63. Williams, "The Trusting Heart," 26.

64. Joshua Fischman, "Type A Situations," *Psychology Today* (August 1988): 22.

65. John C. Barefoot et al., "Suspiciousness, Health, and Mortality: A Follow-Up Study of 500 Older Adults," *Psychosomatic Medicine* 49 (1987): 450–7.

66. Barefoot et al., "Suspiciousness, Health, and Mortality."

67. Donald E. Girard, Ransom J. Arthur, and James B. Reuler, "Psychosocial Events and Subsequent Illness—A Review," *Western Journal of Medicine* 142, no. 3: 358–63, 1985.

68. William H. Hendrix and Richard L. Hughes, "Relationship of Trait, Type A Behavior, and Physical Fitness Variables to Cardiovascular Reactivity and Coronary Heart Disease Risk Potential," *American Journal of Health Promotion* 11, no. 4: 264–71, 1997.

69. Pearsall, *Super Immunity.*

70. Williams, "The Trusting Heart," 26.

71. Eileen M. Mikat et al., "Chronic Norepinephrine Infusion Accelerates Atherosclerotic Lesion Development in Sand Rats Maintained on a High-Cholesterol Diet," *Psychosomatic Medicine* 53 (1991): 211.

72. Robert S. Eliot, *Behavior and Cardiovascular Disease* (Kalamazoo, MI: Upjohn Company, 1989).

73. Eliot, *Behavior and Cardiovascular Disease.*

74. Miller, "What Is Type D Personality?," 8.

75. L. Sher, "Type D Personality: The Heart, Stress, and Cortisol," *QJM* 98 (2005): 323–329, 325.

76. Miller, "What Is Type D Personality?," 8.

77. Sher, "Type D Personality," 325.

78. Miller, "What Is Type D Personality?," 8.

79. Sher, "Type D Personality," 324.

80. Johann Denollet et al., "Personality as Independent Predictor of Long-Term Mortality in Patients with Coronary Heart Disease," *Lancet* 347 (1996): 417–21; and J. W. Pennebaker and H. C. Traue, "Inhibition and Psychosomatic Processes," pp. 146–63 in H. C. Traue and J. W. Pennebaker, eds., *Emotion, Inhibition, and Health* (Seattle, WA: Hogrefe & Huber, 1993).

81. D. Watson and L. A. Clark, "Negative Affectivity: The Disposition to Experience Adverse Emotional States," *Psychological Bulletin* 96 (1984): 465–90.

82. Denollet et al., "Personality as Independent Predictor," 417–21.

83. J. M. Murphy et al., "Affective Disorders and Mortality: A General Population Study," *Archives of General Psychiatry* 44 (1987): 473–80; and R. M. Carney et al., "Major Depressive Disorder Predicts Cardiac Events in Patients with Coronary Artery Disease," *Psychosomatic Medicine* 50 (1988): 627–33.

84. M. A. Mittleman et al., "Triggering of Acute Myocardial Infarction Onset by Episodes of Anger," *Circulation* 92 (1995): 1720–5; and I. Kawachi et al., "A Prospective Study of Anger and Coronary Heart Disease: The Normative Aging Study," *Circulation* 94 (1996): 2090–5.

85. D. K. Moser and K. Dracup, "Is Anxiety Early after Myocardial Infarction Associated with Subsequent Ischemic and Arrhythmic Events?" *Psychosomatic Medicine* 58 (1996): 395–401; and I. Kawachi, D. Sparrow, P. Vokonas, and S. T. Weiss, "Symptoms of Anxiety and Risk of Coronary Heart Disease: The Normative Aging Study," *Circulation* 90 (1994): 2225–9.

86. J. C. Barefoot and M. Schroll, "Symptoms of Depression, Acute Myocardial Infarction, and Total Mortality in a Community Sample," *Circulation* 93 (1996): 1976–80.

87. L. D. Kubzansky et al., "Is Worrying Bad for Your Heart? A Prospective Study of Worry and Coronary Heart Disease in the Normative Aging Study," *Circulation* 95 (1997): 818–24.

88. S. A. Everson et al., "Hopelessness and Risk of Mortality and Incidence of Myocardial Infarction and Cancer," *Psychosomatic Medicine* 58 (1996): 113–21.

89. Underwood, "For a Happy Heart." http://www.newsweek.com/id/55120

90. Ibid.
91. J. Denollet and D. L. Brutsaert, "Personality, Disease Severity, and the Risk of Long-Term Cardiac Events in Patients with a Decreased Ejection Fraction After Myocardial Infarction," *Circulation* 97 (1998): 167–73.
92. Denollet et al., "Personality as Independent Predictors."
93. *Newsweek* (September 27, 2004). Johan Denollet, "The Dangers of Chronic Distress," *Newsweek,* http://www.newsweek.com/id/50927.
94. Roskies, *Stress Management,* 5.
95. Locke and Colligan, *The Healer Within* (Institute of Noetic Sciences, 1986), 140.
96. Ibid., 140–141.
97. Ibid., 140–141.
98. Ibid., 151.
99. Yousfi et al., "Personality and Disease," 627–47.
100. Lydia Temoshok and Henry Dreher, *The Type C Connection: The Behavioral Links to Cancer and Your Health* (New York: Random House, 1992).
101. Locke and Colligan, *The Healer Within,* 134.
102. "Psychoneuroimmunology: Stress Reduction to Prevent Cancer Recurrence," *Medical News Today* (February 28, 2008).
103. "Psychoneuroimmunology," February 28, 2008.
104. Ibid.
105. Phillip L. Rice, *Stress and Health* (Monterey, CA: Brooks/Cole Publishing Company, 1987), 103–4.
106. Tyre, "Combination Therapy," *Newsweek.* (September 27, 2004), 67.
107. Barbara Powell, *Good Relationships Are Good Medicine* (Emmaus, PA: Rodale Press, 1987).
108. Locke and Colligan, *The Healer Within,* 107.
109. Powell, *Good Relationships.*
110. Ibid.
111. Ibid.
112. Friedman, *The Self-Healing Personality,* 85.
113. Locke and Colligan, *The Healer Within,* 108.
114. G. F. Solomon and A. A. Amkraut, "Psychoneuroendocrinological Effects on the Immune System," *Annual Review of Microbiology* 35 (1981): 155–84; G. F. Solomon, N. Kay, and J. E. Morley, "Endorphins: A Link Between Personality, Stress, Emotions, Immunity, and Substance P," pp. 129–44 in N. P. Plotnikoff, R. E. Faith, A. J. Murgo, and R. A. Good, eds., *Enkephalins and Endorphins, Stress and the Immune System* (New York: Plenum Press, 1986); and C. D. Anderson, J. M. Soyva, and L. J. Vaughn, "A Test of Delayed Recovery Following Stressful Stimulation in Four Psychosomatic Disorders," *Journal of Psychosomatic Research* 26 (1982): 571–80.
115. E. M. Sternberg, G. P. Chrousis, R. L. Wilder, and P. W. Gold, "The Stress Response and the Regulation of Inflammatory Disease," *Annals of Internal Medicine* 117, no. 10: 854–66, 1992.
116. E. M. Veys et al., "Evaluation of T Cell Subsets with Monoclonal Antibodies in Synovial Fluid in Rheumatoid Arthritis," *Journal of Rheumatology* 9, no. 6: 821–6, 1998.
117. N. P. Plotnikoff, R. E. Faith, A. J. Murgo, and R. A. Good, *Enkephalins and Endorphins, Stress and the Immune System* (New York: Plenum Press, 1986), v–vi; and Solomon et al., "Endomorphs," 129–44.
118. C. Denko, "Serum Beta Endorphins in Rheumatic Disorders," *Journal of Rheumatology* 9, no. 6: 827–33.
119. J. D. Levine et al., "Hypothesis: The Nervous System May Contribute to the Pathophysiology of Rheumatoid Arthritis," *Journal of Rheumatology* 12 (1985): 406–22.

120. Friedman, *The Self-Healing Personality.*

121. Michael A. Weiner, *Maximum Immunity* (Houghton Mifflin, 1986).

122. Ibid., 61.

123. Friedman, *The Self-Healing Personality,* 89; A. R. Rimon, "A Psychosomatic Approach to Rheumatoid Arthritis: A Clinical Study of 100 Patients," *Acta Rheumatologica Scandinavica,* suppl. 13 (1969): 1–154; R. Rimon and L. Riika-Liisa, "Life Stress and Rheumatoid Arthritis: A 15-Year Follow-Up Study," *Psychotherapy and Psychosomatics* (1985): 43: 38–43; T. W. Smith, J. R. Peck, and J. R. Ward, "Helplessness and Depression in Rheumatoid Arthritis," *Health Psychology* 9 (1990), no. 4: 377–89; A. O' Leary, S. Shoor, K. Lorig, and H. R. Holman, "A Cognitive-Behavioral Treatment for Rheumatoid Arthritis," *Health Psychology* 7 (1988): 527–44; K. Lorig, "Outcomes of Self-Help Education for Patients with Arthritis," *Arthritis and Rheumatism* 28 (1985): 680–5; S. Crown, J. Crown, and A. Fleming, "Aspects of the Psychology and Epidemiology of Rheumatoid Disease," *Psychological Medicine* 5 (1975): 291–9; M. Gringras, "A Clinical Trial of Tofranil in Rheumatic Pain in General Practice," *Journal of International Medical Research* 4 (1976) (suppl. 2): 41–9; W. Scott, "The Relief of Pain with an Antidepressant in Arthritis," *Practitioner* 202 (1969): 802–7; I. Oreskes, "Rheumatoid Factors in an Acute Psychiatric Population," *Annals of Rheumatic Disease* 27 (1968): 60; and G. G. Haydn, "Effect of Imipramine on the Rheumatoid Factor Titre of Psychotic Patients with Depressive Symptomatology," *Annals of Rheumatic Disease* 33 (1974): 274.

124. "Is There an Ulcer Personality?" *Wellness Newsletter* (July 1987): 2; and Sharon Faelten, David Diamond, and the editors of *Prevention Magazine*, "Take Control of Your Life: A Complete Guide to Stress Relief," *Prevention* (Emmaus, PA: Rodale Press, 1988), 206–7.

125. H. Dreher, "The Type C Connection," presentation to the National Institute for the Clinical Application of Behavioral Medicine.

126. Meyer Friedman and Ray H. Rosenman, *Type A Behavior and Your Heart* (Mass Market Paperback, 1982).

127. Hal Straus, *Men's Health* (June 1992): 72.

128. See the discussion of the characteristics of coronary-protected individuals in M. Friedman and D. Ulmer, *Treating Type A Behavior—And Your Heart* (New York: Ballantine Books, 1985), Chap. 3.

CHAPTER 4

Anger, Hostility, and Health

Of the seven deadly sins, anger is possibly the most fun. To lick your wounds, to smack your lips over grievances long past, to roll over your tongue the prospect of bitter confrontations still to come, to savor to the last toothsome morsel both the pain you are given and the pain you are giving back—in many ways it is a feast fit for a king. The chief drawback is that what you are wolfing down is yourself. The skeleton at the feast is you.

—Frederick Buechner

LEARNING OBJECTIVES

- Explore the difference between anger and hostility and the significance of each.
- Define the physiological reactions and health effects that accompany anger and hostility.
- Describe effective techniques for managing and even transforming anger and hostility.

Anger has assumed a whole new importance, particularly when it comes to heart disease. What used to be blamed on "the hurry disease," as researchers called it, has now been more accurately identified. Research has shown that those who hurry out of love for what they are doing have no increased health risk. It is not the hurry itself that is toxic to the heart; instead, the culprit is the often-underlying competitive hostility and anger that is frequently seen as the need to prove oneself.

You can be a heart-healthy Type A as long as, among other things, you're not chronically angry. The impact of anger on health doesn't stop there. The exploding rage you feel when you get really angry brings with it actual physical changes in your body; the health consequences of anger certainly can include high blood pressure and other coronary problems, but the consequences are much more widespread than that. For example, surging stress hormones and chemicals affect many organs and systems other than the heart. When you are chronically angry, as Buechner so graphically stated, "what you are wolfing down is yourself. The skeleton at the feast is you."[1]

"Anger kills," says famed Duke University researcher Redford Williams. "We're speaking here not about the anger that drives people to shoot, stab, or otherwise wreak havoc on their fellow humans. We mean instead the everyday sort of anger, annoyance, and irritation that courses through the minds and bodies of many perfectly normal people."[2]

The Definitions of Anger and Hostility

The terms *anger* and *hostility* are often used interchangeably, but they are not the same.[3] Anger is a transient emotional response that depends on the way one chooses to think about events, usually triggered by perceived provocation or mistreatment. Hostility, on the other hand, is a habitual attitude that may not even require much provocation and is usually associated with cynicism and resentment.[4] Hostile people experience a lot of anger.

What, exactly, is anger? First of all, everyone experiences it. Just watch two toddlers fighting over a favorite set of blocks, a teenager challenging an unreasonable curfew, or an executive whose car gets rear-ended on the way to an important business presentation. If you look closely at each of these examples, the real feeling for each is frustration. In this case, frustration is the primary emotion, and anger is the chosen way of expressing the frustration.

Anger is a temporary emotion. It combines physiological arousal with emotional arousal. It can range in severity all the way from intense rage to "cool" anger that doesn't really involve arousal at all (and might more accurately be described as an attitude, such as resentment).[5] People express anger in all sorts of ways, such as hurling verbal insults, using profanity, slamming doors, or smashing a fist into the nearest available object. Anger can, in fact, often be considered a secondary emotion, that is, a way of expressing blame or communicating discomfort with a more primary emotion such as frustration. When this secondary aspect is realized, one can decide to choose a more healthy way of communicating.

The words we use to describe our anger strongly hint at the turmoil that is going on inside our bodies when we're angry. Social psychologist and anger expert Carol Tavris pointed out some of the most common descriptors:[6]

- His pent-up anger welled up inside him.
- He was bursting with anger.
- I blew my stack.
- She flipped her lid.
- He hit the ceiling.
- Our blood "boils," our muscles tense up, our teeth clench, our stomach feels like it's tied up in knots, and our cheeks feel like they're burning up.

The more angry we become, the stronger and more powerful we feel—and the more pressed we are to "strike out."[7] In fact, that sudden need for power or control may be why anger seems built into us. However, there are usually better ways to gain a sense of control.

The terms *anger* and *hostility* are often used to describe a set of negative emotions, but they differ in duration and intensity. Anger is a temporary emotion that may or may not be accompanied by outward expressions (physical or verbal). Sometimes anger is bottled up; in such a case, there is no outward expression. It's important to realize that the *outward expression* is not the problem—bottled-up anger can be just as unhealthy as anger that is expressed.

Hostility, on the other hand, is not a temporary emotion, but rather an attitude. It is anger that is expressed in aggressive behavior motivated by animosity and hatefulness. "Chronic anger" is usually hostility. Ongoing hostility is usually associated with a cynical and suspicious worldview and sometimes with clinical depression.

"Anger is generally considered to be a simpler concept than hostility or aggression," explain researchers Margaret A. Chesney and Ray H. Rosenman. "The concept of anger usually refers to an emotional state that consists of feelings that vary in intensity, from mild irritation or annoyance to fury and rage. Although hostility usually involves angry feelings, it has the connotation of a complex set of attitudes that motivate aggressive behaviors directed toward destroying objects or injuring other people."[8]

Hostility comes from the Latin word *hostis*, which means "enemy." For the hostile, enemies seem to abound. They are everywhere: at the office, in the elevator, in the grocery store checkout line, on the freeway, in the house on the corner. And, because of the health-damaging effects of hostility, hostile people become their own enemy.

Hostility is an ongoing accumulation of anger and irritation. As psychologist Robert Ornstein and physician David Sobel put it, hostility is "a permanent resident kind of anger that shows itself with ever greater frequency in response to increasingly trivial happenings."[9] Tavris says that "into each life come real problems that people should be angry about. But hostile personality types get equally angry about cold soup and racial injustice. They're walking around in a state of wrath."[10] And, the researchers warn, hostility may go undetected for a long time. One reason for slow detection is that hostile people deny it[11] and often try to hide it (most actually don't really want to be hostile). If asked if they are often hostile, they might angrily reply, "Of course not! What do you take me for, anyway?"

Pioneering researchers like Redford Williams now suspect that the notorious Type A personality may not play the major role once believed in heart disease. Instead, a handful of traits—particularly hostility—may be the actual culprits. According to Williams, about 20 percent of the general population has a level of hostility high enough to be dangerous to health.[12] He describes hostility as having three components:

- **Attitude.** Hostile people are generally cynical toward others.

- **Emotion.** Hostile people express frequent anger, especially over petty incidents or issues.

- **Behavior.** Hostile people display threatening or aggressive behavior.

And for some reason, hostility rarely stands alone; it is often intertwined with cynicism, suspiciousness, and self-centeredness.[13]

Research shows that the most health-harming kind is free-floating hostility, an attitude characterized by being angry or on the verge of anger most of the time, with or without cause. At the best, hostile people are grouchy; at the worst, they are constantly consumed by hatred. Occasional hostility is not the problem; the problem is the constant, slow-burning anger and the willingness to see almost everyone as the enemy.[14]

Manifestations of Anger and Hostility

Anger has as many different causes as there are situations and people in them. A common one is the frustration of physical or psychological restraint—being held back from something we intensely want or want to do.[15] Others include being forced to do something against our will, being taken advantage of, being insulted or ridiculed, or having plans defeated. Sometimes other primary emotions (such as distress, sorrow, or fear) can lead to anger.

Besides individual differences in the way we feel and express anger, there are also some important cultural differences. In a number of Latin and Arab cultures, the free expression of anger is heartily endorsed; two who are angry with each other may fight because they figure that a strong third party (such as a neighbor or family member) will intervene before things go too far. The Utku Inuit in Alaska fall at the opposite end of the spectrum: they ostracize anyone who loses his or her temper, regardless of the reason. Tavris tells of an anthropologist who was shunned for several months by the Utkus when she became angry with some Caucasian fishermen who broke an Inuit canoe.[16]

Between these two extremes are all kinds of middle ground. The Japanese don't display anger as their traditional Western counterparts do; instead of lashing out verbally, the Japanese assume a neutral expression and a polite demeanor when angry. The Mbuti hunter-gatherers of northeast Zaire take it a step farther; when angry, they laugh. Some individual disputes have become "full-scale tribal laugh fests."[17] These differences illustrate how anger is a chosen, expressive (secondary) emotion, and how other expressions might be effectively chosen instead.

Hostility, however, shows up with many associated features. Noted Harvard psychiatrist James Gill has compiled a list of such traits. A hostile person, says Gill, notices with irritation the perceived faults of others, has an intense need to win at games or sports, and gets extremely angry (with self and others) at losing. Much of the hostility seems to come from feeling separate and in competition with others—a feeling that one has to "win" in order to be considered okay. He or she turns most conversations into a debate and argues tenaciously until winning the point. He or she also is extremely demanding and critical, not only of others but also of self, and is extremely sensitive to any kind of criticism or uncomplimentary remark. Even when smiling, the hostile person appears tight and tense, as though ready to quarrel on a second's notice.[18] The key in relating them to hostility, says Gill, is consistency: These aren't occasional attitudes, but habitual and characteristic ways of reacting.

Still another definition of hostility arises from the psychological tests that researchers use to pinpoint it. One of the most standard—and most reliable—is the Hostility Scale, administered as part of the Minnesota Multiphasic Personality Inventory

(MMPI). This scale, called the HO scale or the Cooke-Medley Hostility Scale,[19] has been most used to study the health effects of hostility. Other shorter scales also correlate with heart disease.[20] University of Utah researcher Dr. Timothy Smith administered a wide array of tests to a large group; he then studied how the other tests related to the scores on the MMPI hostility test. Based on his results, he concluded that the traits most related to hostility were suspiciousness, resentment, frequent anger, and a cynical mistrust of other people.[21]

Cynicism refers to the generally negative view that hostile people have toward humankind; they tend to depict others as selfish, deceptive, and unworthy. They tend to have the same kind of attitude toward the world in general, even when their sense of mistrust is not directed at anyone specifically. Redford Williams claims that those with cynical hostility and cynical mistrust are at the greatest health risk of all.[22]

Hostile people tend to have an attitude of paranoia, attributing hostility to others. They often believe that other people are intentionally out to get them, purposely trying to hurt them. If you wonder if you have too much hostility, examine how you tend to project such attributes onto others.

Timothy Smith also noted that people who tested most hostile were less hardy or resilient, experienced more frequent and severe hassles every day, and derived little satisfaction from their daily social contacts.[23] This inability to thoroughly enjoy life sounds very much like depression, and, in fact, clinical depression often takes the form of cynical hostility, particularly in men. Similar to anxious depressive disorders, hostile people often have a nervous system constantly on guard for impending danger. And the health effects, particularly cardiovascular effects, are very similar between cynical hostility and depression.[24]

It's also possible, says Williams, to get a good mental picture of hostility by looking at its opposite, the trusting heart. According to Williams,

> [The] trusting heart believes in the basic goodness of humankind, that most people will be fair and kind in relationships with others. Having such beliefs, the trusting heart is slow to anger. Not seeking out evil in others, not expecting the worst of them, the trusting heart expects mainly good from others and, more often then not, finds it. As a result, the trusting heart spends little time feeling resentful, irritable, and angry. From this it follows that the trusting heart treats others well, with consideration and kindness; the trusting heart almost never wishes or visits harm upon others.[25]

It's like the Law of the Boomerang (also referred to as "karma"): what you throw out is what you get back, and you see what you are looking for and expect. The process becomes a self-fulfilling prophecy—if you expect others to be hostile, your automatic behavior prompts their hostility. On the other hand, if you expect them to be kind, your demeanor toward them is more likely to trigger their kindness. This principle is also sometimes called the Law of Expectations.

Recognizing one's own hostility is sometimes difficult. It is valuable in this discussion to come to know your learned and habitual attitudes by simply asking yourself how you view most people in the world around you: with cynicism or with trust? Is the world to you more hostile or more kind? Do you need to be constantly on guard, or do you feel basically safe?

The Significance of Anger and Hostility

Back when people needed the fight-or-flight response to defend themselves against aggressors, they needed anger. It was important to survival. That surge of energy helped early people defend themselves. Anger enabled them to fight with vigor and great strength.

Our culture evolved much more rapidly than our bodies. We are now a society and a civilization that is expected to deal calmly and rationally with each other. We don't need to fight saber-toothed tigers; our battles are waged in boardrooms and bedrooms. We no longer need the fight-or-flight response as much, but our bodies still respond that way. We call it stress. We seldom need the physical energy of anger, either, but we still get angry. Instead of being a benefit, most regard it as a liability.

In rare cases, anger may play a valuable role in self-defense or in the physical defense of a loved one. Any other time, an angry assault is considered today a violation of both legal and moral ethics; and, while the victim may suffer physical harm, the aggressor almost always gets in trouble.[26]

Research suggests that anger rarely exists in isolation. When researchers at the University of Tennessee studied 87 middle-aged women to determine their anger levels, they found that the women who were angry also tended to be pessimistic, lack social support, be overweight, sleep poorly, and lead sedentary lives. The angriest women were also more likely to have existing health problems and to feel they could do nothing to control their problems.[27] Many of these associated features can be driven by the same neurochemical abnormalities characteristic of clinical depression. The same or similar abnormal neurochemistry is also true of "rage attacks." Such rage can also be part of bipolar ("manic-depressive") disorders.

If what current research indicates is true, hostility may have a powerful (usually detrimental) influence over not only the nervous system, but the body's arsenal of hormones as well. As such, it may play a significant role in premature death, as well as in health and illness. Hostility has such an impact on health, in fact, that the University of Maryland's Theodore M. Dembroski claims it's easy to spot an intensive-care patient in the making: "He's the fellow who mutters and curses to himself if the line at the video store is too long; the one who leans on his horn if you hesitate even a millisecond when the light turns green. He's the hostile man, the one who gets angry over everyday frustrations and expresses those feelings in rude, antagonistic ways."[28]

Causes of Hostility

Where does hostility come from? How do children become hostile? What in our makeup may predispose us toward a hostile attitude? Researchers aren't sure, but they're beginning to find clues by studying the lives and backgrounds of people who are hostile. Genetics plays a predisposing role, but learning, particularly early in life, may be even more important and in fact may activate the genetic vulnerability. Some of this genetic vulnerability to hostility is similar to the same genes and neurochemical mechanisms that predispose individuals to depression[29], and young people with a family history of depression, hostility, or controlling behaviors should aggressively work toward prevention by using some of the anger transformation techniques described below.

In one study conducted by University of Kansas researchers Christine Vavak and Kent Houston, 134 college students were given the Cook-Medley Hostility Scale.[30] They were then asked to complete detailed questionnaires about their self-esteem, their health behaviors, their parents' child-rearing practices, and other background factors.

The students who were most hostile seemed to have had an "oppositional orientation" toward people that was developed during childhood. They came from homes where both parents were strict and coercive, used frequent physical punishment or hostile control, and frequently communicated dissatisfaction with the child. Those who scored high on the hostility scale described parents who were less warm and accepting, who interfered more in the person's desires as a child, were more punishing and less likely to have encouraged independent thinking.[31] Those who were the most hostile (as determined by test scores) were also those who had the lowest self-esteem and those who felt the least degree of acceptance from others. Similarly, another study of the development of hostility in people with coronary disease found it to be related to learned beliefs and attitudes about one's self and others. People who didn't learn self-esteem growing up had a subsequent buildup of negative psychosocial interactions and had poor self-concepts. This poor self-concept was described as hostile in nature and reflects a mistrust of others and a deep sense of isolation.[32]

Finally, the results of at least one sophisticated study indicate that hostility may be more learned than inherited. Researchers came to that conclusion by studying identical twins who had been separated at birth and raised in different families.[33] Researchers learned that hostility often arises from a worldview of a victim, not uncommonly from having experienced the world as a hostile, unaccepting place as a child.

Psychologist Michael J. Strube has seen a pattern of hostility in children as young as age three. One of the main culprits, he says, is "parents urging them to excel, while presenting them with ill-defined goals and little, or ambiguous, feedback."[34]

The Need to Express Anger

Research has shown that, to be healthy, people need to express or transform anger in a managed, wise way. It is a mandate to confront the things that are making us angry and to work through the anger. According to University of Arizona psychologist Roger J. Daldrup, there are two classic ways of expressing anger in an unhealthy way: misdirecting it or suppressing it completely.[35]

Unhealthy Expression of Anger

Misdirected anger, Daldrup says,[36] "is the classic kicking the cat because you're angry at your spouse maneuver. Though people who misdirect their anger seem to be expressing it, they are just burying the real problem and creating more problems along the way."

Originally, many counselors recommended that the healthiest response was to give people the opportunity to act out their aggression, with the philosophy that the ensuing "cathartic" effect would ease the emotions and result in dissipated anger and aggression.[37] In one study, people were given unusually harsh (though bogus) feedback about an essay they had written in an attempt to anger them. These angry people were then given the chance to slam a punching bag for two minutes. The theory of researchers was simple: letting the angry people punch it out for two minutes would reduce their anger and make them less likely to be aggressive later. In fact, the opposite proved true: in a simple contest afterward, those who had punched the punching bag were far more aggressive toward their opponents than angered people who did not pound on a punching bag. The results of the study showed that acting on anger leads to even greater aggression.[38]

At the same time, however, research done by Redford Williams showed that men who openly expressed their anger at the age of twenty-five were more likely to be dead by age fifty than those who did not "get it out" when angry.[39] According to Williams,

> People who "express" their anger are more, rather than less, likely to be more aggressive later and be more, rather than less, likely to have a higher death rate when followed up 25 years later. The simplistic advice, "when angry, let it out," is unlikely, therefore, to be of much help. Far more important is to learn how to evaluate your anger and then to manage it.[40]

The other classic response, complete suppression of anger, doesn't work either because, says Daldrup, it creates what he calls "the keyboard effect." Once a person starts repressing one emotion, he begins repressing them all, something he likens to pressing down the soft pedal on the piano: "That pedal will soften all the notes on a piano, just as dulling one emotion will dull them all. Sadly, people become used to that feeling of dullness, but the anger is still there, destroying your relationships, sabotaging creativity, or interfering with your sex life."[41] Using denial and repression of emotions as a coping strategy, in the long run, has adverse health effects. So is it best to vigorously express anger or to suppress it? As we will see later, there may be another alternative. This was shown, for example, in a classic 40-year study by George Valliant and colleagues at Harvard, where, compared to more adaptive, mature coping styles, chronically using repression and denial to cope were associated with ten times more chronic illness in middle age.[42]

There are many other unhealthy ways of expressing anger, according to Tavris. Some of the most common ones are miscommunicating, emotional distancing, escalating of the conflict, endlessly rehearsing grievances, assuming a hostile disposition, acquiring angry habits, making a bad situation worse, losing self-esteem, and losing the respect of others.[43]

So if both vigorous expression and suppression of anger are harmful to health, what is one to do? What is needed, researchers agree, is the ability to confront the source of anger and express feelings without getting overwhelmed by the anger. As Carol Tavris put it, "The purpose of anger is to make a grievance known, and if the grievance is not confronted, it will not matter whether the anger is kept in, let out, or wrapped in red ribbons and dropped in the Erie Canal."[44]

According to Daldrup, anger becomes frightening (to you and to others) only when it is repressed for a long time and is then expressed with the "force to turn silverware into metal filings."[45] "If you were discharging anger as it came up for you," he says, "there wouldn't be any extra energy attached to it. You'd be able to say 'I disagree with you' or 'I don't like what you are saying' in a straightforward manner without any extra energy attached to it." Instead of doing that, says Daldrup, most people store up—or "stuff"—their anger. "Stuffing is the only way you'll have enough energy for an explosion."[46] So one needs to be honest in communicating their perspective and desires, but not necessarily in a hostile way.

Preliminary research has shown that bottling up anger can lead to many health consequences, among them heart disease, cancer, rheumatoid arthritis, hives, acne, psoriasis, peptic ulcer, epilepsy, migraine, Raynaud's disease, and high blood pressure.[47] Several researchers agree that expressing anger benefits health as long as the expression itself is healthy. The classic idea about expressing anger in screaming and pounding hysteria doesn't stand up under experimental scrutiny, says Tavris. Instead of helping, this kind of reaction "makes you angrier, solidifies an angry attitude, and establishes a hostile habit. If you keep quiet about momentary irritations and distract yourself with pleasant activity until your fury simmers down, chances are that you will feel better, and feel better faster, than if you let yourself go in a shouting match."[48] In her book *Anger: The Misunderstood Emotion*, Tavris adds, "Ventilating is cathartic only when it restores our sense of control, reducing both the rush of adrenaline that accompanies an unfamiliar and threatening situation and the belief that you are helpless and powerless."[49]

The way you deal with anger will have considerable impact on your health, say the researchers. If you get momentarily irritated at something, one approach might be to distract yourself—to concentrate on more pleasant thoughts. However, if you start feeling chronic or continual anger at someone or something, more aggressive action is needed to confront your feelings and work through the anger. "If you're angry at something that is trivial but still infuriating, you can choose to distract yourself," says Tavris, "but if you're continuously angry at someone, you have a problem. You need to look at that problem and work on solving it."[50]

Healthy Expression of Anger

One of the keys to the healthy expression of anger is to face the situation early, before it has a chance to accumulate and fester. Dr. Lenore Walker, one of the nation's top experts on domestic violence, points out that "you can either talk yourself into getting angrier, or you can talk yourself out of it. You have a choice. When you learn to recognize anger and work through it early on, it tends to go instead of grow."[51]

Remember that anger is usually not a primary emotion but more commonly is a chosen way of expressing blame for other feelings, such as frustration. We often think the only alternatives when angry are to either vent it with rage or stuff it. But there is another important alternative. The truth is, anger is not really caused by outside provocation. Instead, the cause of anger is rooted in the way we choose to think about the provocation and thus respond to it. Changing the way one thinks about the provocation can completely dissipate the anger, resulting in no need to either express or stuff it. The anger simply dissipates.

For example, a man who had a heart attack was asked by his physician about the circumstances preceding his chest pain.[52] "It's my boss," he replied. "Every time he comes in the office, he chews us out and puts us down. Everyone hates the guy, and every time he came around, I got chest pain, until finally I had my heart attack. We couldn't say anything to him, because the last guy who got angry with him lost his job!" However, on quiet reflection as to why his boss used such tactics, the employee said, "It's because he is so insecure. He has to put everybody down to make himself look more important and correct."

"I wonder if maybe he's hurting inside," replied his physician, "and just doesn't yet know a better way to get real sense of worth. That must be a painful way to live."

After long discussion, the heart attack patient softened and said, "Maybe you're right. Maybe the guy acts like a turkey because he just doesn't know a better way to deal with his own problems."

"What do you think would happen if, instead of feeding his insecurity with your own anger and subtle putdowns, you chose instead to help heal the insecurity that drives his dumb behavior?" his physician asked.

"I don't think I could do that. I really hate this guy," was the patient's response. Eventually, however, he agreed to try and feel his boss' insecure discomfort for just a few hours and attempt to ease that underlying cause instead of just condemning the behavior that came from it. Before long, this enterprise turned into a day, then a week. Coming back, he said, "This is amazing to me. My anger is just gone. It's hard for me to believe, but I actually feel sorry for him, even a little compassion. Recognizing his insecurity has been very helpful. I've been trying to find some things about him that make him feel valued. That was hard to do at first, but it's easier now. And for what it's worth, he's not putting me down as much any more. And I don't really feel tense around him any more, even when he pulls his old tricks."

This employee had discovered a great secret about dealing with anger:

1. The boss was not the real cause of his anger; instead, his own rigidly judgmental thinking about the boss caused his anger.

2. Coming (with some difficulty) to think differently about his boss, in more understanding ways, dissipated the anger.

3. The key principles here are those of self-assertion: Speak the truth in kindness. That is, be honest about your own point of view, but do it in a way that honors and lifts the other person rather than putting him or her down, either overtly or within yourself. Such helpful expression of anger becomes liberating and empowering for both you and the others involved. The goal of expressing anger in healthy ways, then, is to face it directly, wisely transform it with understanding, and thus get rid of it.

How the Body Reacts: The Health Effects of Anger and Hostility

Anger, whether expressed or repressed, has physical effects very similar to those of chronic stress. According to Carnegie-Mellon historian Peter Stearns, author of *Anger: The Struggle for Emotional Control in America's History*, chronic anger "is an insidious thing, because we aren't even aware that we are repressing. We think we are free to express anger, but we're not as free as we might believe."[53] The results of repressed, chronic, or prolonged anger can be devastating. Such chronic anger usually involves either inherent hostility or the unwillingness to let go of the misery of blaming what someone has done to hurt us. The most recent research shows that the effects of anger are diverse and widespread. Among all personality styles evaluated in a long-term French study, hostility is the most predictive of early mortality (and not just from getting killed by the people who are being provoked).[54]

To understand the broad consequences of anger, consider the wide range of physiological reactions that go with it—effects that have been studied over a long period of time. More than a century ago, psychologist G. Stanley Hall wanted to get a clear picture of how people feel when they are angry, so he gave several thousand people questionnaires that helped examine their responses to anger. The responses were remarkably similar among the 2,184 people who completed the questionnaires. Anger, they said, produced "cardiac sensations, headaches, nosebleed, mottling of the face, dizziness, tears, snarls, or a complete inability to vocalize." Those reactions are probably due in part to the immediate physical changes that accompany anger, much like those described for stress or the classic fight-or-flight response. The heart and respiration speeds up, blood pressure rises, the digestive process slows down, and the muscles tense up, all in readiness for action.

Even the skin is affected by anger. Psychologist Ted Grossbart points out that one of the two most "common human agonies that provide the underlying fuel for skin diseases" is anger.[55] In his research, Grossbart has traced a number of disfiguring skin disorders and rashes—among them acne, eczema, hives, warts, and genital herpes—to anger. When patients are helped to work out their anger, Grossbart says, the skin disorders improve dramatically.

Anger also apparently predisposes its victims to the common cold. Some of the most comprehensive research connecting the two has been conducted at Cornell Medical School and at the Great Lakes Naval Medical Research Unit. Researchers exposed a group of men of similar medical status to the cold virus. Only the ones who were depressed, angry, and frustrated got sick; the rest stayed healthy. Even more important, say the researchers who conducted the studies, was the powerful effect of simply recalling episodes of anger. While simply talking about anger, the researchers say, the patients were more likely to develop nasal congestion, mucoid discharge, and even asthma attacks.[56]

The effect of anger on susceptibility to colds may be because of its effect on immunity, particularly on S-IgA, the antibody in the saliva that helps to protect against the common cold. In one study, volunteers watched videos and looked at pictures designed to make them angry. Researchers found that the anger resulted in a significant reduction in S-IgA for as long as five hours after the emotion of anger was experienced—therefore reducing the volunteers' ability to resist the common cold virus.[57]

Anger has been shown to be a major cause of migraine headaches. In detailed research, a large percentage of migraine sufferers have been those who are unable to express anger verbally. Mismanaged anger, anger that is either suppressed or misdirected, has also been shown to be a major factor in bulimia and anorexia.[58]

Whether expressed or unexpressed, anger has powerfully adverse effects on the heart. Lynda H. Powell, psychologist at Rush-Presbyterian-St. Luke's Medical Center in Chicago, found that women who survived one heart attack but who kept a lid on their anger and had a pattern of reacting slowly to outside events were the ones most likely to suffer fatal heart problems. In commenting on the study, University of California psychologist Margaret A. Chesney said that it challenges traditional thinking: For men, expressing anger and hostility can lead to heart problems. Apparently, the opposite can be true for women: repressing anger and hostility leads to heart disease.[59]

Hostility highly correlates with worsening medical symptoms. A Danish random sample of 3,426 men and 3,699 women (aged forty or fifty years) showed that high symptom load was predicted by cynical hostility as measured by the eight-item Cynical Distrust Scale.[60] Those high in hostility had over twice as many distressing physical symptoms as individuals with lower hostility levels.

Changes in hostility over one's life also play a role in other risk factors for health outcomes. Hostility tends to peak in late adolescence and reach a nadir in middle age, then tends to stabilize into old age.[61] However, a long-term study following the course of hostility from college to middle age showed that those whose hostility increases over those years had double the risk of obesity, inadequate social support, and depression (all health risk factors), as well as reduced life achievements.[62] The same study showed that higher hostility in the late teen years predicted unhealthy behaviors and worse health appraisals thirty years later. This suggests the need for those more angry and hostile in early life to actively pursue strategies to change those patterns. This can be done using some of the suggestions at the end of this chapter and Chapter 22.

Many of the physical problems related to hostility arise because hostility does two things to the body:[63]

1. Hostility causes the constant, unending release of stress hormones, especially norepinephrine, which, when continuous, cause significant pathological changes in a variety of ways.

2. Hostility weakens the parasympathetic branch of the nervous system, which normally functions to calm the body down after an emergency.

To understand why hostility is so harmful to health, it's important to understand what happens in both these scenarios.

Hostility, Hormones, and Neurotransmitters

In essence, chronic hostility causes two kinds of chronic stress reactions: (1) the fight-or-flight response (the body prepares to confront or flee from an enemy), and (2) vigilant observation (the body stays constantly "on guard" in case it should be threatened). Hostility causes both reactions simultaneously—a "double whammy" for the body to deal with continuously.

While stress or a perceived danger may cause these body reactions occasionally or short-term, hostility is a constant, chronic condition. A hostile person goes throughout the entire day in this condition. (Many hostile people don't even get relief at night while sleeping; researchers have shown that stress hormones are secreted throughout the night and eliminated in the urine around the clock.)

To begin with, hostility causes the body to release corticotropin-releasing hormone (CRH), which mobilizes the whole sequence of stress hormones. This hormone instructs the pituitary gland and the adrenal glands to secrete stress hormones like cortisol and catecholamines (including norepinephrine). The result is a classic stress response: blood pressure increases, the heart beats harder and faster, insulin resistance occurs, blood sugars increase from the release of liver starch (glycogen) stores, cholesterol rises, and clotting increases. As you might imagine, all of these are significant coronary risk factors, particularly if operating chronically.

Those reactions are actually helpful when you need to respond to short, acute stress, and they normally shut off after the stressor is gone. However, hostility is chronic and doesn't shut off very reliably. There also is a sudden, possibly lethal reaction connected with hostility as well: The constant on-off of stress hormones that accompanies hostility can trigger both heart rhythm abnormalities (and cardiac arrest) and coronary artery spasm, resulting in a heart attack.[64] This spasm, and the increased clotting, are due not only to hormones like norepinephrine, but also to the effects of hostility and its associated depression of neurotransmitters such as serotonin.

In the central nervous system, increased levels of serotonin relieve stress and calm anger, and decreased levels of serotonin are apparent when control is lost. Genetic deficiency in brain serotonin function also can set a person up to be more depressed or hostile.[65] Serotonin is stored in platelets, the little blood entities that initiate clotting. When brain serotonin falls (as with chronic anger or feeling out of control), a tissue receptor (serotonin type 2) becomes more sensitive; the result is more clotting[66] and blood vessel spasm and ultimately more heart attacks and strokes. A heart attack is caused by the occurrence of three things: artery narrowing (plaque), artery spasm, and then a clot to finish off the occlusion. As you can see, all three are rapidly accelerated with hostility or chronic depression.

Let's take a look at the effects of hostility on some principal stress hormones that can have definite hazardous effects, mostly on the circulatory system.

Epinephrine and Norepinephrine (Catecholamines)   Epinephrine, sometimes called adrenaline, constricts the blood vessels, especially the minute ones in the extremities. At the same time, it causes the heart to work harder and stimulates the heart muscle. As a result, the heart pumps rapidly in high-pressure spurts, driving blood pressure dangerously high.

Sometimes called noradrenaline, norepinephrine also causes the blood vessels to constrict; it is generally released when blood pressure is too low. In addition, persistently high norepinephrine disturbs the platelets and the red blood cells, and it damages the endothelium (the lining of the heart and blood vessels), leading to the influx of lipids into the endothelial wall and creating a place for platelets to adhere—and thereby causing clotting to occur. In carotid artery ultrasound studies, hostile people get more rapid plaque formation and thus more artery narrowing.[67] This is particularly true in individuals with hypertension.[68] Interestingly, meditative stress reduction that lowers these catecholamines reverses the arterial thickening.[69]

Studies have shown that people who are hostile (people traditionally labeled as having Type A personalities) release much more epinephrine and norepinephrine into their systems, and they release much more norepinephrine if confronted with a challenge. In an early study by Friedman and Rosenman (the researchers who pioneered the Type A theory[70]), a group of men were seated at a table. In the middle was an expensive bottle of French wine. Each man was given a pile of puzzle pieces and told that whoever solved the puzzle first would win the bottle of wine.

The men eagerly began trying to put together the puzzle. Soon, loud rock music began to blare out of concealed speakers in the room. The men worked for several minutes, the music blasting, until researchers told them to stop. (No one completed his puzzle because some of the pieces had not been provided.)

Researchers had drawn blood samples from the men at the beginning of the experiment, and they drew samples again after they told the men to stop working on the puzzle. All the men in the study had similar levels of epinephrine and norepinephrine before they started competing for the bottle of wine, but the Type A men—the hostile ones—had much higher levels of norepinephrine after trying to win the contest.[71] Similar effects are seen in runners "who have to win." The extreme competitiveness counters the benefits of the exercise, compared to those who exercise for the fun and value of it.

In a similar experiment, New York City researcher David Glass asked firemen and policemen to volunteer for a study in which they played Pong, a computer game. Each man had the same opponent: a man who was introduced as a fireman or policeman but who was in reality a colleague of Dr. Glass and an expert Pong player. The expert won every game. But it didn't stop there: as he played, he disparaged the opponents—for their lack of skill and their clumsiness—and even impugned their manhood. As in the first experiment, blood samples were taken before the game began and again after it was finished. The Type A men who were most hostile had significantly higher levels of epinephrine in their blood than did the calmer, more easygoing men.[72]

Cortisol   A corticosteroid, cortisol is a potent hormone released by the body in an effort to defend itself. Cortisol inhibits the breakdown of epinephrine and norepinephrine, in essence making it very difficult for the body to calm down after a perceived emergency or threat. To make matters worse, it increases the body's responsiveness to epinephrine and norepinephrine, rendering those hormones more potent. Cortisol also releases chemicals that further damage the endothelium. Finally, in addition to damaging the vessels, cortisol causes an increase in the level of fats, insulin, and sugar in the blood, all known contributors to heart disease. Both cortisol and catecholamines cause insulin resistance, leading to a state called the metabolic syndrome that puts people at high cardiovascular risk. With insulin resistance, the insulin level rises to compensate, and high insulin can also raise both cholesterol and blood pressure.

Prolactin   Prolactin has three effects on the cardiovascular system: (1) it releases calcium into the bloodstream; (2) it makes the blood vessels more vulnerable to the effects of epinephrine and norepinephrine; and (3) it has some role in regulating blood pressure. Prolactin rises in response to a fall in the central neurotransmitter dopamine, which often runs low in depressed, cynical people. The lack of dopamine is one reason why such people have difficulty experiencing joy.

In addition to the specific effects of each individual stress hormone released in response to hostility, the hormones together have synergistic effects:

1. The combined hormones further increase the risk of acute cardiac events.[73]

2. The fluctuation of the hormones released during hostility can trigger spasms of the coronary arteries, resulting in a heart attack.

3. The group of hostility hormones (especially epinephrine, norepinephrine, and cortisol) contribute to premature development of arteriosclerosis.

4. The combination of hormones secreted during hostility interferes with the body's natural messengers that reduce blood pressure. Under normal conditions, tiny regulators (called baroreceptors) in the walls of the blood vessels send messages to the brain to restore blood pressure to normal. Stress and hostility hormones inactivate these baroreceptors, leaving them unable to signal a reduction in blood pressure. As a result, blood pressure stays elevated and can be driven even higher by epinephrine; in addition, the heart rate is less variable (a significant predictor of cardiac events).[74]

5. The stress hormones compromise the immune system, making the individual less resistant to disease. According to researchers at the University of Texas Cancer Center, norepinephrine and other stress hormones block the ability of macrophages (scavenger cells that provide resistance against disease) to kill tumor cells. At the same time, hostility (and depression) is related to increased immune markers of excessive inflammation.[75] This can contribute to excess pain, cardiovascular disease, and more rapid aging.

6. Hormones released in response to hostility interfere with the body's DNA repair system. As a result, the body loses its first line of defense against a number of diseases, including cancer.

All of this combines to end up in the well-demonstrated adverse effects of hostility on health outcomes of many types.[76]

Anger: The Cancer Connection

Studies on the effects of stress on cancer vary between different kinds of cancer. Some conducted as early as the 1950s show a link between anger and some cancers. Most often implicated is chronic anger with an inability to appropriately express that anger. Researchers who were interested in exploring the link between anger and cancer studied the life patterns of approximately 400 cancer patients during the 1950s. There was a common thread among them: Many seemed unable to express anger or hostility in defense of themselves. The same patients were able to get angry in the defense of others, or even in the defense of a cause, but not in defense of themselves. A more recent Michigan study that prospectively followed nearly 700 people for 17 years found a similar pattern: suppressed persistent anger was associated with not only more cancer deaths but also mortality from all causes.[77]

Other studies of cancer patients, especially women with breast cancer, indicate that the style of expressing anger (or the inability to express it at all) seems to have considerable impact on the development and spread of cancer.[78] In one study, researchers interviewed a group of women with breast disease; some had benign breast disease, and others were later diagnosed with breast cancer. Before the diagnoses were made, interviewers made notes on the anger style of each woman. The women who were later diagnosed as having breast cancer had an entirely different anger style than those who had benign breast disease. The cancer victims were much more likely to suppress their anger and then finally explode with anger when they could no longer hold it in. Many didn't express anger at all, and those who did express anger let it go all at once. It is important to know that prospective studies of this kind (first measuring anger, then following over time for the development of subsequent effects) are far more reliable than retrospective studies (looking back with recall) making such comparisons.

So even though women with breast tumors experience more anger than healthy controls, there was a big difference in the way the women expressed their anger. Women in normal health tended to get angry and then forget about it. They were able to confront the situation that made them angry, work quickly through their angry feelings, and move on without anger. The women who had benign breast disease tended to become angry and stay angry. Interestingly, the women with malignant tumors got angry, but either they didn't express it or they apologized for it, even when they were in the right.

A number of other studies have linked suppression of anger with cancer. In Lydia Temoshok's study of malignant melanoma patients[79], those who suppressed anger had fewer lymphocytes at their tumor sites. When Temoshok and her colleagues taught some of the patients different ways to express their anger, tumor growth in those patients stopped. However, results on changing the course of cancer by psychological interventions have not been consistent.[80]

The ability to express anger may even affect survival rates among cancer patients. In one prospective study, researchers found that patients who were able to express negative emotions—anger, hostility, guilt, depression, and aggression—survived longer than the patients who said they had fewer negative emotions.[81]

An Angry/Hostile Heart, an Ill Heart

As you might suspect from the mechanisms above, perhaps one of the most devastating effects of anger is on the heart and the circulatory system. Among all emotional factors, hostility (and its associated depression) is an important determinant of cardiovascular disease.[82] According to research data published in the *New England Journal of Medicine*, mismanaged anger is perhaps the principal factor in predicting cardiovascular disease.[83] According to Redford and Virginia Williams, not all the aspects of a type A personality are harmful to the heart, but one of the aspects that is definitely a risk is anger, particularly if coupled with cynicism and aggression.[84] There is still some controversy over the notion of type A personality as it relates to heart disease risk. It's not the "busy-ness" of type A that is toxic to the cardiovascular system, but rather the toxic factor is the cynical hostility that is often associated with this driven lifestyle. The most toxic mix is hostility, anger, cynicism, antagonism, and mistrust.[85] Heart-harming hostility is characterized by anger-proneness, resentment, suspicion, and the tendency to view photographs of strangers as unfriendly or dangerous.[86] It is also hallmarked by explosive and vigorous vocal mannerisms, competitiveness, impatience, and irritability.

As an example of his concept, Williams points out the person who is stuck in a long line of traffic when he needs to get to an appointment on time. "Anyone will be stressed if he really has to keep an appointment," Dr. Williams explains. The person who is at risk, though,

> . . . may not even have a real deadline or an important appointment to keep, and still becomes angry and hostile in a short period of time. And he'll immediately think that the whole thing is someone's fault—that the police are incompetent because they aren't

directing traffic properly, for instance. He'll get annoyed at the motorists in the other lane, because he thinks they're staring at him. His breathing will become deeper and faster. He may start honking the horn. The anger and resentment just keep building up. He may even try to drive up on the shoulder to get around the other cars.[87]

It's that kind of person, Williams says, who is at risk of a heart attack or other major illness.

The emotion of anger itself can have a direct effect on angina (chest pain) and heart attack. In fact, a study released by the American Heart Association says that people who can't keep their tempers under control and who tend to explode in anger during arguments double their risk of heart attack, especially during the two hours following an episode of intense anger.[88] That risk jumps to triple the risk of heart attack among those who have lower educational levels.[89] The study, led by Dr. Murray Mittleman of Harvard University Medical School, involved more than 1,500 men and women. Research published in the May 2000 edition of *Circulation* found that, compared to individuals with normal anger levels, people who are highly prone to anger are nearly three times more likely to have a heart attack, and even those who have moderate anger have a significant risk of illness and death from coronary heart disease.[90]

In one study, University of Michigan research scientist Mara Julius studied 696 married and single adults for 12 years. As one part of her study, she gave every subject a questionnaire to determine whether he or she was angry and, if so, how the anger was expressed. Of the questionnaire respondents, the ones with the highest blood pressure were those who suppressed anger, expressed anger but then felt guilty, or never protested an unjustified attack. Even more fascinating was Julius's findings on death from high blood pressure: A person with high blood pressure who suppresses anger is five times more likely to die than is a high blood pressure victim without suppressed anger.[91] However, persistent blood pressure effects of anger seem highly dependent on whether the person continues to ruminate on the perceived offense.[92] The article describing this observation is subtitled, "At Least Don't Ruminate on It!" This is important overall advice about anger. Refuse to hang on to it, and it will be far less likely to hang on to you.

Suppressed anger may be a particularly lethal factor. Heart disease rates are significantly higher among both men and women who are unable to express their anger appropriately. One study, which followed 2,500 men for a period of nine years, found that men who suppress their anger are 75 percent more likely to develop heart disease than men who let their anger out or who talk about their anger.

Hostility has a more potent adverse cardiovascular effect than anger alone and is a leading factor in heart disease risk. Researchers studied more than 400 patients at Duke Medical Center to determine coronary artery health and personality traits. More than 80 percent of the men who were classified as both Type A and high in hostility had seriously diseased coronary arteries; only half of the other men did. For women, the risk was even more significant: 50 percent of the hostile Type A women had seriously diseased arteries, while only 12 percent of the others did.[93] Recall that a hostile person who already has coronary disease is much more likely to soon die from it than is a nonhostile person.[94]

Other tests demonstrated that anger causes abnormalities in the wall of the heart similar to those that accompany intense exercise and more intense than those caused by a mental challenge, such as arithmetic.[95] In one study, heart disease patients who merely recalled an event that made them angry experienced a decrease in the amount of blood pumped out by the left ventricle.[96] Research shows that patients with this kind of compromise, compared to those without it, are almost three times more likely to suffer a cardiac event.[97]

Hostility also impacts other coronary risk factors. Williams showed that hostile teenagers are as likely as adults to have high cholesterol. "People with high hostility at nineteen tend to have high cholesterol levels at forty," Williams said in summing up the study, which was presented to the American Heart Association.[98] For the study, Williams and his colleague, Dr. Ilene C. Siegler, studied 830 subjects who took personality tests at the University of North Carolina. They then studied the men and women 20 years later. Those who scored high on a hostility scale while in college tended, 20 years later, to have high levels of total cholesterol in their blood but low levels of HDL (high-density lipoprotein) cholesterol (the beneficial kind).

In addition, high blood homocysteine, which is highly correlated to heart attack risk, is also significantly elevated in hostile people. Elevated homocysteine is also toxic to the nervous system,[99] predicts both brain vascular disease[100] and increased dementia[101] compared to those with normal homocysteine levels. Interestingly, in a Greek study, there was somewhat of a linear relationship between the degree of hostility and the blood level of homocysteine. Specifically, each 10-unit increase in the hostility scale was associated with a rise in homocysteine levels.[102]

A very high predictor of cardiovascular events is the metabolic syndrome, characterized by insulin resistance that then contributes to weight gain, high lipids, and elevated blood pressure. The stress hormones cortisol and catecholamines cause insulin resistance. The development of the metabolic syndrome is much higher in cynically hostile people, and this seems to be an important mediator of the cardiac disease seen in hostility.[103]

Several large-scale and long-term studies have linked hostility to coronary artery disease. In one, again spearheaded by Williams and his colleagues, more than 2,280 Duke University Medical Center patients were studied for signs of Type A behavior and for the trait of hostility. The patients had been referred to the medical center for coronary angiography, a diagnostic procedure for determining the extent of coronary artery obstruction. Researchers found that they could predict which patients would be found to have coronary artery disease by pinpointing which ones were hostile and that hostility served better than overall Type A behavior as a predictor.[104]

In a similar study at Duke University, Williams selected 400 patients admitted to the medical center for coronary arteriography (a study to determine blockage of coronary arteries).[105] Cardiologists let Williams test patients before their arteriogram; each patient was interviewed and given the MMPI. Based on interviews and psychological test scores, Williams determined which of the patients were hostile; then, cardiologists performed the arteriograms.

Williams was fascinated by his findings. In previous studies, Type A personality had always been a predictor of heart disease. It still was, but Williams found that hostility was an even more accurate and powerful predictor. In his study, 70 percent of the patients who were hostile had at least one major blockage of a coronary artery (as compared to

48 percent who were not hostile). Type A people were 1.3 times more likely to have a blockage than were non–Type A individuals, but hostile people were 1.5 times more likely to have blockages than the nonhostile people were.[106] Overall, hostility seemed to be the most influential factor. According to Williams, "Not only did people with higher [hostility] counts have more severe arteriosclerosis, but the [hostility] scores were also associated with arteriosclerosis even more strongly than were Type A scores."[107]

What, then, are the long-term outcomes of hostility? Several prospective studies are convincing. More than 3,000 healthy men between ages of 45 and 55 years were studied for more than eight years in the San Francisco area; all the men were free of apparent coronary artery disease when the study began, and researchers watched them carefully over the years for signs of disease. When the study began, researchers taped interviews with each man and used the interviews to rate each person's potential for hostility. The hostile patients developed heart disease at a much higher rate than those who did not show signs of hostility. Furthermore, the men who reported getting quite angry at least once a week and expressing it outwardly were much more likely to develop heart disease than the hostile men who did not feel anger as often.[108]

In still another study of more than 1,800 factory workers in Illinois, study subjects were carefully followed for more than 20 years. Researchers found that the factory workers who were high in hostility had 1.5 times more heart disease than those who weren't and that hostility was significantly associated with death from all causes over the 20 year period.[109] Interestingly, there was also an increased rate of cancer among the men with high hostility scores.[110] In a smaller but still convincing study, more than 255 young physicians were tested for personality traits and then followed for 25 years. The death rate from heart disease and from all causes in general was six times greater for the physicians who measured high in hostility.[111]

And the problems occur at younger ages. Several follow-up studies involving middle-aged men who had taken the MMPI 25 years earlier showed that the effect of hostility on both coronary disease and mortality was much stronger among younger men than among the middle-aged ones. For younger hostile men, the risk of disease was four to six times greater; for hostile middle-aged men, the risk dropped to 1.5 times. As a result, researchers now theorize that early hostility may most accurately predict premature health problems. As Williams pointed out, "Once middle age is reached, the surviving men with hostility traits may represent a group of biologically hardy survivors."[112] Perhaps a more useful explanation is that people can learn to be less hostile with passing years, which has now proven to reduce the health risk previously present.[113] Even elderly people can learn to reduce hostility, with significant improvement in their health outcomes. In a study at the Ochsner Heart and Vascular Institute in New Orleans, elderly persons with hostility symptoms had greater weight, four times higher anxiety and depression scores ($p < 0.0001$); two times higher scores for multiple, unexplained medical symptoms ($p < 0.0001$); and 17 percent lower scores for quality of life ($p < 0.001$) compared with elderly persons without hostility symptoms. (Note: p values of less than 0.05 are scientifically convincing as being statistically significant. A p value of 0.0001 is very highly statistically significant.) Importantly, in these elderly patients, marked reduction in hostility and improvements in other risk factors occurred following interventions to reduce the hostility and stress reactions.[114] In people who have had heart attacks, both young and old, such interventions can also significantly reduce second attacks and coronary mortality (sometimes by more than 50 percent, which is even more than some medication interventions).[115] Such interventions will be discussed in Chapters 21 and 22.

Learning to respond with less anger may be particularly important for those with a strong family history of heart attacks and strokes. The risk of inheriting cardiovascular disease, once thought to be primarily due to inheriting traditional risk factors such as high cholesterol, has now been shown by Mark Ketterer and his colleagues to be far more related to inheriting the tendency (both neurochemical and learned) to be hostile or depressed.[116] This means that these mental issues more powerfully mediate the inheritance of heart disease than do other medical factors. Ketterer also has shown that one's assessment of his or her own hostility is not nearly as reliable as that of a spouse or close friend, and that, in fact, "denial scores" (spouse/friend assessments minus self-assessments) are even stronger predictors of coronary disease severity and mortality.[117] You need to listen to and trust the opinion of those close to you (even more than your own opinion) as to whether you may be a bit too angry and hostile.

Hostility and Mortality

A number of researchers who have attempted to pinpoint the health effects of hostility have found that it contributes to premature death from many causes, including cancer. In one study, students in law school were given a battery of psychological tests intended to measure hostility. In a 25-year follow-up, researchers found that only 4 percent of the nonhostile lawyers died from any cause, but 20 percent of the hostile attorneys died during the same period.[118] (Why they studied hostility in attorneys is anybody's guess.)

Duke psychologist John Barefoot agrees that hostile or cynical attitudes can lead to premature death. Barefoot and his colleagues followed 500 middle-aged participants for 15 years. All had similar health and lifestyle patterns. Those who scored high on hostility tests had more than six times the death rate of those with low scores. When the researchers followed up on death records at the end of the study, about one-fifth of the participants had died; the survivors were generally the ones with low hostility and less suspiciousness.[119]

The same group followed 968 people who started out with coronary disease and found that, over 15 years, hostility predicted a 33 percent higher mortality rate compared to that of the less hostile.[120]

The Psychological Effects of Anger

The reactions to anger aren't limited to the body. A host of studies shows that anger is linked to an array of psychological symptoms and behaviors, too. A long-term follow-up study interesting to college students showed that if not modified, hostility in the college years leads to sustained hostility in middle age and is highly predictive of poor well-being in those midlife years. Those who were hostile in college were much more likely in later life to have "low social support, achieving less than expected in career and in relationships, risk for depression, and appraisal of life changing for the worse." [121]

In another study, reported in the *American Journal of Health Promotion*, anger was assessed in middle-aged women. Those who were angry generally got inadequate sleep and too little exercise and used a greater than average number of over-the-counter drugs. The angry women in the study also showed lower optimism and a greater number of (and more severe) daily hassles, had less social support, and had lost an important relationship during the previous year.[122] Such anger is frequently associated with clinical depression (particularly bipolar depression), and this seems particularly true for men as well. Similarly, some people with similar neurochemical abnormalities to clinical depression struggle with rage attacks, even with minimal provocation. This can be related to excessive neuron firing in such disorders and may at times need medical treatment.

Which Hurts More: Expressing or Suppressing Anger?

There has been disagreement in the scientific community about which is more dangerous to health: expressing anger or suppressing it. That controversy has been sparked by recent research that shows that anger, regardless of how or whether it is expressed, is detrimental to health. According to Redford Williams, "There is something wrong with being angry: whether you keep it to yourself or let it show; if you have a lot of anger day in and day out, you have a significant increase in risk of premature mortality."[123]

In one study, blood pressure screening was done at the offices of the Massachusetts Division of Employment Security among people who had previously been working but who had involuntarily lost their jobs.[124] Researchers posted an announcement in the hall saying that free blood pressure screening would be performed; volunteers were weighed and asked to be seated for five minutes before blood pressure was taken. While the volunteers waited, they filled out brief questionnaires that sought information on health history and demographics. Questions also determined the style of anger of each respondent.

Three blood pressure readings were taken for each volunteer, and researchers adjusted their data according to age, social class, and obesity. When survey data were controlled for these factors, researchers found a surprisingly consistent result: There was a significant relationship between suppressed anger and systolic blood pressure. The more anger was suppressed, the higher was the blood pressure.

According to studies, suppressed anger is especially dangerous for women—and for more reasons than the increased cancer noted above. Researchers at the University of Michigan conducted an 18-year study of 700 people. They found that women who suppress their anger are three times likelier to die early of any cause than are those who express it. Men, they found, were at higher risk from suppressed anger only if they already had high blood pressure or chronic bronchitis. (Deaths from chronic bronchitis can occur from anger-induced airway spasm.) In commenting on the study, Estelle Ramey, professor emerita of physiology at Georgetown University Medical School, said that women suffer more "when they hold their anger in because they don't have a choice. A man can decide to keep his temper because it's the gentlemanly thing to do. But a woman may have to suppress her anger because she'll trigger male violence if she lets go."[125]

What about the people who sometimes express anger and sometimes repress it? Now research has found that people who have it both ways—who both express and suppress anger—are most prone of all to coronary heart disease.[126]

Fortunately, there is a third alternative that doesn't require either angry expression or suppression. The third alternative goes after the actual cause of the angry feelings: the thinking that causes the anger. We tend to believe that the provoking situation causes the anger. In reality, situations do not themselves make us angry; our chosen thinking about them does. That is, we make ourselves angry about situations by the thinking we choose. It goes like this:

$$\text{Situation} \rightarrow \text{Chosen (or learned) thinking} \rightarrow \text{Feelings}$$

Notice that feelings (such as anger) do not arise directly from the situation but are created by the thinking. Let's illustrate this concept. Suppose a teenager has been rebelling against his parents, provoking them with putdowns and refusing to listen to anything they have to say. The parents get angry, even furious. They react by attempting to take control of him. But it's not working, and their frustration leads to even more anger.

Then, in a moment of quiet reflection and seeking for deeper wisdom, they realize their son is trying to become independent, one of the jobs of the teenage years. He's just not doing it well because he's thinking, "Independence is doing the opposite of what you're told," not realizing that real and rational independence is doing whatever gets the best consequences, whether he was told to do it or not. Wise rationality for the teen would likely include building bridges with those around him, particularly those from whom he could use some support. On the parents' side, once they realize the difficult nature of their son's struggle to understand independence, and that mature independence is also what they want for him, feelings soften. In quiet moments of wisdom, they begin to feel compassion for him (and his natural desire to feel independent) instead of anger. Wanting to empower and lift their child instead of retaliate with their own putdowns, they start searching for ways to gently do that empowering. And suddenly, out of new compassion, the anger is gone. A new, wiser way of thinking, more in line with their values about what great parents do for their children, has created feelings very different from anger. It wasn't the teen causing their anger but rather the judgmental way they chose to think about the teen's actions. And the judgmental way the teen chose to think about his parents was the cause of his retaliatory anger as well.

If the feelings are destructive (making you miserable, hurting relationships, and causing loss of control), the thinking that causes those destructive feelings is usually somewhat irrational or in violation of one's deeper wisdom. This principle is the basis of some of the most effective psychotherapy methods, such as cognitive therapy or rational behavioral therapy.

What is the third alternative for dealing with anger, then? Come to think about the situation in new ways that are more rational and more in line with your deeper wisdom and values. Then the anger tends to dissipate and no longer needs to either be expressed or suppressed.

What does all this boil down to? Anger can compromise health and shave years off life. Redford Williams sums up the situation this way: "Trusting hearts may live longer. For them the biological 'cost' of situations that anger or irritate is lower. . . . So that's what they mean when they say that nice guys finish last. It's because most of the angry, hostile, nasty ones aren't in the race anymore!"[127]

What to Do if Anger Is a Problem

Does all the above mean you can never feel anger? No. Yale oncologist and surgeon Bernie Siegel tells us, "Anger has its place, so long as it is freely and safely expressed rather than held inside where it can have a destructive effect and lead to resentment and hatred." [128] However, the wise way of expressing anger couples it with kindness (avoiding putdowns).

Remember that anger often arises from defending your ego. So how can you get a handle on anger? Try these suggestions:

- Next time you start feeling angry, or when you encounter a situation that you know causes anger, distract yourself. Meditate, listen to a favorite concerto through a pair of headphones, or close your eyes and imagine something you really love (like that border of yellow tulips that breaks through the sodden ground at the edge of your road every spring). Stroke something soothing. If you have a pet, gently caress it. Often in this relaxed, meditative state, new, more rational ways of thinking about the situation will appear. This particularly occurs if you simply label the thinking with something like, "My ego is trying to defend itself by . . . "

- It sounds trite, but it works: When you feel like you're really going to explode, take two or three very deep breaths and count to ten, slowly. Just taking a pause will help you get your perspective so you can express your feelings in a more appropriate way.

- One of the best ways to get a handle on anger is to practice forgiveness. If you need some ideas on how to start forgiving others, see the suggestions in Chapter 14.

- Social connectedness goes a long way toward getting rid of anger. Do what you can to get connected: Find a confidant, get a pet, cuddle. Since connectedness creates stress resilience (see Chapter 8), ask yourself, "Is the way I'm handling this difference connecting us more deeply or disconnecting us?" Remember that handling a conflict well may indeed bring two people to greater understanding than they had before.

- Finally, when you start to feel angry, step back. Take a critical look at your negative thoughts. Think about your thinking, and discover wiser, larger, more rational ways to view the situation. Reason with yourself. See the funny things our egos do to feel important. Then laugh![129]

If ongoing hostility is the problem, in addition to the above suggestions, try some of Diane Ulmer's recommended drills:[130]

- Practice smiling at others and complimenting them.
- Practice giving yourself permission to stay calm when things don't go the way you want.
- Practice laughing at yourself.
- Play fun games.
- Stop using obscenities.
- Look for opportunities to say, "Maybe I'm wrong."
- Volunteer to help people who are less fortunate than you are.

- Learn more about the spiritual practices and teachings of your chosen spiritual tradition.
- And, something mentioned by several researchers, including Redford and Virginia Williams: Pretend that today is your last day.[131]

If ongoing anger seems to be caused by blaming someone or circumstances for hurting you, realize that holding on to that blame is not hurting them but will only eat you alive. The Hindus would say you are giving away your energy, even your spirit, to the one (or circumstances) you are blaming. They might advise, "Call your energy (your spirit) back! Don't give it away any longer." Give up the false notion that they are now controlling you to be so angry. Only your own thoughts are doing that. So let go of the blame, and be the way you want to be regardless of what someone else has done. Take back control of your experience of life. This is the power and value of forgiveness, no matter how grievous the fault. Forgiveness is not giving an undeserved gift to the perpetrator. It is about taking back control of your life and health.

Ellen Goodman, a writer for *The Washington Post,* summed up the sentiment eloquently in a piece about New Year's resolutions. In calling for the resolution to be a civil, social creature, she wrote, This may be a peak period for the battle against the spread of a waistline and creeping cholesterol. But it is also within our willpower to fight the spread of urban rudeness and creeping hostility. Civility doesn't stop nuclear holocaust and doesn't put a roof over the head of the homeless. But it makes a difference in the shape of a community, as surely as lifting weights can make a difference in the shape of a human torso.[132]

WHAT DID YOU LEARN?

1. What is the difference between anger and hostility?
2. What health problems does hostility cause?
3. What are some of the mechanisms of these health costs?
4. What is the primary cause of anger?
5. Is it better to express or suppress anger? What is the third alternative?
6. What can you do when anger appears?

ENDNOTES

1. Frederick Buechner, *Wishful Thinking A Seeker's ABC* (HarperOne; Rev Exp edition 1993).
2. Redford Williams and Virginia Williams, *Anger Kills* (New York: Random House/Times Books, 1993), xiii.
3. T. W. Smith, "Hostility and Health: Current Status of a Psychometric Hypothesis," *Health Psychology* 11 (1992): 139–50.
4. B. E. Hogan and W. Linden, "Anger Responses Styles and Blood Pressure: At Least Don't Ruminate about It!" *Annals of Behavioral Medicine* 27 (2004): 38–49.

5. Carol Tavris, "On the Wisdom of Counting to Ten," pp. 170–91 in P. Shaver, ed., *Review of Personality and Social Psychology*, vol. 5 (Beverly Hills, CA: Sage Publications, 1984).

6. Tavris, "On the Wisdom of Counting to Ten," 173–74.

7. Karen Judson, "Anger: The Shapes of Wrath," *Better Health & Living* (February 1988): 57–8.

8. Margaret A. Chesney and Ray H. Rosenman, *Anger and Hostility in Cardiovascular and Behavioral Disorders* (Washington, DC: Hemisphere Publishing Corporation, 1985).

9. Robert Ornstein and David Sobel, *The Healing Brain* (New York: Simon & Schuster, 1987), 181.

10. M. W. Ketterer et al., "Men Deny and Women Cry, but Who Dies? Do the Wages of 'Denial' Include Early Ischemic Coronary Heart Disease?" *Journal of Psychosomatic Research* 56, no. 1 (2004): 119–23.

11. Ibid.

12. Ibid.

13. Redford Williams, *The Trusting Heart: Great News about Type A Behavior* (New York: Times Books, Random House, 1989).

14. Paul Bagne, "Rude Awakening," *Men's Health* (October 1990): 34–5.

15. Carrol E. Izard, *Human Emotions* (New York: Plenum, 1977), 329–30.

16. Tavris, "On the Wisdom of Counting to Ten," 175–6.

17. Sharon Faelten, David Diamond, and the editors of *Prevention Magazine*, *Take Control of Your Life: A Complete Guide to Stress Relief* (Emmaus, PA: Rodale Press, 1988), 84.

18. Carl E. Thoresen, "The Hostility Habit: A Serious Health Problem?" *Healthline* (April 1984): 5.

19. W. Cook and D. Medley, "Proposed Hostility and Pharisaic Virtue Scales for the MMPI." *Journal of Applied Psychology* 38 (1954): 414–18.

20. M. W. Ketterer et al., "Prospective Study of a Self-Report Type A Scale and Risk of Coronary Heart Disease: Test of the MMPI-2 Type A Scale," *Circulation* 100 (1990): 686–7; and M.W. Ketterer, "The Ketterer Stress Symptom Frequency Checklist: Anger and the Severity of Coronary Artery Disease," *Henry Ford Hospital Medical Journal* 38 (1990): 207–12.

21. T. W. Smith, "Hostility and Health: Current Status of a Psychometric Hypothesis," *Health Psychology* 11 (1992): 139–50.

22. R. Williams, "The Trusting Heart," 71.

23. Ibid., 66.

24. A. Rozanski, J. A. Blumenthal, and J. Kaplan, "Impact of Psychological Factors on the Pathogenesis of Cardiovascular Disease and Implications for Therapy," *Circulation* 99 (1999): 2192–217; and W. Jiang, R. R. K. Krishnan, and C. M. O'Connor, "Depression and Heart Disease: Evidence of a Link and Its Therapeutic Implications," *CNS Drugs* 16 (2002): 111–27.

25. Tavris, "On the Wisdom of Counting to Ten," 173–4.

26. Izard, *Human Emotions*, 333–4.

27. "How Anger Affects Your Health," *Wellness Letter* (January 1992): 5.

28. Diane K. Ulmer, "Helping the Coronary Patient Reduce Hostility and Hurry Sickness: A Structured Behavioral Group Approach," *The Psychology of Health, Immunity, and Disease*, vol. A, 587, in Proceedings of the Sixth International Conference of the National Institute for the Clinical Application of Behavioral Medicine, Hilton Head Island, South Carolina, December, 1994.

29. S. B. Manuck et al., "Aggression and Anger-Related Traits Associated with a Polymorphism of the Tryptophan Hydroxylase Gene," *Biological Psychiatry* 45, no. 5 (1999): 603–14; D. Rujescu et al., "A Functional Single Nucleotide Polymorphism (V158M) in the COMT Gene Is Associated with Aggressive Personality Traits," *Biological Psychiatry* 54, no. 1 (2003): 34–9; I. Giegling, A. M. Hartmann, H. J. Möller, and D. Rujescu, "Anger- and Aggression-Related Traits are Associated with Polymorphisms in the 5-HT-2A Gene," *Journal of Affective Disorders* 96, no. 1–2 (November 2006): 75–81 (E-published June 30, 2006); and S.B. Manuck et al., "Aggression, Impulsivity, and Central Nervous System Serotonergic Responsivity in a Nonpatient Sample," *Neuropsychopharmacology* 19, no. 4 (1998): 287–99.

30. J. C. Barefoot et al., "The Cook-Medley Hostility Scale: Item Content and Ability to Predict Survival," *Psychosomatic Medicine* 51 (1989): 46–57.

31. Brent K. Houston and Christine R. Vavak, "Cynical Hostility: Developmental Factors, Psychosocial Correlates, and Health Behaviors," *Health Psychology* 10, no. 1 (1991): 9–17.

32. C. D. Sofhauser, "Psychosocial Antecedents of Hostility in Persons with Coronary Heart Disease," *Journal of Holistic Nursing* 21, no. 3: 280–300.

33. D. Carmelli, R. H. Rosenman, and G. E. Swan, "The Cook and Medley HO Scale: A Heritability Analysis in Adult Male Twins," *Psychosomatic Medicine* 50, no. 2: 165–74.

34. M. J. Strube, "Performance Attributions and the Type A Behavior Pattern: Causal Sources Versus Causal Dimensions," *Personality and Social Psychology Bulletin*, 14 (1988): 709–721.

35. Roger Daldrup, "How a Good Dose of Anger Therapy Can Restore Peace of Mind," *Your Personal Best* (April 1989): 8.

36. Ibid.

37. B. J. Burshman, R. F. Baumeister, and A. D. Stack, "Catharsis, Aggression, and Persuasive Influence: Self-Fulfilling or Self-Defeating Prophesies?" *Journal of Perspectives in Social Psychology* 76 (1999): 367–76.

38. Redford B. Williams, "Conferences with Patients and Doctors: A 69-Year-Old Man with Anger and Angina," *Journal of the American Medical Association* 282 (August 25, 1999): 8.

39. J. C. Barefoot et al., "The Cook-Medley Hostility Scale: Item Content and Ability to Predict Survival," *Psychosomatic Medicine* 51 (1989): 46–57.

40. R. Williams, "Conferences with Patients and Doctors," 8.

41. Daldrup, "Good Dose of Anger Therapy," 8.

42. G. E. Valliant and C. O. Valliant, "Natural History of Male Psychological Health, XII: A 45-Year Study of Predictors of Successful Aging at Age 65," *American Journal of Psychiatry* 147, no. 1 (1990): 31–7; also G. E. Valliant, *Aging Well* (Boston: Little, Brown, 2000); also Martin Seligman *Learned Optimism* (New York: Knopf, 1990), 179–181.

43. Tavris, "On the Wisdom of Counting to Ten."

44. Ibid.

45. Daldrup, "Good Dose of Anger Therapy," 8.

46. Ibid., 8.

47. Izard, *Human Emotions*, 351.

48. Tavris, "On the Wisdom of Counting to Ten," 170–91.

49. Ibid.

50. Ibid.

51. Lenore Walker, *The Battered Woman Syndrome* (New York: Springer Publishing Company, 1999).

52. N. L. Smith, personal communication, 2004.

53. Peter Stearns, *Anger: The Struggle for Emotional Control in America's History* (Chicago: University of Chicago Press, 1989); cited in Karen Judson, "Anger: The Shapes of Wrath."

54. H. Nabi et al., "Does Personality Predict Mortality? Results from the GAZEL French Prospective Cohort Study," *International Journal of Epidemiology* 37, no. 2 (April 2008): 386–96.

55. Steven Locke and Douglas Colligan, *The Healer Within: The New Medicine of Mind and Body* (New York: E. P. Dutton, 1986), 183.

56. L. D. Kubzansky et al., "Angry Breathing: A Prospective Study of Hostility and Lung Function in the Normative Aging Study," *Thorax*, October 2006.

57. Glen Rein, Mike Atkinson, and Rollin McCraty, "The Physiological and Psychological Effects of Compassion and Anger, Part 1 of 2," *Journal of Advancement in Medicine* 8, no. 2 (1995): 87–105.

58. Tavris, *Anger*, 170–91.

59. Bruce Bower, "Women Take Un-Type A Behaviors to Heart," *Science News* 144 (1993): 244.

60. Ulla Christensen, et al., "Cynical Hostility, Socioeconomic Position, Health Behaviors, and Symptom Load: A Cross-Sectional Analysis in a Danish Population-Based Study," *Psychosomatic Medicine* 66 (2004): 572–577.

61. I. C. Siegler, "Hostility and Risk: Demographic and Lifestyle Variables," pp. 199–214 in A. W. Siegman and T. W. Smith, eds., *Anger, Hostility and the Heart* (Hillsdale, NJ: Lawrence Erlbaum, 1994).

62. I. C. Siegler et al., "Pattern of Change in Hostility from College to Midlife in the UNC Alumni Heart Study Predict High Risk Status," *Psychosomatic Medicine* 65 (2003): 738–45.

63. J. L. Marx, "Coronary Artery Spasms and Heart Disease," *Science* 208, no. 4448 (1980): 1127–30; and E. Braunwald, "Coronary Artery Spasm: Mechanisms and Clinical Relevance," *Journal of the American Medical Association* 246 (1981): 1957–9.

64. Ibid.

65. S. B. Manuck et al., "Aggression, Impulsivity, and Central Nervous System Serotonergic Responsivity in a Nonpatient Sample," *Neuropsychopharmacology* 19, no. 4 (October 1998): 287–9.

66. F. Laghrissi-Thade, "Elevated Platelet Factor 4 and β-thromboglobulin Plasma Levels in Depressed Patients with Ischemic Heart Disease,"*Biological Psychiatry* 42 (1997): 290–5.

67. D. E. Polk, T. W. Kamarck, S. Shiffman, "Hostility Explains Some of the Discrepancy Between Daytime Ambulatory and Clinic Blood Pressure," *Health Psychology* 21, no. 2 (2002): 202–6.

68. M. E. Bleil et al., "Anger-Related Personality Traits and Carotid Artery Atherosclerosis in Untreated Hypertensive Men," *Psychosomatic Medicine* 66, no. 5 (2004): 633–9.

69. A. Castillo-Richmond, "Effects of Stress Reduction on Carotid Atherosclerosis in Hypertensive African Americans," *Stroke* 31, no. 3 (2000): 568–73.

70. Meyer Friedman and Ray Rosenman, *Type A Behavior and Your Heart* (Fawcett, 1974).

71. Karen Judson, "Anger: The Shapes of Wrath."

72. Williams, *The Trusting Heart*, 83–4.

73. Daldrup, "Good Dose of Anger Therapy."

74. R. Virtaaanen et al., "Anxiety and Hostility Are Associated with Baroreflex Sensitivity," *Psychosomatic Medicine* 65 (2003): 751–6.

75. J. C. Stewart, D. Janicki-Deverts, M. F. Muldoon, and T. W. Kamarck, "Depressive Symptoms Moderate the Influence of Hostility on Serum Interleukin-6 and C-Reactive Protein," *Psychosomatic Medicine* 70, no. 2 (February 2008): 197–204 (E-published February 6, 2008).

76. T. Q. Miller et al., "A Meta-Analytic Review of Research on Hostility and Physical Health," *Psychological Bulletin* 119 (1996): 322–48.

77. E. Harburg, N. Kaciroti, L. Gleiberman, and M. A. Schork, "Expressive/Suppressive Anger Coping Responses, Gender, and Types of Mortality Followup," *Psychosomatic Medicine* 65 (2003): 588–97.

78. M. A. Jansen and L. R. Muenz, "A Retrospective Study of Personality Variables Associated with Fibrocystic Disease and Breast Cancer," *Journal of Psychosomatic Research* 28 (1984): 35–42.

79. L. Temoshok et al., "The Relationship of Psychosocial Factors to Prognostic Indicators in Cutaneous Malignant Melanoma," *Journal of Psychosomatic Research* 29, no. 2 (1985): 139–53.

80. L. R. Temoshok and R. L. Wald, "Change Is Complex: Rethinking Research on Psychosocial Interventions and Cancer," *Integrative Cancer Therapy* 1, no. 2 (2002): 135–45.

81. James W. Pennebaker and Harald C. Traue, "Inhibition and Psychosomatic Processes," pp. 152–3 in Harald C. Traue and James W. Pennebaker, eds., *Emotion Inhibition and Health* (Seattle, WA: Hogrefe & Huber Publishers, 1993).

82. M. W. Ketterer, G. Mahr, and A. D. Goldberg, "Psychological Factors Affecting a Medical Condition: Ischemic Coronary Heart Disease," *Journal of Psychosomatic Research* 48, nos. 4–5(2000): 357–67.

83. Ornstein and Sobel, *The Healing Brain,* 181.

84. Redford Williams and Virginia Williams *Anger Kills* (New York: Random House/Time Books, 1993), p. 12.

85. R. B. Williams, Jr. et al., "Type A Behavior, Hostility, and Coronary Atherosclerosis," *Psychosomatic Medicine* 42, no. 6 (1980): 539–49.

86. John Droubay Hardy and Timothy W. Smith, "Cynical Hostility and Vulnerability to Disease: Social Support, Life Stress, and Physiological Response to Conflict," *Health Psychology* 7, no. 5 (1988): 447–459.

87. "The A Is for Anger," *Men's Health* (July 1989): 10.

88. Williams, "Conferences with Patients and Doctors," 8.

89. M. A. Mittleman et al., "Educational Attainment, Anger, and the Risk of Triggering Myocardial Infarction Onset," *Archives of Internal Medicine* 157 (1997): 769–75.

90. Janice E. Williams, "Anger Proneness Predicts Coronary Heart Disease Risk : Prospective Analysis From the Atherosclerosis Risk In Communities (ARIC) Study," *Circulation*, 101 (May 2000): 2034–2039.

91. "Depression, Anger, and the Heart," *Harvard Health Letter* (February 1993): 7.

92. B. E. Hogan and W. Linden, "Anger Response Styles and Blood Pressure: At Least Don't Ruminate About It!" *Annals of Behavioral Medicine* 27, no. 1 (February 2004): 38–49.

93. Locke and Colligan, *The Healer Within,* 183.

94. S. H. Boyle et al., "Hostility as a Predictor of Survival in Patients with Coronary Artery Disease," *Psychosomatic Medicine* 66, no. 5 (September–October 2004): 629–32.

95. A. Rozanski et al., "Mental Stress and the Induction of Silent Myocardial Ischemia in Patients with Coronary Artery Disease," *New England Journal of Medicine* 318 (1988): 1005–12.

96. G. Ironson et al., "Effects of Anger on Left Ventricular Ejection Fraction in Coronary Artery Disease," *American Journal of Cardiology* 70 (1992): 281–85.

97. W. Jiang et al., "Mental Stress-Induced Myocardial Ischemia and Cardiac Events," *Journal of the American Medical Association* 275 (1996): 1651–6.

98. Ilene C. Siegler, Bercedis L. Peterson, John C. Barefoot, and Redford B. Williams, "Hostility during Late Adolescence Predicts Coronary Risk Factors at Mid-Life," *American Journal of Epidemiology* 136, no. 2 (1992): 146–154.

99. S. Seshadri et al., "Association of Plasma Total Homocysteine Levels with Subclinical Brain Injury: Cerebral Volumes, White Matter Hyperintensity, and Silent Brain Infarcts at Volumetric Magnetic Resonance Imaging in the Framingham Offspring Study," *Archives of Neurololology* 65, no. 5 (May 2008): 642–9.

100. M. Kumar et al., "Homocysteine Decreases Blood Flow to the Brain due to Vascular Resistance in Carotid Artery," *Neurochemistry International* 2008 Aug 3. [Epub ahead of print]

101. T. Koike et al., "Raised Homocysteine and Low Folate and Vitamin B-12 Concentrations Predict Cognitive Decline in Community-Dwelling Older Japanese Adults," *Clinical Nutrition* 2008 Oct 1. [Epub ahead of print]

102. D. B. Panagiotakos et al., "Increased Plasma Homocysteine Concentrations in Healthy People with Hostile Behavior: The ATTICA Study," *Medical Science Monitor* 10, no. 8: CR457–62 (E-published July 23, 2004).

103. T. L. Nelson, R. F. Palmer, and N. L. Pedersen, "The Metabolic Syndrome Mediates the Relationship Between Cynical Hostility and Cardiovascular Disease," *Experimental Aging Research* 30, no. 2 (2004): 163–77.

104. Redford B. Williams, Jr., "Hostility, Anger, and Heart Disease," *Drug Therapy* (August 1986): 43.

105. Redford B. Williams, Jr., et al., "Type A Behavior, Hostility, and Coronary Atherosclerosis," *Psychosomatic Medicine,* vol. 42, no. 6 (November 1980): 539–49.

106. Ibid.

107. Ibid.

108. Carl E. Thoresen, "The Hostility Habit: A Serious Health Problem?" *Healthline* (April 1984): 5.

109. Ibid.

110. Williams and Williams, *Anger Kills,* 36.

111. J. C. Barefoot, W. G. Dahlstrom, and R. B. Williams, "Hostility, CHD Incidence and Total Mortality," *Psychosomatic Medicine* 45 (1983): 59–63.

112. R. B. Williams, Jr., "Hostility, Anger, and Heart Disease," 43.

113. Siegler et al., "Pattern of Change," 738–45.

114. C. V. Lavie and R. V. Milani, "Impact of Aging on Hostility in Coronary Patients and Effects of Cardiac Rehabilitation and Exercise Training in Elderly Persons," *American Journal of Geriatric Cardiology* 13, no. 3 (2004): 125–30.

115. Meyer Friedman, "Alteration of Type A Behavior and Its Effect on Cardiac Recurrences in Post-Myocardial Infarction Patients: Summary Results of the Recurrent Coronary Prevention Project," *American Heart Journal* 112 (1986): 653–59; J. A. Blumenthal, M. Babyak, J. Wei et al., "Usefulness of Psychosocial Treatment of Mental Stress–Induced Myocardial Ischemia in Men," *American Journal of Cardiology* 89 (2002): 164–168; also J. A. Blumenthal et al., *Archives of Internal Medicine* 157 (1997): 2213–23.

116. M. W. Ketterer et al., "Familial Transmissibility of Early Age at Initial Diagnosis in Coronary Heart Disease (CHD): Males Only, and Mediated by Psychosocial/Emotional Distress?" *Journal of Behavioral Medicine* 27, no. 1 (2004): 1–10.

117. M. W. Ketterer et al., "Men Deny and Women Cry."

118. Kathy A. Fackelmann, "Hostility Boosts Risk of Heart Trouble," *Science News* 135 (1989): 60.

119. J. C. Barefoot et al., "Patterns of Hostility and Implications for Health," *Health Psychology* 10 (1991): 18–24.

120. S. H. Boyle et al., "Hostility as a Predictor of Survival in Patients with Coronary Artery Disease," *Psychosomatic Medicine* 66, no. 5 (2004): 629–32.

121. I. C. Siegler et al., "Patterns of Change in Hostility from College to Midlife in the UNC Alumni Heart Study Predict High-Risk Status," *Psychosomatic Medicine* 65, no. 5 (September–October 2003): 738–45.

122. Sandra P. Thomas and Madge M. Donnellan, "Correlates of Anger Symptoms in Women in Middle Adulthood," *American Journal of Health Promotion* 5, no. 4 (1990): 267–72.

123. R. Williams, "Conferences with Patients and Doctors," 8.

124. Joel E. Dimsdale et al., "Suppressed Anger and Blood Pressure: The Effects of Race, Sex, Social Class, Obesity, and Age," *Psychosomatic Medicine* 48, no. 6 (1986): 430–6.

125. "Women Who Suppress Anger Die Sooner," *American Health* (July–August 1991).

126. Pennebaker and Traue, "Inhibition and Psychosomatic Processes."

127. Redford Williams, cited in "The A Is for Anger," 11.

128. Bernie Siegel, *Peace, Love and Healing: Bodymind Communication and the Path to Self-Healing* (New York: Harper & Row, 1989), 28.

129. Ibid.

130. Ulmer, "Helping the Coronary Patient," 592; and M. Friedman and D. Ulmer, *Treating Type A Behavior and Your Heart* (New York: Fawcett, 1984).

131. Williams and Williams, *Anger Kills*.

132. Ellen Goodman, "Thoughts for a New Year," *Reader's Digest* (January 1989): 118.

CHAPTER 5

Worry, Anxiety, Fear, and Health

I have had many troubles in my life, but the worst of them never came.

—James A. Garfield

- Define *worry*.
- Understand generalized anxiety disorder, panic disorder, and other common anxiety disorders.
- Define *somaticizing*.
- Discuss the health consequences of chronic anxiety.
- Discuss the irrationality of worry and more productive ways to respond to problems.

Worriers slide into the seat of an airplane, snap the seatbelt closed, and worry that the plane might crash. They worry that a fussy toddler might have contracted chickenpox. They worry that their term paper wasn't good enough or that they'll be fired because they called in sick one too many times.

Worry is something with which most Americans are familiar. According to statistics from a variety of studies, only about a third classify themselves as nonworriers, people who worry less than an hour and a half each day. More than half classify themselves as moderate worriers, people who worry between 10 and 50 percent of the day and may or may not be troubled by worrying. The rest are chronic worriers, people who worry more than eight hours a day.[1]

Andrew Matthews of Louisiana State University says that worry might be a form of increased vigilance against threats, a form of problem solving, or a way to rehearse potentially unpleasant events. If you use it to prepare for and deal with a bad situation, it might be beneficial. Even when used in these somewhat positive ways, there are more effective techniques than worry that will help you prepare for problems. And if worry or other forms of anxiety become excessive, they can harm health.[2]

Definitions of Fear, Anxiety and Worry

We have all experienced **fear,** which usually occurs in response to an external threat. The behaviors of fear are usually avoidance and an attempt to escape. **Anxiety,** on the other hand, can be present even without the external stimulus, and is the result of threats that are perceived to be uncontrollable or unavoidable.[3] The psycho-physiological state of anxiety has emotional, cognitive, somatic, and behavioral components, which combine to create the discomfort of apprehension or worry.[4] Anxiety may help a person generate the energy and attention to cope with a difficult situation, but when it becomes excessive, it may become destructive and be classified as an anxiety disorder.[5]

Worry is the most common form of anxiety. According to clinical psychologist Thomas Pruzinsky of the University of Virginia,

> [Worry is] a state in which we dwell on something so much it causes us to become apprehensive. It differs from the far stronger emotion we call fear, which causes physical changes such as a racing pulse and fast breathing in our bodies. Worry is the thinking part of anxiety.[6]

Worry is a preoccupation with potential dangers or pain in the future. Says Pruzinsky, most people who report to a doctor that they are worried say they worry anywhere from 80 to 95 percent of the day.[7]

Worrying reflects our attempts to cope mentally with our concerns and fears. It's not always bad; worry might be useful if it helps us become more vigilant in the face of real danger or helps us take steps that will keep something negative from happening. Worry becomes harmful when it contributes to our worries becoming reality or when worrying becomes so pervasive that we are immobilized by it.[8] More often than not, what we are worrying about never happens, but the worry makes us feel like we are already living the catastrophe anyway. Worry may be appropriate in a situation where there are real wolves growling at the door, but frequently we create imaginary wolves—and our body then reacts as if they were actually there.

Sometimes worry feels like we are pouring energy into preventing the anticipated catastrophe, but, in fact, the worry may help make the catastrophe more likely to happen. This observation is based on what might be called the "Law of Expectations." For example, if you have to give a talk and you are worrying a lot about it, the energy you spend worrying seems like you are doing something to prepare. In fact, however, your worry is causing you to visualize failure, create unconscious images of being unprepared, or visualize making a fool of yourself. Anytime you visualize failure, it tends to become a self-fulfilling prophecy—the image you "practiced" will come up when it's time for you to speak and will generate behaviors (such as being worried about forgetting, stammering, or being seen as incompetent) that are more likely to lead to failure. Worrying is like visualizing negative performance (versus visualizing positive performance). Highly successful athletes, performers, or speakers often use positive visualization, the process of generating practiced successful images, in order to perform well during actual performance. Worrying is like practicing failure; it is like living the failure, even though it may never happen.

Surveys show that the most common sources of worry for Americans are family and relationships, job or school, health, and finances. According to Jennifer L. Abel, associate director of the Stress and Anxiety Disorders Institute at Pennsylvania State University, most people worry about 5 percent of the time. Chronic worriers, on the other hand, spend an average of about 50 percent of their time worrying; and some, says Abel, worry 100 percent of the time.[9]

Of those chronic worriers, most worry elaborately. In one study demonstrating this point, psychologists compared 24 chronic worriers with 24 people who say they don't worry. The psychologists then gave both groups a scenario: What if you got bad grades? The nonworriers fashioned simple responses: they might get into trouble with their parents or might feel embarrassed for a few days. The chronic worriers, however, were characterized by responses that progressed quickly from bad grades to the more catastrophic possibilities of loss of control, mental illness, pain, deterioration, and even death and hell.[10]

Generalized Anxiety Disorder

Some people have what is called generalized anxiety disorder, a problem often disabling enough to require medication.[11] Generalized anxiety disorder is characterized by:[12]

- excessive worry about many things (as opposed to a specific situational problem).

- worry that is present more than half the time for many months (by definition, more than six months).

- significant body tension and several physical symptoms.

The physical symptoms associated with generalized anxiety disorder are similar to those that are part of panic disorder (see Table 5.1) but are often more prolonged and less dramatic. Generalized anxiety is often also accompanied by symptoms of depression and its associated physical illnesses (see Chapter 6). For example, fatigue, which is often seen with depression, is even more predictive of associated anxiety.[13] Other physical symptoms often seen with depression and especially anxiety include musculoskeletal and back pain, chest pain, heart palpitations, dizziness, numbness or tingling, and trouble swallowing.[14] Of people with major depression, 70 percent also have clinical anxiety problems. Generalized anxiety results in much physical and occupational disability and in high levels of medical care and costs.[15]

According to the National Institute of Mental Health, the anxiety disorders that stem from worry and social anxiety are the United States' most commonly reported mental health problems.[16] And what starts in the mind as worry can have a profound effect on the body.

Panic Disorder

A classic example of mind-body interaction is created when a person experiences spontaneous, usually unprovoked anxiety attacks coupled with several dramatic physical phenomena. The diagnosis requires that at least four of the symptoms listed in Table 5.1 occur simultaneously during these usually brief but frightening attacks. Just as the attacks often come on for no clear reason, they also stop spontaneously after five to thirty minutes. If you or someone you know has one of the symptoms in the list, determine whether any

Table 5.1   Physical Symptoms of Panic Disorder

Cardiopulmonary
Shortness of breath Palpitations (heart pounding, racing, or skipping) Chest pain or pressure
Ear, Nose, and Throat
Dizziness Choking
Gastrointestinal
Abdominal distress (indigestion, nausea, or diarrhea)
Neurological
Numbness and tingling Weakness
Autonomic Nervous System
Sweats Hot flashes or chills Tremors or shakes

Source: R. Spitzer et al., *Diagnostic and Statistical Manual IV* (Washington, DC: American Psychiatric Association, 1998).

of the other listed symptoms also occur during these discrete attacks. If so, it is very likely a panic attack. As noted, these often occur without provocation, often as a spontaneous neurochemical event. Sometimes the feeling of anxiety itself is absent, since it is only one of the potential symptoms.

The problem is that panic disorder, which is very effectively treatable, often goes undiagnosed and thus untreated for prolonged periods of time. If it remains untreated, phobias often develop, usually out of an irrational fear of returning to the place or situation where the first attacks occurred. These phobias can become very disabling, sometimes making a person very fearful to return to work, to drive, or to even leave home.

The medical effects of panic disorder can also be very significant. The physical symptoms of panic disorder can be dramatic and very bothersome, often leading to many tests (usually all with normal results) and multiple medical visits. Some studies suggest that as many as one-sixth of patients seen in a general medical office are having some form of panic attacks that are causing the physical symptoms they come to have evaluated. The symptoms are not imagined but rather are related to abnormal nervous system function, usually involving many of the same neurotransmitter abnormalities that cause clinical depression.

Other Common Anxiety Disorders

Probably the most common anxiety disorder of all frequently goes undetected, often because its very nature causes its victims to hide the fear. Social anxiety disorder is characterized by a sometimes overwhelming, inappropriate fear or embarrassment when under scrutiny by others or even with the attention of an unfamiliar person in a conversation.[17] Flushing, losing focus, and feeling that others are detecting the embarrassment all create more anxiety, sometimes leading the victim to avoid almost all unfamiliar social contact.

Another impressive form of anxiety is obsessive-compulsive disorder, which is characterized by recurrent stressful thoughts (often lacking sense) that are excessively difficult to dismiss. These obsessive thoughts are accompanied by compulsive, repetitive behaviors that are perceived by most others as very excessive, such as some of the following:[18]

- excessive cleanliness
- multiple checking (such as repeatedly checking to see if the front door is locked)
- saving things (without the ability to discard) to the point of severe clutter
- self-inflicted physical trauma, such as picking the skin
- eating disorders, such as anorexia

These compulsive behaviors are often an attempt to take control because the victim feels out of control. The part of the brain that maintains bodily and emotional control (the limbic system) is not functioning correctly in anxiety disorders, and the subsequent feeling of things being out of control elicits controlling behaviors. Controlling behaviors are, for example, a symptom of serotonin deficiency in that part of the brain (and often improve greatly with techniques that improve that serotonin function).

One other anxiety disorder worth mentioning is posttraumatic stress disorder, which is usually triggered by a very traumatic event; the disorder is characterized by flashbacks and nightmares that cause the victim to mentally re-experience the trauma repeatedly.[19] Individuals often avoid circumstances that remind them of the trauma.

All of these "disorders" involve abnormally exaggerated responses of the central nervous system to stimuli; the symptoms listed in Table 5.1, if occurring individually or particularly in combination, are highly likely to have some associated anxiety. For example, in a study done in two general medicine clinics at the University of Utah, if patients had a combination of dizziness and numbness or tingling, 93 percent had an associated anxiety disorder.[20] If these disorders interfere with life, they commonly require medical treatment as well as behavioral reconditioning of the nervous system to respond with more control. Anxiety disorder patients also had much higher-than-normal levels of physical problems.

Somaticizing

Somaticizing is the body's way of turning mental stress, usually anxiety, into physical manifestations. People afflicted with the phenomenon of somaticizing, those whom some experts have come to call the worried well, are usually anxious. "Worried well" is clearly a misnomer because such a person is far from well, but the term implies no clear-cut organ damage on the usual tests to explain the person's physical symptoms. In a classic study of primary care patients, Kurt Kroenke and his colleagues studied patients coming into a primary care clinic, following the medical evaluation of the most common physical symptoms seen (many of which are classic anxiety disorder symptoms). After three years of tests and follow-up, an average of only 17 percent ever received a clear-cut organic diagnosis! The rest (83 percent) went organically "unexplained."[21] It is this very common group of patients that is highly likely to have some of the nervous system dysregulation associated with anxiety and depressive disorders.

The anxious person's biological abnormality lies within the regulation mechanism of the central nervous system. The same neurochemical abnormalities and dysregulation that causes anxiety and depression disorders can at times show up physically without many emotional components. Also, if a person is unwilling to face emotional difficulties, they may subconsciously "somatize" them, or convert them into physical complaints.[22] As many as two-thirds of all patient visits to the doctor may be made by these worried well; and, because some physicians don't recognize the mental basis of the physical complaints, these patients are often sent from one physician to another without being helped.[23] Hosts of studies compiled over the past three decades have shown that addressing the central nervous system issues that underlie somatized physical problems can cut health care costs by an estimated 5 to 80 percent per year.[24]

Psychologist Nicholas Cummings, who founded the Hawaii-based Biodyne Institute, says that "some patients spend as much as $28,000 a year in a fruitless attempt to isolate a physical cause for what is basically an emotional problem . . . . On some days these patients saw four different physicians." Cummings says the emotional problems of anxiety and worry have to be addressed if there is to be an improvement in the patient's condition, and he says he never disputes the reality of patients' difficulties: "I can say with all honesty: 'I know you hurt. But as long as you're here, tell us a bit more about you.'" Cummings adds that addressing the emotional problems often helps when other treatments have failed.[25] This is not to say the medical problems are imagined. Rather the stressed nervous system activates sustained "supersystem" dysregulation (see Chapter 2), and real medical problems emerge.

The nervous system is largely designed to help the body respond to stimuli. That means the nervous system either keeps things in control (by responding to any stressor or perceived threat, whether physical or emotional) or causes the body to respond appropriately (for example, it jump-starts the bowel in response to food). In anxiety disorders, the nervous system is overresponsive (hypersensitive) to all kinds of stimuli—not only emotional, but also excessive pain responses, gut responses, or heart and blood vessel responses. The usual result is physical havoc.

Ultimately, the longer the anxiety (or unrelenting pain or depression) goes unchecked, the more hard-wired the hypersensitive nervous system becomes. Here's what happens: certain neurons, called "inhibitory" neurons, are designed to keep pain and stress responses under control. Chemicals called neurotophins (such as brain-derived neurotrophic factor—BDNF) keep these inhibitory neurons (and also thinking neurons) healthy and functioning well. Under chronic stress—including anxiety—the beneficial neurotrophins are suppressed. As a result, these stress signals, which can be caused by either physical or emotional stress, cause the literal shriveling and malfunction of these inhibitory neurons. The signals designed to keep pain and stress responses in control no longer work.[26] Thus the nervous system starts to become hypersensitive, over-responding to both physical and emotional stimuli. In addition, thinking neurons can also malfunction.

The same neurotrophins (BDNF) suppressed by stress are also needed to keep thinking neurons healthy. Chronic anxiety and pain, then, can lead to less effective cognition when these neurotrophins are suppressed.

Effects of Worry and Anxiety on the Body

Physician Marty Rossman explains that worry "creates negative images about some future event like a deadline or a test. The down side is that chronic worry can overwork and wear down not only the nervous system but also the immune and hormone systems, leading to chronic stress, a state that has been associated with numerous ailments, from headaches to heart disease."[27]

When people somatize an emotion like worry into a physical complaint, they literally feel something physically. However, worry can actually *cause* physical changes that can compromise many body systems, and physical illness can result. The brain has considerable capacity to create bodily responses in line with practiced, visualized expectations. This is the physical expression of the Law of Expectations mentioned above for worried behaviors. This is well demonstrated by the placebo effect: When a person expects to do well with a particular treatment, the brain has a way of eliciting that expected effect, clear down to cellular levels at times. For example, we have already discussed hard-wired changes in the system: If you constantly worry about experiencing more pain, for example, neurotransmitters change in a way that literally signals more pain. On the other hand, if you hopefully expect to experience less pain, that's often exactly what happens: placebos work well in controlling pain—or anxiety—about a third of the time. Medical studies repeatedly find that it's far more effective to give a placebo than to do nothing; that's the reason why good scientific studies of a medical treatment regimen require that treatment be compared to a placebo control (a group of people who are given a placebo).

Worry is literally practicing the visualization of the imagined catastrophe, and the brain has the capacity to elicit physical and behavioral responses that fit with that visualization, thus often creating some of the very problems about which you worry. While we attempt to separate the behavioral or emotional responses from the physical ones, the brain does not differentiate these two so neatly—it tends to elicit an oversensitive physical response at the same time it sends out an oversensitive emotional or behavioral response.

The Association of Anxiety with Common Medical Illnesses

Who gets sick the most? A study of all patients coming in for physical illness at two general medicine clinics at the University of Utah revealed that 47 percent had identifiable anxiety (42 percent also had significant depression, and more than half of all patients coming in had some kind of anxiety or depressive disorder).[28] Linn and Yager found similar numbers in clinics at UCLA.[29] Yet these disorders are present in fewer than 15 percent of the general population. That means that more than half of physically ill general medical patients are coming from the 15 percent of the population that is anxious or depressed! In addition, often what drives a person to see a physician is not the physical symptom itself as much as anxiety about what that symptom means. Once reassured that it is not serious, the problem may be quite tolerable.

High utilizers of medical care are particularly likely to have anxiety and depression disorders.[30] Anxiety disorder includes the entities described above (such as panic disorder, generalized anxiety disorder, obsessive-compulsive disorder, posttraumatic stress disorder, or social anxiety disorder). Any of these anxiety disorders commonly includes, in addition to the symptoms in Table 5.1, other physical symptoms (such as pain[31]) or allergic problems[32] (such as hives). In addition, many very common medical disorders have a high relationship to anxiety.

For example, headaches are the most common pain complaint of patients in general medical clinics. A person with migraine headaches has four times the normal rate of depression but thirteen times more panic attacks than the general population.[33] When carefully evaluated, of people coming to an emergency room or cardiology clinic with chest pain, 40 percent are having panic attacks,[34] and another 25 percent have other kinds of diagnosable anxiety disorders.[35] Treatment of noncardiac chest pain with antidepressant medications (and perhaps stress-reduction techniques) that increase serotonin in the nervous system, even in the absence of depression or anxiety disorders, reduces the chest pain by as much as 80 percent.[36] This suggests that the same neurochemical (namely, serotonin) abnormalities seen with anxiety are important in the chest pain.

Of people with irritable bowel syndrome (the most common disorder seen in gastroenterology clinics), 40 percent are having panic attacks, and 80 to 90 percent are having some form of anxiety or depression disorder.[37] Anxiety is similarly highly associated with dyspepsia, one of the most common upper intestinal symptoms.[38] Treatment of the anxiety, either with medication[39] or stress-reduction techniques,[40] can be very helpful for irritable bowel problems. In fact, antidepressant medications used for anxiety disorders have long been some of the most effective ways to treat these intestinal disorders, even in the absence of depression.[41] Roughly 40 percent of people with esophageal spasm[42] and half of those with heart palpitations[43] are having panic attacks[44] (and the diagnosis is often missed until much later).

Similar very high associations of panic, generalized anxiety, and depression disorders are present with common muscle pain problems such as fibromyalgia[45] or myofascial pain syndrome. For example, chronic back pain (the fourth most common symptom in primary care clinics) is highly associated with anxiety disorders; and, when present, the anxiety precedes the back pain 95 percent of the time.[46] This is not to say that the pain is imagined, but rather that the pain system is overresponsive, just as the stress response system (or bowel system) is overresponsive to stimuli in these disorders.

The reason for these striking associations lies in the fact that migraines, irritable bowel syndrome, fibromyalgia, depression, and anxiety disorders all have similar underlying neurochemical abnormalities in the brain, such as too little of the centrally inhibiting neurotransmitters serotonin, norepinephrine, gamma-aminobutyric acid (GABA), and dopamine but too much of the stimulating neurotransmitters like glutamate and

Substance P.[47] Serotonin and GABA in the brain tend to quiet down the response to a stimulus or stressor. These substances act in the parts of the brain called the limbic system and the hypothalamus, which maintain control of many body systems, preventing those systems from having too little or too great a response. If serotonin function (and that of other quieting neurotransmitters such as GABA) is low, many systems overreact to a stimulus: too much bowel response to food (irritable bowel), too much immune response (multiple allergies or chemical hypersensitivity), too much pain response to a pain signal (headache and fibromyalgia), and too much stress response to a stressor (anxiety disorders). Anxious people tend to diffusely have too much spasm of smooth muscles—those that contract the intestines, bladder, airways, and blood vessels in response to a stimulus. All of these organs can thus become disordered in a very real way in people with anxiety.

These same "overresponsive" disorders are also characterized by too high a level of neurochemicals (such as Substance P or glutamate) that magnify responses to an unpleasant stimulus (like pain). Depressed and anxious people thus tend to have too much pain. This pain is not imagined—rather it is overprocessed and magnified in the nervous system. Normally when a pain signal from peripheral tissue arrives in the brain, the brain sends back a signal to inhibit and control the pain signal. That downward inhibitory tract is driven by the neurotransmitters serotonin, norepinephrine, and dopamine, all of which run low in the central nervous system of abnormally depressed and anxious people. (When central nervous system norepinephrine runs low, it tends to be too high in the periphery, causing some of the damage noted in previous chapters—see Chapter 2.) So the downward inhibitory tract does not work well in anxiety disorders, and the result is overresponsiveness to many stimuli, creating unnecessarily painful symptoms.

Correcting these nervous system chemical abnormalities, both with medications and with other treatments that do not involve drugs, can dramatically improve all these very common "dysregulation" problems. The medications used for these problems are usually antidepressants, so named because they were first used to treat depression, but they often work well for these hypersensitivity disorders even when the symptom of depression is absent. Such medications are not simply symptom-relieving pills; instead they tend to normalize regulation and neurotransmission in the nervous system. Treatments other than medication involve attention to good sleep and exercise and particularly stress-resilience approaches, all of which can improve these same neurotransmitters (see Chapters 21 and 22). Nutrition can also play a role. For example, you need to eat foods that contain tryptophan (such as dairy, nuts, and turkey) to enable your body to make serotonin. Many medications used to treat anxiety don't even work well if these foods are omitted from the diet (see Chapter 20).

Worry and the Circulatory System

Worry has been shown to have significant effects on the heart and circulatory system as a whole. Researchers interested in the effects of worry tested 125 patients for a year following their heart attacks. A real distinction developed between the ones who worried about their condition and the ones who didn't: those who worried were significantly more likely to have arrhythmias (abnormal heart rhythms that can lead to sudden cardiac death).[48]

In fact, cardiologist Robert Eliot catalogues examples of people who have been literally "scared to death." A sudden surge of stress hormones like catecholamines can cause immediate heart muscle damage (necrosis) and abrupt arrythmias that cause sudden death. This was, for example, documented in sudden deaths in the Caribbean after its victims were frightened by a voodoo curse.[49]

Worry has been related to high blood pressure in a number of studies. Some of the most convincing ones involved animals in the laboratory. In one, researchers confined monkeys in a cage in which they had to press a bar once every twenty seconds for twelve hours a day to avoid electrical shocks. After a few months, the monkeys developed high blood pressure. Researchers removed the bar from the cage and stopped delivering electrical shocks. What happened then was the real surprise: the monkeys' blood pressure skyrocketed!

Apparently, the monkeys worried constantly about not being able to avoid the shocks, even though none was delivered. Examinations of the monkeys showed that the arteries to the skin, kidneys, intestines, and muscles were tightly contracted, causing tremendous increases in blood pressure.[50]

A similar thing happened when researchers placed mice in a room with a cat that was confined in a cage. The cat was never let out of the cage and was never allowed or enabled to chase the mice. Within six to twelve months, the mice all developed high blood pressure. They apparently were worried about the cat, and their constant worrying caused high blood pressure.[51]

Worry and Asthma

In primary care medical clinics, two-thirds of those with asthma have an anxiety or depression disorder.[52] From scientific tests, we know that the emotion of worry causes the body to produce the chemical acetylcholine, which causes the airways to contract. When excess acetylcholine is secreted, the effect on the lungs is asthma. The muscles around the bronchioles constrict so tightly that air can no longer flow freely through them. Another important mechanism for anxiety triggering asthma involves the serotonin system, which can also trigger smooth muscle spasm in the airways. Central serotonin function runs low in people with anxiety disorders. When central nervous system serotonin function is low, a serotonin receptor called 5-HT$_2$ up-regulates—that is, becomes more sensitive. When stimulated, this hypersensitive receptor causes smooth muscle spasm, as seen not only in asthma but also in blood vessels,[53] bowel,[54] and bladder[55] (causing such common medical problems as irritable bowel or bladder problems and headaches).[56]

Obviously, then, anxiety can have a significant impact on victims of asthma. In one study, researchers simply told a group of asthmatics that they were being exposed to pollens and other aggravating agents. Then the researchers stood back and watched what happened. More than half of the asthmatics developed a full-blown asthma attack, even though no pollens or other irritants were actually present. Worry that it would happen triggered the attack.[57]

In a similar study, children with asthma were observed to determine the effect of various emotions on their illness. Most saw their parents as overbearing or rejecting, and these children constantly worried that they might not measure up or be accepted. To test a theory, researchers sent the parents on a paid vacation. They left the children with trained observers and watched what happened in the parents' absence. Half of the children improved dramatically without any other treatment. They stopped worrying, and their blood levels of acetylcholine diminished.[58]

One study of asthma patients found that stress-reduction techniques (relaxation and visualization coupled with thinking differently about the stressor) were as effective as airway dilator (relaxant) medication in preventing asthma attacks.

The Effects of Uncertainty

One specific kind of worry, uncertainty, has been shown to create a particularly devastating kind of stress. Uncertainty is defined as not knowing. It's being confronted with a complex situation that the person can't figure out. It's confusion over what is meant by a person or situation. It's a situation that is not predictable and, therefore, a situation in which the individual can't determine how to act. If it gets confusing enough or unpredictable enough, it can cause feelings of futility or helplessness and can lead to considerable distress.[59] The brain seems to require ways of viewing the world (paradigms) that give a sense of how to control whatever comes up. (Even if the constructed world view is erroneous, there is a strong desire to hold onto it and great resistance to giving it up.) When events occur that don't fit the paradigm, the result is uncertainty. Feelings of chaos ensue. If you always feel the need to control what happens, you can become extremely unnerved by the uncertainty. Fear and anxiety result.

It is possible to have an internal sense of control even when you can't control external events. Later we will describe how to be comfortable with—even intrigued by—uncertainty.

Studies involving uncertainty prove the point. One researcher studied a group of 100 patients in a Veterans Administration hospital. Each had rated an upcoming event—treatment, surgery, or the like—as being extremely stressful. When the researcher probed into each patient's situation, however, he found an amazing thing: The patients were not really stressed over the event itself. They were stressed because of uncertainty. They did not have enough information about the event. They didn't feel they knew exactly what was going to happen to them. They didn't really understand the outcome. It was the uncertainty, not the event itself, that caused all the upset.[60] Now, several well-controlled studies of providing information before surgery, detailing what to expect and what to do about it, have been shown to significantly improve surgical outcomes such as complications, time spent in the hospital, and costs. Similarly, for women delivering babies, a woman at the bedside who conveys support and knowledge about what to expect greatly improves obstetrical outcomes[61] (see Chapter 21).

Uncertainty keeps a person in a constant state of arousal, putting a heavy burden on the body's ability to adapt to stress. It's the same reason that predictable pain is so much less stressful: You are capable of learning when it is safe to "lower your guard" and relax. Not knowing when a pain or a shock is coming means having to stay on guard—tensed and stressed—all the time.

A series of studies demonstrates the effect of uncertainty. A report by the British Health Service monitored the prevalence of peptic ulcers during World War II, when England was being bombed frequently by enemy planes.[62] People living in the center of London, where the bombings were regular and predictable, suffered a 50 percent increase in the rate of gastric ulcers. In contrast, the increase in ulcer rate among residents on the outskirts of the city, where the bombings were extremely unpredictable, was six times greater than among the residents of London's central district.

In an experiment in New Jersey, two psychologists divided a group of laboratory rats into two groups.[63] Rats in the first group were given electrical shocks at random and without warning. Rats in the second group were also given electrical shocks, but were warned of the impending shock shortly before each one was delivered. The rats that were given unpredictable shocks developed gastric complications at a significantly greater rate than the rats whose shocks were predictable.

It works likewise with people. A psychologist in New York interviewed college students and kept track of their health histories during the year.[64] He noted not only when the students reported being sick but also the circumstances that preceded and surrounded the episodes of illness. He found that they reported being sick most often following events in their lives that were undesirable. Furthermore, most of the sickness followed events that were not only undesirable but also left the students uncertain about how much control they had.

Other studies show that undesirable life events and uncertainty are a deadly combination. Undesirable life events alone don't usually result in illness nor do uncontrollable life events about which we are uncertain. However, when the two are paired up—when events are both undesirable and unpredictable—there is a "significant impact" on health that usually results in illness.[65]

All of this suggests the value of learning the ways that highly resilient people view uncertainty. The approach is based on hope and on enjoying challenge. Much of future life is uncertain. Trying too hard to control it, particularly when its details are uncontrollable, will be fraught with frustration and then anxiety. Studies of resilient people show that they enjoy a new challenge and fully expect to creatively solve problems as they arrive.[66] The process of uncertainty for them involves an opportunity to learn, to create, and to once again rise to the occasion. Resilient people see chaos as an opportunity to shake off old ruts and move to a new, higher level of capability. Most of us sail along in a comfortable rut until something arises that we can't comprehend with our old world view and habitual responses. This provokes chaos. Three things tend to give a sense of control during chaos: loving support, hope (for something better at the end), and sensing the higher purpose of the chaotic experience (in other words, rising to a wiser, stronger, even more compassionate way of dealing with things.) At the other end of the chaos, we tend to settle into a new (and better) comfortable "rut"—until we face a new chaotic transition in the future. As the cycle repeats, it is part of the process of getting better and better at dealing well with life—and when you see it in this larger context, you can even begin to enjoy the challenge of uncertainty. This is the process of turning distress into eustress (see Chapter 2), and the result is better health.[67]

The Health Consequences of Fear

When worry escalates, the result is fear. Everyone has experienced fear. A swimmer of only moderate skill might be afraid of swift waters; a child might be afraid of the dark. (The swimmer or the child has not yet developed a sense of control— a "comfortable rut"—for dealing with the frightening situations.) A hiker will probably experience fear when hearing the distinctive warning of a rattlesnake; a jogger might feel fear when confronted with the bared fangs of a Doberman pinscher. According to Norman Cousins, "Fear and panic create negative expectations." Then, he says, "One tends to move in the direction of one's expectations."[68] Fear causes the heart to race, the head to spin, the palms to sweat, the knees to buckle, and breathing to become labored. The level of arousal that results is similar to the effects of stress, and the human body can't withstand it indefinitely.

Fear floods the system with stress hormones such as epinephrine. Its most powerful effect is on the heart: Both the rate and strength of contractions increase. Blood pressure soars. The body is stimulated to release other hormones, which act on various other organs and systems. In essence, the body is put on alert. If the fear is intense enough, all systems can even fatally overload.

Medical history is replete with examples of people who were literally frightened to death.[69] Take, for instance, Pearl Pizzamiglio. Fifteen minutes after she started the 11 PM shift at the In-Town Motor Hotel in Chevy Chase, Maryland, Michael Stewart walked in with another man. Stewart handed her a paper bag with a note that said, "Don't say a word. Put all the money in this bag and no one will get hurt." Pizzamiglio put $160 in the paper bag, the men fled, and she called the police. Two hours later, Pearl Pizzamiglio, aged sixty, free of any history of heart problems, was dead of heart failure. Stewart was arrested and charged with murder; the jury decided that, indeed, a simple paper bag and a piece of paper could be considered instruments of death. Stewart had, literally, scared Pizzamiglio to death.

In another incident, Barbara Reyes was spending her Memorial Day weekend floating on a raft on Georgia's peaceful Lake Lanier. The calm of the peaceful, warm afternoon was shattered when a man riding a motorized jet ski roared within a foot of the 40-year-old Reyes. In a panic, Reyes paddled to shore, collapsed, and died. Randolph Simpson, the Gwinnett County coroner who examined Reyes, said, "There's no question she was literally scared to death." The man who roared by on the jet ski was arrested and charged with involuntary manslaughter.

One 45-year-old man died of fright as he stepped to a podium to give a speech. An elderly man sitting on his lawn collapsed and died when a car jumped the curb and appeared to be headed straight for him. Panamanian dictator Omar Torrijos reportedly amused himself by killing a prisoner with an unloaded gun; the sound of the blanks firing was enough to scare the man to death. And in the year 840 AD, Bavarian Emperor Louis died of fright when he saw a solar eclipse. While such examples are unusual, they illustrate the adverse power fear can have.

The physical effects of fear are the same whether the fear is perfectly understandable or illogical. A surge of catecholamines occurs. When dogs are injected with catecholamines, the hormones released in response to fear, they die. Autopsies reveal certain characteristic lesions on the surface of the heart, presumably an effect of the catecholamines. The same lesions are visible under microscopic examination on the hearts of 80 percent of all victims of sudden cardiac death. While much of the evidence on being scared to death is anecdotal, some is very scientific. Consider, for example, the monitoring of Air Force test pilots. Eliot studied scientific documentation from five separate incidents.

In each, Air Force test pilots lost control of their aircraft and were not able to eject. "Their electrocardiograms were being monitored from the ground," Eliot points out. "These people died before they hit the ground, and they died of fright."[70]

One of the most dramatic examples was provided by Bernard Lown, a renowned Harvard cardiologist who witnessed an incredible incident involving a middle-aged woman who had been hospitalized with tricuspid stenosis, a non–life-threatening narrowing of a heart valve. As they were making their rounds one morning, doctors entered this woman's room. Her physician turned to Lown and the other doctors who were gathered around her bedside and announced, "This woman has TS." The doctors then left the room. The woman for some reason decided that TS meant "terminal situation." She began to hyperventilate and sweat profusely, and her pulse shot up to 150. Upon learning of her fear, her doctor tried to explain and calm her, but in vain. She died later the same day of heart failure.[71]

Some of the strongest of all fears are phobias, fears that are irrational and inappropriate. A phobia is an intense fear of an object or situation that would not frighten most people. Victims of phobia become almost immobilized, rearranging their entire life to avoid the feared object or place. One of the most common phobias is agoraphobia, or fear of going out into open spaces (stores, restaurants, theaters—anywhere outside a "safe" place, like home). Other phobias include fear of being trapped in a cramped space, fear of speaking in public, fear of dogs, fear of eating in public, fear of heights, and fear of blood. An estimated 13 million Americans have a phobia of some kind.[72] Many phobias begin first with the unprovoked attacks of panic disorder (a spontaneous neurochemical event). Others can arise from a terrifying traumatic experience.

When a phobic person encounters the feared object or situation, the result is fear—sometimes even a panic attack or phobia attack—and the effect on the body is the same as the well-known fight-or-flight response. In this case, the emphasis is on flight. The most severe physical reactions may occur before an encounter with the dreaded object or situation. The mere anticipation of what might happen is enough to set off the full attack.

The Origins of Fear

Where does fear primarily come from? It is as though we have two minds. One mind, which develops early in life, is caught up in ego issues. The ego sees each of us as separate and competing, and it compares and judges. A great deal of fear comes from the need to protect the ego self: "Am I okay?" "How do I compare?" "Am I acceptable?" "Am I a success or failure?" "Why did they offend me?" Because of the ego, each of us is highly conditioned to see the world through eyes of fear.

On the other hand, we have a deeper, wiser mind and self—one that feels connected and caring; one that sees beauty in the world around us; one that is able to see purpose in whatever comes up. In the face of criticism, the ego mind becomes fearful and angry—but the wise mind accepts the criticism as useful feedback and responds from a place of security with compassion to the concerns of the criticizer. The ego mind feels insecure; the wise mind feels strong and interested and is even able to smile at the funny things the ego does to feel important. You can tell which mind you are coming from at any given moment by whether you are feeling fear or compassion.

Just being aware if the difference between these two minds starts the process of moving from fear to compassion. Simply labeling your fearful thoughts as your ego trying to defend itself moves you to the larger, wise mind and self (it is your larger mind that is doing the labeling). Making this shift in sense of self is the real way to create thinking that gets rid of chronic fear and anxiety. If you'd like to know more about this important process, you might want to read some useful books on this important process—including *The Four Agreements* by Don Miguel Ruiz, *The Seven Spiritual Laws of Success* by Deepak Chopra, and *The New Earth* by Eckhart Tolle.

What to Do About Worry and Anxiety

If you're a worrier, can you stop? Clinical researchers suggest the following techniques:[73]

- Learn to solve problems. According to Dr. Timothy A. Brown, associate director of the Center for Stress and Anxiety Disorders at the State University of New York, most worriers jump from one topic to another without reaching any solutions. To reduce uncertainty, contemplate exactly what you would do if the worst possible scenario occurred—have a plan. Then go to work to create an outcome that is not the worst. For example, if you are constantly worrying about finances, set up a budget or savings plan.

- Create wiser, more rational ways of thinking. Become aware that situations themselves do not stress you—but the way you think about those situations does. Pennsylvania State University's Jennifer L. Abel says that doesn't mean seeing the world through rose-colored glasses. Worriers, she points out, see the world through cracked glasses: "Our goal is to give people clear glasses, so they see things more accurately." More mature, rational thinking about the same situation creates far less anxiety. If anxiety is significantly interfering with your life, counseling can be very helpful in guiding your new thinking process.

- Quiet physical stress by paying attention to your breathing, especially as you feel the "letting go" as you breathe out. Focusing on your breathing helps your irrational thoughts to dissipate. While you are in this more focused state, identify wise ways of responding to the situation—ways you would greatly admire. Then visualize yourself responding in these wiser ways. In your mind's eye, fully experience this new way of thinking and responding. Repeat the visualization for that specific event several times. Then do the same for other worrisome situations. Before long, the new responses begin to feel more natural, more like the real you, and the worry disappears. Visualizing can often best be done in two phases: First, watch yourself in a movielike picture "out there," doing it the new way. Then, when you feel good about that, see yourself doing it in your mind's eye, with all the new sensations and feelings that come from experiencing the new response.

- Let go of catastrophizing. Remember the Law of Expectations: Picturing the catastrophe (worry) is like practicing failure. Practice visualizing success instead. Imagine how a wise, capable person might handle this situation, and then visualize yourself doing it that way.

- Focus on what's going on right now. Stay completely in the present moment, which, after all, is the only moment that is both real and in which you have some sense of personal control. You can't control the past or the future—which is what you worry about the most. Practices that move you into the present moment also allow you to set aside your fearful ego thoughts as you move to the deeper, wiser self.

  Worry is almost always future-oriented. This may explain why practicing "mindfulness" can be so helpful: that is, to focus on what's going on right now in the present moment, not the future or the past, but how to be with whatever is arising here and now. Dr. Jon Kabat-Zinn has demonstrated significantly improved health outcomes from the highly successful stress-reduction program he created at the University of Massachusetts. His program is built primarily around the principle of learning how to stay in the present moment (mindfulness).[74] Methods for learning this are described in detail in his book *Full Catastrophe Living* and also in the works of Thich Nhat Hanh.[75] The Harvard Mind Body Clinic also focuses on learning this technique to elicit the relaxation response.[76] Achieving central nervous system quieting from mindfulness involves practicing meditative methods: It begins with focusing on the breath or a mantralike sound or word and learning to be able to choose where to give your attention (disregarding distractions). Feeling the power of giving attention wherever you choose increases the personal sense of control.

- It seems odd, but it works: Dr. Michael Vasey, assistant professor of psychology at Ohio State University, has joined a number of other researchers in advising people to set aside a worry period, a specific period of time every day (researchers suggest thirty minutes). During that entire period, focus completely on your worry and try to think of solutions to your problems. According to Vasey, "If you practice focusing on worries and thinking of solutions for 30 minutes each day for several weeks, your anxiety starts to taper off. You'll get better at generalizing solutions or realize it's not worth worrying about." Unload the worries: Write down first steps to the solutions, and tomorrow's to-do list, well before going to bed.

- Be sure to get enough sleep (seven to eight hours for most people).

- Exercise regularly. Physical activity dissipates energy that you unnecessarily pour into stressful thoughts, and it raises the neurotransmitters that, when too low, contribute to anxiety.

- Keep in mind that many anxiety *disorders*, such as panic disorder, generalized anxiety disorder, obsessive compulsive disorder, or posttraumatic stress disorder, particularly if depression is also present, may also need a course of medication (usually "antidepressants") to help correct the underlying biochemical abnormalities.

The longer anxiety and worry go without some kind of intervention, the more difficult they are to reverse. Anxiety is very treatable, particularly if treated early, and doing so not only improves symptoms but also helps to prevent its many medical problems.

WHAT DID YOU LEARN?

1. What is somatization?

2. What is the difference between generalized anxiety and panic disorders?

3. In addition to anxiety, what are three or more common physical manifestations of a hypersensitized nervous system?

4. Name two neurotransmitters that quiet responses to stimuli, and name two that magnify such responses.

5. What causes fear even more than the concerning situation itself?

6. What is the difference between ego mind thinking and the thoughts and attitudes of the deeper, wise mind? Which causes most anxiety?

7. Describe five things you can do to reduce anxiety.

ENDNOTES

1. Sharon Faelten, David Diamond, and the editors of *Prevention, Take Control of Your Life: A Complete Guide to Stress Relief* (Emmaus, PA: Rodale Press, 1988).

2. "Worrying Well," *Berkeley Wellness Letter* (June 1993).

3. A. Ohman, "Fear and Anxiety: Evolutionary, Cognitive, and Clinical Perspectives." In M. Lewis & J. M. Haviland-Jones (Eds.), *Handbook of Emotions.* (pp. 573–593). New York: The Guilford Press. (2000).

4. M. E. P. Seligman, E. F. Walker, and D. L. Rosenhan, *Abnormal Psychology*, 4th ed. (New York: W.W. Norton & Company, Inc., 2001).

5. See the discussion of anxiety disorders at the National institutes of Health website, accessed at: http://www.nimh.nih.gov/health/topics/anxiety-disorders/index.shtml

6. Amy H. Berger, "Are You a Chronic Worrier?" *Complete Woman* (October 1987): 58.

7. Ibid.

8. Faelten, Diamond, and the editors of *Prevention, Take Control of Your Life.*

9. Cathy Perlmutter, "Conquer Chronic Worry," *Prevention* (November 1993): 75.

10. "Worrying Well."

11. Susan Ince, "People Who Worry Too Much," *Weight Watchers Women's Health and Fitness News* (1990), 3.

12. R. Spitzer et al., *Diagnostic and Statistical Manual IV* (Washington, DC: American Psychiatric Association, 1998).

13. N. L. Smith and John Shavers, "Physical Symptoms Highly Predictive of Depression and Anxiety," presented at the American Psychosomatic Society annual meeting, *Psychosomatic Medicine* APS abstracts 1996.

14. J. Shavers, *The Identification of Depression and Anxiety in a Medical Outpatient Setting and Their Correlation to Presenting Physical Complaints* (PhD dissertation, University of Utah, 1996).

15. P. P. Roy-Byrne, "Generalized Anxiety and Mixed Anxiety-Depression: Association with Disability and Health Care Utilization," *Journal of Clinical Psychiatry* 57, suppl. 7: 86–91.

16. Berger, "Are You a Chronic Worrier?" 58.

17. Spitzer et al., *Diagnostic and Statistical Manual IV.*
18. Ibid.
19. Ibid.
20. Smith and Shavers, "Physical Symptoms Highly Predictive of Depression and Anxiety."
21. K. Kroenke, et al., "Physical Symptoms in Primary Care. Predictors of Psychiatric Disorders and Functional Impairment," *Archives of Family Medicine* 3 (1994): 774–79; K. Kroenke and A. D. Manglesdorff, "Common Symptoms in Primary Care: Incidence, Evaluation, Therapy and Outcome," *American Journal of Medicine* 86 (1989): 262–66; K. Kroenke and J. G. Rosmalen, "Symptoms, Syndromes and the Value of Psychiatric Diagnostics in Patients Who Have Functional Somatic Disorders," *Medical Clinics of North America* 90 (2006): 603–26.
22. Winifred Gallagher, "Treating the Worried Well," *American Health* (January–February 1988): 36.
23. Carol Turkington, "Help for the Worried Well," *Psychology Today* (August 1987).
24. Ibid.
25. Ibid.
26. V. Maletic, et al., "Neurobiology of Depression," *International Journal of Clinical Practice* 61 (2007): 2030–40.
27. Will Stapp, "Imagine Yourself Well," *Medical Self-Care* (January–February 1988): 27–30.
28. Smith, and Shavers, "Physical Symptoms Highly Predictive of Depression and Anxiety."
29. L.S. Linn and J. Yager, "Recognition of Depression and Anxiety by Primary Care Physicians," *Psychosomatics* 25 (1984): 593–5, 599–600.
30. W. Katon et al., "Distressed High Utilizers of Medical Care," *General Hospital Psychiatry* 12 (1990): 355–62.
31. S. F. Dworkin, M. Von Korff, and L. LeResche, "Multiple Pains and Psychiatric Disturbance: An Epidemiological Investigation," *Archives of General Psychiatry* 47 (1990): 239–44.
32. A. I. Terr, "Environmental Illness: A Clinical Review of 50 Cases," *Archives of Internal Medicine* 146 (1986): 145–49.
33. N. Breslau and G. C. Davis, "Migraine, Physical Health, and Psychiatric Disorder: A Prospective Epidemiological Study in Young Adults," *Journal of Psychiatric Research* 27 (1993): 211–21.
34. T. Dammen, et al. "Panic Disorder in Chest Pain Patients Referred for Cardiological Outpatient Investigation," *Journal of Internal Medicine* 245, no. 5 (1999): 497–507.
35. W. Katon et al., "Chest Pain: Relationship of Psychiatric Illness to Coronary Arteriographic Results," *American Journal of Medicine* 84 (1988): 1–9. Also see R. Mayou, "Non-cardiac Chest Pain and Benign Palpitations in the Cardiac Clinic," *British Heart Journal* 72 (1994): 548–53; and D. Beltman, et al., "Panic Disorder in Patients with Chest Pain and Angiographically Normal Coronary Arteries," *American Journal of Cardiology* 63 (1989): 1399.
36. I. Varia, et al., "Randomized trial of sertraline in patients with unexplained chest pain of noncardiac origin," *American Heart Journal* 140 (2000): 367–72.
37. R. B. Lydiard, M. D. Fossey, W. Marsh, and J. C. Ballenger, "Prevalence of Psychiatric Disorders in Patients with Irritable Bowel Syndrome," *Psychosomatics* 34 (1993): 229–34; and E. A. Walker, P. P. Roy-Byrne, and W. J. Katon, "Irritable Bowel Syndrome and Psychiatric Illness," *American Journal of Psychiatry* 147 (1990): 565–72.
38. G. Magni et al., "DSM-III Diagnoses Associated with Dyspepsia of Unknown Cause," *American Journal of Psychiatry* 144 (1987): 1222–23.
39. P. Poitras et al., "Evolution of Visceral Sensitivity in Patients with Irritable Bowel Syndrome," *Digestive Diseases and Sciences* 47, no. 4 (2002): 914–20; R. E. Clouse, et al, "Clinical Correlates of Abnormal Sensitivity to Intraesophageal Balloon Distension," *Digestive Disease Science* 36 no.8 (1991): 1040–50 and J. E. Richter, et al., "Abnormal Sensory Perception in Patients with Esophageal Chest Pain," *Gastroenterology* 91 no. 4 (1986): 845–52.

40. T. N. Wise, J. N. Cooper, and S. Ahmed, "The Efficacy of Group Therapy for Patients with Irritable Bowel Syndrome," *Psychosomatics* 23(1982): 465–69. Also Poitras, "Evolution of Visceral Sensitivity."

41. D. A. Drossman, "Review Article: An Integrated Approach to the Irritable Bowel Syndrome," *Alimentary Pharmacology & Therapeutics* 13, suppl. 2 (1999): 3–14.

42. R. E. Clouse and P. J. Lustman, "Psychiatric Illness and Contraction Abnormalities of the Esophagus," *New England Journal of Medicine* 309 (1983): 1337–42.

43. A. J. Barsky, P. D. Cleary, R. R. Coeytaux, and J. N. Ruskin, "Psychiatric Disorders in Medical Outpatients Complaining of Palpitations," *Journal of General Internal Medicine* 9 (1994): 306–13.

44. Katon et al., "Chest Pain," 1–9. (Of chest pain patients with normal coronary angiograms, 43 percent had panic disorder and 36 percent had major depression.) Similar results were found by B. Beitman, V. Mukerji, J. W. Lamberti, et al., "Panic Disorder in Patients with Chest Pain and Angiographically Normal Coronary Arteries," *American Journal of Cardiology* 63 (1989): 1399–403.

45. D. L. Goldenberg, "Psychological Symptoms and Psychiatric Diagnosis in Patients with Fibromyalgia," *Journal of Rheumatology* 16, suppl. 19 (1989): 127–30; and T. A. Ahles, M. B. Yunus, and A. T. Masi, "Is Chronic Pain a Variant of Depressive Disease? The Case of Primary Fibromyalgia Syndrome," *Pain* 29 (1987): 105–11.

46. P. B. Polatin, et al., "Psychiatric Illness and Chronic Low-Back Pain. The Mind and the Spine—Which Goes First?" *Spine* 18 (1993): 66–71.

47. I. J. Russell, H. Vaeroy, M. Javors, and F. Nyberg, "Cerebrospinal Fluid Biogenic Amine Metabolites in Fibromyalgia Syndrome and Rheumatoid Arthritis," *Arthritis & Rheumatism* 35 (1992): 550–56.

48. "Heart Attack: Can You Worry Yourself to Death?" *Medical Abstracts Newsletter* (November 1988): 3.

49. Robert S. Eliot, *Is It Worth Dying For? How to Make Stress Work For You—Not Against You* (Bantam, 1989).

50. J. P. Henry, J. P. Meehan, and P. M. Stephens, "The Use of Psychosocial Stimuli to Induce Prolonged Systolic Hypertension in Mice," *Psychosomatic Medicine* 29 (1967): 408–32; R. P. Forsyth, "Blood Pressure Responses to Long-Term Avoidance Schedules in the Restrained Rhesus Monkey," *Psychosomatic Medicine* 31 (1969): 300; and R. P. Forsyth, "Regional Blood Flow Changes During 72-Hour Avoidance Schedules in the Monkey," *Science* 173 (1971): 546.

51. Henry et al., "The Use of Psychosocial Stimuli."

52. Shavers, *The Identification of Depression and Anxiety.*

53. P. M. Vanhoutte, "Serotonin, Hypertension and Vascular Disease," *Netherlands Journal of Medicine* 38, nos. 1–2 (1991): 35–42; and A. E. Doyle, "Serotonin Antagonists and Vascular Protection," *Cardiovascular Drugs & Therapy* 4, suppl. 1 (1990): 13–18.

54. G. Engel, D. Hoyer, H. O. Kalkman, and M. B. Wick, "Identification of 5HT2-Receptors on Longitudinal Muscle of the Guinea Pig Ileum," *Journal of Receptor Research* 4, nos. 1–6 (1984): 113–26.

55. M. L. Cohen, "Canine, but Not Rat Bladder Contracts to Serotonin via Activation of 5HT2 Receptors," *Journal of Urology* 143, no. 5 (1990): 1037–40.

56. A. Srikiatkhachorn and M. Anthony, "Serotonin Receptor Adaptation in Patients with Analgesic-Induced Headache," *Cephalalgia* 16, no. 6 (1996): 419–22; and P. J. Goadsby and J. W. Lance, "Physiopathology of Migraine," *La Revue du praticien* 40, no. 5 (1990): 389–93.

57. T. J. Luparello et al., "The Interaction of Psychologic Stimuli and Pharmacologic Agents in Airway Reactivity in Asthmatic Subjects," *Psychosomatic Medicine* 5 (1970): 500.

58. K. Purcell et al., "Effect on Asthma in Children of Experimental Separation from the Family," *Psychosomatic Medicine* 31 (1969): 144.

59. Phillip L. Rice, *Stress and Health: Principles and Practice for Coping with Wellness* (Monterey, CA: Brooks/Cole Publishing, 1987), 80–81.

60. Ibid.

61. J. Kennell, et al., "Continuous Emotional Support During Labor in a U.S. Hospital: A Randomized Controlled Trial," *Journal of the American Medical Association* 265 (1991): 2197–201.

62. Rice, *Stress and Health,* 80–81.

63. Ibid.

64. Ibid.

65. Ibid.

66. Suzanne Ouellette Kobasa, "How Much Stress Can You Survive?" *American Health* (September 1984): 67.

67. Aaron Antonovsky, *Unraveling the Mystery of Health: How People Manage Stress and Stay Well* (San Francisco: Jossey-Bass, 1987), 36–37.

68. Norman Cousins, *The Healing Heart* (New York: W. W. Norton, 1983).

69. Examples are from Edward Dolnick, "Scared to Death," *Hippocrates* (March–April 1989): 106–8.

70. Ibid.

71. Ibid.

72. Faelten et al., *Take Control of Your Life,* 97.

73. Perlmutter, "Conquer Chronic Worry," 76–80.

74. Jon Kabat-Zinn, *Full Catastrophe Living* (New York: Delacorte Press, 1990).

75. Thich Nhat Hanh, *The Miracle of Mindfulness: A Manual of Meditation* (Boston: Beacon Press, 1976).

76. H. Benson and E. Stuart, *The Wellness Book* (New York: Carol Publishing Group, 1993).

CHAPTER 6

Depression, Despair, and Health

One who expects completely to escape low moods is asking the impossible. Like the weather, life is essentially variable, and a healthy person believes in the validity of his high hours even when he is having a low one.

—Harry Emerson Fosdick

LEARNING OBJECTIVES

- Identify the meaning and prevalence of depression.
- Explain the neurobiology of depression as it affects physical problems.
- Describe the effects of depression on body systems and health outcomes.
- Identify ways to treat and deal with depression.

Life is a series of natural ups and downs. Everyone who lives feels intermittent sadness and grief. While those intermittent sad moods can be depressing, they don't really constitute *clinical* depression.

A Definition

The word *depression* has several meanings:

1. As a normal human affect, it's caused by the disruption of normal life balance, loss, conflict, or trauma.

2. Depression can be a symptom of a physical illness or a side effect of medication.

3. Clinical depression is also a biological syndrome based on neurochemical abnormalities, often genetically based; this is the definition used throughout most of this chapter.

4. Finally, depression can be a combination of all three of the above definitions, and any of these types of depression can also follow a crisis.

Depression as an illness is not a normal reaction, but it can occur even without a clear reason. It is much more than an occasional sad mood. Usually in clinical depression, the pleasure centers in the brain don't work well, and the punishment centers are on overdrive, so even good things feel bad. This phenomenon causes the "perception error" of depression, where everything seems negative.

Sometimes depression involves quitting or just plain giving up. A person who is depressed feels that the present conditions and the future possibilities are intolerable. A more severely depressed person may even "go on strike" from life, doing less and less, losing interest in people, abandoning hobbies, and giving up at work because nothing feels pleasurable or good.[1]

The elusiveness of depression makes it difficult to define: it's not just one single condition with a simple cause. Steven Paul, chief of clinical neuroscience at the National Institute of Mental Health, says that depression is "like a fever, in that it's often an unspecific response to an internal or external insult. Like fever, it has a number of origins and treatments."[2]

Frederick Goodwin, when he was scientific director of the National Institute of Mental Health, says that depression is the richest, most striking example in psychiatry, and possibly in all of medicine, of the relationship between the mind and the body.[3] Another dramatic example of that connection is panic disorder (discussed in Chapter 5), which usually is highly associated with depression.

Rather than being a single illness or condition, many experts believe depression is a group of mood disorders that strike with varying intensity. No one yet has all the answers, but one thing is certain: Depression—together with its neurochemical cousin, anxiety— has some profound effects on who gets sick and, in particular, who comes to see the physician. Many of the neurochemical abnormalities, and thus medical illness connections, are similar in both depression and the anxiety disorders discussed in Chapter 5.

Have you ever wondered if you have clinical depression? The symptoms listed in Table 6.1 provide the clinical criteria that professionals use to diagnose depression; check to see how you stack up against those. Or, better still, answer the questions from the Patient Health Questionnaire (PHQ9) available online at http://www.treatmenthelps.org/treatmenthelps/PHQ9.pdf [4]

The PHQ9 is drawn from the PrimeMD Today questionnaire, which was carefully validated against detailed diagnostic interviews in large numbers of primary care medical patients.[5] The PHQ9 was found to be very reliable for making the diagnosis of clinical depression. Note that depressed mood isn't always the best indicator of depression; in fact, as only one of nine symptoms, it doesn't always have to be present with depression. Note that you must have five or more symptoms at least half the time for at least two weeks in order to be diagnosed with major clinical depression (Table 6.2). The presence of three or four symptoms suggests minor depression. If symptoms of minor depression persist consistently for two years or more, the condition is called chronic dysthymia.

The term *minor* can be misleading when it comes to depression. Minor depression that goes untreated over a long period of time can actually cause more medical problems than a brief period of much more severe depression (the neurophysiological reasons are discussed later in the chapter).

Table 6.1   Patient Health Questionnaire (PHQ9)

Over the last 2 weeks, how often have you been bothered by any of the following problems?				
	Not at All	**Several Days**	**More than Half the Days**	**Nearly Every Day**
• Little interest or pleasure in doing things				
• Feeling down, depressed, or hopeless				
• Trouble falling or staying asleep, or sleeping too much				
• Feeling tired or having little energy				
• Poor appetite or overeating				
• Feeling bad about yourself— or that you are a failure or have let yourself or your family down				
• Trouble concentrating on things, such as reading the newspaper or watching television				
• Moving or speaking so slowly that other people could have noticed. Or the opposite—being so fidgety or restless that you have been moving around a lot more than usual				
• Thoughts that you would be better off dead, or of hurting yourself in some way				

Source: R. L. Spitzer et al., "Validation and Utility of a Self-Report Version of PRIME-MD: The PHQ Primary Care Study," *Journal of the American Medical Association* 282 (1999): 1737–44.

Another important type of depression is the category of bipolar mood disorders, in which the mood fluctuates up and down more precipitously. The "ups" can be too excited, happy, or impulsive in a risky way—but they may also be characterized by agitation, irritability, and anger. In fact, a lot of chronic anger can result from the neurochemistry of depression.

In the PHQ9 test for clinical depression, you will notice several symptoms of dysregulated (too much or too little) basic "vegetative" functions such as appetite, sleep, or movement. A person who eats and sleeps too much may have "atypical depression," which is more likely to be bipolar in its mechanisms.

Table 6.2   DSM-IV Criteria

To diagnose major depressive disorder, for most days in the past two weeks one of the following two symptoms must be present:
• Depressed mood • Loss of interest or pleasure in most activities most days (called anhedonia)
In addition, four of the following symptoms must be present:
• Significant weight loss or gain • Insomnia or sleeping too much • Psychomotor agitation (restless, moving around too much) or psychomotor retardation (moving or speaking so slowly, it's noticeable) • Impaired concentration or decisiveness • Feelings of worthlessness or guilt • Recurrent thoughts of death or suicide • Fatigue or loss of energy

Source: The Diagnostic and Statistical Manual of Mental Disorders, 4th ed. (DSM-IV; Washington, DC: American Psychiatric Association, 1994).

Prevalence and Manifestations of Depression

Approximately 7 percent of all women and 3 percent of all men in the United States have major depression at any given time; another estimated 4 to 5 percent have minor depression; and an estimated 8 percent have major anxiety disorders. The percentages go even higher in winter and are steadily increasing over each decade. The percentage of individuals who have mental disorders at some point during their entire lifetimes is much higher.[6]

During their lifetimes, nearly one-fourth of all women suffer clinical depression.[7] The percentage of teenagers with diagnosed clinical depression has increased more than fivefold over the past 40 years.[8] Teenage depression is more likely to be bipolar, the kind that fluctuates in cycles, an important realization because bipolar problems need to be treated differently than major depression.

Medically, depression is a huge problem. Approximately one-fourth of all primary care medical patients come from the 15 percent of the population with major depression and anxiety disorders. That climbs to almost half of all patients if you include minor depression and anxiety disorders (like chronic dysthymia). An estimated 70 percent of depressed people also have a diagnosable anxiety disorder, and nearly a third have generalized anxiety disorder[9]—a condition characterized by nearly continuous background worry or anxiety. Almost half of the top 10 percent of those who use medical care are people with major depression.[10]

Only about one in three of those who are depressed are recognized and treated, and that drops to fewer than one in four of those with anxiety.[11] (We combine clinical depression and anxiety in this discussion because they so often overlap and because they appear to be caused by some of the same neurochemical abnormalities.) This lack of accurate diagnosis arises largely because depression and anxiety cause so many medical symptoms, and most patients don't want to recognize a "mental" component to their medical illness. The huge numbers of people whose underlying mental problems go untreated repeatedly return with complaints of medical problems. Treating the depression has proven to greatly reduce not only suffering and disability but also medical illness and its attendant costs (see Chapter 21).

People in all walks of life and of all ages suffer from depression. Even well-known people (such as Abraham Lincoln, Ernest Hemingway, Winston Churchill, Sylvia Plath, and Thomas Eagleton) and biblical figures (including Saul and Nebuchadnezzar) have suffered from the "black dog" of depression.[12] Depression occurs among the young— and when it does, it greatly increases the likelihood of physical illness and may lead to drug abuse or tobacco and alcohol dependence during adulthood.[13] Depression seems particularly rampant among downtrodden persons and women. According to Martin E. P. Seligman, "Women are twice as likely to suffer depression as men are, because, on the average, they think about problems in ways that amplify depression. . . . Women tend to contemplate their depression, mulling it over and over, trying to analyze it and determine its source."[14] That may lead to blaming others erroneously for the depressed feelings. Studies show that depression is more prevalent among people with poor social support and a dearth of supportive relationships.[15] Sometimes the biological depression makes such relationships much more difficult. Spouses will comment, "I'm damned if I do and damned if I don't. Anything I do will be seen as negative" (even giving a compliment). And then the disturbed relationship may be blamed for exacerbating the depression. Depression can lead to suicide. Some experts estimate that as many as 15 percent of those with untreated depression eventually resort to self-destruction.[16] The problem may be even more pronounced among the adolescent victims of depression, particularly those who are bipolar. Elliot S. Gershon, when he was chief of the clinical psychogenetics branch of the National Institute of Mental Health, stated

> The chilling fact is that we may be on the verge of an epidemic-like increase of mania, depression, and suicide. The trend is rising almost exponentially and shows no signs of letting up.[17]

His predictions have proven accurate. In 1990, clinical depression was the fourth leading cause of disability; and, in 2003, it was the leading cause of disability among American women. Based on increasing rates, by 2020 depression will be the first or second leading cause of all disability worldwide.[18]

According to several studies of the elderly, depression is often associated with illness, disability, isolation, bereavement, and poverty.[19] Furthermore, according to a study of more than 11,000 people published in the *Journal of the American Medical Association,* people with depression had worse physical, social, and role functioning and were in worse physical health. They suffered more bodily pain than did people with a chronic medical disease such as arthritis, back problems, gastrointestinal disease, or diabetes.[20]

Depressed people have five times the normal disability rates.[21] If you compare the most common chronic medical diseases, only severe heart or pulmonary failure comes close to depression in causing disability. Thus untreated depression causes huge costs to society. About a third of the costs are due to medical effects, but nearly two thirds is from lost productivity in the workplace.[22] Overall, costs of depression in the United

States in 1990 were estimated at $53 billion per year, and only about 10 percent of that was outpatient treatment costs.[23] When workplace costs were added, the figure was $77.4 billion. By 2000, the overall cost had remained relatively stable, despite the fact that depression treatment rates increased by 50 percent during that 10-year period. The increased treatment costs were countered by a fall in the workplace costs when treated workers became more productive.[24] (These figures don't include the costs of treating medical illness caused by undetected depression.)

In a worldwide survey of a quarter million people in sixty countries, depression had the largest effect of all illnesses on producing poor scores for overall health.[25] People with depression have two and a half times more physical illnesses and four times the normal mortality rate[26] (63 percent of that mortality is due to cardiovascular conditions). Additionally, medical patients often feel they are depressed because of the impact of their medical illness; but, interestingly, when the depression itself is treated, the physical problems often greatly improve. Unfortunately, only about 22 percent of those with clinical depression get even minimally adequate treatment.[27] Much of that lack of treatment is due to denial that one has depression or lack of awareness of the significant health and functional impact of depression among those who have it.

Causes of Depression

Most researchers today think that certain brain circuits are fragile and that this renders some people vulnerable to depression. That fragility is determined primarily by the deficient function of the neurotransmitter chemicals (such as serotonin, norepinephrine, and dopamine) that enable brain signals to be transmitted from one cell to the next. That deficiency of brain neurochemical function can often be genetic, and it may explain why depression sometimes runs in families. The familial tendency is real. One early but well-known study of the Amish in Pennsylvania showed that all 26 suicides between 1880 and 1980 were members of only four extended families.[28]

In commenting on the studies and the tendency of depression to run in families, John Mann, director of the laboratory of psychopharmacology at Cornell Medical College, explains, "Serotonin levels are under some genetic control to begin with, and this suicidal tendency appears to be an inherited biochemical trait."[29] To separate the genetic causes from depressed behavior learned from families, studies of identical twins adopted to different families have shown an obvious inheritance pattern, even among those raised by very upbeat families. Nevertheless, the cause is not entirely predetermined by genes, though heredity is an important factor in creating vulnerability to stress.

This interaction between stress and genetics was nicely demonstrated in a lengthy follow-up study in New Zealand. Genes for the "serotonin transporter" that removes serotonin from the connections between nerve cells (neural synapses) were found. Two types of gene alleles (short and long) were identified. Then the effect of stressful events on people with different inherited combinations of these genes was determined. If a person had two short alleles (one from each parent), they were much more vulnerable to stress causing clinical depression than if long alleles were inherited. If two long alleles were inherited, a person was much more stress resilient, with little depression developing despite much situational stress; the protection presumably created better serotonin function. This study seems to show that, rather than arguing over whether depression is inherited or learned by experience, both interact with each other in a very real way. These same serotonin transporter genetics predict suicidality[30] and can affect other mental illnesses as well.[31]

Other gene products related to neurochemicals are also important in determining a predisposition to depression. Examples include those that produce the serotonin receptor called $5\text{-}HT_2$, the dopamine transporter, the chemical COMT that affects the removal of norepinephrine and dopamine, brain-derived neurotrophic factor (BDNF, which helps thinking neurons to stay healthy), and corticotropin-releasing factor. Having one of these gene abnormalities creates some risk; having a combination of them creates a much higher likelihood of depression, particularly when the person is also exposed to stress.[32] Interestingly, these same gene abnormalities predispose a person to suffer an unusual amount of pain.[33]

Older theories (which have been criticized) say that depression primarily occurs as a result of a severe adverse life event or a series of less serious difficulties that gradually erode self-esteem. One scientist who believes that theory is Dr. George W. Brown of the Department of Social Policy and Social Science at the University of London's Royal Holloway and Bedford New College. Brown compiled the results of 10 different studies. They show, he says, that 88 percent of depressed women had experienced some recent severe life event or a "major difficulty" in their lives.[34]

Later, Brown studied that group of results, paying more attention to the details of the adverse life events suffered by the women. He reported a 15-fold difference in the predicted risk of depression between women who had the worst assortment of life events and those who reported no adverse life events at all during the period in which the study took place.[35] Again, these stressful events could be interacting with genetic vulnerability. Another possibility is that the neurochemical problems set up behavior that is more likely to provoke stressful events.

New understanding of the neurochemistry of depression and anxiety recognizes an important role for corticotropin-releasing hormone (CRH), the neuropeptide that activates the adrenal gland in response to stress. Long-lasting CRH and norepinephrine abnormalities can clearly be triggered by early-life traumatic events, which turn on the gene for CRH. The activated brain CRH then causes the nervous system to be excessively sensitive to stimuli and, in essence, to remain on guard for danger, even after the trauma is long gone.[36] The previously activated gene, cranking out CRH, has a hard time turning back off, even though there is no more trauma. If interventions to quiet things down are not used, the sensitized nervous system then overreacts to pain, stress, and other stimuli, sometimes indefinitely. We debate, "Is the depression caused by nature (genetics) or nurture (learned)?" but here we have a case of the nurture turning on the nature.

So which is the cause of depression, inherited neurochemistry or repeated negative experiences that cause both abnormal neurochemistry and a depressed habit pattern? Episodes of depression coming out of the blue, for no reason, certainly make a case for a neurochemical cause. Nevertheless, some further fascinating experiments in mental conditioning again suggest it may be both. Most people have heard of the classical mental conditioning experiments with Pavlov's dogs. Measurements of digestive processes (saliva, enzymes, etc.) were made when the dogs ate food. Then each time they ate, a bell was rung. Before long, the brain became conditioned to expect food when the bell rang; and, in a classic mind-body way, ringing the bell with no food elicited the digestive response (a mental expectation carried to cellular levels). Similarly, under unrelenting stress they cannot control, people and animals show depletion of brain serotonin activity. If the pattern is repeated several times in association with a certain place or situation, long after the stressor is gone, subsequent exposure to the same place or situation will cause a drop in serotonin function and a rise in CRH. Serotonin suppression becomes a conditioned response. (Once again, the body has an immense capacity to produce physiological responses that the brain "expects," including the depressive and physical effects of neurochemical changes.) In the case of learned, conditioned neurochemical changes likely to cause depression, the effect can combine with genetic predisposition to sustain even the biological depression. There is some evidence that repeated depressive episodes can even condition the enzymes that allow genes to express themselves physically to respond so as to lay down "hard-wired" neurological circuits that automatically create a depressed or hypersensitive response that is more resistant to treatment, the so-called kindling phenomenon.[37] Sometimes this phenomenon is called neuroplasticity, a hardwiring of neurons that are conditioned to overrespond to stimuli. The practical implication of this kindling over time is that these depression and anxiety (and pain) disorders need to be treated as early as possible to avoid their becoming hard-wired and thus more difficult to reverse.

This same kindling phenomenon shows up with increases in another neurotransmitter that contributes to depression, Substance P. Substance P is a pain-promoting transmitter that is found in high levels in association with depression and chronic stress and accounts for some of the excess pain and oversensitivity to stimuli seen in depression. Repeated pain conditions a nervous system to produce increasingly more Substance P, resulting in more chronic pain. Since both depression and chronic pain conditions have similar neurochemical abnormalities, one would then expect them to strongly overlap, as they do. Some ask whether the pain causes the depression or the depression causes the excessive chronic pain, but the fact is that both are caused by similar neurochemical abnormalities in the central nervous system.

New concepts currently are developing that suggest some depression could be the result of immune and inflammatory system activation.[38] These observers even speculate that lingering viruses (such as cytomegalovirus) play a role in creating clinical depression,[39] much like the depressed and achy feelings one has with the flu. This becomes confusing in the chicken-and-egg sense; does the inflammatory activation trigger depression, or does depression trigger the inflammatory and immune activation (or do they both trigger each other)?[40] Antidepressant medications reduce the increased inflammation seen with depression.[41] When treated with medications that powerfully reduce inflammation, people with inflammatory arthritis find that their depression improves.[42] Recent proposals have been made to treat depression primarily by reducing the inflammatory response,[43] but adequate studies have not yet been done.

One theory about the cause of depression combines a variety of perspectives. Psychiatrists Hagop Akiskal, Director of the International Mood Center at the San

Diego Veterans Administration Medical Center, and William McKinney, Jr., of the University of Wisconsin proposed the following:

> Assume, first, that a person is genetically susceptible to depression, meaning that certain circuits in the brain areas particularly concerned with pleasure and rewarding experiences are chemically fragile and somewhat easily upset. Give that person some early traumatic experiences and undermine confidence and self-esteem, such as the loss of or separation from a parent at a critical stage of development. Add the kind of psychological stress later in life that echoes the early loss and places unusual demands on the already vulnerable reward system. (Events are particularly likely to affect people with few social supports—family, friends or lovers.) The brain's response to this is felt as a diminished ability to experience emotion, including pleasure. Paradoxically, this lack of emotion, this emptiness, is deeply felt and incredibly painful. At the same time, activity decreases, as do sociability and the opportunity for pleasure and rewards: one tries less, gets less and feels worse.[44]

One other important consideration in the onset of depression is poor nutrition. Amino acids such as tryptophan (which converts to serotonin in the brain) or tyrosine (which converts to norepinephrine) are essential and also require certain vitamins (such as B_6 and B_{12}) that make up the neurochemicals. Deficiencies of these nutrients can also lead to a "chemical" depression.[45] (See Chapter 20 for detailed information on nutrition.) Patients who have responded well to antidepressants, and are then deprived of these nutrients, relapse back into depression while still taking the antidepressant medication.[46] Such medications need these building blocks to work, and people who lack the nutrients may develop depression that responds to their replacement.

Characteristics of Depression

Depression has been called the common cold of mental illness;[47] and, like the common cold, it can have a variety of symptoms that reflect the entire spectrum of severity. In some cases of depression, the few symptoms are quite mild; in others, a host of symptoms are quite severe. Medical symptoms that cannot be clearly attributed to organic disease are especially likely to be due to the neurobiology of depression and anxiety disorders.[48] (See Table 6.3.)

These symptoms are not imagined; rather, they arise from a very real physiological dysregulation that occurs when the midbrain (particularly the mesolimbic system) no longer effectively controls those operations, as happens in persons with depression or anxiety disorders. Normal physical function gets out of balance as do mood and arousal, when the part of the mesolimbic brain that exerts control is not working properly. Again, some chemical neurotransmitters that largely govern function of that part of the brain are serotonin, norepinephrine, and dopamine, the same chemicals that are deficient in persons who suffer depression or anxiety.

The mesolimbic system harbors both the pleasure and punishment centers. When the pleasure center is stimulated electrically, a great euphoria is felt. Animals can become addicted to self-stimulating the pleasure center, even to the point of starving to death while they continue the stimulation. The same effect can be obtained by injecting

Table 6.3 Prevalence of Major Depression and Anxiety Disorders in Medical Patients with Organically Unexplained Symptoms

Symptoms	Unexplained (%)	Depression (%)	Anxiety (%)
Headache	48	53	44
Chest Pain	36	66	66
Back Pain	30	53	40
Joint Pain	26	58	48
Shortness of breath	25	64	44
"Stomach" problems	46	46	40

Source: K. Kroenke and A. D. Manglesdorff, "Common Symptoms in Primary Care: incidence, Evaluation, Therapy and Outcome," *American Journal of Medicine* 86 (1989): 262–66 and K. Kroenke et al., "Physical Symptoms in Primary Care: Predictors of Psychiatric Disorders and Functional Impairment," *Archives of Family Medicine* 3 (1994):774–79.

dopamine (and sometimes serotonin); the natural release of these is the normal way that the pleasure centers are stimulated when pleasurable thoughts occur. When either chemical is deficient, you can't feel pleasure, even in situations that are normally very pleasurable. This anhedonia, the inability to experience pleasure, is the hallmark of a neurobiological depression.

On the other hand, if the punishment center in the midbrain is stimulated, a feeling of great dysphoria (unpleasantness, fear, and loss of control) occurs. When the punishment center in an animal is stimulated, the animal cowers, looks everywhere for danger, and, if the stimulus persists long enough, simply gives up. Because these centers are operated by a different set of neurotransmitters, they continue to work well, even excessively during depression.

What happens, then, for a depressed person? A normally pleasant event feels punishing rather than pleasurable, creating the perception error that makes everything, even good things, look grim. For example, someone gives a compliment; but, instead of feeling good, as was intended, a depressed recipient might even feel bad about it and say to herself, "Why did they feel they had to say that? Do I look needy or something? What do they really want out of me, anyway?" Thus a positive is converted to a negative, and usually people around them don't understand what's going on. It's a vicious cycle, because the distress that results compounds the neurochemical problem, which then intensifies the situational distress. The neurochemical imbalance negatively distorts thought, and the stressful thoughts exacerbate the neurochemical imbalance.

Simply stated, then, the illness called depression usually reflects a disturbance of mood that occurs when the pleasure centers of the brain are not working (or when the punishment centers are working overtime). This illness called depression can be much more, however; and, as mentioned earlier, depressed mood itself can be absent since it is only one component of the syndrome. In depression, the other automatic "vegetative" functions of the middle brain—appetite, sex drive, sleep, metabolism, energy regulation, modulation of hormone, and immune function—are also dysregulated.[49] The stress response itself is dysregulated, causing either too much of a response to a stimulus (anxiety disorder) or too little of a response ("psychomotor retardation").

This mental state can color the way a person feels and thinks until it affects virtually all the activities that are normally considered a part of daily life. The classic mood associated with depression is a combination of helplessness and hopelessness. Often, there is a disturbance in sleep patterns: a person may sleep much more than normal, may sleep at unusual times, may not be able to fall asleep, or may fall asleep easily but then awaken and be unable to fall back to sleep. Partly because of these sleep problems and partly as a result of the depression itself, the person may feel fatigued and lacking energy all the time. Sleep deficiency itself can trigger depression in a genetically predisposed person; when that happens, inadequate sleep and depression become a vicious cycle.

Many times, victims of depression also have eating problems. Some overeat, but many lose their appetite and suffer some weight loss. In many cases, depression leads to complete loss of the pleasure in eating. Many who are depressed sharply increase their alcohol consumption, particularly those who also suffer from anxiety.

In addition, a variety of physical complaints can accompany depression. Most depressed people experience a number of vague physical pains and complaints; some become frantically obsessed with their health and convinced that they are suffering from serious physical diseases. Many lose interest in sex, finding no pleasure in it; others suffer from sexual dysfunction (such as loss of arousal or orgasm).

Many who are depressed struggle with feelings of personal worthlessness; others have vague, usually unjustified guilt feelings. A classic sign is indifference to things that normally held importance in a person's life—family, friends, hobbies, leisure activities, and/or work. Lacking hope, some think about suicide. It may even be possible to predict who is at a higher risk of suicide by measuring some of the neurochemical abnormalities associated with depression.[50] Some of the more meaningful parts of life are lost, along with the ability to savor the things that normally brought great enjoyment— a stroll along a shady street on a Sunday afternoon, a baby's smile, the companionship of good friends.

Researcher Richard Sword has identified what he calls a depression-prone personality, a person who is more likely than others to become depressed. According to Sword, a depression-prone person is ambitious, conscientious, responsible, and hard working; has a high standard of personal honesty and integrity; and sets high standards for others—but even higher standards for him or herself. This person is generally pleasant and seems to be happy, even when inwardly sad. On the other hand, once milder depression develops, anger, irritability, and controlling behavior can increase. Summarizing, National Institute of Mental Health psychiatrist Phillip Gold says that a person with "melancholic depression" has low self-esteem, a sense of hopelessness, intense anxiety about the future, a loss of sleep and appetite, and decreased sexual desire.[51]

In its earlier and most minor forms, inherited neurochemical depression, with its sense of punishment and negative expectations, can tend to put a person more on guard, looking for danger or possible exploitation and disregard by others. This may be manifested as shyness, a feeling of being unaccepted and the need to prove oneself, or hostile cynicism (particularly in men).

Depression and Premenstrual Syndrome

Women with premenstrual syndrome (PMS) have a history of treated depression much more often than do normal healthy women—31 percent, as compared with 6 percent of normal controls. The percent who are depressed also increases when other menstrual complaints are present: 9 percent of women with heavy menstrual bleeding, and 22 percent of women with significant menstrual cramps.[52] Estrogen has an antidepressant effect on several brain neurotransmitters, and a drop in estrogen in the late cycle appears to be associated with a drop in brain serotonin (and endorphin) function in women who are genetically vulnerable to depression. These women are also more vulnerable to postpartum depression, when estrogen levels fall at delivery, and are probably more susceptible to depression at menopause.

If PMS sufferers are followed long enough, the symptoms may begin to extend through the entire cycle, worsening at ovulation or before the period begins. For many, PMS appears to be an early, mild form of depression unmasked by normal hormone changes affecting a vulnerable brain neurotransmitter system. If the PMS is more severe, many of the physical symptoms associated with depression (such as migraine, muscle aches, or bowel symptoms) can appear before the menstrual period and then disappear afterward. Many women find significant relief from PMS with some of the same treatments used for depression—medications that improve serotonin function, exercise, a high-carbohydrate and low-protein diet, stress management and relaxation techniques, and avoidance of stimulants (such as caffeine). Women with PMS are more likely to develop menopausal symptoms, including depression,[53] and estrogen treatment of menopause has an antidepressant effect for many.[54]

Many women with either PMS or depression crave sweets as the symptoms worsen, which is the brain's attempt to boost serotonin levels. In fact, craving sweets is often a signal that serotonin function is deficient. Why? Serotonin is manufactured in the brain from tryptophan, an amino acid in the diet. To get into the brain, tryptophan has to cross the blood-brain barrier, which protects the brain from potentially dangerous substances in the bloodstream. To do that, it has to compete with the other amino acids in dietary proteins. If there are too many other amino acids, tryptophan has trouble getting into the brain, and serotonin production falls. The solution? Eating carbohydrates (either sugars or starches) suppresses competing amino acids and makes it easier for tryptophan to enter the brain. Starches are better than sugars because an excessive rebound in adrenaline often occurs in anxiously depressed people as the sugar level falls a few hours after eating; starches reduce that rebound effect. (White starches like potatoes, however, tend to act more like sugar.) Some physicians use the disappearance of carbohydrate craving as a signal that the dose of antidepressant medication is adequate.

Seasonal Affective Disorder

Winter increases the risk of depression for some people. Experiments at the National Institute of Mental Health have concluded that the ability to deal with stress—and thus to avoid depression—can be significantly influenced by the amount of sunlight received each day. Data from the studies indicate that some people seem better able to cope with stress, change, and challenge during the spring, summer, and early autumn months. As winter approaches and the days grow shorter and darker, many persons become lethargic, anxious, and depressed.[55] Some mechanisms of this seem similar to those that cause winter hibernation in animals.

Investigators at the National Institute of Mental Health noticed that during the winter, when there is less light, some people tend to slow down, gain weight, sleep more, and feel depressed. A few even develop more serious problems than just a mild case of the blues. Some become incapacitated. Some even become suicidal.

Believing that light played a role, investigators exposed persons predisposed to suffer from winter depression to strong artificial, broad-spectrum light for at least five hours a day. For those exposed to light, symptoms of depression and distress were significantly reduced or even completely eliminated.[56] The therapeutic light is broad-spectrum white light; the blue spectrum is the important part. Yellow incandescent bulbs do not work. Since those early studies, the daily regimen has been much simplified and has produced nearly the same benefits. The usual regimen today is exposure to bright lights for 30 to 60 minutes in the early morning.

Researchers who have studied the phenomenon of light have noticed that its effects seem to be influenced by geography. The propensity toward depression is more pronounced in northern climates such as the Scandinavian countries and Canada, where sunlight is limited. By contrast, in sunny areas of the world, as on the Mediterranean coast, people are much less likely to suffer from depression. This winter effect is not uncommon: The seasonal depression effect is seen in nearly 10 percent of the population in New Hampshire and 6 percent in New York, but in only 2 percent of those who live in Florida.[57]

What is the effect of the sunlight? While we're not completely sure, we have been able to glean information by studying animals that hibernate in winter. The seasonal behavior changes in animals—migration and hibernation—seem to be related to a light-sensitive area of the brain, the pineal gland. As days grow shorter, less light is transmitted through the eyes to the brain's pineal gland. In response, the pineal gland releases more of the hormone melatonin, which, among other things, suppresses reproduction and heightens survival adjustments.[58] Melatonin, secreted in response to darkness, is also involved in day-night biorhythms of such things as hormone secretion and sleep cycles by blocking the activating parts of the brain. Taken orally, melatonin induces fatigue and sleepiness (like that of hibernating animals). Injected, melatonin induces depression (probably because it blocks beneficial serotonin receptors.)

Melatonin may therefore be the culprit in the darkness-aggravated depression and sluggishness seen in what researchers have now dubbed seasonal affective disorder (SAD). Symptoms can include pain that is worse in the winter (as with some chronic muscle pain conditions, like fibromyalgia),[59] and even the increased prevalence of infections seen during the winter. Anecdotes indicate that light therapy may be effective to help the increased winter pain, though that has not been rigorously studied. Immune function becomes somewhat dysregulated during the winter in victims of SAD, and it improves with light treatment.[60] Scientists working on the projects say, "The sunlight influence seems to be mediated via the retina, in the eye. It is by looking at the light, not just being generally exposed to it, that one obtains the beneficial results."[61] If a person has a clear-cut winter pattern to their depression, light can sometimes be even more effective than antidepressants or used as a useful adjunct to those medicines. It's important to remember that SAD could be bipolar depression and require different treatment than typical depression.

The Physiological and Anatomical Effects of Depression

Depression obviously has a profound influence on the mind and the emotions, but many studies continue to find that depression has an equally profound influence on the body as well. Researchers have learned that during depression, the body undergoes hormonal and chemical changes similar to those of chronic stress (see Chapter 2). This occurs, says National Institute of Mental Health psychiatrist Phillip Gold, because in depressed people the mechanisms that normally regulate the stress response fail. "Although depressed people often seem to think and react slowly," he says, "they are actually in a highly aroused state, focusing obsessively on their own sense of inadequacy. This state of mind parallels the heightened sense of awareness and focus that plays a positive role in a short-term response to stress, but in depression that intense awareness and focus is turned inward, with psychologically crippling results."[62] This hyperactivity of the brain in depression is demonstrated on functional magnetic resonance imaging (MRI) scans of the brain and likely contributes to the anxiety seen with depression. The response of the brain to the excessive activity in the bodily parts is often accompanied by a shutting down of the prefrontal parts that are involved with thinking and decision making.

Normally, when we are challenged, the brain hypothalamus releases corticotropin-releasing hormone (the CRH mentioned in the genetics discussion, above). This hormone causes the pituitary gland (located near the brain) to stimulate the adrenal gland[63] (located near the kidney) to increase its production of cortisol, a compound that, along with adrenaline, heightens the alerting and protecting systems in the body. When stress passes, or as we adapt effectively to longer term stresses, hormone production diminishes, returning again to normal levels.

However, in certain people subject to serious chronic depression, this endocrine system, once activated, does not seem able to turn itself off. Cortisol and CRH levels remain elevated.[64] In a test of adrenal function, the suppression of hormone activity that should occur after the administration of a compound called dexamethasone fails to occur.[65] Consequently, when depressed, it may take an unduly extended period of time for the individual to recover from the impact of stress; or, in some instances, he may not recover at all without medical intervention.[66]

These stress hormones create structural brain changes that arise from the neuronfunctional abnormalities of depression. Long-term elevations of cortisol and the neuroinflammation seen with depression (that results from reducing protective neurotrophins) start to shrink or even kill neurons in the thinking and memory parts of the brain.[67] On standard MRI brain scans, these areas of the brain continue to shrink in size the longer the depression goes untreated.[68] In 2002, Husseini Manji at the National Institute of Mental Health—and again in 2003, Rene Hen of Columbia University in

New York in the Journal *Science*—reported that antidepressant medication causes regrowth of the damaged cells, which seems to be an important part of how those treatments work.[69] The mechanism of this regrowth appears to be antidepressants that improve brain norepinephrine—and, to a lesser extent, serotonin and dopamine function—that increase the neurotrophin BDNF.[70] (As discussed above, BDNF keeps neurons healthy and creates new ones when needed.) Medications like lithium that treat bipolar depression similarly increase gray matter in the prefrontal (thinking) parts of the brain.[71]

All of these structural brain changes that occur with untreated depression (and the "kindling" that increases over time) may explain why the longer depression goes untreated, the more difficult it is to reverse. This ability to protect the brain through treatment is a good reason for treating depression early.

Nonmedication approaches to treating depression may also have some similar brain structure benefits, though this is less proven. Exercise improves BDNF levels. Counseling to create ways of thinking that improve serotonin (such as getting back an internal sense of control), that improve norepinephrine (such as finding purpose), and that improve the levels of dopamine (feeling loving and connected) may well have similar effects, but that has not yet been as well documented.

As serotonin function in the brain falls, in parallel the endorphin levels drop and pain-promoting Substance P rises.[72] Endorphins are the brain's own chemicals, designed to relieve pain and help us feel good.[73] (Morphine works to relieve pain largely by stimulating the natural endorphin receptors in the brain.) Depression is a state of endorphin deficiency. Other conditions characterized by low endorphin (and sometimes serotonin) levels include chronic pain disorders, migraine, premenstrual syndrome, and some arthritis. This fall in endorphins and rise in Substance P may partly explain why so many people with depression—approximately 60 percent—have recurrent, multiple pain problems. People with more than one pain complaint are six to eight times more likely to have clinical depression than others, and treatment of the depression often solves the pain problem if it has not become too chronic.[74]

Other important mechanisms of this increased pain seen with depression primarily involve defectiveness of the downward inhibitory tracts from the brain down the spinal cord to the sites where pain signals arrive from the body periphery (these tracts were briefly discussed in Chapter 5). That inhibitory tract is manned by the same neurotransmitters that are deficient in depression: serotonin, norepinephrine, and dopamine. The loss of inhibition from the deficiencies of these chemicals in depression results in a host of very common hypersensitivity disorders: irritable bowel syndrome, migraine and tension headaches, neurological symptoms (such as dizziness and tingling), and muscle pain disorders like fibromyalgia. If a person has one of these, he or she is likely to have several others, including depression and anxiety disorders. Improving the norepinephrine, dopamine, and serotonin in the central nervous system reduces pain and improves these hypersensitivity disorders.

One painful condition that deserves attention is fibromyalgia, a common problem characterized by chronic widespread muscle pain that causes fatigue, sleep disturbance, and multiple painful or tender points at sites of muscle insertion. The pain is often exacerbated by mental stress; for many, it's also worse in wintertime. Since the pattern of fibromyalgia is so similar to that of depression, some experts have wondered if the same neurochemical link causes both. For example, Dr. Jon Russell at the University of Texas in San Antonio and others have shown that people with fibromyalgia have three times the normal Substance P (which magnifies pain) in the cerebral spinal fluid and low serotonin, norepinephrine, and dopamine function that inhibits pain—the same as people who have depression.[75] Chronic pain conditions such as fibromyalgia would then be expected to be associated with higher than usual prevalence of depression, and they are. Seventy-one percent of fibromyalgia patients have clinical depression or anxiety, and they also have a strong family history of depression.[76]

Antidepressants,[77] anticonvulsant medication,[78] stress management,[79] and relaxation techniques,[80] with particular attention to improving deep sleep,[81] are helpful in the treatment of fibromyalgia. Also helpful are exercise, a strong physician-patient relationship, and a positive expectation about treatment. Nutritional supplements that increase nervous system serotonin (such as tryptophan or 5-hydroxytryptophan [5-HTP]), increase dopamine (DL-phenylalanine), or stabilize sensitive nerve membranes (omega-3 fatty acids) may help.[82] Fibromyalgia can be very successfully treated early on; however, if left untreated, kindling occurs over time, and the excess pain becomes much more difficult to reverse. This is probably because of similar structural changes in the nervous system over time as was described above for depression. The longer the chronic pain lasts, the harder it is to reverse (just as with depression). Excess Substance P and abnormal serotonin function are also seen in other common pain conditions associated with depression and fibromyalgia, such as migraine and irritable bowel syndrome.

Thus, high rates of underlying depression and panic disorder are also often present in persons who have other, more specific medical problems that combine pain with the smooth muscle spasm discussed in Chapter 5. Examples include irritable bowel syndrome ("spastic colon") patients (23 percent have major depression, and more have milder forms), esophageal motility disorder patients (40 percent are depressed, and 38 percent have panic disorder), patients with migraines (4.2 times normal depression rates and 13 times more panic disorder), and patients with chest pain but normal coronary arteriograms (who have 9 times more depression and 7 times more panic disorder than normal).

There are a number of medical conditions that can mimic depression—so closely, in fact, that a physician may miss the underlying medical condition altogether. According to Gregory Manov and William Guy of the Department of Psychiatry at Vanderbilt School of Medicine and the Tennessee Neuropsychiatric Institute in Nashville, at least five major categories of medical disease can charade as depression.[83] These usually involve inflammation, hormonal, or nutrition problems. But when depressed patients are evaluated for these mimicking medical diseases, they are seldom present. The following can appear—even with careful scrutiny—to be depression:

- **Central nervous system disorders.** Examples include slow-growing brain tumors, multiple sclerosis, brain injuries (including strokes), or dementia.

- **Some endocrine disorders.** These include both hypothyroidism and slowly developing hyperthyroidism. Severe depressive symptoms are also characteristic of Addison's disease and Cushing's syndrome (both diseases of the adrenal gland).

- **Gastrointestinal cancers or inflammation**, such as Crohn's disease (regional enteritis), or ulcerative colitis. Depression may be the only symptom in the early stages of these diseases.

- **Chronic systemic illnesses**, particularly those involving infection or inflammation. Lupus erythematosus is one of the most classic. Chronic infections and infectious diseases (by releasing immune chemicals called interleukins), too, may have direct effects on brain chemistry, leading to serious depression. Such lingering diseases include malaria, tuberculosis, syphilis, viral encephalitis, and meningoencephalitis. Any time an immune response to infections occurs, depressive symptoms are possible. This can cause confusion because depression itself makes a person more prone to infections.

- **Simple nutritional deficiencies**. Most commonly at fault are vitamin deficiencies, such as niacin, folate, and vitamin B_{12}, or deficiencies of amino acids like tryptophan, tyrosine, or phenylalanine. Simple mineral imbalances such as low potassium or magnesium can cause symptoms of depression, too, most often in persons who take diuretics (water pills).

Depression and Longevity

Depression can increase mortality in some obvious ways. As mentioned, severe depression can lead to suicide. Depression, even in milder stages, however, also contributes to a higher risk of getting medical diseases that can be lethal. A long-term study involving over 6,000 people showed that elderly patients with symptoms of depression were 34 percent more likely to develop a new medical disease than were those without depression, predicting significant decline in physical health,[84] and when depression was treated or improved, physical health significantly improved.[85]

Depression can also worsen the plight of people who already have a medical problem. Research shows that, when sick people become depressed, they tend to become sicker, need more medication, and spend more days in the hospital. Worst of all, it can actually reduce survival.[86] Mortality rates are four times the normal rate in depressed persons, not so much from suicide as from increased medical illness (63 percent of it cardiovascular disease). The severity and mortality of almost any disease are substantially worse if the patient is also depressed. This is particularly true for stroke, coronary artery disease, myocardial infarction, heart rhythm disturbances, sudden death, rheumatoid arthritis, certain cancers, multiple sclerosis, Parkinson's disease, epilepsy, kidney disease, psoriasis, acne, and diabetes.[87] The presence of depression powerfully reduces overall health in people with these concomitant diseases.[88]

Depression also shortens life in nursing homes. One group of researchers studied 454 patients who were newly admitted to eight nursing homes in the Baltimore area. Depression at the time of admission raised the risk of death within a year by 59 percent, regardless of physical health. Why? Researchers think several factors may be at work, including poor nutrition, inadequate rest, or impaired immune function among depressed persons.[89]

Just how depression shortens the survival time of patients who are already ill is not exactly known, although we do have some important clues. One came from a study of children who died from asthma attacks; 12 who died were compared with 12 who survived their attacks. According to researchers, "Family and personal characteristics of those who died suggested that depression may have played a role."[90] Depression can also worsen the loving, supportive relationships shown to prolong life (see Chapter 9).

Seven of the children who died—but only two of the ones who survived—came from families marked by marital discord, lack of emotional support, alcoholism, and drug abuse. Eight of the children who died—as compared with three who survived—had talked about death or suicide within a month of the fatal attack.

Researchers who conducted the study and analyzed its results wanted to find out why depression may have contributed to the asthma deaths, so they probed more deeply into the chemistry of depression. According to investigator Bruce Miller, director of the pediatric psychophysiological treatment unit at the National Jewish Center for Immunology and Respiratory Medicine in Denver, depression creates a chemical imbalance in the body that boosts the parasympathetic nervous system. Depression also up-regulates the serotonin 2 (5-HT_2) receptor discussed for asthma in Chapter 5. The result can be deadly for an asthmatic: The parasympathetic nervous system closes the airways.[91] The increased smooth muscle spasm in the airways is much like the increased spasm of the coronary arteries and bowel seen in depression, in which the abnormal 5-HT_2 receptor also plays a role.[92]

When followed prospectively, depressed people have fairly consistently showed greater mortality risk. In one such study, researchers followed up on 1,593 men and women who had been hospitalized for depression at a care facility in Iowa. For a control group, the researchers used randomly selected people of the same age and sex who also lived in Iowa. Follow-up studies began two years after the patients were released from the hospital and continued for 14 years. Death rates among the depressed patients soared for the first two years following hospitalization and remained higher than average throughout the entire study.[93]

In another important large-scale study, Dr. Richard Shekelle of the University of Chicago examined the health of about 2,000 men who were employed by Chicago's Western Electric Company. The men's personalities were first measured in 1958, and then researchers tracked their health for the next two decades. During the next twenty years, those who had scored high on depression in 1958 were more likely than other men to die, including some of cancer. Others also found this depression-death link occurred sometimes from increased infections.[94] It's important to note that this increased risk remained even after the researchers took into account the men's age, occupation, cigarette smoking, and family history of cancer. Researchers found one interesting footnote to the study: the more time that elapsed since the measurement of depression, the weaker was its association with illness and death.[95] In other words, the link between depression and illness/death lessens over time, particularly if the depression has been treated or remitted.

Depression has also been linked to sudden death (usually from heart arrhythmias) in a number of studies. This is particularly true when they were also faced with situational stress. In one of the best-known studies, psychiatrist William Greene and colleagues at the University of Rochester studied 26 employees at Eastman Kodak Company who died suddenly and unexpectedly. Almost all of the employees who died had been depressed before their death—some for only a week, some for several months. Researchers found that the depressed employees suddenly underwent definite arousal; in other words, people who had been living in slow motion or depression suddenly lurched into third gear. The "arousal" that occurred was in the form of an increased workload with its accompanying stress, a conflict in the workplace, or marital stress. The sudden shift from depression to arousal can produce incompatible reactions, leading to arrhythmia, myocardial infarction, or both.[96] The fact is, far and away the greatest cause of the increased deaths among depressed people is cardiovascular disease.[97]

Depression and the Heart

Depression is now considered a major coronary risk factor, comparable in severity to smoking.[98] A number of impressive studies have demonstrated that depression's biological abnormalities can lead to more cardiovascular disease. Researchers in England examined 2,000 patients and an equal number of matched controls. They identified which ones were suffering from chronic mild depression. In prospectively following the study subjects, they found that new coronary artery disease was much more likely to later develop in those who suffered from depression than in those who did not.[99]

In fact, individual symptoms of depression can also predict future heart attacks. In a study of 1,300 graduates of Johns Hopkins Medical School, researchers isolated those for whom depression was a problem. Then they classified the depressed graduates according to their various symptoms of depression. They found that one particular symptom of depression, early-morning fatigue, was more often present among graduates who years later suffered a myocardial infarction than among those who remained healthy.[100]

The effect of depression on the heart is so profound that researchers have been able to predict who would have a heart attack based solely on the presence of depression. In one such prediction, University of Oklahoma Medical School's Dr. Stewart Wolf examined 65 patients who had suffered documented myocardial infarctions and 65 matched control subjects who were healthy and had not had any sign of heart disease.[101] To support his theory, Wolf interviewed all 130 subjects once a month; he also gave each one a battery of psychological tests to determine how depressed each one was. After a series of interviews with each subject, Wolf made his predictions without knowing which ones had previously suffered a heart attack. He chose 10 people who had failed to find meaningful satisfaction in their social and leisure activities (basically, the 10 people who were the most depressed). He predicted (solely on the basis of depression) that they would be among the first to have a heart attack and die. All of the subjects Wolf pinpointed did, indeed, have a heart attack and die. In fact, those 10 were among the first 23 who died during the four years following the predictions.[102]

In another prospective study, death due to heart disease was associated with depression. Robert Anda and his colleagues at the Centers for Disease Control and Prevention in Atlanta studied 2,832 adults, ranging in age from 45 to 57, who entered the study healthy and free of heart disease. As they entered the study, volunteers were asked about their feelings of depression, discouragement, and hopelessness. Researchers then followed them for an average interval of 12 years. They found that those who felt depressed and hopeless suffered four times more deaths from heart disease than those who did not have such feelings.[103]

Other researchers studied heart disease in smokers. Findings showed that potentially fatal blood vessel disease progressed more rapidly among the smokers who were mildly to moderately depressed than among those who were not depressed.[104] One reason may be that depression appears to magnify risk factors associated with heart disease; in other words, depression makes risky behaviors even riskier. For example, diabetes increases coronary risk greatly, particularly if poorly controlled. Depression makes diabetic control much more erratic. This diabetes effect is in part because of the insulin resistance created by depression. This insulin resistance, creating "the metabolic syndrome" that puts people at very high cardiovascular risk, was worsened by depression in several studies.[105] The high levels of cortisol and catecholamines seen with depression make people less responsive to the insulin needed to get sugar into cells.[106] This insulin function is already poor in diabetics and gets twice as bad when they are depressed. In a 10-year study, depressed diabetics had more diabetic complications and over three times as many heart attacks as diabetics without depression.[107] Treating the depression corrects the insulin resistance created by the depression[108] and can significantly lower the high blood sugars.[109]

The negative effects of smoking are 3.4 times greater for people who are depressed. Interestingly, in a study of 3,543 smokers, those who took antidepressant medication that improved serotonin function remarkably had 65 percent fewer heart attacks than the total group.[110] Similarly, an epidemiological study of 52,000 people showed that those taking serotonergic antidepressants had 20 percent fewer heart attacks than did people in the overall community, despite the fact that they were being treated for depression that (when untreated) puts them at higher risk. All of this suggests that central nervous system serotonin abnormalities play a significant role in heart attacks. How that works is now beginning to be understood.

Cardiovascular Mechanisms   Three mechanisms are involved in creating myocardial infarction, or heart attack: plaque, arterial spasm, and finally a clot that finishes the job. All three are significantly accelerated in depression. Depression doubles the negative impact of low-density lipoproteins ("bad" cholesterol) on blood vessels. How could this be? Anxious depression causes an elevation of the stress chemical norepinephrine within peripheral blood vessels. Norepinephrine causes damage to the lining of blood vessels in that it allows any cholesterol present in the blood vessel to create plaque (deposits that narrow the vessels) at a much more rapid rate. This creates a synergy between chronic stress and cholesterol in causing more rapid onset of vascular damage.[111]

Depression creates an additional risk for cardiovascular events both by causing blood vessel (smooth muscle) spasm and by creating more blood clots. Depression's effect on serotonin in the brain is reflected in serotonin problems in the blood-clotting cells called platelets, making them adhere to each other more aggressively, setting off the clotting process that causes the final step in heart attacks and many strokes.[112] Most newer antidepressants that act to improve serotonin levels in the brain also affect serotonin in platelets, producing an antiplatelet effect with less clotting[113] in a similar but different way than aspirin does, thus preventing heart attacks. Antidepressant medications that work by primarily improving norepinephrine levels do not have this platelet-protecting effect.[114] (Also see the discussion of these mechanisms in Chapter 5.)

Depression hits persons who already have coronary artery disease even harder than the general population. A striking example was provided by a study conducted by psychologist Robert M. Carney and his colleagues at the Washington University School of Medicine in St. Louis. For one year the researchers followed 52 persons who had been diagnosed with coronary artery disease.[115] Of the people in the study, 18 percent were seriously depressed before the diagnosis. The researchers used a strict definition for depression, too, taken from the *Diagnostic and Statistical Manual* (revised 3rd edition, or *DSM-IIIR*). To qualify as "depressed," a person had to have suffered extreme sadness or hopelessness, loss of interest or pleasure in most activities, insomnia, loss of energy, or thoughts of suicide for at least two weeks.

Major depression was found to be the best single predictor of serious problems and complications among the heart patients, and it was an even stronger predictor than factors such as age, smoking, severity of artery damage, and levels of cholesterol in the bloodstream.[116] Researchers found that 78 percent of the depressed patients had some cardiac event during the twelve months after the diagnosis, and one died. Only a third of the nondepressed patients had problems.

Similarly, in a Canadian hospital study of more than 200 heart attack patients, patients were given diagnostic interviews a week after entering the hospital and again six months later. Forty percent of the patients had depression, starting before their heart attacks. All else being equal, say the researchers, depression raised the risk of death 3.4 times and the risk of recurrent coronary events 5.7 times.[117] Thus, the mechanisms described above do indeed create cardiovascular havoc.

According to researchers, it's not only increased coronary occlusions that are the problem. The increased stress hormones and activity of the sympathetic nervous system present in depression create more heart rhythm problems (arrhythmias) and thus sudden death. In a prospective study over one year, those depressed at the beginning had five times more ventricular tachycardia than did the nondepressed individuals.[118] (Ventricular tachycardia is a dangerous, rapid heart rhythm that often precedes sudden death, which is death that occurs unexpectedly in a person who previously seemed healthy and exhibited no symptoms of illness.)

A study in New York of 283 myocardial infarction patients found that 45 percent were depressed one week later; 18 percent had major depression, 27 percent had minor depression.[119] (Remember that the symptoms must be present for at least two weeks to make a diagnosis of depression. That means that the above 45 percent were depressed before their myocardial infarction.) Depression was not associated with severity of heart disease, but those who were depressed did have a greater prevalence of other medical problems. Three to four months later, 33 percent were still depressed. After a heart attack, depression was even more predictive of cardiac disability than was the severity of heart damage. Among those who had been working before their heart attack, most who had major depression had not returned to work three months later; only 38 percent eventually returned, as compared with 63 percent of the heart attack victims who were not depressed. Minor depression was not as disabling.

Of interest in this study was the fact that medical problems masked the depression: only 10 percent of those with major depression and 4 percent of all depressed patients had received treatment for depression. Another impressive finding is that, particularly in women, depression appears to predict death from heart disease more accurately than either hostility or Type A behavior; it may also be more important in accelerating the arterial narrowing of atherosclerosis (see the related discussion in Chapter 4).[120] Some of the cardiotoxic type A behaviors, such as cynical hostility (see Chapters 3–4), improve greatly with antidepressant medication. This response implies that some of the neurochemistry of depression (shown to increase heart attacks) probably also underlies the angry, cynical hostility that puts a person at higher risk for heart disease. People with that behavior pattern later develop more clinical depression. In fact, that cynical hostility may be more the way that depression shows up in men.

With depression established as a major coronary risk factor, and based on preliminary results, longer term studies have now begun to determine the outcome of actively treating heart disease patients for depression, and the predicted better outcomes[121] with treatment are beginning to emerge in impressive ways. In two large studies published in recent years in the *Journal of the American Medical Association,* depressed heart attack patients who were treated with serotonergic antidepressants had 43 to 61 percent less cardiac death and fewer heart attacks than those who received a placebo.[122] Those treated with antidepressants that worked by nonserotonin mechanisms were not nearly as protected. These are striking numbers, as good as any cardiac medications used to prevent heart attacks. (The effects of nonpharmacological approaches to these problems will be discussed in Chapter 21.)

The above should demonstrate how important depression is to the heart, not only metaphorically and emotionally, but physically.

Depression and the Immune System

Several years ago, the first phases of an unusually severe Asian influenza epidemic began to creep around the world. In a midwestern college community, people in an enterprising college health center wondered what effect preexisting mental distress would have on those exposed to the flu. Before the epidemic arrived, a large number of college students whose health care was provided by the clinic were screened with the Minnesota Multiphasic Personality Inventory (MMPI), a test that has become a standard for defining mental states. Then they waited for the flu to hit. Those who got influenza returned after three and six weeks for evaluation to see who was still sick (most people recover well by three weeks). Those depressed before the epidemic were significantly more likely to still be sick at six weeks. The same results were found in a similar military study at Fort Dietrich, Maryland.[123]

Other physicians have noted that depressed (or sometimes chronically stressed) patients not infrequently complain of "getting everything that's going around" or of having trouble getting rid of their respiratory or intestinal infection. An interesting British study determined a "stress index" for a group of people, based on the presence or absence of depression symptoms or overwhelming stress. These people were then exposed to tiny amounts of cold viruses in nose drops to see who would actually get a viral infection. Sure enough, those with the high stress index got the colds at a much higher rate.[124] How could that be? What is it about depression and chronic stress that might affect the immunity that protects from such common infections? Are some of the same psychoneuroimmunological mechanisms discussed in Chapters 1 and 2 the culprit? A large part of the nervous system is composed of glia, cells that were thought for years to be simply supporting structures that hold the neurons together. However, it turns out that microglia are very immunologically active, secreting inflammatory cytokines that modulate nerve cell function.[125] With that finding, the immune–nervous system interaction is not surprising.

The increased infections noted above suggest that the immune changes seen in depression are clinically relevant. The immune system has two large components: cellular immunity (which primarily destroys challenging agents like viruses or bacteria) and humoral or antibody immunity (which attracts the cellular components and plays a role in allergies). Both are at times significantly impacted by depression. One of the most significant impacts of depression on immune function is on the activity of natural killer cells, the immune cells that assist the body in its surveillance against tumors and in its resistance to viral disease. A number of studies show that natural killer cell activity is reduced among people who are depressed. Researchers at Boston University School of Medicine, for example, reported lower natural killer cell activity in depressed persons.[126] This can explain why people get more infections when depressed. After the depression is treated, the susceptibility to infection subsides.

Dr. Michael Irwin and his colleagues at the University of California, San Diego, measured the immune function of women whose husbands had recently died. The widows had significantly reduced levels of natural killer cell activity compared to women who were not bereaved. Among the bereaved women, the ones who were depressed had the greatest impairment in natural killer cell activity.[127]

It wasn't just the bereavement that curtailed immune function, then, because the more severely depressed the woman, the more reduced her natural killer cell activity. In reporting on his findings, Irwin commented, "Depression is qualitatively different from grief. People who are depressed feel down, blue, and gloomy persistently. Those who are grieving move in and out of those feelings." In summing up the study results, Irwin confirmed that it was "the severity of their depression," not merely their husbands' death, that seemed to be related to their weakened immune responses.[128]

Researchers also suspect that depression interferes with the ratio of helper and suppressor cells. Helper and suppressor cells are two classes of lymphocytes; the helper cells turn on the immune response, and the suppressor cells turn off the immune response. If the immune system is to function normally, the two kinds of cells have to have a proper ratio. Neither too little immunity (getting infections) nor too much immunity (allergies and autoimmune diseases) is desirable. The higher the ratio of helpers to suppressors, the stronger the immune response; the lower the ratio, the weaker the cellular immunity response. When suppressors severely outnumber helpers, the immune system is suppressed (which is what happens in AIDS, or acquired immunodeficiency syndrome).

The results of a large number of studies show that depression definitely has an influence on the ratio, although the precise results vary. Test results differed somewhat for various reasons: Some of the studies involved patients who were hospitalized, though most did not; in some of the studies, patients were on antidepressant drugs; and so on. In some studies, depressed people had a normal number of suppressor cells but a small proportion of helper cells. In other studies, the people who were depressed had lower numbers of both kinds of cells.[129] When depression is treated, the abnormalities return toward normal.[130]

Psychologist Margaret Kemeny and her colleagues at the University of California School of Medicine in San Francisco studied the helper-suppressor ratio. To test the effect of depression on the immune system, they studied 36 subjects with genital herpes. Kemeny took regular blood samples over a six-month period and monitored outbreaks and recurrences. The people in the study who were depressed showed a drop in both helper and suppressor cells; they had significantly lower levels of suppressor cytotoxic T cells, which are thought to help keep outbreaks from occurring. The depressed people had more recurrences of symptoms and more outbreaks than did others in the study. Kemeny and her colleagues discovered that they could accurately predict which study subjects would have outbreaks based on how depressed they were.[131]

The hormones and chemicals produced in depression may also affect the immune system. One is cortisol. In depression, the adrenal gland often secretes far too much cortisol, which then acts to suppress the immune system.[132] When the adrenals manufacture and secrete these corticosteroids, having "no apparent biological brake,"[133] the immune system begins to slow down. University of Iowa psychiatrist Dr. Ziad Kronfol has done a series of studies in which he has subjected depressed people to standard immunity tests. One finding is consistent: The cellular immune systems of depressed people are less responsive than those of normal people—and even those of people with other mental illnesses.[134]

Now we come to an interesting paradox about the immune abnormality in depression. While decreased cellular immunity may lead to more infections, anxiously depressed patients often have excessive humoral immunity (that is, excessive antibodies), leading to more allergy problems and autoimmune diseases. Studies of people with multiple distressing allergies show that about two-thirds of these people are depressed.[135] Interestingly, when the depression is treated, allergies begin to subside. In fact, in a large (12,058-person) prospective, 31-year follow-up study in Finland, if both the person's mother and the person being studied were allergic, the risk for depression was four times normal.[136] And the severity of the allergies is worse if a person is depressed.[137]

For example, more hives occur when a person is anxiously depressed. Many people with hives experience worse symptoms when stressed. One study found that over one-third of those with hives were depressed.[138] When Japanese hive sufferers were studied, not only for depression but for anxiety as well, the percent went up to 70 percent (compared to 26 percent of controls).[139]

Depression also is a significant factor in activating autoimmune disorders, such as lupus or rheumatoid arthritis.[140] Mental stress itself can activate rheumatoid arthritis[141] in about half the patients. In the other half, mental stress is not much of a factor. Depression is one form of chronic stress. Even animals under chronic stress will overrespond to materials (adjuvant) injected into joints to induce arthritis very much like rheumatoid arthritis. The onset of autoimmune diseases of the thyroid is often preceded by either major stressful events or clinical depression.[142]

Antidepressant medication and neural stabilizers like lithium can help to normalize the abnormal immunity of depression.[143] Both in animals and people, exercise also helps.[144] Those affecting other neurotransmitters in depression, such as dopamine, are not of much benefit for the immune abnormalities.[145] The brain, once again, seems to have great capacity to bring about that which is expected, all the way down to cellular levels (see the later discussions of the effect of optimism versus pessimism in Chapter 16, and of hope in Chapter 14). Immune responses and the well-proven placebo effect are involved in this phenomenon.

Depression and Cancer

Until recently, scientists were convinced that depression could lead to cancer. While researchers argued about how great the effect was—and how strong the link—most agreed that there was a link between depression and cancer. Top medical researchers were convinced that depression either contributed to the development of cancer or caused it to be more severe once it did develop, and a variety of studies seemed to support that conviction.

Then researchers started to waffle. One report found that depression "was associated more strongly with cancer mortality than with cancer incidence suggests that it may promote, rather than initiate, the disease process."[146]

Some research suggests the link between depression and cancer is much less likely. A study published by Alan Zonderman and colleagues in the *Journal of the American Medical Association*[147] says that many factors probably raise the risk of cancer, but depression isn't one of them.

Even with Zonderman's conclusive findings, some scientists think depression may at least contribute to some kinds of cancer (for example, cancers of the immune system, such as lymphoma, and cancers affected by hormones, such as breast cancer) that may be more susceptible to nervous system influence. This may in part be related to damage to DNA seen with depression.[148] University of Miami researcher Karl Goodkin says that depression might affect different types of cancer in different ways. Pointing out that Zonderman and his colleagues didn't specify which kinds of cancer cropped up among their study subjects, "We don't know whether their results are supportive of depression's effect on the incidence of viral tumors or not." Speaking of the danger of lumping together all types of cancer and drawing a single conclusion, he adds that "there may be two strong, opposite effects hidden by mixing all types of cancers."[149]

Feeling Sad, Feeling Bad

The hopelessness, frustration, sadness, and dissatisfaction that constitute depression can quite literally make you feel bad physically. In many studies, the greater the depression, the higher the number of physical symptoms associated with any illness.[150] In fact, both the number of physical symptoms a patient has and the number of medical visits per year are directly proportional to the likelihood of being depressed.[151] The facts and figures from hosts of studies tell the story.[152] Physicians know that high utilizers of medical care (those in the top 10 percent of costs, number of visits, and hospitalizations) have an extremely high likelihood of being depressed (usually prior to all the medical need). One-fourth to one-half of all patients who see primary care physicians are depressed. An estimated three-fourths of all depressed people see physicians because they are physically ill.

During depression, medical problems and discomfort become magnified. Depressed persons are apt to have multiple chronic medical illnesses. They do poorly on self-treatment and self-monitoring of chronic illnesses, such as making sure they inject insulin on schedule.

Depressed people tend to have more aches and pains, too, though researchers debate whether depression causes pain or pain causes depression. However, the fact that the pain tends to greatly diminish, or even disappear, when the depression is treated suggests that the depression (and its associated endorphin and neurotransmitter deficiencies) underlies the pain. More accurately, both chronic pain and depression have the same underlying neurochemistry that magnifies both.

People who are depressed may not do as well in surgery, either. According to a study published in the *American Journal of Public Health*, depressed elderly women who had hip fractures did much more poorly following surgery than did the same type of patients who were not depressed.[153] Surgical complications, prolonged hospitalization, and costs were all significantly higher in those who were depressed.

The person experiencing depression is not the only one who may suffer physical illness as a result; studies show that family members may also have an increase of physical signs and symptoms. In one study, 88 families that each had a depressed member were compared to 88 families that did not; other than the factor of depression, there were no significant demographical differences between the families. The study clearly showed that depression in one member of the family is associated with physical illness in other family members. Before the family member became depressed, these people had no greater incidence of physical illness than those in comparison families, but their episodes of physical illness rose dramatically in the year following the occurrence of depression in the family.[154] This may be because the psychological impact of depressed mothers on children is very significant. The children of inadequately treated depressed mothers have a much higher chance of getting depressed or agitated themselves, compared to those whose mothers are adequately treated.[155]

What to Do About Depression?

At least part of feeling better appears to involve getting control over depression. That may not be as difficult as it seems. Experts estimate that 80 to 90 percent of persons who suffer from depression can be helped substantially. Because of the underlying neurochemical (and conditioned) vulnerability, however, depression tends to be a recurrent illness. Eight years after successful treatment of a first episode, three-fourths of the previously depressed patients will have had a recurrence. Treatment studies show that combined medication and counseling-behavioral treatment is best. If one must choose between one or the other, comparison studies confirm that longer term medication is superior to counseling in preventing recurrence.[156] Medication studies suggest that milder, anxious depression involves more serotonin abnormalities, but more severe, melancholic depression may involve more norepinephrine and dopamine abnormalities.

Treatment is effective and usually shows striking improvement in most of the medical problems associated with depression. Longer term outcome studies are needed to determine how much the treatment of depression substantially prevents many of these associated medical illnesses.

Clearly antidepressant medications improve pain, and the better an agent improves all three of the neurotransmitters—norepinephrine, serotonin, and dopamine—the more relief of pain a person is likely to experience. (Some antidepressants act only on one of these neurotransmitters, while others act on two or three of them.) Norepinephrine seems to be the most important in suppressing pain. You might wonder why increasing norepinephrine in the brain is so useful for improving depression and anxiety when it is a primary stress hormone in the rest of the body. The central nervous system (brain and spinal cord) provides a remarkable feedback system to correct abnormalities in the rest of the body. When norepinephrine gets too high in the rest of the body (stimulating what are called alpha-1 and beta receptors), it stimulates a different kind of receptor (alpha-2) in the central nervous system that shuts down the excess peripheral stimulation. In other words, norepinephrine in the brain quiets stress and pain responses. Norepinephrine in the brain is also the most potent of these three neurotransmitters in improving BDNF and thus improving the function and structure of thinking neurons.[157]

When depression is mild, counseling, exercise, and learning relaxation coupled with stress resilience techniques can be very effective, even without medication. (These resilience techniques will be discussed in Chapter 22) Giving up blame and thus taking back a personal sense of control of one's feelings and responses can improve central serotonin function. Loving relationships can improve dopamine function; and both exercise and meaningful work can improve norepinephrine function. Meditation and deep relaxation techniques can improve GABA function. So all these principles act chemically like antidepressant medications (perhaps not as profoundly). Adequate sleep (usually eight hours—see Chapter 7) is crucial, as is good nutrition (Chapter 20). If the depression primarily occurs in the winter, bright light exposure in the morning can be very useful. If all of these are inadequate, early medical treatment is far more effective than starting late (to avoid the kindling effect mentioned above). Keep in mind that even severe PMS can be a form of depression, and it responds to the same methods of treatment. And common medical problems such as irritable bowel syndrome and migraine are rooted in the same neurochemical abnormalities and usually respond to these same treatments. If all this is starting in childhood or teenage years, is recurrent and with a high family history, the chance of a bipolar depression is much higher and usually needs neural stabilizer medications before any antidepressants are used.

Ongoing research is providing new clues about the malady we call depression, and scientists continue looking for even more effective treatments. One landmark study provided evidence about how pervasive depression can be. The study, conducted by researchers at the University of Washington in Seattle, studied the infants of women who were classified as clinically depressed. According to research director Geraldine Dawson, the infants of mothers who are depressed showed changes in electrical brain activity that led to unusual responses.[158] Simply stated, the infants were prone to depression, too.

Dawson called for further research to determine the exact reasons for the infants' depression. She theorized that the infants may be reacting to nonresponsive mothers or that the depression may be genetic,[159] as discussed above. The mothers' stress hormones can also affect fetal brain development. Motherly neglect in childhood can also activate the genetic vulnerability; for example, by turning on the gene for CRH, as noted above. What is clear, say researchers, is that depression may include a broad circle of influence. Such studies also raise the important question about how depression should be treated in pregnancy—is it safer for the child if a depressed, pregnant mother receives antidepressant medication if counseling is not enough? The evidence thus far suggests the answer may be yes.

While studies like these indicate that depression may be genetic, at least part of the cause of depression is cultural, says San Diego psychiatrist Dennis Gersten. As a response to years of practice, Gersten likens personalities to crystalline structures, like diamonds, quartz, ice, mica, and so on. "Each fractures under predictable lines when stressed," Gersten says. "When the stress is massive enough, each structure will collapse."[160]

It's important to remember that depression can be caused by physical factors—certain prescription drugs (e.g., heart medications, cortisone, oral contraceptives, and antihistamines), premenstrual syndrome, rapid menopause, thyroid problems (perhaps 10 percent of depressed patients[161]), diabetes, rapid-weight-loss diets, lack of exercise, sunlight deficiency, and inadequate nutrient intake (especially of iron, thiamine, and magnesium). If these problems are present, correcting them is important.

The depression-prone personality, Gersten concludes, is one that can fracture under multiple stresses. Those stresses—genetic, psychological, chemical, allergic, and toxic—offer not only a clue to the causes of depression but also a valuable panorama of ways we may prevent it.

WHAT DID YOU LEARN?

1. Describe five or more core symptoms of clinical depression from the Patient Health Questionnaire.
2. Name three important neurotransmitter abnormalities in clinical depression.
3. What are three mechanisms by which depression can increase the incidence of heart attacks and strokes?
4. Describe the paradoxical effects of depression on the immune system: What part is increased, and what part is decreased? What part of the nervous system itself is like immune cells creating inflammation?
5. Name four nonpharmacological things that can be helpful for treating mild depression.

ENDNOTES

1. Bernie S. Siegel, *Love, Medicine, and Miracles* (New York: Harper and Row, 1986).
2. Winifred Gallagher, "The Dark Affliction of Mind and Body," *Discover* (May 1986): 66–76.
3. Ibid.

4. *The Diagnostic and Statistical Manual of Mental Disorders*, 4th ed. (DSM-IV; Washington, DC: American Psychiatric Association, 1994); and "Patient Health Questionnaire, PHQ9" at http://www.treatmenthelps.org/treatmenthelps/PHQ9.pdf (accessed May 31, 2008).

5. R. L. Spitzer et al., "Validation and Utility of a Self-Report Version of PRIME-MD: The PHQ Primary Care Study," *Journal of the American Medical Association* 282 (1999): 1737–44.

6. R. C. Kessler et al., "Lifetime Prevalence and Age-of-Onset Distributions of *DSM-IV* Disorders in the National Comorbidity Survey Replication," *Archives of General Psychiatry* 62 (2005): 593–602.

7. Depression Guideline Panel, *Depression in Primary Care: Volume 1, Detection and Diagnosis* (Rockville, MD: U. S. Department of Health and Human Services, Agency for Healthcare Policy and Research [AHCPR], Publication no. 93–0550, 1993), 23.

8. Joseph Alper, "Depression at an Early Age," *Science* (May 1986): 45–50.

9. Depression Guideline Panel, *Depression in Primary Care*, 47–48.

10. W. Katon et al., "Adequacy and Duration of Antidepressant Treatment in Primary Care," *Medical Care* 30 (1992): 67–76.

11. J. E. Mezzich, K. J. Evanczuk, R. J. Mathias, and G. A. Coffman, "Admission Decisions and Multiaxial Diagnosis," *Archives of General Psychiatry* 41 (1989): 1001–4.

12. Anne H. Rosenfeld, "Depression: Dispelling Despair," *Psychology Today* 13, no. 3 (June 1985): 28.

13. Anna M. Bardone et al., "Adult Physical Health Outcomes of Adolescent Girls with Conduct Disorder, Depression, and Anxiety," *Journal of the American Academy of Child and Adolescent Psychiatry* 37, no. 6 (1997): 594–601.

14. Martin E. P. Seligman, *Learned Optimism* (New York: Alfred A. Knopf, 1991), 75.

15. I. Grant, T. L. Patterson, and J. Yager, "Social Supports in Relation to Physical Health and Symptoms of Depression in the Elderly," *American Journal of Psychiatry* 145, no. 10 (1988): 1254–58.

16. Rosenfeld, "Depression: Dispelling Despair," 28.

17. Alper, "Depression at an Early Age," 45–50.

18. C. J. Murray and A. D. Lopez, "Policy Forum: Evidence-Based Health Policy—Lessons from the Global Burden of Disease Study *Science* 274 (1996): 740–43.

19. G. J. Kennedy et al., "Hierarchy of Characteristics Associated with Depressive Symptoms in an Urban Elderly Sample," *American Journal of Psychiatry* 146, no. 2 (1989): 220–25.

20. Kenneth B. Wells et al., "The Functioning and Well-Being of Depressed Patients," *Journal of the American Medical Association* 262, no. 7 (1989): 914–9.

21. Depression Guideline Panel, *Depression in Primary Care*, 24–5.

22. P. E. Greenberg, R. C. Kessler, et al., "The Economic Burden of Depression in the United States: How Did It Change Between 1990 and 2000?" *Journal of Clinical Psychiatry* 64 (2003): 1465–75.

23. P. E. Greenberg, L. E. Stiglin, S. N. Finkelstein, and E. R. Berndt, "The Economic Burden of Depression in 1990," *Journal of Clinical Psychiatry* 54 (1993): 405–18.

24. P. E. Greenberg, R. C. Kessler, et al., "The Economic Burden of Depression in the United States: How Did It Change Between 1990 and 2000?" 1465–75.

25. S. Moussavi et al., "Depression, Chronic Diseases and Decrements in Health: Results from the World Health Surveys," *Lancet* 370 (2007): 851–8.

26. W. R. Coryell, R. Noyes, and J. Clancey, "Excess Mortality in Panic Disorder: A Comparison with Primary Unipolar Depression," *Archives of General Psychiatry* 39 (1982): 701–3.

27. R. C. Kessler et al., "The Epidemiology of Major Depressive Disorder: Results From the National Comorbidity Survey Replication (NCS-R)," *Journal of the American Medical Association* 289 (2003): 3095–105.

28. Gallagher, "The Dark Affliction of Mind and Body," 66–76.

29. Ibid.

30. M. Anguelova, C. Benkelfat, and G. Turecki, "A Systematic Review of Association Studies Investigating Genes Coding for Serotonin Receptors and the Serotonin Transporter: II. Suicidal Behavior," *Molecular Psychiatry* 8, no. 7 (2003): 646–53.

31. D. A. Collier et al., "A Novel Functional Polymorphism within the Promoter of the Serotonin Transporter Gene: Possible Role in Susceptibility to Affective Disorders," *Molecular Psychiatry* 1, no. 6 (1996): 453–60; and V. E. Golimbet et al., "Serotonin Transporter Polymorphism and Depressive-Related Symptoms in Schizophrenia," *American Journal of Medical Genetics* 126B, no. 1 (2004): 1–7.

32. R. S. Duman and L. M. Monteggia, "A Neurotrophic Model for Stress-Related Mood Disorders," *Biological Psychiatry* 59, (Issue 12), (2006): 1116–27.

33. D. Buskila, "Biology and Therapy of Fibromyalgia. Genetic Aspects of Fibromyalgia Syndrome," *Arthritis Research & Therapy* 8 (2006): 218.

34. Clive Wood, "Who Gets Depressed?" *Advances in Mind-Body Medicine* 4, no. 2 (1989): 61–5.

35. G. W. Brown, A. Bifulco, and T. O. Harris, "Life Events, Vulnerability, and Onset of Depression: Some Refinements," *British Journal of Psychiatry* 150 (1987): 30–42.

36. C. B. Nemeroff, "The Persistent Neurobiological Consequences of Early Life Trauma: Implications for the Pathopyshiology of Mood and Anxiety Disorders," American Psychosomatic Society 59th Annual Scientific Meeting March 10, 2001, Monterey CA.

37. R. M. Post, "Transduction of Psychosocial Stress into the Neurobiology of Recurrent Affective Disorder," *American Journal of Psychiatry* 149 (1992): 999–1010.

38. L. Capuron and R. Dantzer, "Cytokines and Depression: The Need for a New Paradigm," *Brain, Behavior, and Immunity* 17, no. 1 (2003): 119–24.

39. P. Trzonkowski et al., "Immune Consequences of the Spontaneous Pro-Inflammatory Status in Depressed Elderly Patients," *Brain Behavior and Immunity* 18, no. 2 (2004): 135–48.

40. G. Fricchione, R. Daly, M. P. Rogers, and G. B. Stefano, "Neuroimmunologic Influences in Neuropsychiatric and Psychophysiologic Disorders," *Acta Pharmacologica Sinica* 22, no. 7 (2001): 577–87.

41. G. Kenis and M. Maes, "Effects of Antidepressants on the Production of Cytokines," *International Journal of Neuropsychopharmacology* 5 (2002): 401–12.

42. S. D. Mathias et al., "Health Related Quality of Life and Functional Status of Patients with Rheumatoid Arthritis Randomly Assigned to Receive Etanercept or Placebo," *Clinical Therapy* 22 (2000): 128–39.

43. Ibid.

44. Rosenfeld, "Depression: Dispelling Despair," 30.

45. A. Neumeister, "Tryptophan Depletion, Serotonin, and Depression: Where Do We Stand?" *Psychopharmacological Bulletin* 37, no. 4 (2003): 99–115.

46. P. L. Delgado et al., "Tryptophan-Depletion Challenge in Depressed Patients Treated with Desipramine or Fluoxetine: Implications for the Role of Serotonin in the Mechanism of Antidepressant Action," *Biological Psychiatry* 46 (1999): 212–20.

47. D. L. Rosenhan and M. E. P. Seligman, *Abnormal Psychology* (New York: Norton, 1984), 307.

48. K. Kroenke and A. D. Mangelsdorff, "Common Symptoms in Ambulatory Care: Incidence, Evaluation, Therapy, and Outcome," *American Journal of Medicine* 86, no. 3 (March 1989): 262–6.

49. Depression Guideline Panel, *Depression in Primary Care*, 18, 49, 50, 64, 80.

50. E. R. Braveman and C. C. Pfeiffer, "Suicide and Biochemistry," *Biological Psychiatry* 20 (1985): 123–4.

51. Christopher Vaughan, "The Depression-Stress Link," *Science News* 134 (1988): 155.
52. J. Bancroft, D. Rennie, and P. Warner, "Vulnerability to Perimenstrual Mood Change: The Relevance of a Past History of Depressive Disorder," *Psychosomatic Medicine* 56 (1994): 225–31.
53. E. W. Freeman, M. D. Sammel, P. J. Rinaudo, and L. Sheng, "Obstetrics Premenstrual Syndrome as a Predictor of Menopausal Symptoms," *Gynecology* 103(5 Pt 1) (2004): 960–6.
54. I. Rudolph et al., "Influence of a Continuous Combined HRT (2 mg Estradiol Valerate and 2 mg Dienogest) on Postmenopausal Depression," *Climacteric* 7, no. 3 (2004): 301–11.
55. T. Silverstone and C. Thompson, eds., *Seasonal Affective Disorder* (London: Clinical Neuroscience Publishers, 1989).
56. D. A. Oren and N. E. Rosenthal, "Seasonal Affective Disorders," pp. 551–67 in E. S. Paykel, ed., *Handbook of Affective Disorders*, 2nd ed. (London: Churchill Livingstone, 1992); and M. Terman, "On the Question of Mechanism in Phototherapy for Seasonal Affective Disorder: Considerations of Clinical Efficacy and Epidemiology," *Journal of Biological Rhythms* 3 (1988): 155–72.
57. M. Terman et al., "Seasonal Symptom Patterns in New York: Patients and Population," pp. 77–95 in T. Silverstone and C. Thompson, eds., *Seasonal Affective Disorder* (London: Clinical Neuroscience Publishers, 1989).
58. Michael Freeman, "Don't Be SAD," *Medical Self-Care* (January–February 1989).
59. R. M. Gallagher et al., "Myofascial Face Pain: Seasonal Variability in Pain Intensity and Demoralization," *Pain* 61, no. 1 (April 1995): 113–20.
60. S. Kasper et al., "Immunological Correlates of Seasonal Fluctuations in Mood and Behavior and Their Relationship to Phototherapy," *Psychiatry Research* 36 (1991): 253–64.
61. Frederic Flach, *Resilience* (New York: Fawcett Columbine, 1988).
62. Vaughan, "The Depression-Stress Link," 155.
63. Blair Justice, *Who Gets Sick: Thinking and Health* (Houston, TX: Peak Press, 1987), 106–8.
64. C. B. Nemeroff, "The Persistent Neurobiological Consequences of Early Life Trauma."
65. Depression Guideline Panel, *Depression in Primary Care: Volume 2, Treatment of Major Depression, Clinical Practice Guideline Number 5* (Rockville, MD: U. S. Department of Health and Human Services, Agency for Healthcare Policy and Research (AHCPR), Publication no. 93–0551, 1993).
66. Flach, *Resilience.*
67. J. D. Bremer et al., "Hippocampal Volume Reduction in Major Depression," *American Journal of Psychiatry* 157 (2000): 115–8.
68. Y. I. Sheline et al., "Untreated Depression and Hippocampal Volume Loss," *American Journal of Psychiatry* 160 (2003): 1516–8.
69. This is also confirmed by E. J. Nestler et al., "Neurobiology of Depression," *Neuron* 34 (2002): 13–25.
70. H. K. Manji et al., "Enhancing Neuronal Plasticity and Cellular Resilience to Develop Novel, Improved Therapeutics for Difficult-to-Treat Depression," *Biological Psychiatry* 53 (2003): 707–42. Also O. Berton et al., "Essential Role of BDNF in the Mesolimbic Dopamine Pathway in Social Defeat Stress," *Science* 311, no. 5762 (February 10, 2006): 864–8 and N. M. Tsankova et al., "Sustained Hippocampal Chromatin Regulation in a Mouse Model of Depression and Antidepressant Action," *Nature Neuroscience* 2006.
71. Manji et al., "Enhancing Neuronal Plasticity and Cellular Resilience to Develop Novel, Improved Therapeutics for Difficult-to-Treat Depression."

72. Depression Guideline Panel, *Depression in Primary Care,* 23.

73. Justice, *Who Gets Sick,* 100, 102–3.

74. Depression Guideline Panel, *Depression in Primary Care,* 51–2.

75. I. J. Russell, "Fibrositis/Fibromyalgia Syndrome," in B. M. Hyde, ed., *The Clinical and Scientific Basis of Myalgic Encephalitis/Chronic Fatigue Syndrome* (Ottawa: Nightingale Research Foundation, 1992); H. Vaeroy et al., "Elevated CSF Levels of Substance P and High Incidence of Raynaud Phenomenon in Patients with Fibromyalgia: New Features for Diagnosis," *Pain* 32 (1988): 21–6; and R. M. Murphy and F. P. Zemlan, "Differential Effects of Substance P on Serotonin-Modulated Spinal Nociceptive Reflexes," *Psychopharmacology (Berlin)* 93 (1987): 118.

76. J. I. Hudson et al., "Fibromyalgia and Major Affective Disorder: A Controlled Phenomenology and Family History Study," *American Journal of Psychiatry* 142 (1985): 441–6.

77. L. M. Arnold, P. E. Keck, Jr., and J. A. Welge, "Antidepressant Treatment of Fibromyalgia: A Meta-Analysis and Review," *Psychosomatics* 41, no. 2 (2000): 104–13.

78. L. J. Crofford et al., "Pregabalin for the Treatment of Fibromyalgia Syndrome. Results of a Randomized, Double-Blind, Placebo-Controlled Trial," *Arthritis and Rheumatism* 52 (2005): 1264–73.

79. B. B. Singh, B. M. Berman, V. A. Hadhazy, and P. Creamer, "A Pilot Study of Cognitive Behavioral Therapy in Fibromyalgia," *Alternative Therapies in Health and Medicine* 4, no. 2 (1998): 67–70.

80. L. A. Rossy et al., "A Meta-Analysis of Fibromyalgia Treatment Interventions," *Annals of Behavioral Medicine* 21, no. 2 (1999): 180–91.

81. M. B. Scharf et al., "Effect of Gamma-Hydroxybutyrate on Pain, Fatigue, and the Alpha Sleep Anomaly in Patients with Fibromyalgia," *Journal of Rheumatology* 25, no. 10 (1998): 1986–90.

82. I. Caruso, P. Sarzi Puttini, M. Cazzola, and V. Azzolini, "Double-Blind Study of 5-Hydroxytryptophan Versus Placebo in the Treatment of Primary Fibromyalgia Syndrome," *Journal of International Medical Research* 18, no. 3 (1990): 201–9; and P. S. Puttini and I. Caruso, "Primary Fibromyalgia Syndrome and 5-Hydroxy-L-Tryptophan: A 90-day Open Study, Rheumatology Unit, L Sacco Hospital, Milan, Italy," *Journal of International Medical Research* 20, no. 2 (1992): 182–89.

83. Gregory Manov and William Guy, "Medical Disorders That May Present as Depression," *Physician and Patient* (January 1985): 46–51.

84. B. Han, "Depressive Symptoms and Self-Rated Health in Community-Dwelling Older Adults: A Longitudinal Study," *Journal of the American Geriatric Society* 50(9) (2002): 1549–56.

85. B. Han and M. Jylha, "Improvement in Depressive Symptoms and Changes in Self-Rated Health among Community-Dwelling Disabled Older Adults," *Aging Mental Health* 10, no. 6 (November 2006): 599–605.

86. Linda C. Higgins, "Depression May Shorten Survival," *Medical World News* (July 10, 1989): 20.

87. G. I. Keitner et al., "12-Month Outcome of Patients with Major Depression and Comorbid Psychiatric or Mental Illness," *American Journal of Psychiatry* 148 (1991): 345–50; P. J. Lustman, L. S. Griffith, and R. E. Clouse, "Depression in Adults with Diabetes: Results of a Five-Year Follow-Up Study," *Diabetes Care* 11 (1988): 605–12; and R. M. Carney, et al., "Depression as a Risk Factor for Mortality after Acute Myocardial Infarction," *American Journal of Cardiolology* 92, no. 11 (2003): 1277–81.

88. S. Moussavi et al., "Depression, Chronic Diseases, and Decrements in Health: Results from the World Health Surveys," *Lancet* 370 (2007): 851–8.

89. Barry W. Rovner et al., "Depression and Mortality in Nursing Homes," *Journal of the American Medical Association,* 265 (1991): 993–6.
90. Higgins, "Depression May Shorten Survival," 21.
91. Ibid., 21.
92. A. Schins et al., "Increased Coronary Events in Depressed Cardiovascular Patients: 5-HT2A Receptor as Missing Link?" *Psychosomatic Medicine* 65, no. 5 (2003): 729–37.
93. D. W. Black, G. Winokur, and A. Nasrallah, "Mortality in Patients with Primary Unipolar Depression, Secondary Unipolar Depression, and Bipolar Affective Disorder: A Comparison with General Population Mortality," *International Journal of Psychiatric Medicine* 17 (1987): 351–60.
94. Janice K. Kiecolt-Glaser and Ronald Glaser, "Psychological Influences on Immunity," *Psychosomatics* 27 (1986): 621–24.
95. Howard S. Friedman, *The Self-Healing Personality* (New York: Henry Holt and Company, 1991), 61.
96. W. A. Greene, S. Goldstein, and A. J. Moss, "Psychosocial Aspects of Sudden Death," *Archives of Internal Medicine* 129 (1972): 725–31; R. M. Charney et al., "Ventricular Tachycardia and Psychiatric Depression in Patients with Coronary Artery Disease," *American Journal of Medicine* 95 (1993): 23–8; and E. M. Levy et al., "Biological Measures and Cellular Immunological Function in Depressed Psychiatric Inpatients," *Psychiatry Research* 36 (1991): 157–67.
97. L. R. Wulsin and B. M. Singal, "Do Depressive Symptoms Increase the Risk for the Onset of Coronary Disease? A Systematic Quantitative Review," *Psychosomatic Medicine* 65, no. 2 (2003): 201–10.
98. J. Barth, M. Schumacher, and C. Herrmann-Lingen, "Depression as a Risk Factor for Mortality in Patients with Coronary Heart Disease: A Meta-Analysis," *Psychosomatic Medicine* 66, no. 6 (2004): 802–13; R. M. Carney , K. E. Freedland, and A. S. Jaffe, "Depression as a Risk Factor for Coronary Heart Disease Mortality," *Archives of General Psychiatry* 58, no. 3 (2001): 229–30; S. Yusuf, INTERHEART Study Investigators, et al., "Effect of Potentially Modifiable Risk Factors Associated with Myocardial Infarction in 52 Countries (the INTERHEART study): Case-Control Study," *Lancet* 364, no. 9438 (2004): 937–52; A. Rosengren, INTERHEART investigators, et al., "Association of Psychosocial Risk Factors with Risk of Acute Myocardial Infarction in 11119 Cases and 13648 Controls from 52 Countries (the INTERHEART study): Case-Control Study," *Lancet* 364 (2004): 953–62; and David S. Sheps et al., "The INTERHEART Study: Intersection Between Behavioral and General Medicine," *Psychosomatic Medicine* 66 (2004): 797–98.
99. Donald E. Girard, Ransom J. Arthur, and James B. Reuler, "Psychosocial Events and Subsequent Illness—A Review," *Western Journal of Medicine* 142, no. 3 (1985): 358–363.
100. Ibid.
101. James J. Lynch, *The Broken Heart The Medical Consequences of Loneliness* (New York: Basic Books, 1977).
102. Ibid.
103. R. Anda et al., "Depressed Affect, Hopelessness, and the Risk of Ischemic Heart Disease in a Cohort of U.S. Adults," *Epidemiology* 4, no. 4 (1993): 285–94.
104. Ibid.
105. F. Okamura et al., "Insulin Resistance in Patients with Depression and Its Changes during the Clinical Course of Depression: Minimal Model Analysis," *Metabolism* 49 no. 10 (2000): 1255–60; M. Chiba et al., "Tyrosine Hydroxylase Gene Microsatellite Polymorphism Associated with Insulin Resistance in Depressive Disorder," *Metabolism* 49, no. 9 (September 2000): 1145–9; R. Rosmond and P. Björntorp, "Endocrine and Metabolic Aberrations in Men with Abdominal Obesity in Relation to Anxio-Depressive Infirmity," *Metabolism* 47,

no. 10 (1998): 1187–93; A. Winokur et al., "Insulin Resistance After Oral Glucose Tolerance Testing in Patients with Major Depression," *American Journal of Psychiatry* 145, no. 3 (March 1988): 325–30; and P. Bjorntorp, *Diabetic Medicine* 16, no. 5 (May 1999): 355–7.

106. G. P. Chrousos, "The Role of Stress and the Hypothalamic-Pituitary-Adrenal Axis in the Pathogenesis of the Metabolic Syndrome: Neuro-Endocrine and Target Tissue-Related Causes," *International Journal of Obesity and Related Metabolic Disorders* 24, suppl 2 (June 2000): S50–5.

107. M. de Groot et al., "Association of Depression and Diabetes Complications: A Meta-Analysis," *Psychosomatic Medicine* 63, no. 4 (2001): 619–30. Also see R. E. Clouse, *Psychosomatic Medicine* 63 (2001): 103.

108. F. Okamura et al., "Insulin Resistance in Patients with Depression and Its Changes during the Clinical Course of Depression: Minimal Model Analysis," *Metabolism* 49 (2000): 1255–60; also F. Okamura, "Insulin Resistance in Patients with Depression and Its Changes in the Clinical Course of Depression: A Report on Three Cases Using the Minimal Model Analysis," *Internal Medicine* 38, no. 3 (1999): 257–60.

109. P. J. Lustman et al., "Fluoxetine for Depression in Diabetes: A Randomized Double-Blind Placebo-Controlled Trial," *Diabetes Care* 23, no. 5 (2000): 618–23; also P. J. Goodnick et al., "Use of Antidepressants in Treatment of Comorbid Diabetes Mellitus and Depression as Well as in Diabetic Neuropathy," *Annals of Clinical Psychiatry* 4101, no. 13 (2001): 31–41.

110. W. H. Sauer et al., "Selective Serotonin Reuptake Inhibitors and Myocardial Infarction," *Circulation* 104 (2001): 1894–98.

111. S. B. Manuck, J. R. Kaplan, and K. A. Matthews, "Behavioral Antecedents of Coronary Artery Disease and Atherosclerosis," *Atherosclerosis* 6 (1986): 2–14.

112. J. I. Haft and Y. S. Arkel, "Effect of Emotional Stress on Platelet Aggregation in Humans," *Chest* 70 (1979): 501–5; and S. Cohen, J. R. Kaplan, and S. B. Manuck, "Social Support and Coronary Heart Disease: Underlying Psychologic and Biologic Mechanisms," in S. A. Shumaker and S. M. Czajkowski, eds., *Social Support and Cardiovascular Disease* (New York: Plenum, 1992).

113. V. L. Serebruanny et al., "Selective Serotonin Reuptake Inhibitors Yield Additional Antiplatelet Protection in Patients with Congestive Heart Failure Treated with Anticedent Aspirin," *European Journal of Heart Failure* 5 (2003): 517–21.

114. B. G. Pollock, "Evaluation of Platelet Activation in Depressed Patients with Ischemic Heart Disease after Paroxetine or Nortriptyline Treatment," *Journal of Clinical Psychopharmacology* 20 (2000): 137–40.

115. R. M. Carney et al., "Major Depressive Disorder Predicts Cardiac Events in Patients with Coronary Artery Disease," *Psychosomatic Medicine* 50 (1988): 627–33.

116. Ibid.

117. Nancy Frasure-Smith, Francois Lesperance, and Mario Talajic, "Depression Following Myocardial Infarction: Impact on Six-Month Survival," *Journal of the American Medical Association* 270 (1993): 1819–25. (See also the editorial by Williams and Chesney in the same issue.)

118. R. M. Carney et al., "Ventricular Tachycardia and Psychiatric Depression in Patients with Coronary Artery Disease," *American Journal of Medicine* 95 (1993): 23–8.

119. Margaret A. Chesney, "Social Isolation, Depression, and Heart Disease: Research on Women Broadens the Agenda," *Psychosomatic Medicine* 55 (1993): 434–5.

120. Ibid.

121. Redford B. Williams and Margaret A. Chesney, "Psychosocial Factors and Prognosis in Established Coronary Artery Disease," *Journal of the American Medical Association* 270 (1993): 1860–1.

122. A. H. Glassman et al.,"Sertraline Treatment of Major Depression in Patients with Acute MI or Unstable Angina." [The SADHART Trial], *Journal of the American Medical Association* 288 (2002): 701–9; and S. M. Czajkowski and the Writing Committee for the ENRICHD Investigators, "The Effects of Treating Depression and Low Perceived Social Support on Clinical Events after Myocardial Infarction: The Enhancing Recovery in Coronary Heart Disease Patients (ENRICHD) Randomized Trial)," *Journal of the American Medical Association* 289 (2003): 3106–16.

123. J. B. Imboden, A. Cantor, L. E. Cluff, "Convalescence from Influenza. A Study of the Psychological and Clinical Determinants," *Archives of Internal Medicine* 108 (1961): 393–9.

124. S. Cohen, D. A. Tyrell, and A. P. Smith, "Psychological Stress and Susceptibility to the Common Cold," *New England Journal of Medicine* 325 (1991): 606–12.

125. C. L. Raison, L. Capuron, and A. H. Miller, "Cytokines Sing the Blues: Inflammation and the Pathogenesis of Depression," *Trends in Immunology* 27, no. 1 (2006): 24–31.

126. S. E. Locke et al., *Life Change Stress and Human Natural Killer Cell Activity* (research report, Department of Biological Sciences and Psychosomatic Medicine, Division of Psychiatry, Boston University School of Medicine, 1979).

127. M. Irwin et al., "Immune and Neuroendocrine Changes during Bereavement," *Psychiatric Clinics of North America* 10 (1987): 449–65.

128. Ibid.

129. "Depression and Immunity," *Harvard Medical School Mental Health Letter* (1986): 8.

130. A. V. Ravindran, J. Griffiths, Z. Merali, and H. Anisman, "Lymphocyte Subsets Associated with Major Depression and Dysthymia: Modification by Antidepressant Treatment," *Psychosomatic Medicine* 57, no. 6 (1995): 555–63.

131. Margaret Kemeny et al., "Psychological and Immunological Predictors of Genital Herpes Recurrence," *Psychosomatic Medicine* 5 (1989): 195–208; also Justice, *Who Gets Sick,* 157.

132. "Depression and Immunity," 8.

133. Steven Locke and Douglas Colligan, *The Healer Within: The New Medicine of Mind and Body* (New York: E. P. Dutton, 1986), 66.

134. Ibid., 68.

135. A. I. Terr, "Environmental Illness: A Clinical Review of 50 Cases," *Archives of Internal Medicine* 146 (1986): 145–9.

136. M. Timonen et al., "Presence of Atopy in First-Degree Relatives as a Predictor of a Female Proband's Depression: Results from the Northern Finland 1966 Birth Cohort," *Journal of Allergy and Clinical Immunology* 111, no. 6 (2003): 1249–54.

137. M. Kovacs, A. Stauder, and S. Szedmak, "Severity of Allergic Complaints: The Importance of Depressed Mood," *Journal of Psychosomatic Research* 54, no. 6 (2003): 549–57.

138. S. G. Consoli, "Psychological Factors in Chronic Urticaria," *Annales de Dermatologie et de Venereologie* 130, spec. no. 1 (2003): 1S73–7.

139. M. Hashiro and M. Okumura, "Anxiety, Depression, Psychosomatic Symptoms and Autonomic Nervous Function in Patients with Chronic Urticaria," *Journal of Dermatological Science* 8, no. 2 (1994): 129–35.

140. A. J. Zautra et al., "Immune Activation and Depression in Women with Rheumatoid Arthritis," *Journal of Rheumatology* 31, no. 3 (2003): 457–63.

141. A. J. Zautra, N. A. Hamilton, P. Potter, and B. Smith, "Field Research on the Relationship Between Stress and Disease Activity in Rheumatoid Arthritis," *Annals of the New York Academy of Science* 876 (1999): 397–412.

142. V. J. Pop et al., "Are Autoimmune Thyroid Dysfunction and Depression Related?" *Journal of Clinical Endocrinology & Metabolism* 83, no. 9 (1998): 3194–7.

143. J. Lieb, "Lithium and Antidepressants: Inhibiting Eicosanoids, Stimulating Immunity, and Defeating Microorganisms," *Medical Hypotheses* 59, no. 4 (2002): 429–32.

144. S. Kubesch et al., "Aerobic Endurance Exercise Improves Executive Functions in Depressed Patients," *Journal of Clinical Psychiatry* 64 (2003): 1005–12; and A. Moraska and M. Fleshner, "Voluntary Physical Activity Prevents Stress-Induced Behavioral Depression and Anti-KLH Antibody Suppression," *American Journal of Physiology–Regulatory, Integrative, and Comparative Physiology* 281, no. 2 (2001): R484–9.

145. A. Mizruchin et al., "Comparison of the Effects of Dopaminergic and Serotonergic Activity in the CNS on the Activity of the Immune System," *Journal of Neuroimmunology* 101, no. 2 (1999): 201–4.

146. B. Bower, "Science News of the Week/Depression and Cancer: A Fatal Link," *Science News* 132 (1987): 244.

147. Alan B. Zonderman, Paul T. Costa, and Robert R. McCrae, "Depression as a Risk for Cancer Morbidity and Mortality in a Nationally Representative Sample," *Journal of the American Medical Association* 262, no. 9 (1989): 1191–200.

148. M. Irie, S. Asami, M. Ikeda, and H. Kasai, "Depressive State Relates to Female Oxidative DNA Damage via Neutrophil Activation," *Biochemical and Biophysical Research Communications* 311, no. 4 (2003): 1014–18.

149. Karl Goodkin, quoted in S. Hart, "Depression and Cancer: No Clear Connection," *Science News* 136 (1989): 150.

150. K. Bolla-Wilson and M. L. Bleecker, "Absence of Depression in Elderly Adults," *Journal of Gerontology* 44, no. 2 (1989): 53–5.

151. N. L. Smith, "Physical Symptoms Predictive of Depression and Anxiety," American Psychosomatic Society annual meeting, May 8–10, 1996, Williamsburg, Virginia, *Psychosomatic Medicine* abstracts 1996, and J. Shavers, *The Identification of Depression and Anxiety in a Medical Outpatient Setting and Their Correlation to Presenting Physical Complaints* (PhD dissertation, University of Utah, 1996).

152. Wayne Katon, "Depression: Somatization and Social Factors," *Journal of Family Practice* 27, no. 6 (1978): 579–80.

153. Jana M. Mossey, Elizabeth Mutran, Kathryn Knott, and Rebecca Craik, "Recovery After Hip Fractures: The Importance of Psychosocial Factors," *Advances in Mind Body Medicine* 6, no. 4 (1991): 23–5.

154. Magdalena Sobieraj, Jeanine Williams, John Marley, and Philip Ryan, "The Impact of Depression on the Physical Health of Family Members," *British Journal of General Practice* 48 (1998): 1653–5.

155. M. Weismann et al., "Remissions in Maternal Depression and Child Psychopathology," *Journal of the American Medical Association* 295 (2006): 1389–98.

156. E. Frank et al., "Three Year Outcome for Maintenance Therapies in Recurrent Depression," *Archives of General Psychiatry* 47 (1990): 1093–99.

157. V. Maletic et al., "Neurobiology of Depression: An Integrated View of Key Findings," *Clinical Practice* 61, no. 12 (2007): 2030–40.

158. G. Dawson, et al., "Infants of Depressed Mothers Exhibit Atypical Frontal Brain Electrical Activity During Interactions with Mother and with a Familiar, Nondepressed Adult," *Child Development* 70 (1999): 1058–66.

159. Ibid.

160. Dennis Gersten, "Depression: Is It a Product of Our Culture?" *Brain/Mind Bulletin* 16, no. 6 (1991): 6–7.

161. "Ten Physical Reasons You May Be Depressed," *Prevention* (June 1992): 69–76.

CHAPTER 7

Insomnia and Sleep Deprivation: Health Effects and Treatment

Not poppy, nor mandragora,
nor all the drowsy syrups of the world
shall ever medicine thee
to that sweet sleep which thou ow'dst yesterday.

—William Shakespeare

LEARNING OBJECTIVES

- Define *insomnia* and *sleep deprivation*.
- List the major types and causes of insomnia.
- Understand the factors in the development of chronic insomnia.
- List the behavioral, psychological, and physiological effects of insomnia.
- Understand the treatment of insomnia.

As often happens with new mothers, Maria found her sleep frequently interrupted after the birth of her baby; soon, she began to get irritable, and eventually she became depressed. Even after the baby finally began sleeping through the night, Maria continued to have trouble sleeping. To make matters worse, she also started having aching muscles and stomach problems. Thinking she could at least do something about her sleeping problems, she tried some over-the-counter sleeping aids (antihistamines) but was disappointed when they didn't seem to help much.

Months later, when seeking medical help for her muscle aches and stomach problems, she mentioned the insomnia to her physician. Maria was somewhat surprised when her physician focused on treating the insomnia, not the pain. He started with some short-term medication to help her sleep but also taught her some long-term relaxation and stress resilience techniques. Maria was amazed: the techniques not only relieved her fatigue and irritability but also resolved her physical problems as well.

Sleep Needs and Definitions

We all recognize sleep as a natural, periodic state of rest during which consciousness of the world is suspended. Body repair and growth occurs better during sleep, and dreams seem to help incorporate new experience into our functional paradigms. Insomia is defined as inadequate or poor-quality sleep because of one or more of the following: difficulty falling asleep; waking up frequently during the night with difficulty returning to sleep; waking up too early in the morning; or unrefreshing sleep.

Sleep needs vary greatly from person to person. Some people are "short sleepers," requiring less than six hours a night, though that is quite uncommon. Others are "long sleepers," requiring nine hours or more. Most people need seven to eight hours of sleep at night to feel good all the next day.

So, how do you determine how much sleep you need? You need enough sleep to provide full restoration and function for the next day. In other words, you need to feel fully rested and energized enough to meet the demands of the day. If you "hit the wall" in the afternoon, need caffeine, or get drowsy when you slow down, you are clearly not getting enough sleep at night. And don't think you can simply make up for it with a couple of quick naps during the day: Napping during the day causes the quality of night sleep to deteriorate. Using stimulants to compensate for sleep loss is not a great idea. You may temporarily function better with the caffeine, but the medical problems of sleep deprivation ultimately will catch up with you.

Tiredness is the number one reported symptom in general medical clinics. Tiredness can be either true fatigue (an exhausted feeling not relieved well by rest) or excess day sleepiness (feeling drowsy when slowing down, which usually responds to adequate rest). It's important to make the distinction because the two have different causes. Fatigue is usually caused by medical illness (about 10 percent), sleep deprivation (about 20 percent), or mental disorders like depression and anxiety disorders (about 70 percent). Excessive sleepiness in the day is almost always caused by inadequate night sleep—either too few hours or poor-quality sleep. Thus, much of the tiredness people experience today is due to sleep deprivation—simply, they don't spend enough time asleep in bed.

About 70 years ago, Americans became hooked on the notion that a person's worth was based on their measurable productivity—the numbers they generate, hours worked, income, status, and so on—and thus the conundrum of "having too much to do." This notion has caused great distress. For example, in America old people are seen as having lesser value because they are "less productive." That's not always true elsewhere. (For example, look at some Asian cultures, where the measure of worth has more to do with wisdom, character, vision, and the insights necessary to nurture and empower the young in meaningful ways.) It's possible we may be killing ourselves mentally and spiritually, and even physically, with this excessive productivity notion. Too many tend to think that sleep is a waste of time or that they have too many other "more important" things to do instead. That kind of thinking leads to sleep deprivation and is likely to be very costly to both health and quality of life. The National Sleep Foundation surveys find that 50 percent of Americans are sleep deprived, with 30 percent averaging less than six hours sleep per night.

Table 7.1   Epworth Sleepiness Scale (ESS)

For each situation described below, rate your chance of dozing while doing the activity: (0 = would never doze; 1 = slight chance of dozing; 2 = moderate chance of dozing; 3 = high chance of dozing)	
Situation	**Chance of Dozing**
Sitting and reading	
Watching television	
Sitting inactive in a public place—for example, a theater or meeting	
As a passenger in a car an hour without a break	
Lying down to rest in the afternoon	
Sitting and talking to someone	
Sitting quietly after lunch (with no alcohol)	
In a car, while stopped in traffic	
Total Score	

Source: Modified from M. W. Johns, "A New Method for Measuring Daytime Sleepiness: The Epworth Sleepiness Scale," *Sleep* 14 (1991): 540–5.

If you wonder if you are getting enough sleep, take the Epworth Sleepiness Scale in Table 7.1. Be very honest in your appraisal.

If your score is 1 to 6, congratulations! You are probably getting enough sleep. A score of 7 to 9 is not bad, but you may need to consider more sleep. If your score is above 9, you have pathological sleepiness. If increasing your hours of sleep time is not enough to correct this score, you may have poor-quality sleep and should look into the reasons (which usually requires medical evaluation).

Getting enough sleep is far more important to physical health than many realize, yet far too many people don't get adequate sleep. More than one-third of all Americans complain of trouble sleeping, and half of those feel that their inability to get enough sleep interferes significantly with their health or their ability to function. The frequency of insomnia increases with age: after age 50, more than half of all Americans are unable to get the sleep they need.[1] For one-fourth of the troubled sleepers—approximately 9 percent of the population—the insomnia is chronic and unrelenting. Twenty-four percent of young adults (aged 18 to 29) doze off while driving. (Such dozing causes more accidents than alcohol.)

That's not all: The total annual cost of sleep problems to Americans is startling— one careful and conservative 1994 estimate placed the total cost of insomnia (including lost productivity) in the United States between $92.5 and $107.5 billion per year.[2] To put that in perspective, that's more than the cost in 2008 of heart disease (at $87 billion a year) or cancer (at $66 billion a year).[3]

As a society, Americans now sleep less than their counterparts of previous generations. A Stanford study spanning more than seventy years shows that, since 1910, the average time of sleep among Americans has decreased nearly one and a half hours per night.[4]

(Presumably nighttime lighting, television, and the desire to be more productive have cut sleep hours from the natural amount needed to provide adequate rest.) Those hours may not seem like much, but other studies show that a sleep deficit of just two hours per night has significantly detrimental effects on health, as will be discussed later in this chapter.

When patients in two general internal medicine clinics were recently surveyed, physicians found that 43 percent have bothersome sleeping problems—and "problems with sleep" was the third most common medical symptom listed by the patients (fatigue was first).[5] However, while almost half of any patient population may have problems sleeping, few of those ever mention their sleep problems to their physician. Another survey found that 69 percent of people with chronic insomnia had never let a physician know about the problem. Only 5 percent of patients with insomnia came to the physician specifically to get help for their insomnia, and an additional 26 percent mentioned it only incidentally while being evaluated for other problems.[6] Obviously, a very common and significant problem often remains undetected!

Research shows that there is a significant gender difference when it comes to insomnia. Women are more prone to insomnia than men—and are more susceptible to the mood-altering effects of sleep loss. This gender difference is even truer at menopause, particularly among women who experience hot flashes.[7] Insomnia is the most common bothersome menopausal symptom, and experience shows that estrogen replacement therapy reduces the number of nighttime awakenings.

There are three general kinds of insomnia:

1. Trouble falling asleep

2. Trouble staying asleep (either waking up too early or waking up multiple times during the night)

3. Perception of inadequate sleep (not feeling refreshed after sleep)

Each of these types of sleep disturbance has different causes, and each calls for different types of treatment.

Types and Causes of Insomnia

Different patterns of insomnia tend to have varying causes:

- **Initiatory insomnia,** or trouble falling asleep, may be caused by anxiety disorders or poor "sleep hygiene." Poor "sleep hygiene" can occur when a person or an environment is not conducive to sleep—for example, the room may be noisy, too light, too warm, or too cold, or the person's core body temperature may be too high. Another very common cause of trouble falling asleep among teens and young adults is "sleep phase delay"—a problem with one's internal sleep clock. This is generally the case when a person wants to go to bed late (between 2 and 3 AM) and get up late (between 10 and 11 AM). This will be discussed in more detail later.

- **Early awakening**—waking up at 3 or 4 AM and not being able to go back to sleep— is most commonly caused by clinical depression. Aging can also contribute, particularly if there is a need to go to the bathroom during the night.

- **Multiple awakenings**—waking up numerous times during the night, often with difficulty going back to sleep—may be caused by a medical problem, such as heart failure, acid reflux, or obstructive sleep apnea (with loud snoring). Depression also commonly causes multiple awakenings.

- **Daytime sleepiness,** as opposed to simple fatigue, is often caused by inadequate time in bed but can also be caused by poor sleep quality from primary sleep disorders, an underlying medical problem, or the sleep phase delay common in teenagers that was mentioned earlier. These potential causes need to be ruled out before assuming that the sleepiness is simply caused by too little time in bed. (Primary medical sleep disorders are discussed briefly later in this chapter.)

Far more than half of the people who come to primary care medical clinics with sleep problems also have problems with anxiety or depression. It is important to remember that sleep deprivation itself can, in turn, precipitate or contribute to a major depression or anxiety episode in a person who is under stress or who is genetically predisposed to depression or anxiety problems.

Factors in the Development of Chronic Insomnia

Three major types of factors play a role in the development of chronic insomnia:[8]

1. **Predisposing factors.** These include a genetic predisposition to hyperarousal, depression, anxiety, or insomnia; some psychological coping styles; learned habits; the inability to relax; and age.

2. **Precipitating factors.** Acute insomnia (that may later become chronic) may be caused by a series of stressful events, a psychiatric or medical illness, environmental disturbances, or certain kinds of drugs used to treat unrelated medical or psychiatric conditions (a few drugs cause sleep disturbances as a side effect).

3. **Perpetuating factors.** Perpetuating factors include mentally conditioned anxiety or arousal upon going to bed, poor sleep hygiene, a chronically stressed lifestyle, drugs used to treat medical or psychiatric conditions, or certain psychiatric disorders. Mental conditioning is the primary cause.

Alcohol, caffeine, and tobacco are also important perpetuating factors. These substances disturb sleep in various ways:

- Caffeine and other stimulants inhibit the neurochemistry of sleep, disturbing the natural chemical balances in the brain that promote sleep. If one is not sleeping well, these should not be taken after 2 PM.

- Alcohol causes what's known as "rebound"; it initially causes drowsiness, but as it wears off, it causes rebound arousal a few hours later in the middle of the night.

- Nicotine has a two-phase effect on sleep; at low levels, it is relaxing; but at high levels, it inhibits sleep.

- Activating medications, such as some antidepressants or medications used for attention deficit disorder (stimulants such as amphetamines or methyphenidate) can interfere with sleep if taken late in the day.

- Older benzodiazepine sleeping pills or herbs that are used over an extended period of time may create a rebound effect; instead of promoting sleep, they may actually cause arousal. (Most newer sleeping pills have been designed to eliminate this effect.)

- Herbs used "for energy" often contain high doses of caffeine and other stimulants.

Mental Conditioning and Perpetuating Factors

Regardless of which precipitating factor contributes to insomnia, other components quickly enter the equation to create a "learned" (conditioned) insomnia. In other words, cognitive and behavioral components soon pitch in to create chronic insomnia, independent of what originally caused the problem. If treatment is to be effective, it is critical to understand what goes into that "conditioning" or learned response, particularly if the insomnia is chronic.

Mental conditioning is an essential part of life and allows us all to be able to effectively function through the day. For example, automatic conditioned responses come into play every time you tie your shoes or drive a car; those responses are triggered by the situation. When you are exposed to a situation to which you have responded in a certain, repeated way—such as seeing your untied shoelaces—the expected automatic response is elicited once again, usually both behaviorally and physiologically.

That's what happens with "repetitively practiced" insomnia as well. An initial stressor, particularly in a predisposed individual, can cause a few days of sleeplessness. For example, you may be making an important presentation at the end of the week, and thoughts about what you need to do and how well you need to perform may be racing through your mind. The more frustrated you get—and the more you worry about your possible poor performance or lack of well-being the next day—the harder you "try to sleep." (Remember: "Trying" to do anything is arousing—and anything that is arousing causes you to stay awake.) You may then decide to do something active in order to avoid wasting time—so you get up, go over your presentation a few times, and then watch some television.

As this pattern repeats itself for a few nights, a mentally conditioned effect is created. Gradually, you create an expectation, or mental "picture," of what is going to happen when you go to bed—you will become anxious, do all these other things in bed, and be unable to sleep. Once this conditioning has been established, it automatically takes over. As soon as you see your bed at bedtime, your mind automatically elicits its established response: You are frustrated, anxious, and unable to sleep, even though you're no longer dealing with the upcoming presentation. That frustrated, anxious response (or doing a lot of other things in bed) is "just what happens" when you're exposed to the bed, even when you are extremely tired.

Approaches to treating chronic insomnia that neglect this conditioning effect, which has usually become the predominant perpetuating factor, will be less effective than those methods that include reconditioning—learning a different behavior (relaxation and sleep) in response to the bed and bedtime. (We'll discuss more about how to do this later.)

Why Do We Sleep?

The National Sleep Foundation describes at least two reasons we sleep:

1. Repair and restoration. During deep stages of sleep is when most growth hormone is secreted. This is needed for repair of the microinjuries (for example, from muscle use) we all sustain daily. Growth hormone deficiency, which occurs with loss of deep stages of sleep, causes aches and symptoms similar to depression. Also during sleep is when restoration occurs for many of the neurotransmitters that keep the nervous system running well. For example, sleep deprivation causes a decrease in central nervous system serotonin, which then can also worsen pain, depression, and anxiety.

2. Integration of experience. Particularly during REM (rapid eye movement, or dream) sleep, we seem to organize new memory and to incorporate the day's experiences into our worldview. Deprivation of REM sleep can sometimes cause psychosis-like symptoms.

Five Stages of Sleep

Stages I and II are light sleep—dozing. Brain waves here show moderate activity. Much of the night is spent in stage two.

Stages III and IV are deep sleep, when much restoration occurs. Brain waves here consolidate into large "delta waves," indicating that many neurons are firing in rested synchrony with each other.

The fifth stage, REM sleep, is when we dream and is almost the opposite of deep sleep. The brain waves look much like they do when we are awake, but we are paralyzed so as not to act out the dreams. "REM sleep disorders" are characterized by some loss of this paralysis: walking, talking, and even doing seemingly purposeful but often bizarre things while sleeping. Other significant sleep disorders will be discussed near the end of this chapter.

Behavioral and Psychological Effects of Insomnia

Sleep deprivation leads to some significant reductions in functioning, particularly in concentration, memory, well-being, enjoyment, coping, and motivation. Persistent sleep loss also causes an increased number of mistakes and boosts the incidence of irritability and depression.[9]

Accidents

When compared to people who do not have insomnia, chronic insomniacs have four times the incidence of automobile accidents—a rate comparable to that caused by alcohol.[10] Falling asleep at the wheel causes half of all accidents that result in fatal injuries, and insufficient sleep is the primary cause of falling asleep at the wheel.[11]

The problem isn't limited to the highways. A strikingly large percentage of catastrophes caused by human error—including the nuclear disasters at Chernobyl and Three

Mile Island—and many accidents in the workplace occur when operators are sleep-deprived or working on night shifts. Night shifts aren't the only problem, either; more than half of sleepy day shift workers have accidents, too.[12]

People with sleep problems also have 2.4 times more alcoholism than average,[13] which in turn also increases the rate of both industrial and automobile accidents.

Depression

There is a major link between depression and insomnia in both directions: 70 to 90 percent of all depressed patients have insomnia,[14] and people with insomnia have 35 times the rate of depression as people who sleep well.

Insomnia often precedes depression, rather than simply being a consequence of depression. A well-designed study of almost 8,000 adults found that those with successfully treated insomnia had only 1.6 times the risk of subsequently developing clinical depression when compared to people who had never suffered with insomnia. However, those with unresolved, continuous insomnia had nearly 40 times the likelihood of developing subsequent major depression.[15] Over time, about 40 percent of untreated, chronic insomniacs develop major depression or anxiety disorders.

It doesn't take months of full-blown insomnia to cause a problem. Symptoms of depression can be caused by depriving normal people of just two hours less sleep than they need to feel good for as few as five nights.[16] When the sleep problem is corrected, the depression is usually relieved. (Perhaps the current "epidemic" of clinical depression may be compounded by the fact that the average American now gets that 1 1/2 hours less sleep than Americans did a century ago, as was mentioned earlier.) More than 2,000 children in Holland, ages 4 to 16 years, were studied to determine the long-term effects of sleep deprivation while young. After adjusting for related social factors, those who slept less when young had 43 percent more depression and 51 percent more aggressive behavior disorders at ages 18 to 32 than those who got good sleep as children.[17]

Part of the reason for depression among those with sleep problems is that changes in day-night sleep cycles affect the brain chemicals that regulate mood. Research shows that people who have lived for months without clocks or external cues to light and dark cycles become depressed.[18] These mechanisms may account in part for the symptoms of depression that occur with jet lag and that often happen with changes in work schedules. Findings of some compelling research suggest that those who tend to get depressed should avoid jobs that require changes in work shifts. Shift work can indeed become hazardous to health because it increases not only accident risk but also cardiovascular disease and mood disorders.

Quality of Life and Function Issues

Lack of sleep has a significant impact on function, especially in the workplace.[19] People who suffer from insomnia are often simply too tired to perform their assigned tasks effectively. When workers are tired, mistakes occur, and the rate of industrial accidents soars.

People who chronically don't get the sleep they need may also simply not show up at work—and if they do, they are generally far less productive than their colleagues.

Insomnia is the second most powerful predictor of job absenteeism and lost productivity and is an even more powerful predictor of absenteeism than is job dissatisfaction.

The effects of insomnia spill over into most aspects of life, affecting both the quality of life and the stability of relationships. A study of 691 untreated insomniacs revealed that:[20]

- 83 percent were "easily upset, irritated, or annoyed"
- 78 percent were "too tired to do things"
- 59 percent had "trouble remembering things"
- 43 percent were "confused in their thinking"

Other proven complications of insomnia include reduced life satisfaction, unsatisfying relationships, reduced ability to cope, and reduced enjoyment of life.[21] Quality of sleep is also a powerful predictor of academic performance.[22]

Economists have known for decades about the "point of diminishing returns," which comes from studies of productivity in workers relative to the time and effort spent on the job. With more effort, productivity goes steadily up—to a certain point. And then, with more time and effort, productivity goes back down. When that happens—because of fatigue, burnout, and mental clumsiness—the point of diminishing returns has been reached. One then becomes more productive by reducing the time spent working back to where adequate rest allows for renewed energy, sharpness, and creativity. All these enhance the joy of life. And perhaps much of the purpose of life has to do with discovering what brings joy. One occasionally needs to ask, "Is all this I'm doing enhancing the joy or getting in the way of it?"

Physiological Effects of Sleep Deprivation

Sleep loss can cause physiological havoc in several body systems.[23]

Metabolic

Studies involving animals have shown that sleep deprivation causes malnutrition and weight changes.[24] Lack of sleep causes increased stress hormones, which in turn causes insulin resistance, which then causes central obesity. One study showed that the number of hours of sleep deprivation were proportional to the body mass index—a standard measure of obesity. Children who sleep fewer than 12 hours a day between the ages of six months and two years are twice as likely to be obese at age three as those who sleep more than 12 hours.[25] Malnutrition may also occur in humans, along with increased pain and changes in other body systems. Compared to good sleepers, people with insomnia are hospitalized twice as often, are admitted to nursing homes twice as often, and have more than twice as many medical office visits.[26]

Pain

Pain increases significantly as sleep decreases. In one study that has since been repeated twice with the same result, normal volunteers who were deprived of deep-stage sleep for a period of only several days developed muscle aches and pains similar to those of fibromyalgia,[27] a common muscular pain disorder caused by hypersensitivity of the pain system. Those aches and pains were relieved when the volunteers' sleep was allowed to return to normal.

The study was prompted by the fact that most people with fibromyalgia have sleep disturbance characterized by loss of deep-stage sleep, which also occurs in people with depression and those with chronic fatigue syndrome.[28] Researchers and physicians have noted that when sleep problems are corrected, patients with fibromyalgia usually experience improvement of muscle pain.[29] Exercise also reduced the increased pain caused by sleep loss, as did some medications that improve deep sleep.

Loss of deep-stage sleep also often accompanies other chronic pain problems. Insomniacs have two to three times the incidence of headaches, gastrointestinal pain, muscle pain, and back and neck pain as noninsomniacs.[30] There is also a strong link between pain and depression in both directions: when depressed people are persistently deprived of deep sleep, they experience greater aches and pain, and two-thirds of chronic pain patients have major depression.

Some people become obsessed with cause and effect: Which comes first, the pain or the insomnia? Does the pain cause the insomnia, or does the insomnia cause the pain? A study of recurrent headaches (usually occurring during the day) showed a high incidence of treatable sleep problems,[31] suggesting similar neurochemical abnormalities contributing to both.

Focusing on the result may be more appropriate. Clinical experience shows that treating the insomnia (or the underlying anxiety/depression, if present) significantly relieves pain and reduces other medical problems. Clinical experience also shows that attempts at treating chronic pain without restoring deep-stage sleep are likely to fail.

Immune System Function

When people in experiments are deprived of sleep, the immune system stops functioning as it should.[32] When that happens, the body is not able to defend itself against invasion by bacteria, viruses, and other microorganisms, and illness, disease, and infection can result.[33] This may account in part for the fact that the body wants more sleep when infected—and why colds and other infections are more readily picked up when people have not had enough sleep.

Studies also show that sleep deprivation reduces the protective response provided by immunization.

Hormonal Changes

Research also demonstrates that when people are chronically deprived of the sleep they need, hormonal changes occur in the body.[34] Especially impacted are thyroid and growth hormones, which are necessary for the repair of body tissues. Insulin resistance occurs, causing diminished blood sugar control and weight gain.

Nervous System Changes

The nervous system changes that occur with inadequate sleep are usually mild, but they can include tremors and increased gag and deep tendon reflexes. There is also an increased potential for seizures and a worrisome loss of respiratory response to low oxygen levels.[35] As noted above, sleep deprivation also creates neurochemical changes in the brain (such as a decrease in norepinephrine and serotonin concentrations) that can lead to depression and anxiety disorders, which in turn can cause a multitude of medical problems (see Chapters 5 and 6). In general, sleep deprivation causes the nervous system to become irritable. That's entirely understandable: *you* likely become irritable without enough sleep.

Mortality

Mortality is 30 percent higher among people who sleep less than six hours a night (compared to those who sleep seven to eight hours a night). Inadequate sleep (less than six hours of sleep a night) also diminishes the protective effects of other good health practices, such as not smoking and getting regular exercise. A study of health-oriented churchgoers in California showed that the protective effects of avoiding smoking, alcohol, and unhealthy foods were lost when people did not get enough sleep.[36]

Treatment of Insomnia

Appropriate treatment depends on the pattern of insomnia and how long the insomnia has been a problem.

Transient insomnia is insomnia that has lasted for only a few nights. It can usually be successfully treated by improving sleep hygiene and relaxation (as detailed below) and, if necessary, using a short-term sleep medication. For example, a short-acting sedative used by night shift workers creates both better function and improved daytime sleep.[37] The idea is to be aggressive in early treatment to prevent chronic insomnia.

Short-term insomnia is insomnia that has lasted for as long as three weeks. It should be treated the same as transient insomnia—by improving sleep hygiene, using relaxation, doing stimulus control (see below), and using short-term sleep medication—as well as by identifying and dealing with the precipitating stressor. Active treatment in the early stages of short-term insomnia can successfully prevent the conditioning that leads to chronic insomnia, which is much more difficult to treat.

Chronic insomnia is defined as sleep problems that have consistently occurred for more than three weeks. The treatment of chronic insomnia, which is much more difficult than the treatment of shorter-term sleep problems, involves treating the underlying psychological or medical condition, as well as all the methods used for shorter-term insomnia, and undergoing behavioral reconditioning. A sleep medication may be used for as little as a few days to as long as three weeks to facilitate the mental reconditioning process. The downside of using medication, however, is that it can be tempting to continue the medication without doing the work of the behavioral reconditioning.

The integrated approach to chronic insomnia involves combining both medication and behavioral reconditioning. Older sleep medications generally work well during the first three weeks and then tend to lose effectiveness. Behavioral methods work more slowly at first, as they are being learned, but then increase substantially in effectiveness after the first two weeks—just as the effectiveness of the medication is declining. Some newer sleep medications are considerably less likely to lose effect, to create dependency, or to cause rebound problems when stopped.[38]

In a study of older patients, researchers compared three groups of people with chronic insomnia: those who were treated with medication alone, those who were treated with behavioral reconditioning alone, and those who were treated with a combination of medication and behavioral reconditioning.[39] After eight weeks, patients who underwent only the behavioral reconditioning were doing better than those who received only the medication, but the patients who had the most significant improvement were those who had a combined treatment of both behavioral reconditioning and medication.

One plausible explanation for these results makes a lot of sense. Behavioral therapies recondition what happens when the person goes to bed, promoting relaxation and sleep. Medication facilitates the reconditioning by causing sleepiness; after a few days of taking the medication, the person expects to be sleepy and get deeply relaxed when going to bed. The new behavioral reconditioning (particularly regularly practiced deep relaxation techniques and stimulus control) then maintains the improved sleeping pattern.

Successful treatment of chronic insomnia generally requires several types of behavioral reconditioning. Some behavioral therapies, such as stimulus control, are more effective for helping people get to sleep. Other types of behavioral therapies, such as progressive muscle relaxation, work better to deepen the quality of sleep.[40] Several types are explained in greater detail below.

When stress is a significant component of the sleep trouble, cognitive behavioral therapy (see Chapter 22) can be highly effective, even more so than the progressive muscle relaxation described below. This therapeutic approach, in addition to the behavioral techniques described below, focuses on coming to think in more rational, productive ways about the situational stressors.

Specific Behavioral Strategies for Treating Insomnia

Some of the more effective behavioral strategies for treating insomnia include sleep hygiene, stimulus control, relaxation methods, thought stopping, exercise, and paradoxical intention.[41]

Sleep Hygiene   All people with insomnia can benefit from improving their sleep hygiene, which includes some of the following techniques:

- Do something enjoyable and relaxing in a routine, ritualistic way before you go to bed.

- Set your troubles and concerns aside. For example, if you're facing a hectic day, plan out on paper how you'll tackle all your demands well before going to bed, and then forget about it. If you're afraid you might forget an important detail, call your own voice mail and leave yourself a reminder.

- Wake up at the same time seven days a week, and go to bed on time so that you get enough hours of sleep. Use an alarm to get up on time, no matter how much sleep you get that night.

- Avoid taking naps; naps almost always disturb the pattern of night sleeping.

- Expose yourself to plenty of bright light early in the day, particularly as soon as you wake up.

- Avoid caffeine after 2 PM, and avoid alcohol after supper. (Alcohol initially helps you fall asleep; but you become aroused as it wears off, which interferes with sleep in the middle of the night).

- Warm your body by taking a bath or exercising four to six hours before you go to bed. As your body cools down four hours later, you will get sleepy.

- Avoid going to bed either hungry or full. A small snack can help promote sleep. Starches and foods containing tryptophan (such as walnuts and milk) increase the amount of the brain chemical serotonin, which promotes sleep. Avoid fluids after supper.

Stimulus Control   Reinforce your bed as a sleep stimulus by limiting any nonsleep behaviors in or around bed. For example:

- Use the bed only for sleep, relaxation, and sex. Don't read, eat, watch television, study, or catch up on work from the office in bed (or in the bedroom).

- Go to bed only when you are feeling drowsy.

- If you haven't fallen asleep within ten to fifteen minutes after you get into bed, get out of bed, leave the bedroom, and read something dull somewhere else in the house until you are drowsy.

- Make sure the conditions in your bedroom are optimal for sleep. Your room should be dark and quiet, your room should be the right temperature (a room that is either too warm or too cool can interfere with sleep), your nightclothes and sheets should not be binding, and your bed should be comfortable and supportive (a mattress that is either too firm or too soft can also interfere with sleep).

Relaxation Methods   Any kind of stress arouses both the mind and the body. Relaxation methods train you to mentally quiet the arousal of stress, inducing the relaxation response. With practice, you can produce deep relaxation rather quickly; this ability not only helps you fall asleep quickly, but also helps to quiet stress responses that occur during the day.

Some relaxation methods can be learned within a few days; others may take as long as three or more weeks to learn. As you use these methods over time, you can get very good at doing them quickly. Different people respond differently to each method, and each person will likely have a preference for a particular method that is based on the way he or she mentally processes information. For example, some people process information best if they have visual cues; others do best if they hear or feel the information. If you have difficulty learning a particular method after three weeks, your practitioner should have you learn a different method.

The relaxation methods most commonly used in the treatment of insomnia include the following:

- **Focused attention on your breath.** Using slow, diaphragmatic breathing (the kind where your abdomen rather than your chest rises as you breathe), feel the air bringing in life-giving energy as you inhale, then feel it carrying away all the unnecessary things as you exhale. The breath is actually a powerful tool for releasing stressful thoughts and becoming calmly focused in the moment. See how long you can keep doing this without reverting back to your usual thoughts. When those thoughts return, just briefly notice them, and let them go again as you focus your attention back on the breath.

- **Progressive muscle relaxation.** This helps people stay asleep and feel more refreshed. Specific muscle groups are tightened and then relaxed, with the tightening and relaxing of muscle groups progressing over the entire body. For example, using the in-breath to tense and the out-breath to relax, start at one foot, then one leg, then the other side, and slowly progress up each part of the body to the face and head. By focusing attention on the difference between how tension and relaxation feel, you can learn how to create relaxation from tension. This then can become a metaphor for life's stresses: converting tension to focused, relaxed responses.

- **Imagery.** Mentally go to a beautiful, relaxing place (a mountain meadow, a quiet beach, a hearthside . . .). Experience this mentally in great detail; use all your senses in creating this image. Smell the smells of this place. Hear the sounds; feel the textures and temperature, and look around you at the beauty. As you do so, the entire mind and body relax, much like being on vacation with nothing to do but soak up the beauty and peace.

- **Self-hypnosis.** Progressively deepening relaxation is used to help the body "let go" of the tension it uses for protection. Some common methods of self-hypnosis include using a mental escalator, slowly counting down, or imagining a heavy and warm feeling in the arms and legs, then eyelids.

- **Mindfulness meditation.** Total attention is focused on one specific thing. For example, complete attention may be focused on a pattern of breathing, a harmonious sound (even music), slow and progressive counting, or the details of an image.[42] Some like to focus on a word, a phrase, or a thought that has symbolic meaning.[43] Meditation, however, is best done well before bedtime, not to induce drowsiness but to create a background calming. Meditation often increases alertness and focus.

Thought Stopping   Thought stopping is a technique that helps people whose minds are crowded with "racing" or worrisome thoughts.[44] Its foundation lies in the understanding that mental distress is caused not so much by events themselves as by the thoughts about those events. With simple training, you can learn to control those kinds of thoughts.

A technique called cognitive psychotherapy can help you change thoughts about underlying anxieties and requires professional work over a period of time. A simpler technique that can help improve your sleep involves what is called "rapid thought stopping":

- Learn and practice one of the relaxation methods above, identifying a quieting focus that works for you.

- As soon as your thoughts start to race or you have an unwanted thought, mentally say with definitive emphasis, "Stop!" Redirect your attention instead to the relaxing thought that you've planned ahead of time. You might use your breath, muscle relaxation, mindfulness, or imagery to redirect your thoughts. You need to have something calming and familiar on which to shift your focus.

- If the unwanted thoughts reappear, repeat the process as needed, saying, "Stop!" more softly each time.

- Keep in mind that racing thoughts could be a symptom of a mood disorder (such as bipolar) that might need medical attention.

Exercise   Exercise has a double benefit: it improves your ability to handle stress, which can interfere with sleep, and it changes your core body temperature in a way that promotes sleep.[45] When compared to people who are not fit and do not exercise, those who are physically fit get to sleep more quickly, wake up less often during the night, have more slow-wave sleep, and feel more rested when they wake up in the morning.[46]

Here's what happens: Normally, core body temperature falls at bedtime, and this drop in core body temperature causes a feeling of sleepiness. Exercise (or a hot bath) raises the core body temperature at first but then induces a rebound drop in temperature approximately four to six hours later. This means that, if you want to improve your sleep, you should exercise (or take a hot bath) about four to six hours before you want to go to bed and fall asleep (about 3 to 6 PM for most people). Be careful: if you exercise in the morning, you may get drowsy in the afternoon.

Rhythmic aerobic exercise is best for inducing sleep. Avoid any rigorous or hostile competition, which may undermine the stress-reduction effect of the exercise. As far as exercise is concerned, there's an important caveat to remember: exercise increases deep sleep—but only if you are careful to replace body fluids after you exercise.[47]

Paradoxical Intention   Oddly enough, trying to stay awake can make you sleepy. Why? The act of trying to stay awake apparently reduces the anxiety that is associated with trying to fall asleep.

Sleep Restriction   This is surprisingly effective at times, particularly for those who lay awake in bed a lot. First, calculate the number of hours you actually sleep on an average night. On following nights, you are allowed to stay in bed only that number of hours. This consolidates your sleep into deeper, more restful types. Once you are sleeping 80 percent of the limited time you are in bed, and as drowsiness increases, you can slowly increase the time you spend in bed (gradually increase the time in 20- to 30-minute increments). Repeat this process until you achieve a full night's quality sleep. This may take two to three weeks to achieve but is very effective.

Choosing Behavioral Techniques

How does one choose which of these behavioral techniques to use? All sleep problems can benefit from good sleep hygiene.

If the problem is *falling asleep:*

- If you feel awake as soon as you go to bed: use stimulus control and perhaps sleep restriction.

- If you are physically tense and anxious: use cognitive behavioral therapy and progressive muscle relaxation.

- For mind racing: Use thought stopping and mindfulness practice.

If the problem is *staying asleep:*

- Use stimulus control and sleep restriction.

- Breathing and progressive muscle relaxation can deepen sleep.

These techniques are often called cognitive behavioral therapy, or CBT. Sleep research shows that "CBT, alone or in combination with pharmacotherapy, is more effective than pharmacotherapy alone or a placebo for the treatment of sleep-onset insomnia. CBT alone was equal or superior to a combination of CBT and pharmacotherapy on most outcome measures. CBT yielded the largest number of normal sleepers after treatment, and maintained therapeutic gains at long-term follow-up."[48] Medications alone tend to work while they are taken, but sleep problems tend to recur when the medications are stopped. However, CBT maintains benefits even after it is no longer formally being done.

Using Medication to Treat Insomnia

The studies that compared the effectiveness of behavioral and drug treatment (described earlier) suggest that medication is best used for periods of less than three to four weeks. For one thing, older sleep medications tend to lose effectiveness after about three weeks. Additionally, using some of the older sleep medications for a long period can perpetuate the insomnia because of habituation, rebound anxiety, or insomnia when the medication is stopped. Some of the newer sleep medications, however, cause no drowsiness or impairment the next day and pose little risk of withdrawal or rebound insomnia. Nevertheless, if really necessary, such medications are best used in the short term to prevent or help solve the conditioning problems of insomnia. Keep in mind that getting good sleep is more important than toughing it out without treatment.

Several kinds of medications are used to treat sleep problems, with varying success.

Over-the-counter sleep aids that contain antihistamines are generally not a good idea because of side effects, which can include:

- daytime drowsiness

- drying and slowing of the bowels

- dizziness

- reduced coordination

- weight gain

- paradoxical agitation or delirium (particularly in the young)

Herbal sleeping medications act like tranquilizing drugs and need to be treated as such. Remember that some herbs touted as promoting sleep are not effective. For example, a study by the National Institutes of Health showed that kava and valerian root were no better than placebos as sleep aids.

Some antidepressants can be very useful if sleep problems are accompanied by anxiety or depression. In addition, antidepressants are not habit forming. They work better for awakening-type insomnia. However, other antidepressants can interfere with sleep.

Melatonin is a natural, sedating neurotransmitter that the body secretes in response to darkness as part of normal sleep cycling and body rhythms. Studies have found that people with insomnia, especially the elderly, frequently have low blood levels of melatonin—often half that of people without insomnia.[49] Melatonin has not been very effective for most insomnia, though a medication called ramelteon, which acts like a very powerful form of melatonin, is effective (particularly when combined with CBT). Ramelteon has also been shown to be very safe. Neither melatonin nor ramelteon is particularly sedating; instead, they work by suppressing arousal.

There is a particular situation in which melatonin or ramelteon can be very useful. Short-term use of these medications can reset the timing of sleep rhythms when needed for the circadian rhythm disorders discussed below. The doses taken are well above the naturally secreted melatonin levels. The usual dose of melatonin used in these studies is 2 to 3 mg, which is seven to ten times the normal amount secreted by the brain. Taking such a dosage is probably not wise over a prolonged period of time because it may disrupt necessary normal body rhythm cycles. Long-term side effects of even low doses of melatonin are not known. Higher doses of melatonin (but not ramelteon) can cause depression, and studies show that melatonin contributes to the winter depression known as seasonal affective disorder (SAD).[50]

Herbal sedatives and tranquilizers need to be used with the same caution as any other drug. Unfortunately, the side effects of these preparations are often not known, and in some cases information about quality controls in manufacturing is not available.

Amino acids such as tryptophan, together with vitamin B_6 to help convert it to serotonin, can occasionally be helpful.

Other Primary Medical Sleep Disorders

It's important to differentiate between the kind of insomnia that has been discussed in this chapter and other primary sleep disorders, which are characterized by excessive daytime sleepiness. These other disorders usually have some characteristic hallmarks. They require different kinds of treatment than those described above as effective for insomnia, and sufferers should seek medical evaluation.

Obstructive Sleep Apnea

The tipoff to this is loud snoring accompanied by pauses in breathing (apnea) while asleep. Obstructive sleep apnea (OSA) can cause a multitude of serious health problems, including hypertension, cardiovascular disease, heart rhythm problems, and swelling of the legs. When a person with OSA becomes deeply relaxed, the airways also relax and close off, obstructing air flow into the lungs. The resulting low oxygen and high carbon dioxide causes recurrent arousals in the nervous system all night, blocking deep sleep and resulting in a system that starts to overrespond to stimuli, including pain. Anyone who snores and feels sleepy in the day should consider being tested for this very common condition.

Restless Legs Syndrome

The tipoff here is a crawling, creeping sensation in the legs that causes the legs to be constantly moving. This occurs most commonly before falling asleep at night. Restless legs syndrome can also interfere with deep sleep, but it is readily treatable medically. It seems to be caused, at least in part, by low central dopamine function and occasionally by iron deficiency.

Circadian Rhythm Disorders

In addition to shift work problems and jet lag, circadian rhythm disorders include sleep phase delay (often seen in teenagers and young adults) and sleep phase advance (often seen in the elderly). The brain's internal sleep clock is largely controlled by melatonin secreted in response to darkness and by morning sunlight. Light stimulates the tiny suprachiasmatic nucleus (SCN, consisting of about 20,000 neurons in the hypothalamus of the brain), which causes increasing arousal during the day. On the other hand, another place in the hypothalamus increases the drive to sleep, which intensifies the longer you go without sleep. These forces (SCN arousal and sleep drive) balance each other through the day until it gets dark. In darkness, melatonin is secreted by the pineal gland to shut off the arousing SCN, allowing the sleep drive to take over. When it gets light again, melatonin falls, the SCN turns back on, and people wake up.

Sleep phase delay is important to distinguish from insomnia because its treatment is quite different and usually fairly simple. In sleep phase delay, the melatonin appears to be secreted too late. This disorder consists of the whole sleep cycle being shifted back a few hours—for example, feeling naturally inclined to fall asleep about 2 or 3 AM and to wake up around 10 or 11 AM if allowed to stay in bed (and usually sleeping well in between). This can easily be confused as insomnia. Sleep phase delay is treated for one to two weeks with either ramelteon or melatonin, plus light. If melatonin is used, usually 1 1/2 mg is taken at supper and 3 mg taken half an hour before the new, desired bedtime, followed by using bright light (sunlight or a bluish, bright light box) for sixty minutes at the desired wake-up time. The sleep phase will usually shift to a more socially acceptable time frame fairly soon following this treatment.

Sleep phase advance (for example, falling asleep at 7 to 8 PM and awakening at 4 AM) is treated in the opposite way: bright light for an hour about 7 PM and melatonin on awakening in the early morning.

Such simple corrections of sleep cycles pay big dividends in quality of life.

Conclusions Regarding Sleep

Insomnia and sleep deprivation are significant medical problems that need to be taken seriously. First and foremost, be sure you get enough time in bed—whatever it takes for you to be alert all day (without the need for caffeine). If you start having sleep problems that can't be resolved by fairly simple measures, tell your physician right away—the longer you struggle with sleep problems, the more likely you are to develop long-term or chronic insomnia as the brain becomes "conditioned" to expect them. Make sure you share any depression or anxiety problems with your physician as well; these problems exist in about half of all cases of chronic insomnia, can cause significant health problems if untreated, and are usually very treatable.

The most effective treatment for insomnia is usually an integrated approach that uses both short-term medication and behavioral reconditioning. Both medication and behavioral treatment are effective regardless of the duration of the insomnia, but behavioral reconditioning (CBT) is especially important in the treatment of chronic insomnia.

In nature, insomnia is often a protective mechanism. Dolphins, for example, are able to let only half of their brain sleep at any given time; the "awake" half of the brain watches for sharks while the other half sleeps. We can learn a tremendous lesson from nature: As humans, we often create our own "sharks" out of the stresses we are faced with on a daily basis. The lesson? A deep sense of inner peace may be one of the most effective ways to promote restful sleep.

WHAT DID YOU LEARN?

1. How can you tell if you are getting enough sleep?

2. Describe three patterns of insomnia?

3. Find an example of each of the factors listed below in the development of chronic insomnia.

   A. Predisposing:

   B. Precipitating:

   C. Perpetuating:

4. What are three behavioral effects of insomnia?

5. What are three physiological effects of insomnia?

6. Describe three primary sleep disorders other than insomnia.

7. Identify and discuss at least four behavioral methods to treat insomnia.

ENDNOTES

1. G. D. Mellinger, M. D. Balter, and E. H. Uhlenhuth, "Insomnia and Its Treatment: Prevalence and Correlates," *Archives of General Psychiatry* 42 (1985): 225–32.

2. M. K. Stoller, "Economic Effects of Insomnia," *Clinical Therapeutics* 16 (1994): 263–87.

3. "An Unhealthy America: The Economic Burden of Chronic Disease," accessed 11/08 at http://www.chronicdiseaseimpact.com/ebcd.taf?cat=disease&type Also see P. E. Greenberg, L. E. Stiglin, S. N. Finkelstein, and E. R. Berndt, "The Economic Burden of Depression in 1990," *Journal of Clinical Psychiatry* 54 (1993): 405–18 (also 419–24).

4. Reported in the National Commission on Sleep Research, *Wake Up America: A National Sleep Alert,* vol. 1 of Executive Summary and Executive Report (Washington, DC: National Commission on Sleep Research, 1993), 17–37. Also H. S. Friedman et al., "Psychosocial Predictors of Longevity: The Aging and Death of the Termites," *American Psychologist* 50 (1995): 69–78.

5. N. L. Smith, "Physical Symptoms Highly Predictive of Depression and Anxiety," American Psychosomatic Society annual meeting, Williamsburg, Virginia, May 8–10, 1996, *Psychosomatic Medicine* abstracts 1996, and J. Shavers, *The Identification of Depression and Anxiety in a Medical Outpatient Setting and Their Correlation to Presenting Physical Complaints* (PhD dissertation, University of Utah, 1996).

6. Gallup Organization, *Sleep in America: A National Survey of U.S. Adults* (Washington, DC: National Sleep Foundation, 1991).

7. J. Shaver, E. Giblin, M. Lentz, and K. Lee, "Sleep Patterns and Stability in Perimenopausal Women," *Sleep* 11 (1988): 560–1.

8. A. J. Spielman, L. S. Caruso, and P. V. Glovinsky, "A Behavioral Perspective on Insomnia Treatment," *Psychiatric Clinics of North America* 10 (1987): 541–53. Also H. M. Bearpark, "Insomnia: Causes, Effects and Treatment," pp. 588–613 in R. Cooper, ed., *Sleep* (London: Chapman and Hall Medical, 1994).

9. M. Kuppermann et al., "Sleep Problems and Their Correlates in a Working Population," *Journal of General Internal Medicine* 10 (1995): 25–32.

10. A. I. Pack, "The Prevalence of Work-Related Sleep Problems," *Journal of General Internal Medicine* 10 (1995): 57. Also see Gallup Organization, *Sleep in America*; M. B. Balter and E. H. Uhlenhuth, "New Epidemiological Findings About Insomnia and Its Treatment," *Journal of Clinical Psychiatry* 53, suppl. (1992): 34–3; P. K. Schweitzer et al., "Consequences of Reported Poor Sleep," *Sleep Research* 21 (1992): abstract, 2; and M. S. Aldrich, "Automobile Accidents in Patients with Sleep Disorders," *Sleep* 12 (1989): 487–94.

11. D. Leger, "The Cost of Sleep-Related Accidents: A Report for the National Commission on Sleep Disorders Research," *Sleep* 17 (1994): 84–93; and Pack, "The Prevalence of Work-Related Sleep Problems."

12. P. Lavie, "Sleep Habits and Sleep Disturbances in Industrial Workers in Israel: Main Findings and Some Characteristics of Workers Complaining of Excessive Daytime Sleepiness," *Sleep* 4 (1981): 147–58.

13. F. Hohagen et al., "Prevalence and Treatment of Insomnia in General Practice: A Longitudinal Study," *European Archives of Psychiatry and Clinical Neuroscience* 242 (1993): 329–36.

14. Ibid.

15. D. E. Ford and D. B. Kamerow, "Epidemiologic Study of Sleep Disturbances and Psychiatric Disorder: An Opportunity for Prevention?" *Journal of the American Medical Association* 262 (1989): 1479–84.

16. T. Wehr, "Manipulations of Sleep and Phototherapy: Nonpharmacological Alternatives in the Treatment of Depression," *Clinical Neuropharmacology* 13, suppl. 1 (1990): S54–65.

17. A. M. Gregory et al., "Parent-Reported Sleep Problems During Development and Self-Reported Anxiety/Depression, Attention Problems and Aggressive Behavior Later in Life," *Archives of Pediatrics and Adolescent Medicine* 162 (2008): 330–5.

18. S. H. Onen, F. Onen, D. Bailley, and P. Parquet, "Prevention and Treatment of Sleep Disorders Through Regulation of Sleeping Habits," *Presse Medicale* 23 (1994): 485–9.

19. P. V. Leigh, "Employee and Job Attributes as Predictors of Absenteeism in a National Sample of Workers: The Importance of Health and Dangerous Working Conditions," *Social Science & Medicine* 33 (1991): 127–37.

20. M. B. Balter and E. H. Uhlenhuth, "The Beneficial and Adverse Effects of Hypnotics," *Journal of Clinical Psychiatry* 52, suppl. (1991): 16–23.

21. Stoller, "Economic Effects of Insomnia."

22. M. W. Johns, H. A. F. Dudley, and J. P. Masterson, "The Sleep Habits, Personality and Academic Performance of Medical Students," *Medical Education* 10 (1976): 158–62; and

D. Blum et al., "Relation Between Chronic Insomnia and School Failure in Preadolescents," *Sleep Research* 19 (1990): abstract, 1.

23. Ford and Kamerow, "Epidemiologic Study of Sleep Disturbances and Psychiatric Disorder," and M. H. Bonnet, "Sleep Deprivation," pp. 55–68 in M. H. Kryger, T. Roth, and W. C. Dement, ed., *Principles and Practice of Sleep Medicine* (Philadelphia: W. B. Saunders, 1994).

24. C. A. Everson and T. A. Wehr, "Nutritional and Metabolic Adaptations in Prolonged Sleep Deprivation in the Rat," *American Journal of Physiology* 264, 2, pt. 2 (1993): R376–87.

25. E. M. Taveras et al., "Short Sleep Duration in Infancy and Risk of Childhood Overweight, *Archives of Pediatrics and Adolescent Medicine* 162 (2008): 305–11.

26. Stoller, "Economic Effects of Insomnia," and S. Weyerer and H. Dilling, "Prevalence and Treatment of Insomnia in the Community: Results From the Upper Bavarian Field Study," *Sleep* 14 (1991): 392–8; J. D. Kales et al., "Biopsychobehavioral Correlates of Insomnia. V. Clinical Characteristics and Behavioral Correlates," *American Journal of Psychiatry* 141 (1984): 1371–6. Similar results were found in L. C. Johnson and C. L. Spinweber, "Quality of Sleep and Performance in the Navy: A Longitudinal Study of Poor Sleepers," pp. 13–28 in C. Guilleminault and E. Lugaresi, eds., *Sleep/Wake Disorders: Natural History, Epidemiology and Long Term Evolution* (New York: Raven Press, 1983).

27. H. Moldofsky et al., "Induction of Neurasthenic Musculoskeletal Pain Syndrome by Selective Deep Sleep Stage Deprivation," *Psychosomatic Medicine* 38 (1976): 35–44.

28. C. L. Whelton, I. Salit, and H. Moldofsky, "Sleep, Epstein-Barr Virus Infection, Musculoskeletal Pain and Depressive Symptoms in Chronic Fatigue Syndrome," *Journal of Rheumatology* 19 (1992): 939–43.

29. H. Moldofsky, "Sleep and Fibrositis Syndrome," *Rheumatic Disease Clinics of North America* 15 (1989): 91–103. Also H. Moldofsky, "Fibromyalgia, Sleep Disorder and Chronic Fatigue Syndrome," *CIBA Foundation Symposium* 173 (1993): 262–79; and H. Moldofsky, P. Scarsbrick, R. England, and H. Smythe, "Musculoskeletal Symptoms and Non-REM Sleep Disturbance in Patients with 'Fibrositis Syndrome' and Healthy Subjects," *Psychosomatic Medicine* 37(1975): 341–51.

30. Kuppermann et al., "Sleep Problems and Their Correlates in a Working Population."

31. A. H. Calhoun et al., "The Prevalence and Spectrum of Sleep Problems in Women with Transformed Migraine," *Headache* 46, no. 4 (April 2006): 604–10.

32. Bonnet, "Sleep Deprivation," 57.

33. C. A. Everson, "Sustained Sleep Deprivation Impairs Host Defense," *American Journal of Physiology* 265, 5, pt. 2 (1993): R1148–54.

34. A. Baumgartner et al., "Neuroendocrinological Evaluations During Sleep Deprivation in Depression. I. Early Morning Levels of Thyrotropin, TH, Cortisol, Prolactin, LH, FSH, Estradiol, and Testosterone," *Biological Psychiatry* 28 (1990): 556–68; A. Baumgartner, D. Riemann, and M. Berger, "Neuroendocrinological Evaluations During Sleep Deprivation in Depression. II. Longitudinal Measurement of Thyrotropin, TH, Cortisol, Prolactin, GH and LH During Sleep and Sleep Deprivation," *Biological Psychiatry* 28 (1990): 569–87; and Bonnet, "Sleep Deprivation," 56–7.

35. Bonnet, "Sleep Deprivation," 56–68.

36. J. E. Enstrom, "Health Practices and Cancer Mortality Among Active California Mormons," *Journal of the National Cancer Institute* 81 (1989): 1807–14.

37. M. H. Kryger, *Principles and Practice of Sleep Medicine* (Philadelphia, PA: Saunders, 1994).

38. H. Y. McClusky et al., "Efficacy of Behavioral Versus Triazolam Treatment in Persistent Sleep Onset Insomnia," *American Journal of Psychiatry* 148 (1991): 121–6. Compare A. D. Krystal et al., "Sustained Efficacy of Eszopiclone over 6 Months of Nightly

Treatment: Results of a Randomized, Double-Blind, Placebo-Controlled Study in Adults with Chronic Insomnia," *Sleep* 26 (2003): 793–9; and T. Roth et al. "An Evaluation of the Efficacy and Safety of Eszopiclone over 12 Months in Patients with Chronic Primary Insomnia," *Sleep Medicine* 6 (2005): 487–95.

39. C. Morin et al., "Cognitive-Behavioral Therapy and Pharmacotherapy for Late-Life Insomnia: A Placebo-Controlled Trial," *Sleep Research* 22 (1993): abstract, 21.

40. C. A. Espie et al., "A Controlled Comparative Investigation of Psychological Treatments for Chronic Sleep-Onset Insomnia," *Behaviour Research and Therapy* 27 (1989): 79–88.

41. D. J. Buysse and C. F. Reynolds, "Insomnia," pp. 375–433 in M. J. Thorpe, ed., *Handbook of Sleep Disorders* (New York: Marcel Dekker, 1990); and A. J. Spielman et al., "A Behavioral Perspective on Insomnia Treatment."

42. J. Kabat-Zinn, L. Lipworth, and R. Burney, "The Clinical Use of Mindfulness Meditation for the Self-Regulation of Chronic Pain," *Journal of Behavioral Medicine* 8 (1985): 163–90; and J. Kabat-Zinn, *Full Catastrophe Living* (New York: Delacorte Press, 1990): 362–7.

43. J. Kabat-Zinn, L. Lipworth, R. Burney, and W. Sellers, "Four Year Follow-Up of a Meditation-Based Program for the Self-Regulation of Chronic Pain: Treatment Outcomes and Compliance," *The Clinical Journal of Pain* 2 (1986): 159–73.

44. M. Davis, E. R. Eshelman, and M. McKay, "Thought Stopping," pp. 91–7 in *The Relaxation and Stress Reduction Workbook* (Oakland, CA: New Harbinger Public, 1988).

45. P. Hauri and S. Linde, *No More Sleepless Nights* (New York: John Wiley, 1991): 130–31.

46. J. D. Edinger et al., "Aerobic Fitness, Acute Exercise and Sleep in Older Men," *Sleep* 16 (1993): 351–9.

47. A. Montmayeur, A. Buguet, H. Sollin, and J. R. Lacour, "Exercise and Sleep in Four African Sportsmen Living in the Sahel: A Pilot Study," *International Journal of Sports Medicine* 15 (1994): 42–5.

48. G. D. Jacobs, E. F. Pace-Schott, R. Stickgold, and M. W. Otto, "Cognitive Behavior Therapy and Pharmacotherapy for Insomnia: A Randomized Controlled Trial and Direct Comparison," *Archives of Internal Medicine* 164 (2004): 1888–96.

49. I. Haimov et al., "Sleep Disorders and Melatonin Rhythms in Elderly People," *British Medical Journal* 309 (1994): 167.

50. J. S. Carman, R. M. Post, R. Buswell, and F. K. Goodwin, "Negative Effects of Melatonin on Depression," *American Journal of Psychiatry* 133 (1976): 1181–6; and A. J. Lewis, N. A. Kerenyi, and G. Feuer, "Neuropharmacology of Pineal Secretions," *Drug Metabolism and Drug Interactions* 8 (1990): 247–312.

CHAPTER 8

The Disease-Resistant Personality

The mind is its own place, and in itself can make a heaven of hell, a hell of heaven.

—John Milton

LEARNING OBJECTIVES

- Identify major stress buffers.
- Define the personality traits that help people resist disease.
- Identify healthful choices that will promote disease resistance.
- Describe personal qualities and coping styles highly associated with happiness and health.
- Suggest techniques to implement these qualities.

Too often we ask ourselves why someone became ill instead of how someone managed to stay well. As Pennsylvania State University's Evan G. Pattishall reflected, if we study twenty-five people who are exposed to the influenza virus and five of them get sick, "we tend to study the five who developed influenza, when we should be exerting even more effort studying the twenty who didn't become ill."[1]

Howard S. Friedman echoed that sentiment when he wrote, "Each week the prestigious *New England Journal of Medicine* publishes a 'Case Record of the Massachusetts General Hospital,' detailing the pathology of an unusual or informative patient's case. There is no corresponding 'Case History of a Person Who Remained Well Throughout a Long Life.'"[2]

Researchers have long known that certain groups of people enjoy "remarkable good health and longevity." Among them are "Mormons, nuns, symphony conductors, and women who are listed in *Who's Who*. This suggests that something in the way these people live, possibly even such abstractions as faith, pride of accomplishment, or productivity, plays a role in diminishing the ill effects of stress."[3] About half a century ago, Abraham Maslow studied "self-actualizers" to determine their common characteristics, ways of thinking, and approaches to life in the hope that others might learn from them and have the same experience. (See Appendix A.) The self-actualizers were highly functioning people who were making valuable contributions and who were fulfilled, happy, and healthy. This emphasis on studying healthy people requires a significant shift in perspective. In the same way, knowing what to do, rather than what *not* to do, is a great step forward in creating healthy behaviors.

The way we behave powerfully influences health. Whether we smoke cigarettes, sip wine before dinner, start the day with a brisk walk, and eat fatty foods all affect our health. But could something other than these physical behaviors play a role in our ability to withstand stress and stay healthy? Researchers believe so. And the key may lie in personality and the way we think because these are apparently major determinants in how well we are able to resist stress.

The Role of Stress Resilience in Health

Chapter 2 details the way in which stress affects health. However, if stress research has shown one thing, it is that stress alone won't cause illness. How a person *reacts* to stress does determine whether that person becomes ill or stays well. In other words, your unique way of looking at things determines what impact stress has on you—and, to a large extent, determines your ability to stay healthy.

The decades of research that have focused on the human stress response and its associated ills have posed a fascinating question: Why do some people who are submitted to chronic stress fall ill while others sail through unscathed? One of the researchers intrigued by that question was Suzanne Ouellette Kobasa, who taught psychology in the City University of New York's graduate school. She was familiar with the research that drew definite connections between stress and illness—but she believed there had to be a middle ground. Kobasa knew that it is impossible to avoid stress altogether; some stressful events (such as the death of a loved one) are completely beyond our control. Even if it were possible to completely avoid stress, she concluded that such would be "a prescription for staying away from opportunities as well as trouble. Since any change can be stressful, a person who wanted to be completely free of stress would never marry, have a child, take a new job, or move."[4]

Kobasa had other concerns, too. The popular notion regarding stress and illness, she believed, ignored "a lot of what we know about people. It assumes we're all vulnerable and passive in the face of adversity. But what about human resilience, initiative, and creativity? Many come through periods of stress with more physical and mental vigor than they had before."[5]

The more she pondered the stress-illness connection, the more engrossed Kobasa became with the people who didn't get sick under stress—and the more intent she became on discovering why. In 1975, she mobilized a group of her colleagues and went to work on a study of what she calls "the walking wounded of the stress war": a group of high-powered business executives faced with personal and career upheaval. They found that the stressor itself was not nearly as important to who suffered illness as were the attitudes the people had toward the stressor and the approach they took to deal with it. (Kobasa and her team then described their results in terms of the differences between stress "hardiness" and stress vulnerability, which are discussed in more detail below.)

Watching general population groups during stress demonstrates the importance of our attitude toward stress and our subsequent response. The Irish are one example. When the Irish were transplanted by the thousands to the eastern seaboards of America during the last century, their standard of living improved dramatically. Conditions were much cleaner, and they had plenty of food to eat (in contrast to Ireland, where they had faced starvation). In spite of the improved conditions and nutrition, the death rate from tuberculosis among the Irish who had moved to America soared. While the transplanted Dubliners were better housed and better fed, the tuberculosis death rate was 100 percent higher than it was during the same period in Dublin, where the conditions were much worse. Why did the Irish die of tuberculosis despite such dramatically improved conditions? Simple: Many of them had not wanted to migrate to America, and they were unprepared for the discrimination they faced.[6]

In another example, when the American Indians were forced off the Plains and onto reservations (often within only a few miles of where they had lived), they had much better sanitation and a higher standard of living in their new situations. Considering physical conditions alone, they should have enjoyed much better health. But that didn't happen. Again, deaths from tuberculosis increased.[7] Why? The Indians were being uprooted from the land of their forefathers. Their traditions were in danger. They felt powerless—and they gave in. Curiously, when people give in to their struggles, their immune system protecting them from diseases like tuberculosis "gives in" also.

A third example is the Bantu natives of South Africa. They were moved in droves from their native villages into Johannesburg, where sanitation was dramatically better and where food and housing were vastly improved. Thousands became ill with tuberculosis. When hundreds of the dying were permitted to return to their native villages to die, the tuberculosis bacillus was then spread throughout the villages, but the people who had remained in the villages didn't get sick.[8]

Was it the move alone that made these populations sick? To answer that question, consider the Chinese and Hungarian refugees who overcame great odds and dangerous political upheaval to immigrate to the United States. Although their new home represented a place vastly different than the one they left, they thrived. Why? Rather than seeing this upheaval as negative, they viewed their new lives as an opportunity and a challenge.[9] This difference in perception about the changes with which they were confronted (when compared to the Irish, the Indians, and the Bantu) created very different health outcomes.

The effect is even more pronounced in populations in which one segment has a different outlook than another. Take, for example, a group of Portuguese who immigrated to Canada for employment reasons. The men who immigrated saw the move as a chance for a better job and a new future; their health actually *improved* after their move to

Canada. Their wives saw the move as a disruption of their valued family ties in Portugal, and they were more likely to get sick.[10]

Stress Buffers

Some things have been identified as "stress buffers," or elements that alleviate the harmful effects of stress. Some of these findings have been controversial, but researchers have generally shown that social support, a sense of control, physical fitness, a sense of humor, self-esteem, optimism, problem-solving coping styles, and Kobasa's "hardiness" personality all help to buffer stress.[11]

In her revolutionary studies on stress and illness, Kobasa and her colleague Salvatore Maddi commented, "We could not believe that the same human imagination responsible for urbanization and industrialization was somehow incapable of coping with the . . . ensuing pressures and disruptions. It seemed obvious that the individual differences in response to stress were important."[12]

With that attitude, Kobasa and her colleagues decided to expand their stress and illness studies beyond the original group of Illinois telephone company executives. Would the same principles hold true in other populations?

Others have done similar studies, and their findings have been remarkably consistent with Kobasa's. Lawrence Hinkle and his associates in the departments of medicine and psychiatry at New York Hospital's Cornell Medical Center conducted a series of studies over a 20-year period. They found that personality traits had a definite bearing on health. They concluded that those with "a good attitude and an ability to get along with other people" enjoyed the lowest frequency of illness.[13]

In another study, two psychiatrists, an endocrinologist, and a cancer specialist in New York teamed up to determine the stress reactions and hormonal changes that occurred when people were faced with a truly life-threatening situation. To test their theories, they picked a group who did face a life-threatening situation: 30 women who were undergoing biopsies for breast tumors at Montefiore Hospital and Medical Center.

To determine the amount of "distress" each woman was suffering, researchers did tests to determine how much cortisol each woman secreted. (Cortisol is a hormone secreted by the adrenal gland in response to stress.) Researchers measured the amount of cortisol each day for the three days preceding each woman's biopsy. At the end of the study, the researchers concluded that the crisis of possibly having cancer wasn't what determined how much or how little distress each woman experienced. Instead, the determining factor was each woman's "psychological defenses" or coping style—especially her outlooks and beliefs. For example, the lowest amount of adrenal hormone was secreted by a 45-year-old woman who consistently used faith and prayer to deal with life's stressful events. The woman who fared the next best was a 54-year-old who had a healthy philosophical acceptance of adversity.

What we're saying is this: being resilient is a greater determining factor than the stressor itself. Some key components that improve well-being in the face of stress include caring love (being committed to the fulfillment of the other), responsible free will (creating your own life experience and influencing events), integrity (being true to core values), challenge (enjoying growth), and hope (feeling positive expectation). The studies cited throughout this book confirm that these same resilient qualities have powerful effects on measurable health. Later we'll discuss the fact that these same principles also underlie spiritual well-being (see Chapter 14). These same characteristics thus mediate the crossover between mental, physical and spiritual well-being.

Gender Differences

Interestingly, there appear to be differences in the way men and women handle stresses—and the differences appear to be tied even more to emotion, personality, and sociology than to biology. The differences are especially linked to gender role socialization among men.[14]

According to researchers, many emotions are largely learned behaviors; and, as discussed elsewhere in this book, the efficient handling of emotions is a key to good health. It is generally accepted among those who study disease resistance that men are not as efficient as women in dealing with emotions and that ineffective emotion management is implicated in each of the four causes of death for which men's death rates are twice as high as women's: accidents, suicide, cirrhosis of the liver, and homicide.[15] Those same researchers suggest that significant reductions in death rates among men could be achieved if men learned healthier ways of handling their feelings.[16]

The following are particular areas of emotion toward which men are socialized that can harm health—and areas in which changes could promote disease resistance.

Anger and Hostility

Studies show that men are more likely than women to have cynical hostility and poorly controlled anger.[17] Unfortunately, boys tend to learn harmful lessons about anger and aggression during childhood. For one thing, parents tend to better accept expressed anger in their sons than in their daughters.[18] Furthermore, the gender role socialization for boys actually encourages them to be aggressive when they get angry.[19] Boys are often given "messages" in the media, as well as from their peers and often even from their parents, that it is appropriate to settle arguments by wrestling, hitting, kicking, pushing, or shoving. In many cases, physical aggression is required for boys to earn respect from peers both at school and in the neighborhood.[20]

During the developmental period when girls are learning that it's good to express emotions (other than anger), boys are learning that anger shows masculinity and toughness—but that expressing other emotions demonstrates weakness and cowardice. As shown in Chapter 4, the health effects of anger and hostility are devastating, and men who are not able to overcome early socialization are at risk as a result.

Depression and Grief

Most of the major studies on depression have focused on women—possibly because only an estimated 13 percent of men struggle with major depression at some time during their lives.[21] Many now believe, however, that depression among men is undiagnosed and underreported, probably because men are socialized not to complain about (or admit to) sadness or guilt.[22] Instead, men are prone to see their physicians about the less stigmatized symptoms of depression, such as fatigue or irritability. In men, depression often appears with increased hostility, cynicism, and controlling behavior. The connection here is interesting from a health standpoint because both depression and cynical hostility are coronary risk factors and respond to similar treatments. One large study found that physicians failed to properly diagnose depression in almost two-thirds of men who were actually depressed.[23]

The cause of depression in men is much the same as that in women: similar neurobiological abnormalities and similar situations that provoke depression, such as the incomplete mourning of a loss—including death, divorce, the end of a significant relationship, the loss of a job, or retirement (which often represents the loss of status or financial security). Unfortunately, though, men are taught as boys to "keep a stiff upper lip" and to avoid crying—at least in public. They are much less likely than women to reach out and discuss their feelings with their male friends;[24] in fact, one prominent scholar contends that alexithymia (having no words for emotions) is so common among men that it is considered normal.[25] If it is a factor, alexithymia may well prevent men from successfully resolving their grief after a major loss.

Substance Abuse and Misuse

Studies consistently show that men have much higher rates of substance abuse and misuse than do women.[26] Studies also show that men turn to substance abuse/misuse to assuage difficult or painful feelings, and the type of substance they use depends on the feelings or type of pain they are trying to deal with.[27]

There are other factors as well. For example, drinking alcohol is sometimes considered an integral part of becoming a man in the United States; there is frequently a firm association between alcohol use and manliness. Because there is such widespread acceptance of alcohol use among men, they rely on alcohol more often than do women to cope with stressors. As a result, men in the United States are twice as likely to engage in heavy drinking episodes (having more than five drinks in one sitting),[28] and heavy episodic drinking is the leading cause of death among America's undergraduate college students.[29]

Called "chemical coping," using alcohol and other substances to cope with stress may steer a person away from using the real coping described below.

Personality Traits That Keep Us Well

The cumulative results of studies conducted over the past three or four decades—Kobasa's as well as others—show beyond a doubt that certain personality traits keep us well, boost our happiness, and improve our immune systems. Perhaps most convincing was a study of 650 children in Hawaii.

In their book *Vulnerable But Invincible*, researchers Emmy Werner and Ruth Smith report their study of the 650 children who were born and reared on the island of Kauai in Hawaii. The children in the study were followed from a few months before their birth until they were in their early twenties. Each was assessed at regular intervals with a battery of interviews, questionnaires, and examinations; researchers monitored the health records of each child closely.[30]

By all standards, these children were at high risk. All were born into poor families and lived in chronic poverty. Many were born to single mothers, some of whom were depressed or schizophrenic. Of those who did have fathers in the home, the fathers were semiskilled or unskilled laborers. More children were born prematurely than would have been expected; many were victims of severe perinatal stress. The mothers had little formal education (none had graduated from high school). The families themselves were plagued by a multitude of problems.

The stresses didn't end there. As psychologist Robert Ornstein and physician David Sobel put it:

> [These children] came of age in the years 1955 to 1979—a time of unprecedented social change. They had to deal with the influx of many newcomers from the U.S. mainland during the long war in Southeast Asia and later with the burgeoning of tourism. They witnessed the assassination of one president and the resignation of another. They were the first generation to deal with the invasion of the home by television. They faced unprecedented choices since they had access to contraceptive pills and mind-altering drugs.[31]

The combination of these biological and social stresses took their toll on some of the children. By the age of ten—the first major interval used by the researchers—at least half of the children were in serious trouble. They were in ill physical health, had serious behavioral problems, and had learning disabilities that impacted their ability to progress through the school system.

By the age of eighteen, the next major follow-up period, an additional 25 percent—or three-fourths of all the children in the study—had very serious problems. Those who didn't have profound psychological problems often had learning disabilities, behavioral problems, and poor health.

That didn't surprise anyone. After all, these kids had started out under the most dreadful conditions and had grown up in an environment charged with unrelenting stress. What did surprise researchers was the group of kids—approximately one-fourth of the group studied—who, despite all the stress, rallied. They prevailed with strong psychological adjustment, good health, and enviable school records. Ornstein and Sobel describe three of them:

> Life did not start out well for Michael. His mother was sixteen years old, unwed, and lived with her mother and grandmother. She managed to hide her pregnancy from her own mother until the third trimester when she married a nineteen-year-old boy. The child's biological father was very much against the marriage. The mother did not receive any medical care until the seventh month of pregnancy, and Michael was born prematurely and weighed only four pounds ten ounces. Michael spent the first three weeks of his life in an army hospital. At two, Michael's adoptive father was sent with the army to Korea, where he remained for two years. At age eight, Michael's parents divorced and his mother left, leaving him with his father and three younger siblings.
>
> Early life was also not easy for Kay. She was born to seventeen-year-old unmarried parents. They had both been asked to leave school because of the pregnancy, and the father was without a job. Family Court sent Kay's mother to a Salvation Army Home to

have her baby; placing her for adoption was considered but rejected, and the parents were eventually married when Kay was six months old despite objections from their parents. Kay's parents later separated.

Mary got off to a rough start as well. Her mother's pregnancy occurred after many unsuccessful attempts to conceive and a previous miscarriage. Her mother was very much overweight and had various minor medical problems during pregnancy. She was hospitalized three times for severe false labor and eventually was in labor for more than twenty hours. During Mary's childhood her parents experienced financial difficulties, and her mother found it necessary to work outside the home for short periods. Between Mary's fifth and tenth birthdays, her mother had several major illnesses, surgeries, and two hospitalizations for "unbearable tension," nervousness, annoyance with her children, and fears that she might harm them.[32]

How did things turn out for the three? Despite everything, they grew up to be healthy, well-adjusted, successful adults. Michael ranked at the top of his class and was awarded a college scholarship. Well-liked by his peers, he was described as confident, persistent, self-assured, dependable, and realistic. Kay did well also. She was an alert, healthy, affectionate, and robust baby; as a child, she had above-normal grades in school and was described as agreeable, relaxed, and mentally normal. As an adult, she was described as poised, sociable, self-assured, respectful, and accepting of others, as well as a person who made good use of the abilities she had. She planned to go into the entertainment field and to marry. Mary was described as having high self-esteem, persistence, concern for others, and an outgoing personality; she was willing to open herself up to new possibilities after only initial hesitancy. She planned to enroll in college, and was keeping her future career goals open. At eighteen, Mary described herself this way:

> If I say how I am it sounds like bragging—I have a good personality and people like me. . . . I don't like it when people think they can run my own life—I like to be my own judge. I know right from wrong, but I feel I have a lot more to learn and go through. Generally, I hope I can make it—I hope.[33]

What made the difference? *Hope* seemed to be a key attitude with the children who prevailed over their difficult circumstances. So did *perseverance*. They were what Indiana psychiatric social worker Katherine Northcraft calls "transcenders"—people who, "in the worst of times, envision themselves as elsewhere, imagining that they can do great things despite their surroundings."[34] Also, despite difficult family situations, these resilient children developed *strong bonds* with a parent, grandparent, sibling, or other caretaker, usually early in life (almost always during the first year). When they felt confused or troubled, they sought help—but they were also children who eagerly *accepted challenge*. These children had personalities that kept them healthy and enabled them to overcome adversity. They were, in Kobasa's terms, "hardy."

Where do resilient traits come from? No one knows for sure. Some of them may be inborn. Werner found that most of the resilient children in her study had been alert, sociable, even-tempered, responsive infants. "There seems to be a group of children who temperamentally and probably constitutionally have a better chance of making lemonade out of lemons," she believes. Does that doom the rest—those who are introverted, shy, or difficult? Not necessarily, she says—it's just that "it's easier for those who are more outgoing to find support."[35]

According to psychologist Ann Masten, associate director of the University of Minnesota's Institute of Child Development, the fact that Werner's resilient children had a strong adult figure is important. "When resilient adults talk about how they made it, virtually everyone mentions a key adult," she explains. That adult doesn't have to be a parent. In fact, in her study of more than 200 resilient children, many found inner strength through bonds they developed with a neighbor, family friend, teacher, minister, or other respected adult.[36]

Hardiness

Kobasa studied a large group of Illinois Bell Telephone executives who lost their jobs when the telephone company monopoly divested and many new companies emerged. She found that some of the newly jobless thrived—often even coming out of it better than before ("stress hardy")—while others were blown away by the difficulty ("stress vulnerable"). She then analyzed and compared how differently the two types approached life's problems. Her later studies of other groups found the same differences.

What were the common elements in those who did well? According to Kobasa, it's hardiness, "a set of beliefs about oneself, the world, and how they interact. It takes shape as a sense of personal commitment to what you are doing, a sense of control over your life, and a feeling of challenge."[37]

Kobasa defines the key components of hardiness as "the three C's": commitment, control, and challenge. Commitment is an attitude of purpose and meaning, making a difference to what is happening around you; control is the belief that you can influence events instead of becoming a victim; and challenge is the belief that change brings a chance for growth instead of the fear that change is threatening.[38]

Commitment   Commitment—an attitude of curiosity and involvement in what is happening around you—means a commitment to yourself, your work, your family, and the other important values in your life. If spiritually inclined, it is a trusting commitment to the sources of one's spiritual empowerment. It is not a fleeting involvement but a deep and abiding interest. People who are committed in this way have a deep involvement with their work and their families, a deep sense of meaning, and a pervasive sense of direction in their lives. In one study involving students at Harvard Medical School, students best able to withstand stress were personally committed to a goal or mission of some kind.[39] Altruism is an important quality associated with commitment (see Chapter 15).

A sense of commitment may drive us to a hectic pace filled with plenty of pressures; however, it is healthy because there is a drive to live life to its fullest, and there is a sense of mission in the work. The important element, say some researchers, is commitment to an ideal greater than oneself.[40] For some people, that commitment comes in the form of commitment to a religion; for others, it's a commitment to political reform or to a certain philosophy. Some healthy people have a deep sense of commitment to something as simple as a hobby. Each of these involves making a positive difference to something outside of one's self or to making something happen that is important to you. Thus, commitment involves a deep sense of *purpose and meaning*—both to one's life and work and to what is happening at the moment.

A perfect example is Mohandas K. Gandhi, a man who by all standards was a driven workaholic. He went on countless fasts, depriving himself of nourishment, and spent months in prison—one of the most stressful scenarios possible. Yet he was strong and healthy until his assassination at the age of 77. Many believe it was because of his unwavering commitment to become one of the world's great leaders and to win political freedom for his homeland. Similarly, older people who retire *to* something that makes a difference in their world thrive much better than those who simply retire *from* something they want to escape.

Control   There is a wonderful paradox about control: the more you try to control the external world, the more out of control it begins to feel. (For example, try to control someone in your family who's acting belligerent.) A healthy sense of control is not about controlling the world out there.

The flip side of the paradox is this: the more you accept what's out there and let go of trying to control external factors, choosing to respond in ways you would deeply admire, you then feel an internal sense of control. If you were to imagine how someone of great wisdom, strength, and goodness would respond to what has happened, and the more you try to respond that way, the more you feel the kind of internal control we are talking about. A strong sense of internal control involves integrity to your deepest values. It requires taking full responsibility for how you respond.

This kind of control is the belief that you can cushion the hurtful impact of a situation by the way you look at it and react to it. The kind of control that keeps you healthy is the opposite of helplessness. It involves a deep sense of choice about how to be in this present moment with what is here. You can't control the past or the future. What you *can* control is how you are going to be and act right now. It's the refusal to be victimized. It is not the erroneous belief that you can control your environment, your circumstances, or other people; that kind of an attitude leads to illness, not health. The control that keeps you healthy is a belief that you can control yourself and your own reactions to what life hands you. This internal locus of control not only creates resilience (stress hardiness), but also has significant health effects (see Chapter 18).

In the Harvard Medical School study discussed earlier, the healthiest students were the ones who approached problem solving with a sense of control; the least healthy were those who were passive.[41] The healthiest and hardiest people are those who focus on what they can control, ignoring the rest. Hope and control are closely linked for these individuals: they believe that through skill, planning, diligent attention to detail, and kindness, every problem has a solution.

We all want to be able to predict what will happen to us, but we can't reliably do so. We all crave a sense of mastery,[42] but the only way to feel that mastery is to stop blaming external events for controlling your life, feelings, or behavior and to accept responsibility for how you respond. The moment you point your finger in blame, your sense of control disappears. A sense of control—a belief that you can control your *own* behavior, not necessarily that you can control the people and events around you—promotes health. It endows you with the belief that even if everything around you gets bad, you will still be fine.

Challenge   Challenge is the ability to see change as an opportunity for growth and excitement. Excitement is critical because boredom puts people at a high risk for disease.[43] People who are constructively challenged are more healthy, and a German philosopher mused that one of the two biggest foes of human happiness is boredom. Excitement—and, as a result, challenge—surrounds the good kind of stress (eustress) that *improves* health.

A person who is not healthy and hardy views change with helplessness and alienation. A healthy, hardy person can face change with confidence, self-determination, eagerness, and excitement. Change becomes an eagerly sought-after challenge, not a threat. Joan C. Post-Gorden, psychologist at the University of Southern Colorado, says that healthy people don't even see the negatives because they thoroughly expect a positive outcome.[44] Once again, this describes an attitude of hope.

That healthy view of challenge is exemplified by Mary Decker Slaney, a world-class runner who broke four world records.[45] The stress of competition is crushing—yet she stayed healthy and kept competing. When asked why, she responded, "I love it. Running is something I do for myself more than anything else." Those positive emotions and personal triumph demonstrate a great sense of healthy challenge and commitment. And since every life is filled with obstacles, it stands to reason that the way we view those obstacles, whether as crushing problems or as challenges to be eagerly met, determines in part how healthy we are.

A sense of challenge can be powerful. Research showed that among more than 60 HIV-positive gay men, those who treated their HIV-positive status as a challenge (even an opportunity to refocus their lives on that most important to them) and then developed strategies to fight it had improved natural killer cell activity. University of Miami psychiatrist Karl Goodkin, who spearheaded the study, observed that an active coping style, along with good social support, led to improvement of natural killer cell activity and immunity.[46]

The enjoyment of challenge goes well beyond stress hardiness. It is also a key component in human happiness. In a classic study of the great—even joyful—moments in people's lives, Mihaly Csikszentmihalyi found the moments did not come at times devoid of stress but rather at times when one was responding to a challenge with a sense of "flow": feeling control, often in connection with others, creatively rising to the occasion with a certain sense of handling the challenge in a great way.[47] It was the "We did it!" moments that were the great ones.

Coherence and Connectedness   Adding to Kobasa's "three C's" is coherence—a "pervasive, enduring though dynamic feeling that one's internal and external environments are predictable and that there is a high probability that all things will work out as well as can be reasonably expected."[48] This might also be called *hope*.

Another additional C of resilience is *connectedness*. Other research verifies that stress-resistant personality traits include the ability to relate well to others and the ability to interact in a strong social network. The most vulnerable people are those who are socially isolated. The healthiest Harvard Medical School graduates sought out other people, were actively and empathically engaged with other people, and had strong social networks.[49] Resilient connectedness also includes a sense of connection with nature and the cosmos, oneness with one's sources of spiritual strength, and, indeed, connecting with one's deepest, wisest self. The health effects of this connectedness will be further explored later (see Chapters 9–12).

Healthful Choices

People with a disease-resistant personality seem to make healthier lifestyle choices, which could be a factor in their ability to resist disease. For one, they tend to exercise regularly; 80 percent of the healthiest Harvard Medical School students engaged in regular aerobic exercise, while only 20 percent of the ill students did.[50] Scientists at the Institute for Brain Aging and Dementia (at the University of California, Irvine) have also shown that exercise increases the brain neurotrophic chemicals that help thinking nerve cells work better.[51]

The healthy students also relax for at least fifteen minutes a day.[52] The more formal practice this relaxation takes, the better, but any form helps (see Chapter 21). In the Harvard study, healthy students limit refined sugars in their diet and used a minimum of "substances" (things they considered to be drugs or drug-like, including stimulants like nicotine and caffeine).[53] By engaging in more consistent health behaviors "hardy" people under stress are physically more resistant to disease and illness."[54]

Thus, hardiness or stress-resistant personality traits may combine with healthy behaviors to result in enhanced resistance to disease. "When individuals have high health concern they are more likely to engage in appropriate health behavior if they are at the same time high in hardiness," one researcher concluded. "When hardy people become concerned about their health, they are more likely than nonhardy people to engage in appropriate health-protective behaviors."[55]

The hardy (or disease-resistant) personality is summed up in a profile provided by Ornstein and Sobel:

> A small, neat man in his mid-50s, Chuck L. introduced himself as someone who enjoys solving problems. In the company, his specialty is customer relations, even though he was trained as an engineer. His eyes light up as he describes the intricacies of investigating customer needs and complaints, determining the company's service capabilities and obligations, formulating possible solutions that appear fair to all parties, and persuading these parties to agree. He thinks customer relations work is more demanding as the company streamlines and approaches reorganization. Asked in a sympathetic manner whether this is making his job unmanageable, he notes an increase in stress but adds that the work is becoming all the more interesting and challenging as well. He assumes that the role he plays will become even more central as the company's reorganization accelerates. He looks forward to this and has already formulated plans for a more comprehensive approach to customer relations.
>
> Chuck doesn't seem to neglect family life for all his imaginative and energetic involvement at work. He married in college, and the couple has two grown children. His wife has returned to school to finish a college degree long ago interrupted.

Although her absence from the home causes Chuck some inconvenience, it is clear that he encouraged her. He is full of plans about how he can preserve a close home life. Should he find too much time to himself, he imagines he will get involved in useful community activities.

In the past, Chuck's family life has hardly been uneventful. His daughter's two-year-old son died; then her husband divorced her, and she returned home for a year. This was a difficult time not only for her but for Chuck and his wife, who felt their daughter's pain and sense of failure in a very personal way. Chuck describes the long talks they had. Although he mentions their crying together, it is also clear that he was always searching for a way, a formula, to relieve mutual pain. He encouraged his daughter to pick up the pieces of her life, learn from what had happened, and begin again. He tried to help his wife see that she had little responsibility in what had happened and that it was not the end of the world. He told himself the same thing. This difficult time, in his view, drew the three of them closer together.[56]

Note how Chuck's resilient approach to difficult problems consisted of creating deeper *connectedness*, *hope*, and a sense of *internal control* ("We can deal well with this").

In a comprehensive year-long study of college students, researchers at Boston University School of Medicine concluded that there's a definite series of events that precedes illness. Here's what they believe happens:[57] A person perceives a distressing life situation. For whatever reason, he or she is not able to resolve the distressing situation effectively. As a result, the person feels helpless and anxious; those feelings of helplessness weaken the immune system and the resistance to disease, and the person becomes more vulnerable to disease-causing agents that are always in the environment.

The traits of a disease-resistant personality interrupt this cycle and, therefore, help prevent illness. With resilience, a sense of control and challenge replaces helplessness. When one expects to somehow deal well with the challenge, hope replaces hopelessness, and both anxiety and vulnerability subside. There's a real difference between the way healthy people and ill people look at things.[58] Healthy people, for example, tend to maintain reasonable personal control in their lives. If a problem crops up, they look for resources and try out solutions. If one doesn't work, they try another one. People who are frequently ill, on the other hand, leave decisions up to others and try to get other people to solve their problems. Their approach tends to be passive. We of course are speaking regarding general patterns here. Anyone exposed to enough of a pathogen can get sick. Certainly this pattern does not imply that anyone with illness has a vulnerable personality. The issue is who gets sick the most, and what can we do to best prevent that.

Researchers have observed that healthy people are generally committed to a goal of some kind, and they typically spend at least a few hours every week doing something that provides a sense of challenge or enhances their sense of meaningful participation in life. What they do holds personal significance for them. People who are ill, on the other hand, often report being bored; they are not able to find things that interest them. Healthy people generally seek out other people and are actively involved with them. Ill people, on the other hand, tend to be more socially isolated.

In discussing people who were able to overcome disease and heal themselves, *Psychology Today* editor Marc Barasch said that if "there is a thread that stands out, it is that each person, some readily, some reluctantly, wound up doing the opposite of what sick people are supposed to: Rather than only trying to 'get back to normal,' they embarked on a voyage of self-discovery. Like early circumnavigators, they seemed to cling to an instinctive faith that the only way home was forward, into the round but unknown world of the self."[59]

What all these experts are describing is resilience and hardiness. Following the initial phase of their landmark study at Illinois Bell, Kobasa and Maddi began training the telephone executives in hardiness; that is, they began helping them develop disease-resistant personalities. Specific health benefits came to the people who received the training. They not only enjoyed more job satisfaction but also had reduced anxiety, less depression, fewer physical ills (such as headaches), lower blood pressure, and better sleep.[60]

An entire spectrum of studies verifies the findings: People with the traits of a "disease-resistant" personality do, indeed, enjoy better health. They have fewer episodes of illness, even when people around them have contagious diseases. The results of preliminary studies show that a resilient personality may even help boost recovery from illness. In fact, scientists have identified what they call a "self-healing personality"—and they say it's characterized by enthusiasm, alertness, responsiveness, energy, curiosity, security, and contentment. Scientists say "self-healing" people have a continual sense of growth and resilience; achieve balance in meeting their biological needs, gaining affection, and having self-respect; are good problem solvers; have a playful sense of humor; and have good relationships with others.[61] The large concept is that resilience in the face of mental stress translates in body systems to resilience when confronted with the stress of organic causes of disease.

Positive Psychology

The millennial issue (2000) of the prestigious journal *American Psychologist* focused on a fresh approach to human psychology. Rather than the traditional emphasis on mentally ill people and how to treat such mental illness, the article drew on seminal work studying highly effective, happy, and mentally healthy people. The focus was on determining the common elements of such well-being and happiness. Rather than getting rid of what makes people suffer, how might we promote, even from an early age, patterns of responding to life through key principles that make life worth living? Five years later in the same journal, Martin Seligman, Christopher Peterson, and their colleagues reviewed the progress that had been made with this approach.

Some psychologists had been skeptical that negative personality characteristics were difficult to change so were basically "locked in." Research on how to best make the change to the positive qualities is just beginning. Much of the new positive psychology research had been first directed toward clearly identifying the healthy traits to foster. Much has been accomplished in this regard.

As part of their work, Seligman and Peterson published for the American Psychological Association a book describing these proven qualities; it was thought that their book, *Character Strengths and Virtues: A Handbook and Classification* (the CSV),[62] could do for well-being research what the *Diagnostic and Statistical Manual of Mental Disorders* had done for mental illness. Six virtues and 24 character strengths were well validated across 40 countries and were nearly universally recognized as the keys to human happiness and well-being. These are shown in Table 8.1.[63] These characteristics confirm the core resilience principles and further break them down into subcomponents, allowing more directed implementation. The review in 2005 also described

Table 8.1   Classification of Six Virtues and Twenty-Four Character Strengths

Virtue and Strength	Definition
1. Wisdom and knowledge	Cognitive strengths that entail the acquisition and use of knowledge
Creativity	Thinking of novel and productive ways to do things
Curiosity	Taking an interest in all of ongoing experience
Open-mindedness	Thinking things through and examining them from all sides
Love of learning	Mastering new skills, topics, and bodies of knowledge
Perspective	Being able to provide wise counsel to others
2. Courage	Emotional strengths that involve the exercise of will to accomplish goals in the face of opposition (external or internal)
Authenticity	Speaking the truth and presenting oneself in a genuine way
Bravery	*Not* shrinking from threat, challenge, difficulty, or pain
Persistence	Finishing what one starts
Zest	Approaching life with excitement and energy
3. Humanity	Interpersonal strengths that involve "tending and befriending" others
Kindness	Doing favors and good deeds for others
Love	Valuing close relations with others
Social intelligence	Being aware of the motives and feelings of self and others
4. Justice	Civic strengths that underlie healthy community life
Fairness	Treating all people the same and according to notions of fairness and justice
Leadership	Organizing group activities and seeing that they happen
Teamwork	Working well as member of a group or team
5. Temperance	Strengths that protect against excess
Forgiveness	Forgiving those who have done wrong
Modesty	Letting one's accomplishments speak for themselves
Prudence	Being careful about one's choices; *not* saying or doing things that might later be regretted
Self-regulation	Regulating what one feels and does
6. Transcendence	Strengths that forge connections to the larger universe and provide meaning
Appreciation of beauty and excellence	Noticing and appreciating beauty, excellence, and/or skilled performance in all domains of life
Gratitude	Being aware of and thankful for the good things that happen
Hope	Expecting the best and working to achieve it
Humor	Liking to laugh and tease; bringing smiles to other people
Religiousness	Having coherent beliefs about the higher purpose and meaning of life

Source: C. Peterson and M.E.P. Seligman, *Character Strengths and Virtues: A Handbook and Classification* (New York: Oxford University Press/Washington, DC: American Psychological Association, 2004).

some simple online interventions that have been shown to increase some of these qualities and to then significantly improve measures of both happiness and depression.[64] These interventions included practices as simple as:

- Write a letter of gratitude to someone who is particularly kind.
- Each day write down three things that went well and provide a causal explanation.
- Take a test to identify personal strengths, and then use one of these in a new way each day.

The increased happiness and reduced depression created by these simple one-week interventions lasted for six months, but the increase was even greater if the interventions were continued for longer than a week. However, in a field this young, much more research on implementing these positive principles is needed. What has been done so far does seem to show that old habits can be lastingly changed if one is motivated to do so. As you might suspect, the changes occur much more quickly if the methods used are experiential (practicing doing or visualizing the changes) rather than only thinking or talking about them. (See the six-step process at the end of this chapter.)

One extraordinary proof of the impact of these principles of resilience on long term health outcomes came with George Vaillant's remarkable 35 year study of 185 men who had been Harvard students[65] (a 45 year extension to age 65 included 178 men).[66] As sophomores in college, their typical styles for dealing with stress were studied (coping styles). Their styles of responding were categorized into four groups: (1) Denial (just don't deal with it); (2) Blaming (victimizing: it's out there being done to me); (3) Repression (including a tendency to intellectualize or explain away); (4) Mature and adaptive. (We all tend to use each of these methods from time to time, but the study identified their predominant style.) The students were then followed prospectively for 35 years. In their forties, they tended to cope the same way; which tells us that unless we consciously change they way we respond to life, we tend to just keep doing the way we learned as youth. Then at age 53 their physical health was assessed. Of those using the first three less adaptive styles, 37 percent had some form of chronic physical illness or death. Of those responding in mature, adaptive ways, only 3 percent had chronic illness.[67] At age 65 the pattern was similar. This 12 fold difference makes one ask what are the key elements of this remarkably protective coping style, and can one learn to do that and change from less mature styles? The answer appears to be yes, the style can be changed if consciously and experientially pursued (See Chapter 22). Sounding almost repetitious with the above, the key elements of this health-giving "mature, adaptive style" appear to be (1) An internal locus of control (integrity to one's deep wisdom and values regardless of external pressures); (2) A sense of connectedness; (3) A sense of purpose and meaning (both for one's life and for the events currently occurring; including high altruism); (4) hope (optimism and positive expectation); and (5) constructive humor.[68] Also of great interest was the role of loving parents in teaching this style of responding.[69]

Practices and Methods for Increasing Resilience

Despite the research and scientific backup, disease resistance is an extremely individual thing. What works for one person might not necessarily work for another, so we need to exercise great caution and resist the tendency to create universal "formulas." In expressing that thought, Friedman wrote, "Self-healing personalities have an inherent resilience, but they are not identical. They share an emotional equilibrium that comes from doing the right combinations of activities appropriate for the individual."[70]

Bernie Siegel, Yale cancer surgeon, sums up the entire personality/wellness picture by advising people to take control over their own lives and to have hope:

> If there's one thing I learned from my years of working with cancer patients, it's that there is no such thing as false hope . . . hope is real and physiological. It's something I feel perfectly comfortable giving people—no matter what their situation. I know people are alive today because I said to them, "You don't have to die."
>
> If statistics say that nine out of ten people die from this disease, many physicians will tell their patients, "The odds are against you. Prepare to die." I tell my patients, "You can be the one who gets well. Let's teach you how."[71]

Is it possible to develop hardiness? Researchers believe so. Kobasa herself has two exercises she recommends to people who are trying to develop a more disease-resistant personality.

The first is called compensating through self-improvement. What it entails, she says, is an important strategy that helps you overcome stressful situations that you can't control by experiencing personal growth in an area you can control. Here's how it works: Say the company you work for is purchased by a larger corporation, and your division is abolished as part of the merger. Or say a favorite brother-in-law is killed in a traffic accident. You can't control either of those things so, says Kobasa, you compensate. How? You might learn to pilot a small-engine plane, write the family history you've been researching for a decade, or learn a difficult foreign language that has always interested you. Simply stated, you focus your energies on a new challenge instead of on the stress you can't control. This strategy, she says, helps you feel confident and in control.

Kobasa's second strategy is what she calls reconstructing stressful situations. In essence, it's a clever way of "rewriting" your own history—only this time, you come out the winner. Here's how: Start by mentally recalling a stressful event that happened to you; the more stressful the better, the more recent the better. Rehearse the whole thing in your mind, and concentrate on remembering as many details as you can. Now, write down three ways the event could have been worse. You might even feel some gratitude that it didn't turn out worse. Finally, write down three ways it could have been better; in other words, what could you have done to improve the situation? What did you learn from this? (In other words, is there something of value—a *purpose*—in this experience that makes you wiser?)

This kind of an exercise does three things for you, says Kobasa. First, it helps you realize that things weren't as bad as they could have been (a realization that, in itself, can help change your perspective on stress). Second, it gives you ideas about what to do better next time (ideas that can help relieve stress about the future). Third, and most important, it gives you a sense of control by teaching you that you can influence the way things turn out.

Following are some additional suggestions on what you can do to increase your resilience:

- Do whatever you can to develop creativity, to find new ways of looking at things, or to transform confusion into order. The creative expressions you make through writing, playing a musical instrument, dancing, or painting can also help you work through inner strife.

- When confronted with a challenge, rely on keen insight. Ask tough questions; be a careful observer; use brainstorming techniques to come up with as many ways as possible to look at the situation. You can learn from the experience of others, but trust what inherently feels right to you.

- If you start to feel stressed, break your problems down into smaller "chunks" that you can face more easily. Take on the easiest challenges first; those help you gain confidence and make the next problem easier to solve.

- Change your perspective on problems: Instead of seeing them as negatives, try finding the positives—the exciting challenges that can result. An upcoming professional examination is an undisputed stress; however, look at studying for it as a chance to hone your skills, increase your knowledge, and give yourself an edge for success in the job market.

- Do whatever you can to build your network of social support. If a friend has failed you, that's okay—start now to cultivate a circle of even better friends. Laugh together. Develop a sense of humor, a sense of compassion, and empathy. Whatever happens, stay involved with the people around you—start a study group, join a church committee, get involved in a political campaign, or volunteer at your child's school.

Take time now to study carefully Appendix A, Appendix B, and Appendix C at the end of this book. They are placed there, instead of in this chapter, so you can easily return to them repeatedly and contemplate what you've learned. The qualities listed there derive from careful studies of "self actualized" people, "highly effective people" and of the high-functioning but misunderstood "Type B" personality (the person who is protected from heart disease). Meditate on what specific situations would look like to you if you were looking through resilient eyes. Note how seeing the experience from this hardy standpoint changes it for you.

1. If you know (or can imagine) someone very much like the resilient people described in this chapter or in the appendixes, and if you admire the way they handle challenging situations, then do the following: Imagine what that person would do in the challenging situation before you. Picture that person doing it.

2. Write down in some detail what you admire and would want to emulate about the way that person responds. Your words create newness. Choose them wisely. What you admire and capture in writing reflects your own deeper wisdom and values about the way a good, wise, capable person would respond, and initiates an active process. Trust this.

3. Visualize yourself doing it that way. First, try seeing it "out there" like a movie, until it feels good to you. Finally, put yourself into the movie, mentally experience behaving in this resilient way; this time, look out from within yourself at the situation.

4. Mentally experience responding to the challenge with a sense that you are in *control* of your response, handling it in a way that increases *connectedness*, seeing the larger *purpose* of this and *hopeful* of handling it wisely and well. Note that the very process of visualizing doing it well creates a sense of control and hope. (Throughout this book, you will see that the four italicized mental principles in this step are highly associated with not only resilience, but also better health.)

5. Repeat this mental visualization experience four or five times (to get through differ-ent levels of memory).

6. Go through the same process for other situations, until you begin to respond in this way almost automatically.

   Developing resilience means developing an internal sense of control—of recognizing that you are ultimately the one in charge of your experience of whatever you encounter. One of the best tips comes from psychiatrist Steven Wolin and developmental psycholo-gist Sybil Wolin: "Get revenge by living well instead of squandering your energy by blaming and faultfinding."[72]

WHAT DID YOU LEARN?

1. Describe Kobasa's "three C's" of stress hardiness and what they mean.

2. What is positive psychology, and how does it differ from the traditional psychologi-cal approach?

3. What are four mental principles highly associated with better health outcomes?

4. Which of the characteristics of self actualized people or effective Type B from the appendixes are most appealing to you? How do you plan to further develop those characteristics?

5. Describe a visualization process you could use to experience responding in resilient ways to stressful situations.

ENDNOTES

1. Evan G. Pattishall, "The Development of Behavioral Medicine: Historical Models," *Annals of Behavioral Medicine* (November 1989): 43–8.

2. Howard S. Friedman, *The Self-Healing Personality* (New York: Henry Holt and Company, 1991), 99.

3. Claudia Wallis, "Stress: Can We Cope?" *Time* (June 6, 1983): 48–54.

4. Suzanne Ouellette Kobasa, "How Much Stress Can You Survive?" *American Health* (September: 1984): 67.

5. Ibid., 67.

6. W. F. Adams, *Ireland and Irish Emigration to the New World* (New Haven, CT: Yale University Press, 1932); and G. J. Drolet, "Epidemiology of Tuberculosis," in B. Goldberg, ed., *Clinical Tuberculosis* (Philadelphia, PA: F. A. Davis, 1946).

7. L. J. Moorman, "Tuberculosis on the Navajo Reservation," *American Review of Tuberculosis* 61 (1950): 586.

8. J. B. McDougal, *Tuberculosis—A Global Study in Social Pathology* (Baltimore, MD: Williams & Wilkins, 1949).

9. L. E. Hinkle, "The Effect of Exposure to Culture Change, Social Change, and Changes in Interpersonal Relationships on Health," pp. 9–44 in B. S. Dohrenwend and B. P. Dohrenwend, eds., *Stressful Life Events: Their Nature and Effects* (New York: Wiley, 1974).

10. E. Roskies, M. Iida-Miranda, and M. G. Strobel, "Life Changes as Predictors of Illness in Immigrants," pp. 3–21 in C. D. Spielberger and I. G. Sarason, eds., *Stress and Anxiety* (Washington, DC: Hemisphere, 1977).

11. Robert J. Wheeler and Monica A. Frank, "Identification of Stress Buffers," *Behavioral Medicine* 14, no. 2 (1988): 78–9.

12. Joshua Fischman, "Getting Tough," *Psychology Today* (December 1987): 26–8.

13. Blair Justice, *Who Gets Sick: Thinking and Health* (Houston, TX: Peak Press, 1987).

14. W. H. Courtenay, "Counseling Men in Medical Settings in the Six-Point HEALTH Plan," pp. 59–91 in G. R. Brooks and G. E. Good, eds., *The New Handbook of Psychotherapy and Counseling with Men* (San Francisco, CA: Jossey-Bass, 2001).

15. D. R. Williams, "The Health of Men: Structured Inequalities and Opportunities," *American Journal of Public Health* 93, no. 5 (2003): 724–31.

16. Sandra P. Thomas, "Men's Health and Psychosocial Issues Affecting Men," *Nursing Clinics of North America* 39 (2004): 259–70.

17. J. C. Barefoot et al., "Hostility Patterns and Health Implications: Correlates of Cook-Medley Hostility Scale Scores in a National Survey," *Health Psychology* 10 (1991): 18–24.

18. D. W. Birnbaum and W. L. Croll, "The Etiology of Children's Stereotypes about Sex Differences in Emotionality," *Sex Roles* 10 (1984): 677–91.

19. H. Lytton and D. M. Romney, "Parents' Differential Socialization of Boys and Girls: A Meta-Analysis," *Psychology Bulletin* 109 (1991): 267–96.

20. B. Murray, "Boys to Men: Emotional Miseducation," *American Psychological Association Monitor on Psychology* 30, no. 7 (1999): 38–9.

21. G. E. Good and N. B. Sherrod, "Men's Problems and Effective Treatments: Theory and Empirical Support," pp. 22–40 in G. R. Brooks and G. E. Good, eds., *The New Handbook of Psychotherapy and Counseling with Men* (San Francisco: Jossey-Bass, 2001).

22. M. C. Miller, "Stop Pretending Nothing's Wrong," *Newsweek* 24, no. 141 (June 16, 2003): 71–2.

23. M. K. Potts, M. A. Burnam, and K. B. Wells, "Gender Differences in Depression Detection: A Comparison of Clinician Diagnosis and Standardized Assessments," *Psychological Assessment* 3, no. 4 (1991): 609–15.

24. C. C. Cooper, "Men and Divorce," pp. 335–52 in G. R. Brooks and G. E. Good, eds., *The New Handbook of Psychotherapy and Counseling with Men* (San Francisco: Jossey-Bass, 2001).

25. R. F. Levant, "Toward the Reconstruction of Masculinity," pp. 229–51 in R. F. Levant and W. S. Pollack, eds., *A New Psychology of Men* (New York: Basic Books, 1995).

26. R. C. Kesler et al., "Lifetime and 12-Month Prevalence of DSM-III-R Psychiatric Disorders in the United States: Results from the National Comorbidity Survey," *Archives of General Psychiatry* 51 (1994): 8–19.

27. B. Schaub and R. Schaub, *Healing Addictions: The Vulnerability Model of Recovery* (Albany, NY: Delmar, 1997).

28. Williams, "The Health of Men."

29. G. W. Wechsler, et al., "Correlates of College Student Binge Drinking," *American Journal of Public Health* 85 (1995): 921–26.

30. Emmy E. Werner and Ruth S. Smith, *Vulnerable but Invincible: A Longitudinal Study of Resilient Children and Youth*, 3rd ed. (Adams Bannister Cox Publishers, 1989).

31. Robert Ornstein and David Sobel, *The Healing Brain* (New York: Simon & Schuster, 1987), 228–30.

32. Ibid., 228–9.

33. Ibid., 229.
34. Kenneth Pelletier, *Sound Mind, Sound Body: A New Model for Lifelong Health* (New York: Simon & Schuster, 1994), 57.
35. Susan Chollar, "The Miracle of Resilience," *American Health* (April 1994): 74.
36. Ibid., 74.
37. Fischman, "Getting Tough."
38. Joan Borysenko, *Minding the Body, Mending the Mind* (Reading, MA: Addison-Wesley, 1987), 24.
39. Raymond B. Flannery, "The Stress-Resistant Person," *Harvard Medical School Health Letter* (February 1989): 1–3.
40. Friedman, *The Self-Healing Personality,* 110.
41. Flannery, "The Stress-Resistant Person."
42. Friedman, *The Self-Healing Personality,* 106.
43. Friedman, *The Self-Healing Personality,* 111.
44. Darius Razavi et al., "Psychosocial Correlates of Estrogen and Progesterone Receptors in Breast Cancer," *Lancet* 335 (1990): 931–3.
45. Friedman, *The Self-Healing Personality,* 114.
46. K. Goodkin et al., "Active Coping Style Is Associated with Natural Killer Cell Cytotoxicity in Asymptomatic HIV-1 Seropositive Homosexual Men," *Journal of Psychosomatic Research* 36, no.7, (1992): 635–50; also see C. L. Mulder et al., "Active Confrontational Coping Predicts Decreased Clinical Progression Over a One-Year Period in HIV-Infected Homosexual Men," *Journal of Psychosomatic Research* 39, no. 8 (1995): 957–65.
47. Mihaly Csikszentmihalyi, *Flow: The Psychology of Optimal Experience* (New York: Harper Perennial, 1991).
48. Paula Tedesco-Carreras, "Maintaining Mental Wellness," National Student Nurses Association, *Imprint* (February/March 1988): 38.
49. Flannery, "The Stress-Resistant Person."
50. Flannery, "The Stress-Resistant Person."
51. A. A. Russo-Neustadt et al., "Physical Activity and Antidepressant Treatment Potentiate the Expression of Specific Brain-Derived Neurotrophic Factor Transcripts in the Rat Hippocampus," *Neuroscience* 101, no. 2 (November 7, 2000): 305–12; also, Zhe Ying, "Exercise Restores Levels of Neurotrophins and Synaptic Plasticity Following Spinal Cord Injury," *Experimental Neurology* 193 (2005): 411–9.
52. Flannery, "The Stress-Resistant Person."
53. Raymond E. Flannery, Jr., "Towards Stress-Resistant Persons: A Stress Management Approach to the Treatment of Anxiety," *American Journal of Preventive Medicine* 3, no. 1 (1987): 26.
54. T. Edward Hannah, "Hardiness and Health Behavior: The Role of Health Concern as a Moderator Variable," *Behavioral Medicine* (Summer 1988): 59–62.
55. Ibid.
56. Robert Ornstein and David Sobel, *Healthy Pleasures* (Reading, MA: Addison-Wesley, 1989), 280–81.
57. M. A. Jacobs, A. Spilken, and M. Norman, "Relationship of Life Change, Maladaptive Aggression, and Upper Respiratory Infection in Male College Students," *Psychosomatic Medicine* 31, no. 1 (1969): 31–44.
58. Flannery, "The Stress-Resistant Person," 5–6.
59. Marc Ian Barasch, "The Healing Path: A Soul Approach to Illness," in *Proceedings of the Sixth International Conference of the National Institute for the Clinical Application of*

Behavioral Medicine, The Psychology of Health, Immunity, and Disease, Hilton Head Island, vol. B (December 1994): 9.

60. Fischman, "Getting Tough."

61. Howard S. Friedman and Gary R. VandenBos, "Disease-Prone and Self-Healing Personalities," *Hospital and Community Psychiatry* 23, no. 12 (1992): 1178.

62. C. Peterson and M E. P. Seligman, *Character Strengths and Virtues: A Handbook and Classification* (New York: Oxford University Press/Washington, DC: American Psychological Association, 2004).

63. Martin Seligman et al., "Positive Psychology Progress: Empirical Validation of Interventions," *American Psychologist* 60 (2005): 410–21.

64. Online information and participation in such interventions is available at the following web-sites: www.positivepsychology.org; www.apa.org/science/postivepsy/html; and www.bus.umich.edu/Positive/

65. G. E. Vaillant, "Natural History of Male Psychologic Health: Effects of Mental Health on Physical Health," *New England Journal of Medicine* 301, no. 23 (1979): 1249–54; also G. E. Vaillant, "Natural History of Male Psychological Health. III. Empirical Dimensions of Mental Health," *Archives of General Psychiatry* 32, no. 4 (Apr 1975): 420–6.

66. G. E. Vaillant and C. O. Vaillant, "Natural History of Male Psychological Health, XII: A 45-Year Study of Predictors of Successful Aging at Age 65," *American Journal of Psychiatry* 147(1) (1990): 31–7.

67. G. E. Vaillant, "Natural History of Male Psychologic Health: Effects of Mental Health on Physical Health," 1249–54; also see G. E. Vaillant, "Natural History of Male Psychological Health, IV: What Kinds of Men Do Not Get Psychosomatic Illness," *Psychosomatic Medicine* 40, no. 5 (1978): 420–31.

68. G. E. Vaillant, *Aging Well* (Boston: Little, Brown, 2000); also, Martin Seligman, *Learned Optimism* (New York: Knopf, 1990), 179–81.

69. Linda G. Russek and Gary E. Schwartz, *Feeling of Parental Caring Predict Health Status in Midlife: A 35-Year Follow-up of the Harvard Mastery of Stress Study* 20 (1997): 1–13.

70. Friedman and VandenBos, "Disease-Prone and Self-Healing Personalities."

71. Bernie S. Siegel *Love, Medicine and Miracles* (New York: Harper & Row, 1986), 28–9; also, "Mind Over Cancer," 64.

72. Chollar, "The Miracle of Resilience," 75.

CHAPTER 9

Social Support, Relationships, and Health

Help thy brother's boat across, and lo!
thine own has reached the shore.

—Hindu Proverb

LEARNING OBJECTIVES

- Define *social support.*
- Understand why there have been inconsistencies in studies of social support and health.
- Identify the sources of social support.
- Understand how social support protects health and how isolation has the potential to harm health.
- Discuss the implications of social support on the health of the cardiovascular system.
- Understand the importance of touch to health.

For most of us, life centers around our relationships with the significant people in our lives—our family members, other loved ones, and close friends. Within our culture and society, it's not unusual to have a broad array of friends garnered from many different places. You've probably inherently known that life is easier and more comfortable when you have people you can depend on. What may not be so obvious is what science is now telling us: the existence and quality of these relationships and the support they provide has substantial impact on not only our psychological well-being but our physical health and longevity.[1]

A number of interesting studies bear this out. One of the best known was conducted by a group of researchers in Alameda County, California, who gathered data on more than 7,000 people over a nine-year period. At the end of the study, they found the common denominator that most often led to good health and long life is the amount of social support a person enjoys.

The people with many social contacts—a spouse, a close-knit family, a network of friends, church, or other group affiliations—lived longer and had better health. People who were socially isolated had poorer health and died earlier. In fact, those who had few ties with other people died at rates two to five times higher than did those with good social ties.[2] The link between social ties and death rate held up regardless of gender, race, ethnic background, or socioeconomic status.[3] "Some well-loved people fall ill and die prematurely," researchers concluded; "Some isolates live long and healthy lives. But these occurrences are infrequent. For the most part, people tied closely to others are better able to stay well."[4]

Furthermore, people with strong social ties not only live longer, healthier lives, but they tend to enjoy themselves more, too. More than 3,000 elderly people who were tested on pleasure and well-being were also asked about their social connections. Social isolation had an "amazingly" strong correlation with a low sense of pleasure and well-being. Those with the strongest social connections also had the strongest sense of well-being and pleasure.[5]

The importance of social relationships actually begins at birth, as infants are cared for and develop attachment to their parents and other consistent caregivers. An important determinant of both physical and mental health is demonstrated in the bond between an infant and a caregiver: The healthiest infants have a secure bond with at least one caregiver, express distress when separated from the caregiver, and receive appropriate attention from the caregiver in response to that distress—and those are the infants who are most likely to survive to adulthood. The security of that relationship enables a child to develop a sense of self-worth, to see others as supportive, and to accept others as a source of affection and comfort. On the other hand, when a caregiver's response is chronically inadequate or is poorly matched to the infant's needs, the attachment disorder that develops impacts the child's emotional and physical health and can lead to premature death.[6]

Writing in *The Sciences,* the journal of the New York Academy of Sciences, California physician and epidemiologist Leonard Sagan made a sobering observation of the state of social connectedness in our nation. The United States, he wrote, spends far more per capita on health care but has far lower life expectancies than Greece, Spain, and Italy. The difference, he believes, "exists because of the decreasing level of natural family support in America. Many of us badly need an activity that boosts our sense of social support and our connections with other people."[7]

Dr. Kenneth Pelletier of the Stanford Center for Research in Disease Prevention says that "a sense of belonging and connection to other people appears to be a basic human need—as basic as food and shelter. In fact, social support may be one of the critical elements distinguishing those who remain healthy from those who become ill."[8]

Studies involving large samples demonstrate that the protection of social support comes in many different forms and through a number of different channels: marriage and family, ties to friends and neighbors, civic engagement (both individually and collectively), relationships with coworkers, and trust all seem to be independently and robustly related to happiness, health, and life satisfaction.[9] The strongest associations between social support and health are related to psychological health; those who have the greatest social support are at the lowest risk for psychological distress, especially depression.[10] Social support seems to boost psychological health by increasing the sense of self-worth, belonging, and purpose. A variety of studies indicate that strong social ties help protect psychological well-being by mitigating the effects of stress, reducing symptoms of depression, and easing anxiety.[11]

Even though the results are less well documented, and while researchers aren't sure why, it has become apparent that social support also affects physical health, both in terms of mortality and in the onset and progression of disease.[12]

As a positive influence, social support and personality are considered the two best predictors of recovery from illness or other assault to the body's ability to defend itself.[13] According to the research, social support influences behaviors that impact health—such as diet, the amount of exercise you get, whether you smoke cigarettes, and whether you drink alcohol (as well as how much you drink). The amount of social support you enjoy also appears to have an impact on biological processes, such as neuroendocrine responses, immune responses, and changes in blood flow. In their negative influence, these behavioral and biological influences together may directly or indirectly lead to stroke, coronary heart disease, coronary artery disease, cancer, infectious diseases, allergies, autoimmune diseases, and liver disease.

Sidney Cobb, president of the Society of Psychosomatic Medicine, claims that the notion of social support as an element of health is not new. What is new, he says, is the collection of hard evidence that demonstrates the case—proof positive that social support can indeed protect people in crisis from what he calls a "wide variety" of diseases. Adequate social support, Cobb says, has been proven to protect against or mitigate the effects of conditions "from low birth weight to death, from arthritis through tuberculosis to depression, alcoholism, and other psychiatric illness. Furthermore, social support can reduce the amount of medication required, accelerate recovery, and facilitate compliance with prescribed medical regimens."[14]

Social Support Defined

As defined by most researchers, social support is the degree to which a person's basic social needs are met through interaction with other people. It's the resources, both tangible and intangible, that other people provide. It's a person's perception that he or she can count on other people for help with a problem or for help in a time of crisis. For some, strong social support depends on a large, diverse system of people to whom they can turn; for others, equally strong social support can come from a small but intimate and reliable circle of friends. And you don't have to actually get help from those people to benefit from their support—just knowing they are there, and that you *can* turn to them for help, brings the benefits of social support.[15] Social support is *not* the same as a support group; support groups are structured groups that generally use structured self-help meetings and are most often run by mental health professionals.

Leading researchers who have studied the effect of social support on heart disease say it involves five components:[16]

- Being cared for and loved, with the opportunity for shared intimacy
- Being esteemed and valued; having a sense of personal worth

- Sharing companionship, communication, and mutual obligations with others; having a sense of belonging
- Having "informational" support—access to information, appraisal, advice, and guidance from others
- Having access to physical or material assistance

The resources that your social network provides may come in the form of tangible, instrumental aid such as lending you money, driving you to your doctor's appointment, doing your grocery shopping, or helping assume responsibility for your children while you are sick. But another kind of resource is equally important: it's the emotional, "intangible" kind of help such as affection, understanding, acceptance, and esteem.[17]

Researchers often use six criteria to determine the level of overall social support available to any one individual. Those include the amount of attachment provided by a spouse or lover, the level of social integration (usually related to friends or a group of people), feelings of self-esteem and worth, assurance that others can be depended on to provide help, presence of a "higher" figure (such as a parent or mentor), and the opportunity to nuture.[18]

According to research, you probably don't derive health benefits from a single, isolated, personal encounter or relationship. More likely, the health benefits of social support are cumulative, resulting from recurring patterns of love, affection, nurturance, and the other positive effects and emotions that stem from social ties.[19] The greater the number of positive social relationships you have over a prolonged period of time, the greater the benefit to your health and longevity. In a similar way, it is a recurrent pattern of stress, isolation, and negative interaction that is most likely to impact health in a negative way, not a single episode or relationship.[20]

According to University of Michigan researchers James S. House and Robert L. Kahn, three factors comprise social resources:[21]

1. Social network—the size, density, durability, intensity, and frequency of your social contacts
2. Social relationships—the existence of relationships, number of relationships, and type of relationships
3. Social support—the type, source, number, and quality of your resources

It's important to realize that you can live alone and still have solid social support—the size of your household isn't the determining factor. The greater factors in social support are having close friends who provide you with positive experiences, socially rewarding roles, and an important ability to cope with difficult situations and events in your life.[22]

Sources of Social Support

Social support can come from family members, friends, professional associates, members of the church congregation, neighbors, people who belong to the same bowling league or bridge club, and so on. The people who make up one's social support network are the people with whom one associates and to whom one could turn in time of need.

Sources of social support vary, depending on gender, age, and other factors. In one study, 900 people selected at random from six states were interviewed. All were aged 65 and older; none was living in an institution. Almost half were married, and more than half (64 percent) were retired.[23]

The main source of social support for married men was their wives—but the same didn't hold true for women. The married women in the study relied more heavily on other family members and friends than they did on their husbands. According to the results of the study and the findings of other researchers, women seem to get their greatest health benefits from contact with other women. Those with the best health had close female friends or relatives. There may be a number of reasons why this is true, and one of them, according to sociologists at the University of Texas at Austin, may be evidence showing that "women are just more effective at providing support" than are men.[24] When it came to "instrumental" support—the rendering of physical help and the sharing of responsibilities—women used family helpers, agency personnel, and paid helpers more than men did.[25]

Research has also exploded some long-held myths about elderly people and social support. For years, the elderly were often regarded as being "takers," the ones who gained from a network of social support. Recent research, however, dispels that myth. A national survey involving more than 700 elderly adults demonstrated that their health and vitality have more to do with what they contribute to their social support network than what they receive from it.[26]

It's also important to consider both gender and age in considering the importance of specific kinds of social support. An Australian study looked at more than 11,000 men and women between the ages of 18 and 95, all of whom were twins. The study found that seven kinds of social support were consistently important: support from spouse, twin, children, parents, other relatives, friends, and helpers. The importance of support from a twin remained constant across ages and for both men and women. As they grew older, the women found support from spouse, parents, and friends slightly less important than did the men; the men found support from relatives and helpers to be more important as they got older. Both men and women relied substantially on support from children as they grew older. Interestingly, women were more likely to have an important confidant when young, but the importance of that relationship grew less significant as they got older. Not so for the men in the study: the importance of having a confidant grew more important for the men.[27]

An important source of social support for both men and women of all ages is the sense of belonging to a neighborhood. "Belonging" to a neighborhood can encompass factors like interaction with other people in the neighborhood and/or community, the nature and quality of social contacts in the neighborhood, emotional attachment to neighbors and/or the community, the belief that people in the neighborhood can be effective in making positive changes, participation in community organizations, feelings of safety and security, and a positive environment (such as a neighborhood or community with low crime rates). A sense of belonging to a neighborhood generally increases the longer a person lives in one place; it is more likely in rural or remote areas and suburbs and least likely in urban areas. Research shows that a strong sense of belonging to a neighborhood reduces stress, improves mental and physical health, and increases the likelihood that people are physically active.[28] Neighborhood quality is especially important in promoting the well-being, both physical and mental, of children.[29]

Research also suggests that for both men and women, socioeconomic status plays a role in the amount of social support that is available—or even the amount that is perceived. Low socioeconomic status tends to be associated with certain stressors, such as financial strain, crowded living conditions, and fear of crime, all of which are stressors that also cause lower levels of perceived social support. These same stressors can foster a distrust of others, which naturally leads to reduced social support.[30]

How Does Social Support Protect Health?

Researchers have looked at the role of social support in health for almost three decades, and there have been inconsistencies in their findings. A number of factors can cause those inconsistencies.[31]

- Social support and social networks are measured differently from one study to another.

- The association between social support and health may be bidirectional—in other words, someone in poor health may not have strong social support because the health condition itself prevents the person from developing a good social network.

- The effects of social support may vary because of a wide variety of characteristics, such as gender, age, cultural setting, socioeconomic status, disease, or stage of disease, and these may vary from one study to another.

- The associations between social support and health rely on a number of mechanisms, all of which are not clear.

- There need to be clearly defined theoretical paradigms to be used in designing the studies and analyzing the data.

- Many studies automatically adjust certain variables, which may not help understand the effects of social support on health.

One thing is certain: the way that social support impacts health is a complex one, and that complexity in itself has caused some of the inconsistency in research findings. Furthermore, there can be some difficulty in measuring and conceptualizing "social support." For example, there are real differences between perceived support, the quality of support, received support, emotional support, and structural support.[32] There can also be differences based on gender: One study of heart disease in Finland found that men—but not women—with the lowest amount of social support were at highest risk for cardiovascular disease.[33] While some researchers enthusiastically endorse social support as a beneficial factor for good health and longevity, others are not as eager, and some say that findings are simply inconclusive.

Important future directions for the study of social support and health include a variety of areas such as matching people with support based on their needs, mutual coping and support-giving dynamics, identifying properties of groups that can provide a sense of social support, and determining the negative effects that may exist in social relationships and how they impact health.[34] Two research streams that seem particularly promising are (1) an examination of how supportive social ties have a positive influence on health, and (2) how social strain has a negative impact on health and well-being. "Social strain" might include situations in which a person cannot provide assistance, either from lack of knowledge or from being unwelcome to do so; a person tries to help but is inept; the person going through difficulty causes psychological distress (such as shame, resentment, or sadness) for the potential helper; the give-and-take aspects of the relationship are too unbalanced; the person needing help makes unreasonably high demands; or the person wanting to help is overwhelmed by too many roles. These two streams need to include input from gerontology, physiology, psychology, and psychiatry, among many other fields, and need to examine the relation between social factors and disease.[35]

While these caveats are important to consider, there are simply too many large-scale studies with convincing results to ignore the work that has been done connecting social support and health. No one knows for certain how social support works to protect health, but some theories by prominent researchers who have done the most specialized work in the field of social support seem to be standing up to close scrutiny:[36]

1. Social support enhances health and well-being no matter how much stress a person is under; the enhancement may result from an overall positive feeling and a sense of self-esteem, stability, and control over one's environment.

2. Social support acts as a buffer against stress by protecting a person from the diseases that stress often causes.

Still other researchers believe that a strong social network and healthy social ties gradually lead to a greater, more generalized sense of control. An impressive array of studies has shown that a sense of control improves and protects health, whereas a feeling of little control can have serious health consequences.

Regardless of how social support protects health, we know that it does. Psychologist Joan Borysenko writes, "The consequences of emotional abandonment are no less serious than those of physical abandonment. Babies in foundling homes that are fed and changed on schedule but starved emotionally often develop a syndrome called "hospitalism," or failure to thrive. No one is present to coo when the baby coos, to smile when the baby smiles, to mirror back its existence to the child. As a result of this loneliness, the babies' pituitary glands fail to produce sufficient growth hormone and the children wither away despite adequate nutrition. Many of these children die before reaching toddlerhood, and those who do survive are often severely damaged psychologically."[37]

Early researchers who struggled to determine what sort of patient has disease found striking similarities in the circumstances of people with conditions as diverse as depression, tuberculosis, high blood pressure, multiple accidents, and even complications in pregnancy. The people who were ill usually lacked a strong supportive network or had experienced a recent disruption in their traditional sources of social support.[38]

Unfortunately, the number of people in this category seems to be increasing. In comparing people in the United States today with those of earlier generations, a disturbing trend is evident. People today are more likely to live alone, less likely to be married, and less likely to belong to a social organization.[39] The result is a generation of people with weaker social ties—and poorer health.

Besides buffering the effects of stress and protecting health, strong social ties might give people still another edge in good health. Research at the University of Oregon shows that people with more social ties and stronger social support engage in a greater number of health-promoting and preventive behaviors—and fewer risk-taking behaviors. The study, which involved 2,603 adults, showed that the link is strongest among older people.[40]

There's more: The range of problems that people bring to friends and neighbors is much broader than those brought to doctors, says Dr. Eva Salber, professor emeritus of Duke University's School of Medicine. Fewer than 5 percent of all physician visits are for psychological problems, she says, "because we learn that if we want a doctor's attention, we must focus on a physical symptom. A woman might tell her doctor she has a bladder infection," but she'll tell a friend "that she's lost her job, had a fight with her husband, and has a bladder infection." What it boils down to, says Dr. Salber, is that "the great majority of human ills are never seen by a doctor. The real primary care is provided by one's family, close friends, and neighbors."[41] These natural helpers—friends, family, and neighbors—may "very well prove to be our most important untapped resource," she adds. That can be especially true for people who are unable to effectively use the medical resources normally available, either because of poverty, lack of transportation, language barriers, or disabilities.

The act of confiding may be one of the most important health boosts of all. Research into the importance of various kinds of social support to health found that interactions with confidants mattered the most; in other words, they had the greatest impact on health.[42] University of Texas psychologist James W. Pennebaker has done some of the most impressive research in the area of confiding. Apparently all kinds of health benefits are associated with confiding. In his pioneering book, *Opening Up: The Healing Power of Confiding in Others,*[43] Pennebaker sums it up simply by saying, "Not disclosing our thoughts and feelings can be unhealthy. Divulging them can be healthy."

As mentioned earlier, there is a difference between the genders when it comes to the importance of confidants. Both men and women report feeling less lonely when their interactions with confidants are more intimate and satisfying. Interestingly, women report confiding in both men and women—but men overwhelmingly report intimate and satisfying confidant relationships with women and significantly less intimate relationships with other men.[44]

In recounting more than two decades of specialized research into the health benefits of confiding, Pennebaker says his initial interest was piqued by a polygrapher in San Francisco.[45] The polygrapher, who was examining a 45-year-old bank vice president for embezzlement, explained to Pennebaker that the banker's physiological signs—such as heart rate and blood pressure—were very high at first, which is normal for both guilty and innocent people confronted by the threatening dilemma of taking a polygraph test. When quizzed about the details of the embezzlement, however, his vital signs skyrocketed so dramatically that he broke down and confessed to embezzling $74,000 over six months.

That in itself was not dramatic, says Pennebaker. The surprise came later, when the bank official was retested—standard procedure to test the possible deception of a confession. This time the man was completely relaxed. His breathing was slow and relaxed; his heart rate and blood pressure were not only normal, but extraordinarily low; and his palms were dry.

"You can appreciate the irony of this situation," Pennebaker writes. "This man had come into the polygrapher's office a free man, safe in the knowledge that polygraph evidence was not allowed in court. Nevertheless, he confessed. Now, his professional, financial, and personal lives were on the brink of ruin. He was virtually assured of a prison term. Despite these realities, he was relaxed and at ease with himself. Indeed, when a policeman came to handcuff and escort him to jail, he warmly shook the polygrapher's hand and thanked him for all he had done. This last December, the polygrapher received a chatty Christmas card written by the former bank vice president with a federal penitentiary as the return address.

"Even when the costs are high," Pennebaker concludes, "the confession of actions that violate our personal values can reduce anxiety and physiological stress.... Revealing pent-up thoughts and feelings can be liberating, even if they send you to prison."[46]

The healthful aspects of confiding can also occur when the confession is written, says Pennebaker. In an experiment that demonstrated the power of written confession, Pennebaker and his former colleagues at Southern Methodist University asked a group of student volunteers to write about their experiences for fifteen minutes a day over a total of four days.

The students could choose to write either about superficial topics or about a traumatic experience. The students who chose to write about a traumatic experience were instructed to describe their emotions about the event, describe the facts surrounding the event, or write about both the facts and their emotions. Researchers then attempted to determine how often the students got sick by noting how often they visited the student health center. Researchers compared the number of visits in the two and a half months before the students wrote with the number of visits in the five and a half months after they wrote.

All of the students who participated in the experiment visited the health center at the same rate before writing. After writing, those who wrote both the facts and their feelings about a traumatic experience visited the health center 50 percent less often than those who simply wrote about a superficial topic—or those who wrote either the facts or their feelings.

Interestingly, says Pennebaker, writing about a traumatic experience didn't make the students feel better right away. In fact, just the opposite was true—"at first, they were depressed."[47]

In a subsequent study, Pennebaker and Martha E. Francis recruited 41 university employees to write for 20 minutes once a week for four consecutive weeks.[48] The employees wrote about personal experiences, either traumatic or nontraumatic.

During the month that the employees were writing, those who wrote about traumatic experiences had a 28.6 percent decrease in absentee rates; those who wrote about nontraumatic experiences had a 48.5 percent increase in absentee rates. Pennebaker and Francis followed up with blood tests that showed significant health benefits from writing about traumatic experiences.

Although heart rate and blood pressure almost always increase significantly during the act of confiding, they decrease significantly afterward. It's a long-lasting effect, too: people who confide continue to show smaller increases in blood pressure when under stress or when confronted with a challenging task—a benefit that can make big differences in overall health.

There are other health benefits associated with confiding, says Pennebaker, but perhaps the one most associated with good health is immunity.[49] People who confide enjoy better functioning of the immune system. Those who don't confide face a myriad of immune system disorders; their white blood cell counts are "seriously disturbed." Natural killer cells are weakened and decrease in number; T cells can't do their job. Almost without exception, Pennebaker says, the people in his studies who began confiding enjoyed enhanced immune function. They showed improvement in physical symptoms; they visited the doctor less often.

Best of all, Pennebaker says, immune system enhancement related to confiding lingers. In one test, students who wrote about troubling experiences they had never before confided experienced significant improvement in immune function as a result—and the improvement from that one session tended to persist for six weeks following the confiding experience.[50]

Part of the benefit from writing about feelings is that it doesn't require feedback—in other words, we're not restricted by how others react. "One reason why writing is so potent is that usually when we start to tell somebody about some personal thing," Pennebaker explains, "we're watching their face very closely to see how they react. If we see any sign that the other person is shocked or disapproving, we immediately start to change the story."[51]

Want to try it yourself? To get started, follow Pennebaker's guidelines for effective written confession:

- To get started, write continuously about the most upsetting or traumatic experience of your entire life. Keep writing until you can't think of anything else to say.

- Don't worry about spelling, grammar, or sentence structure; work on a free flow of your feelings and the facts as you remember them.

- Go beyond the surface—discuss your deepest thoughts and feelings about the experience.

"You can write about anything you want," says Pennebaker. "But ideally, it should be about something you have not talked about with others in detail. It is critical, however, that you let yourself go and touch those deepest emotions and thoughts that you have. In other words, write about what happened, how you felt about it at the time it occurred, and how you feel about it now."[52]

The Ties That Bind

Social ties—good friendships, good relationships with family members, the presence of people we know we can lean on—play an important part in our good health. A scientific panel convened by the U. S. government found that social support not only reduced mortality but was key in protecting health as well. According to the panel, there is a close relationship between the number and strength of an individual's social relationships and an individual's health and longevity. Panel experts say that strong social support can be shown to reduce complications in pregnancy, aid in recovery from surgery, reduce the need for medications in some chronic illnesses, combat the symptoms of stress, protect against a variety of emotional and psychological problems, and help to keep patients in needed medical treatment and promote adherence to needed medical treatment regimens.[53] Social support has also been shown in several studies to promote positive health practices.[54]

Information continues to pour in as studies are completed that demonstrate that, indeed, something very important is happening. "The ties that bind," as we so often call them, are also apparently the ties that can keep us healthy and help us live a long, happy life.

In a long-term study, almost 3,000 adults in Tecumseh, Michigan, were studied for 10 years. At the beginning of the study, each adult was given a thorough physical examination to rule out any existing illness that would force a person to become isolated. Researchers then watched these people closely for the next 10 years, making special note of their social relationships and group activities. Those who were socially involved were found to have the best health. When social ties were interrupted or broken, the incidence of disease increased significantly. Researchers particularly noticed that certain conditions seemed related to marginal social ties. Among them were coronary heart disease, cancer, arthritis, strokes, upper respiratory infections, and mental illness. In fact, researchers concluded, interrupted social ties actually seemed to suppress the body's immune system.[55]

Those who conducted the study called close personal relationships a "safety net." They stated that people without such a safety net fall vulnerable to a wide variety of diseases far more frequently than people who are surrounded by the comfort of good social relationships.

Apparently, the impact of social relationships on immunity may be affected by how early in life the social support occurs and how long-lasting social relationships are. A brief disruption in social support (such as a brief separation) may have impact on immunity, but it is likely to be a short-term effect. Disruption in social support that occurs early in life (stress on the fetus during pregnancy or separation from the mother at birth, for example) or that is more long-lasting causes more long-term impact on immunity—sometimes lasting longer than two years. Studies show that it is often difficult to restore normal immunity after that kind of serious impact.[56]

We seem to derive an odd sort of comfort from other people—a comfort that can literally influence us biologically. One researcher observed that the menstrual cycles of close friends and roommates in a college dormitory appeared to be related, but randomly selected girls on the same campus showed no similarities in cycles.[57]

In another experiment, researchers from Walter Reed Army Institute studied a group of three crewmen who worked closely together on a lengthy B-52 flight. The crew members were studied for both physical and emotional symptoms and disorders, and blood tests were taken as part of the study. Researchers found that the levels of 17 stress-related hormones peaked in all three crewmen at the same time each day.[58]

One note of caution: some types of "social support" can actually be detrimental instead of beneficial. Researchers caution that several situations can actually harm your health in the long run:[59]

- People who are constantly stressed or ill may actually cause you to suffer along with them. If they require more help than you can realistically provide, you may end up feeling anxious and depressed as you try to provide assistance.

- People who are involved in unhealthy behaviors that you are trying to avoid—such as substance abuse—may get in the way of your own recovery.

- People you feel "obligated" to can actually exact a heavy psychological toll. This is especially true if you find that you need to conform to someone else's beliefs or ideas. Carefully assess the relationship if you constantly feel the need to repay someone for his or her efforts on your behalf.

- Watch out for support systems that are oppressive, rigid, or unhealthy or that demand conformity. These kinds of systems can actually be worse than having little or no social support at all.

Battle Stress

The importance of the support factor was demonstrated even more clearly in a comprehensive study conducted by the U. S. Office of the Surgeon General. As part of the study, researchers looked at the way World War II troops reacted to the intense stress of battle. Researchers decided that the sustaining influence of other people is what kept troops from crumbling under the stress of battle. Soldiers who benefited from "group identification," "group cohesiveness," or "the buddy system"—those who had strong social support—were able to withstand even intense battle stress. Those in the small combat groups who were sustained by other members suffered the lowest casualties.

Those who did not feel the cohesiveness of a small group, who were not encouraged to come together in "the buddy system," or whose small group was disrupted during combat were the ones who mainly suffered psychiatric breakdown in battle. These soldiers—the lonely, isolated ones—were the ones who suffered the greatest casualties.[60]

Epidemiologist Leonard Syme, who was one of the researchers instrumental in the study of the 7,000 Alameda County, California, residents, confirmed the importance of social support in helping people deal with "battle stress"—not the kind encountered in combat, but the kind real people contend with every day. He remarked that "people who have a close-knit network of intimate personal ties with other people seem to be able to avoid disease, maintain higher levels of health, and in general, to deal more successfully with life's difficulties."[61]

Unemployment

Can social support help ease the problems associated with unemployment? Apparently it can. In one study, researchers looked at 110 men who were forcibly unemployed when a plant closed.[62] The men were given thorough examinations at various times before and after the plant closing. Examiners measured levels of serum cholesterol, symptoms of illness, symptoms of depression, and the degree of social support each man had from his family and his friends.

The result was a firm testimony of social support. The men who had little social support during the study were significantly more likely to get sick, become depressed, and suffer from elevated levels of serum cholesterol. The men who had good social support from their friends and family members and who had plenty of opportunity for social interaction were significantly more healthy, despite the stress of losing their jobs.

Pregnant Women Under Stress

Another study looked at pregnant women who were undergoing stressful life events. Researchers studied 170 women, assessed how stressful the life events were, both before and during pregnancy, and also determined how much social support each woman had. (A number of other "psychosocial assets" were also measured.) Researchers then recorded the outcome of each of the pregnancies.

Again, social support seemed to be the key: Only 33 percent of the women under stress had complications during pregnancy if they felt they had strong social support. Among the stressed women who perceived that their social support was weak, 91 percent had complications during pregnancy.[63]

Women who have children with chronic diseases or disabilities have a particular need for strong social support—especially if the child has few skills that allow for any independence. As caregivers, these mothers are responsible not only for meeting the needs of the child but for meeting other social demands as well. The availability of strong social support, especially from family members, enables mothers to adjust to such a range of demands.[64]

Relocation and Disruption

Part of the stress from relocation is connected to unfamiliar geographic territory, but another (and perhaps even more significant) part is related to the loss of familiar friends. It is, in a real sense, a loss of social support.

Experiments in the animal world have demonstrated how important it is to be surrounded by friends. In one experiment, chickens were injected with neoplasms (which would have been expected to cause cancer). The chickens that remained in their familiar pecking order stayed healthy; the chickens that were housed with unfamiliar chickens developed cancer.[65]

The same thing holds true for people. When people are uprooted and forced to move away from familiar people or places, they often get sick. People who have moved or who have otherwise experienced great disruption in their situations are sicker more often and absent from work at a higher rate than their coworkers.

Researchers were able to observe the effect of disruption by watching the coal miners and their families who moved from small valleys in Appalachia to the company towns created when coal mines were reopened. By looking at the family names of the workers, it was possible to determine how many had relatives living in the towns to which they had come.

Researchers found that those who moved to towns where they did not have family members had a significantly higher rate of absenteeism due to sickness. The coal miners who moved to towns where they had kinfolk were able to stay significantly healthier. The only real factor that distinguished the two groups was the amount of social support they had.[66]

These findings have particular significance for the elderly, whose disrupted social ties are a common part of daily life associated with bereavement, retirement, or a change in residence. Researchers have noted that these changes tend to cause severe depression among the elderly—but that people are able to maintain good health and avoid depression if they have even one close supportive confidante.[67]

A fascinating study conducted on the Sinai peninsula in Israel sheds light on social support in general but also gives particular insight into the phenomenon of relocation, disrupted ties, friendships, and the presence of kinfolk.[68] In 1972, a civilian community named Ophira (Sharm-el-Sheik in Arabic) was established at the southernmost tip of the Sinai peninsula, primarily by families with a pioneering spirit who had wanted to build a town in the desert. Geographically, Ophira was quite isolated. The closest Israeli town of any size, Eilat, was more than 200 miles away.

Because of its distance from Eilat, the town of Ophira quickly became self-contained and self-sufficient, both physically and psychologically. Not only were residents of the town self-sufficient, but they were also unusually similar to each other, partly because the living conditions in the community were so uniform. All the people in town lived in a single housing complex. There was only one shopping center, one school, and one medical center with one doctor and one nurse, so everyone in town also shared the same support services.

Ten years after it was established, Ophira was disbanded as part of the Camp David accords with Egypt that ordered evacuation of the Sinai peninsula. The residents of Ophira, who had lived as such a tightly knit group for 10 years, were forced to evacuate—and were relocated over a widely scattered area throughout Israel. Some of the Ophira residents were relocated to rural areas, and others moved to urban areas.

Researchers interested in the effect of the relocation assessed the residents six weeks before the final evacuation and again two years later. A questionnaire and a variety of tests were given to the residents who participated in the study; researchers focused on 18 husband/wife pairs (a total of 36 people) similar in age, ethnic background, educational level, and occupational status.

Several interesting findings emerged:

1. The demoralization and distress that stem from stressful life events (such as relocation) are long-lasting, not temporary. Sophisticated psychological tests given to Ophira residents showed that the stress associated with the relocation was basically as severe after two years as it was six weeks before the actual evacuation. Researchers concluded from their findings that an individual's adjustment to stress at the time it occurs is a good predictor of how adjusted he or she will be two years later.

2. Each individual in the study was asked to list his or her friends, both six weeks before evacuation and two years later. As could be predicted, the first list of friends—the one made six weeks before the relocation—consisted almost entirely of other Ophira residents. The list made two years later, predictably, contained an entirely new group of friends, with only one or two Ophira residents still included. In almost all cases, the lists were almost exactly the same size at two years as they had been at six weeks! Even though the friends themselves changed, the size of the network remained about the same, which led researchers to conclude that people actively work to shape their own friendship networks. (Previous theories had suggested that the size of one's friendship network is largely dependent on environment and circumstances, not the result of any effort.)

3. A strong social relationship with kinfolk (or family members) seemed to be a better predictor of health and adjustment than a strong relationship with friends.

Few of the couples in the study had kinfolk in Ophira. Likewise, few of the couples moved to areas where their kinfolk were. But those who had strong ties with their kinfolk tended to maintain them and gain strength from them regardless of where they lived. Unlike friends, family members seem to be a source of strength even at distances.

In summing up the general protective nature of social ties, California psychiatrist Robert Taylor said, "When people have close relationships, they feel less threatened, less alone, more confident, and more in control. Knowing you have people you can turn to in times of need can provide some very important feelings of security, optimism, and hope—all of which can be great antidotes to stress."[69]

Love Stronger, Live Longer

Larry Dossey, MD, co-chair of the newly established Panel on Mind/Body Interventions at the National Institutes of Health, says about one of the most celebrated emotions, "The power of love to change bodies is legendary, built into folklore, common sense, and everyday experience. Love moves the flesh, it pushes matter around—as the blushing and palpitations experienced by lovers attest. Throughout history, 'tender, loving care' has uniformly been recognized as a valuable element in healing."[70]

The results of a variety of studies prove that if we want to live longer, we surround ourselves with at least a few good people who can act as friends and confidants. That finding has consistently held true across the board, regardless of how studies have been set up or what population was studied. Healthy people with good social support are at consistently lower risk for mortality than are their isolated counterparts.[71] Again, that finding holds true across the board. Some studies show results for both men and women. Others have studied only women and show that women with good social support have much less disease than those who are more isolated.

Social support is such a powerful factor in mortality that it even lowers mortality among those who are unhealthy (such as survivors of heart attacks). In one study of more than 2,500 elderly men and women, researchers asked each how many sources of social support they had. The researchers then observed those who were eventually hospitalized for heart attack.

The differences were stark. Only 12 percent of those with two or more sources of social support died in the hospital. However, 23 percent of those with only one source of social support died while still in the hospital, and 38 percent of those who said they had no source of social support died in the hospital. The results applied to both men and women even after taking into account differences in the severity of the heart attack, illness due to other diseases, the presence of traditional risk factors (such as cigarette smoking and high blood pressure), and symptoms of depression.

"It appears that being married or unmarried, living with someone or living alone, are not as critical to surviving a heart attack as just having someone to turn to for emotional support," the researchers concluded. "And this support seems to work like a drug—the higher the dose, the greater the protective effect."[72]

In a paper presented by residents from Portland's Kaiser Permanente Center for Health Research at the Society of Behavioral Health Meetings, the strength of social networks was shown to predict mortality at 2-, 5-, 10-, and 15-year follow-up visits.

The Alameda County Study

In the Alameda County, California, study discussed at the beginning of this chapter, the residents were initially studied for nine years.[73] First, researchers separated people into two groups: those who lived lonely lives (without many friends or relatives) and those who had rich resources of family and friends. To determine which category a person fit into, researchers looked at marital status, a person's contact with friends and relatives, church membership, organizational affiliations, political activities, and group activities (such as membership in a garden club or bridge club or participation on a bowling league).

Then researchers wanted to make sure they were comparing the right set of statistics, so they accounted for things that might artificially shorten life. They made allowances for factors such as obesity, cigarette smoking, alcohol consumption, lack of exercise, harmful health practices, and poor health at the beginning of the study.

Researchers then painstakingly sifted through all the data, examining the records of the state health department and cross-checking death certificates. As a final check, the researchers checked each name to determine which category the individual had initially been classified in—lonely or friendly.

The results were convincing: The people who had been classified as lonely and isolated were dying at three times the rate of those who had stronger social ties.[74] To put it simply, people with many social contacts had the lowest mortality rates; those with the fewest contacts had the highest rates.

The results of that study, as well as many others, show that people with social ties—no matter what the source—live longer than isolated people. This holds true regardless of cigarette smoking, alcohol consumption, obesity, sleeping and eating habits, and medical care.[75]

As part of the follow-up to the initial Alameda County study, researchers continued to monitor health and death records for the next eight years; as a result, they had access to complete records for a 17-year period. When later analyses of the data were made, the same results held true: People with the strongest social ties had the lowest mortality rates. Those rates were lowest for the people with the best social contacts even after allowances were made for age, sex, race, health status at the beginning of the study, depression, health practices, and the way people viewed their own health.[76]

According to the researchers who analyzed the data from the study, the types of social ties seemed to vary in importance to health, depending on the person's age. At the beginning of the study, the participants ranged in age from 38 to 94 years. For those under 60, marital status seemed the best way to predict health and mortality. For those over 60, ties with close friends or relatives, or both, seemed to be more important to health and long life than did marital status.[77]

The North Carolina Study

In another study involving more than 100 communities in North Carolina, researchers looked at black men of all ages. The highest death rates—regardless of the men's age—occurred among those who were "socially disorganized." Social disorganization in the study was characterized by family instability, separation, divorce, single-parent families, and many illegitimate children.[78]

The Swedish Study

A study of Swedish men who were all 50 years old at the beginning of the study showed that good social support and strong social networks decreased mortality from all causes.[79] In the study, the men who did the worst were those who felt a lack of social and emotional support, those who were dissatisfied with their social activities, and those who lived alone.

The Japanese Studies

Some of the most fascinating evidence regarding social ties and mortality involved a group of studies of Japanese people. A number of studies showed that people in Japan—even though they smoke cigarettes, have high blood pressure, endure crushing stress, and live in polluted and crowded cities—live longer than we do. In fact, despite those normally unhealthy factors, they enjoy the longest life expectancy in the world. And, even though those same factors are characteristically considered to be factors leading to heart disease, the Japanese enjoy relative immunity from heart disease. Researchers who strived to figure out why finally decided that the Japanese are protected from ill health and death by their unusually close ties to friends, family members, and community. University of California, San Francisco, School of Medicine researcher Ken Pelletier believes that the longevity of the Japanese is due to the emphasis they place on the community. The social aspect of human companionship, Pelletier believes, is one of the most important factors in health.[80]

Dr. S. Leonard Syme of the Department of Epidemiology and Public Health at Yale University teamed up with researchers from the University of California, Berkeley, to study the situation in greater depth. Syme and his colleagues studied 12,000 Japanese men in three different groups: (1) men who still lived in southwestern Japan, (2) men who had emigrated from Japan to Hawaii and who had resisted a Westernized lifestyle, and (3) men who had emigrated from Japan to the San Francisco Bay area.[81]

To their surprise, researchers found the highest life expectancy and the lowest rate of heart disease among the group in which they least expected it: the men who had immigrated to San Francisco. The men who had immigrated to San Francisco had formed the closest social ties, the closest family ties, and the strongest social networks. Researchers found that the Japanese men in the San Francisco area stayed heavily involved with Japanese people, moved into Japanese neighborhoods, formed close friendships with other Japanese people, attended Japanese-language schools in addition to English-language schools, and returned to Japan for further schooling.

Research from a variety of studies shows, in essence, that people who are socially isolated—the unmarried, divorced, and widowed; people with few friends; and people who have few church or social contacts—are three times as likely to die of a wide variety of diseases than those who have happy, fulfilling social lives.[82]

A number of studies show that social support may even increase the longevity of people infected with HIV (human immunodeficiency virus). Long-term HIV survivors have been studied to determine what nutritional, medicinal, and other factors may contribute to the ability of the immune system to resist the onslaught of the disease for a prolonged period of time. Research has found that those with low social support are much more prone to depression, other mental health problems, and poorer physical health, while those who maintain strong social support have much better physical health. Some of the ways HIV patients are able to maintain strong social support include positive ways of dealing with family, renegotiating the friendship group, helping others with HIV infection, and developing a relationship with a higher power.[83]

Social Connections and the Heart

Researchers who studied the Japanese men (cited earlier) found that those who had immigrated to the San Francisco Bay area were the ones with the lowest incidence of heart disease. The unique and intense social ties they formed in San Francisco seemed to offer protection against heart disease. The Japanese men had significantly lower heart disease, even though they had the same high serum cholesterol levels as their Western counterparts, often ate Western foods, smoked cigarettes, and had high blood pressure.[84]

Even the most simple social support appears to affect the heart. In one ambitious study (the Enhancing Recovery in Coronary Heart Disease Patients, reported in the *Journal of the American Medical Association*), it was determined that social isolation is a "special hazard" for people with heart disease, according to Harvard University's Lisa Berkman, one of the study's lead investigators.[85] One particular study shows how simple that support can be. Researchers at the University of Pennsylvania gave a series of college women stressful tasks to do. As the students struggled to complete the stressful tasks, researchers measured their blood pressure and heart rates. The women who brought a friend along had significantly lower blood pressure and heart rates while under stress than the women who faced doing the stressful task by themselves.[86]

Exactly how social connections strengthen the circulatory system—and how loneliness harms it—are still mysteries. The most prominent theory is that social support somehow influences the regions of the brain that either calm the body or put it on high alert. The cascade of hormones that floods the body on alert can do significant damage to the circulatory system as it makes arteries less flexible, causes inflammation, and increases blood pressure, factors that contribute to heart disease.[87]

Some examples: A study in Chicago showed that blood pressure averaged 30 points higher among people who lacked good social connections. Heart attack survivors who said they were lonely were four times more likely to die during the three years following their heart attacks than were people with abundant social connections. Swedish men who underwent bypass surgery were twice as likely to die within five years if they felt lonely at the time of the surgery. Similarly, older people hospitalized for heart failure were three times as likely to have a heart attack or die within the year if they expressed a lack of social support; interestingly, the impact was greater on women than on men.[88]

Another theory is that social support somehow mitigates inflammation, a factor in heart disease as well as a number of other diseases. Eric B. Loucks of the Harvard School of Public Health studied more than 3,000 participants in the Framingham Heart Study; their average age was 62. He and his team measured blood concentrations of four inflammatory markers, including interleukin-6 (IL-6). Study participants were also asked about their social support—their marital status, the number of relatives in whom they could confide private matters, the number of close friends in whom they could confide private matters, their involvement in religious meetings or services, and their participation in groups (such as senior centers). There was a "statistically significant difference" between the men who had strong social support and those who did not: the ones with little social support had the highest levels of IL-6 and other inflammatory markers.[89]

Still another theory is that people with strong social support are less likely to engage in heart-harming behaviors. For example, people who have strong social support are less likely to smoke, one of the key risk factors for heart disease, says University of Minnesota researcher Chris J. Armstrong. And married men with strong social support are also more likely to engage in regular physical exercise, an accepted way to reduce the risk of heart disease.[90]

Whatever the link, it has probably always been there—it was just a matter of looking for it, says Dr. Tim Gardner, professor of surgery at the Hospital of the University of Pennsylvania. "We haven't looked at the impact of behavior on health as much as we should," he says. "Especially within the scientific community, the emphasis has been on new drugs." [91]

The Roseto Study

A landmark study in the 1960s in Roseto, Pennsylvania, confirms other research and theories that social support and social ties protect the heart. Roseto is a close-knit Italian American community nestled among other traditional eastern communities. Researchers interested in the lifestyle of the community residents followed their health status and rates of death for years. They found that the residents of Roseto had average incidences of exercise, cigarette smoking, obesity, high blood pressure, and stress. In addition, their diets were higher in fat, cholesterol, and red meat than is the average American diet. Despite all this, the men in Roseto had only about one-sixth the incidence of heart disease and deaths from heart disease as random population groups in the United States. The rates for Roseto's women were even better.

Researchers concluded that the protective factor was the people's strong sense of community and their strong social ties. Stewart Wolf, a professor of medicine at Temple University School of Medicine in Philadelphia and one of the study's researchers, said:

> More than any other town we studied, Roseto's social structure reflected old-world values and traditions. There was a remarkable cohesiveness and sense of unconditional support within the community. Family ties were very strong. And what impressed us most was the attitude toward the elderly. In Roseto, the older residents weren't put on a shelf; they were promoted to "supreme court." No one was ever abandoned.[92]

Researchers continued to watch the residents of Roseto. They found that, when the younger generations began changing (moving away, marrying "outsiders," severing the close emotional ties to the "old neighborhood"), the physical health of the Rosetans began to deteriorate. By the mid-1970s, the mortality and heart disease rates of the Rosetans were comparable to that in surrounding Pennsylvania communities.

Community members had tremendously strong social ties, and their hearts were protected. When the social ties started to vanish, so did the protection. "The experience clearly demonstrates that the most important factors in health are the intangibles—things like trust, honesty, loyalty, team spirit," Wolf concluded. "In terms of preventing heart disease, it's just possible that morale is more important than jogging or not eating butter."[93]

Indeed, studies have shown that human interaction itself has a biological value: Human interaction causes changes in blood pressure, heart rate, and blood chemistry. Those changes promote good health for the heart.

The British Study[94]

Dr. Roberto De Vogli and his colleagues at University College London studied more than 9,000 British civil servants who completed a questionnaire about their four closest social relationships. They were asked specifically how much practical and emotional support they received from the people closest to them. Researchers then followed participants for 12 years to determine whether any had nonfatal heart events. Those who had a high level of negativity in their close personal relationships, signaling a lack of social support, were 1.34 times more likely to suffer a coronary event.

Authors of the study point out that negative social relationships, especially in marriage, are associated with depression, "often in combination with reduced self-esteem and/or higher levels of anger. These emotional reactions have been found to influence coronary heart disease through the cumulative 'wear and tear' on organs and tissues caused by the alterations of autonomic [involuntary] functions, neuroendocrine changes, disturbances in coagulation [clotting of the blood], and inflammatory and immune responses."

Type A Studies

A number of studies show that social support may actually help reduce or modify risk factors. One well-known risk factor for heart disease is the type A personality—a person who is time-oriented, hard-driving, stressed, and competitive. While there is not yet any scientific evidence, researchers have suggested a general hypothesis that type A personality might actually be caused by low social support.[95] If such is the case, then social support could carry double significance: boosting social support might not only help prevent type A personality traits but could help protect against heart disease in other ways.

In an attempt to find out what factors might help modify the risk to people with type A personality, researchers at Duke Medical Center interviewed 113 patients (most of them men) who had come to the hospital for coronary angiography (X-rays of the heart that reveal how much blockage exists in coronary arteries).[96]

All the men in the study were given psychological tests to determine if they were type A personality or type B personality (a much more easy-going, relaxed type of personality, much less prone to coronary heart disease). The patients were also given a questionnaire to help determine whether they had strong or weak social support. Finally, patients had a coronary angiography.

When researchers analyzed data from all of the tests and questionnaires, they found that the type A personalities who had strong social support were on a par with the type B personalities in terms of coronary disease. The type A personalities who were isolated or had weak social support had the most severe coronary artery disease. The study indicates "that social support moderates the long-term health consequences of the type A behavior pattern."[97]

Other Studies

Even with established heart disease, social support can be a healing and protective factor. The National Heart and Lung Institute did a five-year study of angina pectoris among men at the Sackler School of Medicine at Tel Aviv University. Even when coronary risk factors were present, the men who had loving wives and strong social relationships did significantly better than those who did not have good social relationships.[98]

In another study, researchers at Yale studied men with coronary heart disease; they looked at how much social support the men in the study enjoyed and focused their interest on men who had survived myocardial infarction. Their findings add dramatically to the evidence that strong social support can help prevent heart disease. They found that good social support actually reversed the effects of stress and distress on cardiac symptoms. Social support acted not only as a powerful preventive but also as a healer. The effects of social support were greatest in the first six months following myocardial infarction.[99]

A series of studies that spanned more than a decade demonstrates that social support is an important factor to recovery following heart attack. The first study showed that socially isolated men had a greater risk of death during the recovery period following myocardial infarction. The second study showed that those who were unmarried and did not have a confidant had substantially worse survival rates in the five years following a heart attack. The third study showed that people who lived alone were significantly more likely to have follow-up coronary events—both fatal and nonfatal—during the four years after the initial heart attack.[100]

The Best Health Bet—Good Social Ties

One reason social support promotes good health is that it appears to improve immune function.[101] In the same way, a lack of strong social support—as a result of a small or weak social network, loneliness, bereavement, stressful social relationships, marital strain, or divorce, for example—appears to adversely affect immunity and can result in health problems.[102] According to researchers, "We are not yet at a point where we can claim that immune changes account for a proportion of the [disease and death] risk associated with social integration, social support, and relationship discord. However, it should be clear that psychological and behavioral interventions targeted at close relationships should be included in the arsenal of methods we consider as we strive to improve physical as well as psychological well-being."[103]

A review of a number of studies shows that interpersonal relationships reverse the adverse effects of both short- and long-term stress. Well-documented studies show that stress generally decreases the number and function of natural killer cells and lowers the percentage of T cells. Strong interpersonal relationships, however, protect the functioning of the immune system—even in the face of stress.[104]

In several studies of college students, researchers measured the secretion rate of immunoglobulin A (s-IgA) into the students' saliva; s-IgA is an important immune defense against upper respiratory infections caused by both viruses and bacteria. In one part of the study, researchers found that students under stress secreted significantly less s-IgA than did students not under stress. Students under stress were not as able to resist or fight infection. However, researchers also found that students who had good social ties and valued warm personal relationships secreted more s-IgA at all points than did the other students in the study. The students who were socially connected were always in a better position to fight infection, regardless of whether they were under stress.[105]

Still other research shows that strong social support might help protect against the common cold. "We know that people with good and diverse social relations live longer," wrote Carnegie Mellon University psychologist Sheldon Cohen, whose team of researchers set out to determine if that same support might help protect against common infections, such as the cold. His researchers studied 276 healthy volunteers between the ages of 18 and 55 who were not pregnant and did not have HIV infection. Each person in the study was given nasal drops that contained one of two rhinoviruses, and then they were monitored to see which ones developed colds.[106]

The team counted the number of "social roles" each person in the study filled; these roles were things such as parent, child, employee, or church member. The more roles the person had—hence, the broader the network of social support—the greater the ability to resist the common cold. When exposed to the cold virus, 62 percent of those with three or fewer roles got a cold; 43 percent of those with four or five roles got sick; and only 35 percent of those with six or more social roles got the sniffles.[107] Those with more social roles also produced less mucus, shed fewer virus particles, and had more effective ciliary clearance of the nasal passages if they did get a cold.[108] The positive effects of social support (and the negative effects of stress) held up even after typical risk factors for respiratory infection (such as cigarette smoking) were removed.

Cohen wishes he knew *why* social support has the effect it does, but he figures it must change something measurable in the body, such as in the brain, the immune system, or the hormonal system. While we know that "stress and social conflict are associated with greater susceptibility to colds, we haven't learned anything about the psychological or biological pathways that mediate [cause] this effect." Cohen also concedes that his study relied on measurements in the mucus and blood, but he points out that "the action" is in such internal organs as the thymus and the spleen. Once scientists find out exactly what's happening there, he says, "there are a myriad of possibilities."[109]

Ohio State University psychologist Janice Kiecolt-Glaser tested groups of people with psychological profiles designed to determine how lonely they were. Those who were lonelier—those with the lowest levels of social support—also suffered in other ways: Their immune systems did not function as well as their counterparts who had good social support. The lonelier people in the studies had significantly lower levels of natural killer cells, an important part of the immune system that helps control viruses and cancerous tumor formation. Kiecolt-Glaser reported that the lonelier people in her study were less capable of fighting cancer because of immune system weakness.[110]

Increasing social support and reducing loneliness seem to help strengthen the immune system significantly. In a study of 30 elderly patients in retirement homes, researchers took blood tests at the beginning of the study and continued to measure immune system components throughout the test. Volunteers visited the patients in the retirement home three times a week for one month. There was a significant increase in both antibodies and natural killer cell activity, proving that there had been a real boost in the immune system.[111]

Possibly because of the immune system boost, social support seems to have significant impact on a number of disease conditions. Take cancer, for example. Some studies show no correlation between isolation and cancer, but others show a link between social isolation or disruption and cancer.

Lawrence LeShan studied the personalities and emotional life histories of more than 300 cancer patients. When he compared the life histories and emotional circumstances of cancer patients with those of healthy patients, he noticed a pattern in more than 60 percent of the cancer victims—but in only 10 percent of the healthy people: Early in life, these patients learned to perceive relationships as dangerous, to be invested in only at the risk of much pain and rejection. To protect themselves, they kept relationships with others on a superficial basis. They held back emotionally and felt isolated and different from others, though they appeared to be functioning well.[112]

Usually in adolescence or early adulthood, "A relationship came along that seemed relatively safe. Slowly this new relationship became the central focus of life. Then, for one reason or another, the loved one was lost. A spouse died, children grew up and moved away, or a divorce occurred. Cancer developed following the loss."[113]

Social support may even help determine the outcome of cancer. One study that supports that theory was conducted at the Stanford University Medical School and was reported to professionals gathered for annual meetings of the American Psychiatric Association; similar studies in Michigan, Georgia, Sweden, and Finland have produced comparable results.

For the Stanford study, professor of psychiatry David Spiegel followed 86 breast cancer patients for 10 years.[114] During the first year, the women were randomly divided into two groups. The first group of 36 received traditional medical treatment. The second group of 50 received weekly 90-minute group therapy sessions in addition to traditional medical treatment. At the end of 10 years, those who had received therapy lived for approximately 37 months following diagnosis, whereas those who did not receive therapy lived an average of only 19 months.

Spiegel originally designed the research to refute the notion that the mind plays a role in the course of disease. What he did find was the powerful effect of social support. Taking care to describe his findings, Spiegel commented that "we did not find that any psychological variables—like mood—were associated with survival time. It was only participation in the groups that seemed to make a difference."[115]

Describing himself as "stunned" at the study results, Spiegel said the magnitude of the effects on the body was "much greater than anything I expected."[116] William Breitbart, assistant professor of psychiatry at Memorial Sloan-Kettering Cancer Center, says the important factor is "an intervention addressing two factors: social support and feelings of hopelessness and isolation."[117]

Several other research groups have had similar findings. A study conducted by Jean Richardson of the University of South California found that lymphoma patients who participated in counseling and home visits outlived that ones who didn't.[118]

Spiegel says that social support may influence health because of the "grandmother effect": People who feel that others care about them are more likely to eat well, sleep well, exercise, and avoid harmful habits, thus maximizing the body's ability to cope with illness. It's also possible, he says, that people who interact well with family and friends also have better relationships with their healthcare providers.[119]

In commenting on the study, Spiegel expressed concern that some cancer patients might be made to feel "responsible" for their illnesses or be labeled a "failure" because they did not defeat the disease. The effect of the social support, he maintains, "comes not by denying the illness or wishing it away, but by more successfully managing one's life in terms of family relationships, relationships with physicians, and one's own feelings about having a terminal illness, and dealing with these factors as directly as possible."[120]

In fact, Spiegel says, it's important to face the issues head-on. "It doesn't demoralize patients to talk about these things," he says. "The less hidden the problem, the better. Isolation is a symbol of death. The more isolated patients feel, the more helpless and already dead they feel. This is a time to strengthen social networks, not let them wither."[121]

"We're trained to treat crying as bleeding," Spiegel says of treatment teams, "to apply direct pressure to stop it. But if a strong emotional response is appropriate," it should be allowed, he says. Otherwise, people facing life-threatening events are made to feel that their very normal reactions are not, in fact, normal at all, and that such reactions are not acceptable. His mantra might be well-taken by all who are providing social support: "If you see somebody crying, don't just do something—stand there."[122]

In a similar study headed by UCLA psychiatrist Fawzy I. Fawzy, researchers provided a 90-minute weekly group therapy session for one group of malignant melanoma patients; the other group received no therapy.[123] The therapy sessions, which continued for six weeks, focused on education about melanoma, stress management, coping and problem-solving skills, and psychological support.

Six years after their initial diagnosis and treatment, the people in the support group had a 60 percent reduction in death rate as compared with the other patients—and approximately half as many recurrences of the melanoma.[124]

Similar findings emerged from separate studies involving people with breast, lung, and colorectal cancer. Researchers in each of the studies found that social support and a sense of control were important to coping with serious illness.[125]

An interesting study shows that social support may impact patients differently, depending on the cancer site and the extent of the disease. In the 17-year study, socially isolated women were shown to have a significantly higher risk of dying of cancer of all sites and of smoking-related cancers. Cancer incidence was not associated with social connections among men, but men with few social connections had significantly poorer survival rates from cancer.[126]

Social support has been found to impact recovery from stroke. In a longitudinal study conducted in New Haven, Connecticut, those who were isolated or who did not have good social support before experiencing the stroke had significantly poorer function six months after having the stroke. They also suffered greater impairments in daily living activities and were more likely to be placed in a nursing home. Other studies have found that good social support following a stroke makes a substantial difference in recovery.[127]

Research results indicate that social support may also have a positive effect on diabetes. One study involved 263 black diabetes patients between the ages of 16 and 89 at two outpatient clinics in Pretoria, South Africa; the majority were women, and most had type 2 diabetes. Researchers looked at not only the tangible aspects of social support, such as the provision of assistance, but also considered the existence of close, caring relationships. Those with the strongest relationships and the best social support were also the ones who had the best control of their diabetes (measured by metabolic control and blood pressure, which is one aspect of diabetes management).[128]

Social support can even affect the unborn. To test what kind of impact social support had on newborns, researchers studied single adolescent Navajo mothers at the University of Arizona. Questionnaires and detailed interviews enabled researchers to categorize the mothers-to-be into three different groups—those who had low social support, medium social support, and high social support. Researchers then followed the women through their pregnancies and deliveries.[129]

The teenagers who had only medium or low social support delivered babies who were significantly more prone to complications. The mothers with medium or low social support also had four times the rate of neonatal complications when compared with the mothers with high levels of social support![130]

Controlled tests by researchers at Baylor College of Medicine showed that the presence of a female companion who provided continuous emotional support throughout labor and delivery was a significant benefit. When such a woman was present, Caesarean section rates dropped from 18 percent to 8 percent. The need for epidural anesthesia dropped from 55 percent to 8 percent, and the average labor was shortened by about two hours. Finally, the need for prolonged hospitalization of the babies after birth was significantly decreased.[131]

The amount of social support given to a mother can even influence the way she bonds to her infant. In one study, researchers evaluated how much social support mothers had from family members and friends; they then rated how well the mothers and infants had become attached to each other. Among the women with good social support, only 10 percent had problems bonding with their infants. Among the women with poor social support, however, more than half—55 percent—had inadequate or insecure bonding with their infants.[132]

Convinced of the need for good social support? If you need to strengthen your own social connectedness, try the following suggestions:

- Start by making your needs known; let others know that you're interested in strengthening your friendships and your circle of support.

- If you've got a pet (sometimes a great source of support in itself!), seek others who share your love of pets. You might look for a dog park, for example—and strike up conversations with others who are there.

- Look for groups to join. Many corporations offer groups for people who share the same interests (such as stress management); also, you can often find groups through your community or church. Find a group that you feel comfortable in and that deals with a subject you're interested in learning more about.

- Consider enrolling in special courses (such as how to create furniture from willows or how to administer cardiopulmonary resuscitation) or adult education classes offered through your local school district. These classes are usually widely varied in subject—almost everyone can find something of real interest. Or consider going back to school after you finish your degree; take the classes that really interest you but that may not have applied to your major course of study.

- Join a gym, community fitness facility, or other exercise group—or even start a walking club at your dormitory, in your neighborhood, or at work. Exercise itself is great for alleviating stress, and you'll also benefit from a new group of friends who share your interests.

- Find a cause you're committed to, and volunteer; you might consider a political election, a cleanup campaign, or a religious activity. Most universities and communities have many volunteer positions available, and they are often listed in local newspapers or on the community or county website. You'll find more information about all aspects of volunteer work in Chapter 15.

- Plan now for what you'll be doing a year from now, ten years from now, and during your retirement years. Too often, people restrict their social connections to the workplace; once they retire, they become isolated and lonely. Make active decisions now to help you stay involved.

Remember, too, that social support involves both give and take: sometimes you're on the receiving end, but many times you're on the giving end, too. It's important to nurture friendships and other sources of support—and to let others know that you will be there for them when they need a little help.

If you feel you need to expand your circle of friends, remember: it's never too late. You can generally improve family relationships and develop friendships by considering the following:[133]

- Find out how others perceive you. Ask a trusted friend or family member for honest feedback about how you come across to others. If you find out there is room for improvement, work on those areas that might make you seem unapproachable.

- Work on a healthy self-image. Both extremes—arrogance or vanity and constant self-criticism—will make you unattractive to most potential friends.

- Avoid the tendency to complain. Constant complaining is a drain for everybody, including you. Adopt a positive outlook, and remember to foster your sense of humor.

- Listen to others. Having compassion and understanding can only happen if you genuinely listen to the other person.

- Leave your competitive nature behind. Some of the people you have always considered to be rivals might actually turn out to be the best friends.

- Don't overwhelm people. As you start to build a friendship, keep your contacts genuine but brief. Respect boundaries, and keep the relationship on a positive level for both of you.

Touch: A Crucial Aspect of Social Support

As important as social support is to health, perhaps one of its most powerful components is also one of its simplest: People who touch others and are touched themselves seem to enjoy the best health!

Observations made by researchers nearly four decades ago as they watched groups of monkeys provided us with some of the best information we have on the power of touch. University of Wisconsin researchers Harry and Margaret Harlow compared monkeys who were raised together in cages with monkeys whose only social contact came through seeing, hearing, and smelling other monkeys.[134]

The Harlows found that the monkeys who did not have touch, or actual body contact with other monkeys, grew up with a variety of emotional abnormalities. While young, the monkeys seemed especially prone to self-mutilation; as they grew older, their self-aggression turned into aggression against other monkeys. Perhaps most striking was the example of how mothers behaved toward their young: The mothers who grew up without touch showed less warmth and affection toward their offspring. Some even killed their own babies.

The same thing happens with humans. One simple experiment demonstrated the impact of touch on babies who were having blood drawn. Some were held skin-to-skin by their mothers; the others were swaddled in a blanket. Those who were being hugged had lower heart rates and cried 82 percent less than those who were left in their blankets lying in a crib.[135]

Countless studies have borne out the deleterious effects on people who are deprived of touch. One landmark study of victims of child abuse spanned three generations of families in which child abuse had occurred. The most powerful predictor of child abuse was not necessarily whether the abuser had himself been abused—but, instead, whether the abuser had been deprived of touch and its associated pleasure.[136]

The skin is the earliest sensory organ to develop. Many researchers argue that it is also the most important.[137] According to one health reference,[138] a piece of skin the size of a quarter contains more than 3 million cells, 12 feet of nerves, 100 sweat glands, 50 nerve endings, and 3 feet of blood vessels. Overall, the skin has about 50 receptors per 100 cm^2, or a total of 900,000 sensory receptors. "Viewed from this perspective," reports the book, "the skin is a giant communication system that, through the sense of touch, brings messages from the external environment to the attention of [the body and the mind]."[139]

Some researchers have shown that touch is stronger than either verbal or emotional contact—and that touch affects nearly everything we do.[140] Cornell University researcher Diane Ackerman points out that "massage therapy"—the act of reaching through the holes in isolettes to stroke and massage premature babies—literally saves their lives. Ackerman cites a previously published article in *Science News* confirming that preemies who are touched are "better able to calm and console themselves." Eight months after being released from the hospital, the preemies who benefited from massage therapy, says Ackerman, are healthier, have better weight gain, and have fewer physical problems than the infants who were not touched regularly.[141]

Although the research linking touch to emotional behavior occurred nearly four decades ago, the first research linking touch to physical health happened—by accident—nearly seventy years ago. Anatomist Frederick Hammett did an experiment in which he removed rats' thyroid and parathyroid glands, and he was astonished when some of the rats survived. Careful research led him to the discovery that the rats who survived the surgery came from colonies where they had been regularly "petted and gentled" by their keepers. They were six times more likely to survive the operation than were rats that had not been touched regularly—and were also much less timid, apprehensive, and highstrung.[142]

According to researchers, touch has both physical and emotional benefits. For example, studies show that touch subdues heart irregularities; people who have a certain type of irregular heartbeat have a more normal heartbeat in the minute after they are touched as their pulse is being taken. Touch also can relieve depression; in one study, daily massage improved depression and anxiety scores in children and adolescents who were hospitalized for depression.[143]

A fascinating look at stroke survivors compared those who worked with a physical therapist to those who underwent physical therapy with a robotic device. A team of researchers at the Rehabilitation Institute of Chicago evaluated stroke survivors who had been partially paralyzed on one side of the body for more than six months; each participated in a dozen 30-minute therapy sessions on a treadmill while wearing a harness to support their body weight. Those who worked with the physical therapists—in other words, those who were touched by another human being instead of by a robot—had twice the improvement in walking speed and had significant improvement in the ability to stand on one leg (a measure of progress in stroke victims).[144]

What does all of this mean? People who enjoy regular, satisfying touch—a pat on the back, a hug—enjoy health benefits as a result. Their hearts are stronger, their blood pressure is lower, their stress levels are decreased, and their overall tension is reduced. So try these simple ways to add more touch to your life: acknowledge your children with a hug, kiss, or gentle squeeze of the arm; shake hands when greeting someone; hold a friend's hand while you talk; have a massage; get a manicure; have someone else wash your hair; or volunteer to rock babies at a local hospital.[145] Having good relationships with other people seems to help us resist infection. It seems to protect us against disease. It helps protect us against stress, and it makes us healthier physically and mentally. It can even help us live longer.

Truly, no man is an island. Only by surrounding ourselves and becoming involved with others can we live the longest, healthiest, happiest life possible.

WHAT DID YOU LEARN?

1. Just what does the phrase *social support* mean?
2. What did you learn from the Alameda County, California, study on social support?
3. What are the strongest associations between social support and health?
4. What are your own major sources of social support?
5. What do we know about social connections and heart health?
6. What did the Roseto Study teach us about social support?

ENDNOTES

1. Jennifer E. Graham, Lisa M. Christian, and Janice K. Kiecolt-Glaser, "Close Relationships and Immunity," pp. 781–93 in Robert Ader, ed., *Psychoneuroimmunology*, 4th ed., vol. 2 (New York: Elsevier, Inc., 2007).
2. Sheldon Cohen, "Social Relationships and Susceptibility to the Common Cold," in Carol D. Ryff and Burton H. Singer, eds., *Emotion, Social Relationships, and Health* (New York: Oxford University Press, 2001).
3. Ibid.
4. Marc Pilisuk and Susan Hillier Parks, *The Healing Web* (Hanover, NH: University Press of New England, 1986).
5. Thomas R. Blakeslee, "Social Ties and Good Health," http://www.attitudefactor.com, revised 2008.
6. Harry T. Reis, "Relationship Experiences and Emotional Wellbeing," in Carol D. Ryff and Burton H. Singer, eds., *Emotion, Social Relationships and Health* (New York: Oxford University Press, 1998), 23.
7. Allan Luks and Peggy Payne, *The Healing Power of Doing Good* (New York: Fawcett Columbine, 1992).
8. Kenneth Pelletier, *Sound Mind, Sound Body: A New Model for Lifelong Health* (New York: Simon & Schuster, 1994), 137–8.
9. J. F. Helliwell and R. D. Putnam, "The Social Context of Well-Being," *Philosophical Transactions of the Royal Society of London. Series B: Biological Sciences* 359, no. 1149 (September 2004): 1435–6.
10. Teresa Seeman, "Social Support and Social Conflict," *John D. and Catherine T. MacArthur Research Network on Socioeconomic Status and Health,* http://www.mases.ucsf.edu/Research/Psychosocial/notebook/socsupp.html, accessed May 2008.
11. I. Kawachi and L. F. Berkman, "Social Ties and Mental Health," *Journal of Urban Health* 78, no. 3 (September 2001): 458–67.
12. Sheldon Cohen, "Psychosocial Models of the Role of Social Support in the Etiology of Physical Disease," *Health Psychology* 7, no. 3 (1988): 269–97.
13. "Up Close and Personal," *British Medical Journal* 321, no. 7253 (July 8, 2000): 92.
14. Pilisuk and Parks, *The Healing Web.*
15. MayoClinic.com, "Developing Social Support: How to Cultivate a Network of Friends to Help You Through Rough Times," http://www.cnn.com/HEALTH/library/MH/00041.html, accessed May 2008.

16. Terrence L. Amick and Judith K. Ockene, "The Role of Social Support in the Modification of Risk Factors for Cardiovascular Disease," pp. 260–61 in Sally A. Shumaker and Susan M. Czajkowski, eds., *Social Support and Cardiovascular Disease* (New York: Plenum Press, 1994).

17. Deborah Preston and Jorge Grimes, "A Study of Differences in Social Support," *Journal of Gerontological Nursing* 13, no. 2 (2003): 36–40.

18. Corey M. Clark, "Relations Between Social Support and Physical Health," from http://www.personalityresearch.org/papers/clark.html, updated November 2005.

19. Carol D. Ryff and Burton H. Singer, "Introduction: Integrating Emotion into the Study of Social Relationships and Health," in Ryff and Singer, *Emotion, Social Relationships, and Health.*

20. Reis, "Relationship Experiences."

21. Cohen, "Social Support and Physical Illness."

22. C.L. Keyes et al., "Social Support and Health-Related Quality of Life among Older Adults—Missouri, 2000," *Morbidity and Mortality Weekly Report [MMWR] Weekly* 54, no. 17 (May 6, 2005): 433–437.

23. Preston and Grimes, "A Study of Differences."

24. Editors of *Prevention* magazine and the Center for Positive Living, *Positive Living and Health: The Complete Guide to Brain/Body Healing and Mental Empowerment* (Emmaus, PA: Rodale Press, 1990), 165.

25. Preston and Grimes, "A Study of Differences."

26. C. E. Depner and B. Ingersoll-Dayton, "Supportive Relationships in Later Life," *Psychology and Aging* 3, no. 4 (December 1988): 348–57.

27. W. L. Coventry, N. A. Gillespie, A. C. Heath, and N. G. Martin, "Perceived Social Support in a Large Community Sample," *Social Psychiatry and Psychiatric Epidemiology* 39 (2004): 625–6.

28. Anne F. Young, Anne Russell, and Jennifer R. Powers, "The Sense of Belonging to a Neighbourhood: Can It Be Measured and Is It Related to Health and Well Being in Older Women?" *Social Sciences and Medicine* 59, no. 12 (December 2004): 2627–37.

29. Lori J. Curtis, Martin D. Dooley, and Shelley A. Phipps, "Child Well-Being and Neighbourhood Quality: Evidence from the Canadian National Longitudinal Survey of Children and Youth," *Social Sciences and Medicine* 58, no. 10 (May 2004): 1917–27.

30. L.C. Gallo et al., "Socioeconomic Status, Resources, Psychological Experiences, and Emotional Responses: A Test of the Reserve Capacity Model," *Journal of Personality and Social Psychology* 88 (2005): 386–99.

31. Elaine D. Eaker, "Social Support and Physical Health: Understanding the Health Consequences of Relationships" (book review), *American Journal of Epidemiology* 161, no. 3 (2005): 297–8.

32. Bert N. Uchino, *Social Support and Physical Health: Understanding the Health Consequences of Relationships* (New Haven, CT: Yale University Press, 2004).

33. George.A. Kaplan et al., "Social Connections and Mortality from All Causes and from Cardiovascular Disease: Prospective Evidence from Eastern Finland," *American Journal of Epidemiology* 128, no. 2 (August 1988): 370–80.

34. Peggy A. Thoits, "Stress, Coping, and Social Support Processes: Where Are We? What Next?" *Journal of Health and Social Behavior* 35 (1995), 53–79.

35. Maurice B. Mittelmark, "Social Ties and Health Promotion: Suggestions for Population-Based Research," *Health Education Research* 14, no. 4 (August 1999): 447–51.

36. Sheldon Cohen and S. Leonard Syme, eds., *Social Support and Health* (London: Academic Press, 1985).

37. Joan Borysenko, *Fire in the Soul* (New York: Warner Books, 1993), 83.
38. Meredith Minkler, "The Social Component of Health," *American Journal of Health Promotion* (Fall 1986): 33–8.
39. "Social Isolation Pessimism: Link to Poor Health," *Medical Abstracts Newsletter* (October 1988): 5.
40. Judith H. Hibbard, "Social Ties and Health Status: An Examination of Moderating Factors," *Health Education and Behavior* 12, no. 1 (1985): 23–4.
41. Tom Ferguson, "The Invisible Health Care System," from http://www.healthy.net/scr/Article.asp?Id=1016, January–February 1988.
42. Reis, "Relationship Experiences."
43. James W. Pennebaker, *Opening Up: The Healing Power of Confiding in Others* (New York: William Morrow and Company, 1990), 67.
44. Ryff and Singer, "Introduction."
45. Pennebaker, *Opening Up,* 68.
46. Ibid., 69.
47. Martha E. Francis and James W. Pennebaker, "Putting Stress into Words: The Impact of Writing on Physiological, Absentee, and Self-Reported Emotional Well-Being Measures," *American Journal of Health Promotion* 6, no. 4 (March/April 1992): 280–7.
48. Ibid.
49. Pennebaker, *Opening Up,* 71.
50. Ibid., 71.
51. "Writing as a Means of Healing," *HealthFacts* 16, no. 145 (1991): 1.
52. Henry Dreher, "The Healing Power of Confession," *Natural Health* (July–August 1992): 80.
53. Leonard A. Sagan, *The Health of Nations* (New York: Basic Books, 1987).
54. N. E. Mahon, A. Yarcheski, and T. J. Yarcheski, "Social Support and Positive Health Practices in Early Adolescents: A Test of Mediating Variables," *Clinical Nursing Research* 13, no. 3 (August 2004): 216–36.
55. Hafen and Frandsen, *People Who Need People* (Cordillera Press, 1987), 136.
56. Ryff and Singer, "Introduction."
57. James Lynch, *The Broken Heart* (New York: Basic Books), 86.
58. Ibid., 87.
59. MayoClinic.com., "Developing Social Support: How to Cultivate a Network of Friends to Help You Through Rough Times," http://www.cnn.com/HEALTH/library/MH/00041.html, accessed May 2008.
60. Ibid.
61. Emrika Padus, *Positive Living and Health: The Complete Guide to Brain/Body Healing and Mental Empowerment* (Emmaus, PA: Rodale Press, 1990).
62. Minkler, "The Social Component of Health," 33–38.
63. Ibid., 33, 38.
64. T. V. Horton and J. L. Wallander, "Hope and Social Support as Resilience Factors of Psychological Distress of Mothers Who Care for Children with Chronic Physical Conditions," *Rehabilitation Psychology* 46 (2001): 382–99.
65. Animal studies from Pilisuk and Parks, *The Healing Web.*
66. Pilisuk and Parks, *The Healing Web.*
67. Ibid.
68. Peter Steinglass, Eli Weisstub, and Atara Kaplan De-Nour, "Perceived Personal Networks as Mediators of Stress Reactions," *American Journal of Psychiatry* 145, no. 10 (October 1988): 1259–63.
69. Hafen and Frandsen, *People Who Need People* (Cordillera, 1987), 137.

70. Larry Dossey, *Healing Words* (San Francisco: Harper San Francisco, 1993), 109.

71. Cohen, "Social Support and Physical Illness."

72. "Surviving a Heart Attack: Emotional Support Is Key," *Mental Medicine Update* (Spring 1993): 2.

73. S. Leonard Syme, "Coronary Artery Disease: A Sociocultural Perspective," *Circulation* 76, suppl. I (1987): 1–112; and Steven Locke and Douglas Colligan, *The Healer Within* (New York: E. P. Dutton, 1986), 89.

74. Ibid.

75. Cohen, "Social Support and Physical Illness."

76. Teresa Seeman et al., "Social Network Ties and Mortality among the Elderly in the Alameda County Study," *American Journal of Epidemiology* 126, no. 4 (1987): 714–23.

77. Ibid.

78. Robert Ornstein and David Sobel, *The Healing Brain* (New York: Simon & Schuster, 1987), 121.

79. Teresa Seeman, "How Do Others Get Under Our Skin? Social Relationships and Health," pp. 1988, 26 in Ryff and Singer, *Emotion, Social Relationships, and Health.*

80. Editors of *Prevention* magazine and the Center for Positive Living, *Positive Living and Health,* 163.

81. Hafen and Frandsen, *People Who Need People* (Cordillera, 1987), 138.

82. Meade, "How to Enrich Your Relationships," 86–89.

83. Julie Barroso, "Social Support and Long-Term Survivors of AIDS," *Western Journal of Nursing Research* 19, no. 5 (October 1997): 554–82.

84. Hafen and Frandsen, *People Who Need People* (Cordillera, 1987), 138.

85. "Enriching Mental Health Good for the Heart," *Harvard Health Letter* 14, no. 1 (September 1, 2003).

86. Thomas W. Kamarck, Stephen B. Manuck, and J. Richard Jennings, "Social Support Reduces Cardiovascular Reactivity to Psychological Challenge: A Laboratory Model," *Psychosomatic Medicine* 52 (1990): 42–58.

87. Harvard Medical School, "Making Connections Good for the Heart," *Harvard Health Publications* (December 19, 2006).

88. Ibid.

89. "Social Connections: Could Heartwarming Be Heart-saving?" *Science Daily* (May 2, 2005); also American Heart Association (May 2, 2005), "Social Connections: Could Heartwarming Be Heart-saving?" *ScienceDaily.* Retrieved October 15, 2008, from http://www.sciencedaily.com/releases/2005/05/050502144309.htm.

90. Charlene Laino, "Social Ties Guard Against Heart Disease," *WebMD,* November 8, 2004. Accessed May 2008 from http://www.webmd.com/balance/news/20041108/social-ties-guard-against-heart-disease

91. Ibid.

92. Hafen and Frandsen, *People Who Need People* (Cordillera, 1987), 140.

93. Ibid., 141.

94. Adapted from "Chronic Arguing With Your Spouse May Raise Your Heart Disease Risk," *Archives of Internal Medicine* 167, no. 18 (2007): 1951–7.

95. Clark, "Relations Between Social Support and Physical Health," 95; "Friendship: Heart Saver for Type A's," *Men's Health* (November 1987): 4.

96. "Friendship: Heart Saver for Type A's," 4.

97. Ibid.

98. Hafen and Frandsen, *People Who Need People* (Cordillera, 1987), 143.

99. Alan F. Fontana, Robert D. Kerns, Roberta L. Rosenberg, and Kathleen L. Colonese, "Support, Stress, and Recovery from CHD: A Longitudinal Causal Model," *Health Psychology* 8, no. 2 (1996): 175–93.

100. Seeman, "How Do Others Get Under Our Skin?"

101. Graham, Christian, and Kiecolt-Glaser, "Close Relationships and Immunity," 781.

102. Ibid., 792.

103. Ibid., 793.

104. S. Kennedy, J. Kiecolt-Glaser, and R. Glaser, "Immunological Consequences of Acute and Chronic Stressors: Mediating Role of Interpersonal Relationships," *British Journal of Medical Psychology* 61 (1988): 77–85.

105. Cohen, "Social Relationships and Susceptibility."

106. S. Cohen et al., "Social Ties and Susceptibility to the Common Cold," *Journal of the American Medical Association* 277, no. 24 (June 24, 1997): 1940.

107. Sheldon Cohen, "Psychological Stress and Susceptibility to Upper Respiratory Infections," *American Journal of Respiratory and Critical Care Medicine* 152 (1995): S53–8.

108. S. Cohen et al., "Social Ties and Susceptibility to the Common Cold."

109. Ibid.

110. Editors of *Prevention* magazine and the Center for Positive Living, *Positive Living and Health.*

111. Blair Justice, *Who Gets Sick* (Houston, TX: Peak Press, 1987), 134.

112. Barbara Powell, *Good Relationships Are Good Medicine* (Emmaus, PA: Rodale Press), 1987.

113. Ibid.

114. David Spiegel and Rachel Kimerling, "Group Psychotherapy for Women with Breast Cancer: Relationships Among Social Support, Emotional Expression, and Survival," pp. 196, 197 in Ryff and Singer, *Emotion, Social Relationships, and Health,* 196–7.

115. Spiegel and Kimerling, "Group Psychotherapy," 196, 197.

116. Ibid., 197.

117. "Can the Right Attitude Cure Cancer?" *Patient Care* (June 15, 1991): 208–9.

118. J.L. Richardson et al., "The Effect of Compliance with Treatment on Survival Among Patients with Hematologic Malignancies," *Journal of Clinical Oncology* 8 (1987): 356–64.

119. "A Strong Circle of Friends," *Consumer Reports,* February 1993.

120. Spiegel, "A Psychosocial Intervention."

121. "Can the Right Attitude Cure Cancer?"

122. David Spiegel, "Effect of Psychosocial Treatment on Survival of Patients with Metastatic Breast Cancer," *Lancet,* ii (1989), 888–91.

123. Fawzy I. Fawzy, "Malignant Melanoma: Effects of an Early Structured Psychiatric Intervention, Coping, and Affective State of Recurrence and Survival Six Years Later," *Archives of General Psychiatry* 50 (1993): 681–9.

124. Ibid.

125. K. O. Ell, J. E. Mantell, M. B. Hamovitch, and R. H. Nishimoto, "Social Support, Sense of Control, and Coping Among Patients with Breast, Lung, or Colorectal Cancer," *Journal of Psychosocial Oncology,* 7, no. 3 (1989): 63–89.

126. Kathleen Ell et al., "Social Relations, Social Support and Survival Among Patients with Cancer," *Journal of Psychosomatic Research* 36, no. 6 (1992): 531–41.

127. Seeman, "How Do Others Get Under Our Skin?"

128. W. Thomas Boyce, "Stress and Child Health: An Overview," *Pediatric Annals* 14, no. 8: 539–42.

129. Margaret Westaway, John Seager, Paul Rheeder, and Danie Van Zyl, "The Effects of Social Support on Health, Well-Being, and Management of Diabetes Mellitus: A Black South African Perspective," *Ethnicity and Health* 10, no. 1 (February 2005): 73–89.

130. Boyce, "Stress and Child Health."

131. J. Kennell et al., "Continuous Emotional Support During Labor in a U. S. Hospital: A Randomized Controlled Trial," *Journal of the American Medical Association* 265 (1991): 2197–201.

132. Boyce, "Stress and Child Health."

133. MayoClinic.com., "Developing Social Support: How to Cultivate a Network of Friends to Help You Through Rough Times," http://www.cnn.com/HEALTH/library/MH/00041.html, accessed May 2008.

134. Albert L. Huebner, "The Pleasure Principle," *East/West* (May 1989): 14–9.

135. "Skin-to-Skin Contact and the Benefit of Human Touch," *C–Health,* http://chealth.canoe.ca, posted May 16, 2008.

136. Huebner, "The Pleasure Principle."

137. Ibid.

138. Barbara Montgomery Dossey, Lynn Keegan, Leslie Gooding Kolkmeier, and Cathie E. Guzzetta, *Holistic Health Promotion: A Guide for Practice* (Rockville, MD: Aspen, 1989), 255.

139. Diane Ackerman, "The Power of Touch," *Parade Magazine* (March 25, 1990): 4–6.

140. Ibid.

141. Ibid.

142. Robert Ornstein and David Sobel, *Healthy Pleasures* (Reading, MA: Addison-Wesley, 1989).

143. *Mayo Clinic Health Letter* (June 1994): 7.

144. *Stroke* (June 2008).

145. *Mayo Clinic Health Letter.*

CHAPTER 10

Loneliness and Health

We are, most of us, very lonely in this world; you who have any who love you, cling to them and thank God.

—Author Unknown

- Define *loneliness,* and distinguish how it is different from being alone.
- Identify national trends in being alone.
- Understand the factors that contribute to loneliness.
- Identify the health consequences of loneliness.
- Understand the importance of good friends.
- Discuss the health benefits of pet ownership in alleviating loneliness.

The dayroom on the fourth floor of the nursing home was sparkling clean. The television was on. The sun streamed in. There were only two patients in the room, each in a wheelchair. The woman slumped in her chair. Her hair was dull; I could hardly see her face. She rolled her chair toward where I sat on a couch talking with the psychiatrist, stopped, looked us over, turned, and wheeled away.

The man, who, I was told, was over a hundred years old, was dressed in a blue polka-dot shirt and gray pants. Nurses came in to check on him from time to time, touching his shoulder, adjusting his wheelchair. He didn't come near us. From afar, he tapped out a rhythm with his hand on the arm of the chair. Every once in a while, he let out a sound. At first, I thought he was whining.

Did he feel fatherless?

Was his freedom unbearably curtailed?

Not this man. He had been kissed and stroked and fussed over.

"Loneliness," Dr. Cath had said, "has to do with an individual's failure to create an inner, soothing presence." This man, for whatever reasons, had not failed. He was not whining. As I came closer, I heard, distinctly, the rhythm and the pitch.

He was singing.[1]

What Is Loneliness?

Loneliness—a condition that has been shown to affect both health and long life—is a feeling of isolation that results when we have suffered the loss of a loved one, feel misunderstood or useless, feel unloved, or spend too much time alone. But loneliness can also be present when we're surrounded by people. As the popular saying goes, a person can be "lonely in a crowd." Loneliness is generally defined as the failure to attain satisfying levels of social involvement; and, as such, it is one of the most common types of distress people feel.[2] It strikes regardless of gender, income, ethnicity, or education.

Instead of defining loneliness by the number of people who surround us, it's more accurate to define loneliness as the lack of sympathetic or friendly relationships—people upon whom we can depend for support in times of difficulty.[3]

According to psychologist and cell biologist Joan Borysenko, "To be isolated is the greatest tragedy for a human being and the most generic form of stress."[4] According to research at Kent State University, loneliness is connected less with the number of people in our lives than to satisfaction with those relationships. Loneliness occurs when we believe that current relationships fall short of our ideal.[5]

Feelings of loneliness are worse when the lonely person is surrounded by people who don't seem to be lonely—people who seem to have secure interpersonal attachments—or when the lonely person suffers from a sense of low self-esteem.[6] Although loneliness can stem from lack of attachment to someone else, loneliness can be just as intense if there is a sense of not belonging within an accepting community.[7] Loneliness is not the same as being alone; you can feel lonely when surrounded by people if those people don't meet your expectations.

Loneliness has been characterized as an "unpleasant experience that occurs when a person's network of social relationships is significantly deficient in either quality or quantity."[8] And loneliness can be more than just unpleasant; it can be profound. One prisoner during the Korean War endured extreme physical torture and starvation with surprising stamina. His worst point came, however, when he was placed in solitary confinement and separated from the friends he had made during his confinement in the prison camp. "I was captured and tortured," he remembers, "and after a while I could stand it. But I couldn't stand even a few days of this," he said, referring to his loneliness.[9]

A questionnaire about loneliness that appeared in five U. S. newspapers was answered by more than 22,000 people over the age of 18. The survey confirmed that feeling lonely is associated with greater health risks. What was a little surprising was that loneliness is not necessarily a consequence of living alone. In fact, almost one-fourth of the survey respondents who lived alone fell into the "least lonely" category. (Survey results, however, showed that they had more friends on average than people who lived with other people.)

The loneliest respondents were people who lived with their parents, possibly because of psychological conflict or social stigma that leads to feelings of rejection.

Another important quality of loneliness is the way in which its impact tends to increase with age. The toll of loneliness may be fairly mild and unremarkable early in life, but that toll grows increasingly more serious over time.[10] One reason, of course, may be the fact that the number of stressful experiences also tends to increase over time: A university student isn't likely to face the job, marriage, parenting, and physical stresses of someone in her forties or fifties.

Loneliness versus Aloneness

Loneliness is quite different from merely being alone. The number of persons with whom we surround ourselves is not what counts—what counts is the satisfaction we get from our relationships and whether we perceive that we are isolated.[11] Many feel lonely within a marriage or when surrounded by a group of people if they are unsatisfied with the sense of connection they get from others. On the other hand, people who are alone much of the time may not necessarily feel "lonely" because of the fulfillment they get from the relationships they do have in their lives.

Loneliness is generally characterized by three conditions: isolation (distance from or absence of a romantic partner); feelings of being disconnected (not having close friends); and feelings of not belonging (not being accepted by or not identifying with valued social groups).[12] Obviously, all three of these conditions can occur regardless of whether a person is alone.

These are some of the factors that help determine whether someone who is "alone" is also "lonely":

- General attitude. People either react to being alone by being sad and passive or by developing "creative solitude": spending time reading, listening to music, working on a hobby, studying, writing, playing a musical instrument, or some other creative endeavor.

- Boredom. Researchers concluded from the survey that some loneliness stems from simple boredom.

- Attitude toward self. Researchers concluded that a person must feel secure with him- or herself in order to be content when alone.

Associate Professor of Psychology David A. Chiriboga has this advice: "When you find yourself alone, see it as an opportunity to discover yourself. Take it as a challenge. Find out what you want to be, where you want to go, and what gives you pleasure. Anyone can be an interesting person. All you have to do is look inside yourself." And, he concludes, people who are loving—who completely accept themselves and others—can be happy and content whether they are in a crowd of people or quietly at home by themselves. In a study of more than 9,000 people reported in the *Journal of Community and Applied Social Psychology,* researchers found that living alone can be healthy if those who live alone seek outside contacts (such as friends and extended family members) and limit their alcohol intake.

Anne Morrow Lindbergh wrote in *Gift from the Sea*:

> I find there is a quality to being alone that is incredibly precious. Life rushes back into the void, richer, more vivid, fuller than before. It is as if in parting one did actually lose an arm. And then, like starfish, one grows it anew; one is whole again, complete and round—more whole, even, than before, when the other people had pieces of one.[13]

Trends in Being Alone

Although being alone doesn't necessarily mean people are lonely, many people who are alone are lonely. And there are more people than ever living alone—according to U. S. Census figures, more than 31 million Americans are projected to be living alone, a 40 percent increase from 1980.[14] Between 1950 and 1980, the figure rose by 385 percent.

According to the 2000 U. S. Census, the number of Americans living alone (more than 27 million) has now exceeded the number of households comprised of the classic nuclear family: a married couple and their natural children. Approximately 26 percent of all households in America are now comprised of a single individual, while only 22 percent consist of a married couple and their natural children.[15] The number of single-person households in the United States grew 21 percent in the 1990s, eclipsing the growth rates for all other types of living arrangement.

The increase in single-person households continues a trend that started decades ago. In 1950, just 9.3 percent of American households consisted of people living alone, according to the U. S. Census Bureau. A number of trends and factors help explain why so many Americans in such increasing numbers are living alone.

1. According to the U. S. Census Bureau, half of all marriages in the United States will end in divorce.

2. In the United States, there has been a trend away from marriage. People are waiting longer to get married, and many are not marrying at all. According to figures released by the U. S. Census Bureau, the median age of first marriage was 27.1 years for men and 25.8 years for women in 2005 (the latest year for which figures are available), up from 23.2 and 20.8 years, respectively, in 1980.[16]

3. Household size is getting smaller. The average household size in the United States was 4.1 members in 1930; that figure dropped to 2.8 in 1980.[17] In 2005, the average household size had declined to 2.57 people.[18]

4. Mobility is increasing. In the United States, one in five persons changes residence every year; almost half the U. S. population relocates within any five-year period. According to the U. S. Census Bureau, more than 22 million Americans moved from one state to another between 1995 and 2000.[19] Young, educated people move—often long distances—in search of employment and more favorable environments. Poor people move—usually short distances—as the economic and ethnic characteristics of their neighborhoods force them out. We are free—free to relocate to another

area, free to quit our job, free to quit our family, free to move on. The changing face of America reflects this "freedom"; the individual is in many ways replacing the family as the basic unit of society.[20]

Other trends have led to the alone and lonely trend in the United States. Fewer face-to-face business transactions are completed; computers write letters, make telephone calls, and handle all financial transactions. People sit alone in front of the television set and video/DVD machine instead of going out into the community to watch movies, go to the theatre, attend plays, or patronize the arts. Our larger cities, especially, have become impersonal—and the high crime rate in many cities discourages people from leaving home for purely social reasons.[21]

Reasons for Loneliness

There are very personal reasons for being lonely. Researchers have divided these into five separate categories:

1. Being alone (coming home to an empty house)

2. Needing friends (feeling different, being misunderstood)

3. Forced isolation (being housebound, being hospitalized, having no transportation)

4. Being unattached (having no spouse, having no sexual partner)

5. Dislocation (being far from home, being in a new job or school, moving too often, traveling often)[22]

Whatever the reason, many Americans feel lonely. Estimates reveal that more than 35 million are lonely each month. Nearly one-fifth of the U. S. adult population feels lonely at least once a month, and one in ten feels overwhelming loneliness at least once a week.

Research also shows that education may play a role in loneliness. In a study involving the effects of loneliness on heart attack, Dr. William Ruberman and his colleagues found that the best-educated people had the least amount of social isolation. On the other hand, poorly educated people had the most job stress and the most social isolation—and the highest risk of dying.

Although Ruberman and his associates considered social isolation to be the most potent factor in the increased death rate among their study subjects, they believe that poor education may also result in less access to good health care and the tendency to neglect self-care practices.[23]

Causes of Loneliness

According to researchers with the Department of Health and Human Services, loneliness has two basic causes: (1) predisposing (general cultural values, the characteristics of the situation, or the characteristics of the individual), and (2) precipitating (what happens following a specific event, such as a move to a new community or the breakup of a love relationship). The following causes are the most common.[24]

Personal Characteristics

Many lonely people have distinctive social characteristics that make it difficult for them to form and maintain relationships. They may be extremely shy, for example, and may find it very difficult to introduce themselves, participate in groups, enjoy parties, make phone calls to initiate social activities, and so on. They may lack self-esteem or may be excruciatingly self-conscious. Researchers have found a strong relationship between loneliness and self-concept, as well as the individual's concept about his or her relationships with both same-gender and opposite-gender peers: the lower that belief in self and the ability to relate to others, the greater the loneliness.[25] Many lonely people are unable to be assertive, and some feel they are controlled by others.

Lonely people also tend to have distinct patterns of interaction. Some believe that real loneliness begins with the inability to communicate.[26] When they are conversing with someone else, they respond slowly to the other person's statements, change the subject often, talk more about themselves, and ask few questions of the other person. A researcher who studied these patterns says that lonely people are "self-focused and non-responsive." Lonely people tend to spend less time with confidants and often have trouble developing the kind of intimacy that helps them build those deeply connected types of relationships.

Lonely people often had problems relating to their parents, too. Many lonely people say their parents did not give emotional nurturance, failed to give guidance or support, and did not encourage their children to strive for relationships or popularity. Many lonely people remember their parents as remote, untrustworthy, and disagreeable.

Characteristics of the Situation

Certain situations have everything working against them as far as fostering relationships and becoming involved in meaningful social networks. Some constraints are very basic—time, distance, and money. The student who carries a full course load and a heavy work schedule may have little time for sleep, let alone for making friends. The fire spotter who lives in a remote part of the forest has few opportunities to socialize. The single parent on a tight budget may not be able to afford the babysitter who would allow time for social activities.

Constraints can also limit the number of "eligible" people. For example, a person may not be surrounded by people considered appropriate as friends. An elderly person may live in an apartment building full of young married couples, or a Hispanic family may be the only one of that ethnic group on the block. This kind of "situational" isolation sometimes makes it difficult to initiate relationships.

Cultural Values

American culture encourages us to be independent, individualistic, and eager to travel our own paths. Those who rely on others or lean on people for help, even in critical difficulties, are often seen as weak, so people try to handle things on their own—something they confuse with being self-reliant. In addition, as mentioned, we have become a highly mobile, urban society; many people who live in condominiums or townhouses in crowded urban areas could not tell you the name of their next-door neighbors.

The Nature of Social Relationships

Lonely people tend to have fewer social contacts and relationships than people who are not lonely. They spend less time with other people, and are likely to spend their time with people they are not close to rather than with good friends. Children who are lonely often have poor relationships with their mothers; adults who are lonely are apt to lack meaningful relationships with other adults.

The quality of relationships is important as well. People who have shallow, withdrawn relationships are much more likely to feel lonely (even when surrounded by throngs of people) than are those who have deep, intense, and close friendships with others.

Relationships That Don't Meet Needs

A person might have ten close relationships with others and still be lonely. For most people, relationships have to provide a feeling of personal attachment and social integration; they have to provide nurturance, reassurance of one's worth, a sense of reliable alliance, and guidance. Relationships that meet those needs are more likely to keep a person from feeling lonely.

Precipitating Events

Countless events in life (many of which are beyond our control) can make us feel lonely, rejected, alone, and inadequate. The most frequent precipitators of loneliness are the death of a spouse, divorce, geographical moves, leaving family and friends to begin college or start a new job, the breakup of a romantic relationship, and a fight with a good friend or family member. Serial relationships also exaggerate feelings of loneliness, as does alcohol abuse.

Risk Factors for Loneliness

No one is immune from loneliness. Depending on one's needs, relationships, and life circumstances at any given time, anyone may fall prey to loneliness. However, two groups are at higher risk for loneliness overall: teenagers and people over age 80.

It shouldn't surprise many that people over 8 are at risk. As people mature, they tend to become more satisfied with their relationships, and loneliness is not as common—until people experience the death of friends, loved ones, and spouses. As people age, they typically suffer more losses; besides the death of friends and family members, they suffer losses such as the stress of relocating after spending years in a community, the loneliness that results when children leave home, and the isolation that can result when friends become seriously ill.[27]

According to one study, more than half of all seniors report feeling lonely;[28] another study places the figure at more than a third.[29] The exact percentage isn't what's important: the important thing is that loneliness is rampant among the elderly and that its effects on health are serious, especially among the elderly as immunity declines. The most powerful predictions of loneliness among the elderly include living alone, poor understanding by friends and family members, unfulfilled expectations of contacts with friends, and depression. Interestingly, it's not the frequency of contacts with friends and family members that counts—instead, it's whether expectations were fulfilled and the contact was satisfying.[30]

Some think that teenagers are the most socially active. It's true that they usually have more opportunity for social interaction, but many teenagers also have unrealistic expectations about what friendships should involve. Therefore, their needs aren't met, and they feel lonely. Teenagers who get pregnant may have an especially difficult time with loneliness. A 12-year longitudinal study looked at the social relationships and psychological status of young adult women who had been pregnant as teenagers as compared to similar young adults who did not have their first child until in their twenties. Those who had their first child while still teenagers struggled with greater loneliness, depression, and lack of self-esteem.[31] Another study had similar findings: Adolescent mothers recruited from primary health care practices in various midwestern cities found a strong correlation between early pregnancy, loneliness, and depression.[32]

Also, people who are happily married are less lonely than people who are single. Among single people, those who have never been married are less lonely than those who have been divorced or widowed.

Loneliness tends to be less of a problem for women than men, although women are more willing to admit they are lonely. Women fare slightly better because they tend to form deep and intimate relationships; they generally remain friends with people, even though time and distance separate them. Their conversations are more personal and intimate; women tend to discuss feelings, whereas men tend to discuss things (such as the structure at the office or the results of last night's football game).

As one researcher put it, "In public, the loneliness of men is more visible than the loneliness of women. Men make friends less easily as they grow older; women seem to continue to replace the friends they have lost. Most older men lack what social scientists call the social skills for making friends with other men and have had little experience in making friends with women."[33]

People with certain kinds of family structure are also more prone to loneliness than others. In doing research on loneliness, psychologists commented on many people who described a family life in which one or more of the following was true:

> The parents clung tightly to one another and shut out both the world and the child. The parents had no friends; there were no models in the home of what it meant to have friends. There was a sense of being stranded, both shut out from the clinging marriage and alone in the rest of the world. Nobody ever came to dinner. Nobody ever called or went to the movies. Nobody confided in anyone. The family seems, to people who talk this way, the most antisocial unit imaginable, less a haven than a dungeon. Some children growing up in families like these become compensatory—filling their lives with other people, looking for other families to "adopt" themselves into, marrying young. Others repeat the patterns they learned at home, isolating themselves, walling themselves off from intimate connections, ignoring the thirst.[34]

People with lower incomes are more likely to be lonely than those at middle- or high-income levels, probably because there are fewer opportunities for socializing due to economic restrictions. Other groups at higher risk for loneliness are recent widows, couples who are separating or getting a divorce, students changing schools, people starting new jobs, people who are moving, unemployed people, people who live alone, prison inmates, patients with chronic or terminal illness, children of divorced parents, and women whose children have left home (commonly called the "empty nest syndrome").[35] Research shows that childlessness itself is not as great a factor as marital status, however: Those in middle and old age who are married demonstrate far less loneliness, regardless of whether they have children.[36] Other studies also show that those middle-aged people who are single or divorced not only have a higher risk of loneliness than those who are married but also suffer greater social isolation, more frequent depression, more pronounced hopelessness, and lower emotional support than those who are married.[37]

The Health Consequences of Loneliness

Loneliness carries with it a big risk for health problems. The social isolation that accompanies loneliness is a significant risk factor for disease—and is comparable to obesity, sedentary lifestyle, and possibly even smoking.[38]

Both short-term and chronic loneliness are major risk factors for illness and premature death from a number of causes; they have been shown in studies to be linked to unhealthy behaviors, major depression, and diminished immune function.[39] Psychologist James J. Lynch, scientific director of the Psychophysiological Clinic at the University of Maryland Medical School, says loneliness is "the greatest unrecognized contributor to premature death in the United States."[40] Widespread evidence indicates that those who are lonely are less healthy and die earlier than those with strong social involvement;[41] those who are socially isolated are twice as likely to die during any given period than those who enjoy good social relationships.[42] In a 1992 study by researchers at Duke University Medical Center, scientists studied patients with coronary artery disease. Those who were isolated—unmarried and without a close friend or confidant—had a 50 percent death rate within five years, as compared to only a 17 percent death rate among the heart disease patients who had a spouse, a close friend, or both.[43]

Loneliness—and the stress that accompanies it—has been connected to not only premature death[44] but a host of physical and mental disorders as well. Loneliness has been shown to be important in three factors that can cause disease: unhealthy behaviors,[45] excessive reaction to stress, and inadequate or inefficient ability of the body to repair and maintain its normal physiological processes.[46] University of Chicago research indicates that loneliness undermines health by disrupting sleep and by altering cardiac function.[47]

Good social support has been linked to a lower risk of depression, heart disease, and alcoholism.[48] Loneliness, on the other hand, has been definitely linked to disease; people who are not lonely have a better chance of staying healthy or recovering from disease than people who are lonely. Studies have shown that those who are lonely are more likely to get sick in the first place when exposed to pathogens, like bacteria and viruses, presumably because of the impact of loneliness on the immune system. Those who have only one to three satisfying relationships run more than four times the risk of becoming ill when exposed to pathogens than do those with less loneliness and more social relationships.[49]

Researcher Louise Bernikow reports:

> Loneliness can, indeed, make you sick. Heart disease and hypertension are now generally thought of as loneliness diseases, exacerbated by a person's sense of abandonment by the world, separation from the rest of humanity. Most addictions are also considered loneliness diseases, which the medical profession is beginning to recognize but which recovering alcoholics, drug addicts, even smokers have been long aware of. Most addicts admit that their best friends have been booze, drugs, or tobacco.[50]

One reason for the link between loneliness and illness may actually be genetic. Research conducted at UCLA found that certain genes were more active in people who were lonely and socially isolated—and they are genes that impact immunity and tissue inflammation, both of which are factors in disease. While a certain amount of inflammation helps the body fight disease, too much inflammation damages tissues and causes disease. The research from this and other studies indicates that loneliness causes a spike in inflammation throughout the body. It also indicates that those who are lonely have weaker genes that are responsible for producing the cells that fight viruses and produce immune antibodies.[51]

Dr. Steven Cole, who directed the study, commented, "What this shows us is the biological impact of social isolation reaches down into some of our most important basic internal processes—the activity of our genes." And the important factor, he said, is not how many friends you have. "What counts, at the level of gene expression, is not how many people you know, it's how many you feel really close to over time."[52]

Apparently one of the crucial factors in determining whether loneliness will make you sick is what it means to you to be lonely; one study of immigrants to Israel from the former Soviet Union showed that those who suffered distressing effects of loneliness were the ones who saw their loneliness as negative.[53] Research shows that the effects of loneliness on the immune system, which can lead to the development of cancer, not only depend on how an individual perceives the loneliness but also appear to unfold over a relatively long period of time.[54] In one study, California Department of Health Services epidemiologists Peggy Reynolds and George A. Kaplan used data from the Alameda County study, which involved 7,000 healthy adults. What they found was that socially isolated women had a significantly greater chance of developing cancer and dying from it.[55]

But what interested the researchers most was the fact that the determining factor seemed to be the women's perception of loneliness—what being lonely meant. Some of the women had many social contacts but still felt isolated; Reynolds and Kaplan found those women had 2.4 times the normal risk of dying from cancers of the ovary, uterus, and breast. Then there were the women who had few social contacts and felt isolated: they were five times as likely to die from the same cancers.[56]

Early attachment to a consistent caregiver is critical to the health and well-being of infants and children. Infants who fail to develop attachments sometimes do not survive. Those who do survive are believed to be more likely to develop psychopathic personalities (personalities that render them unable to care and be responsible for others).[57] The resulting loneliness leads to a variety of physical and mental health problems and sometimes prema-ture death. People with strong attachments, on the other hand, suffer far less loneliness—and are less vulnerable, less helpless, more likely to have the confidence to take risks, more likely to have the confidence to move in new directions, and more creative.[58]

Attachment—both the social ties it brings and the loneliness in its absence—appears to be an extremely important health factor. Dr. James House, a sociologist at the Institute of Gerontology at the University of Michigan, has done an in-depth review of a series of studies conducted in the United States, Sweden, and Finland. The studies exam-ined various health issues in relationship to how lonely people were, with loneliness cal-culated in terms of whether a person was or was not married, had contacts with extended family, had a strong network of friends, was active in a church, or had any other social affiliations. In cooperation with a team of two other researchers who also examined the studies, House concluded that loneliness constitutes a "major risk factor" for health—rivaling the effects of "well-established health risk factors such as cigarette smoking, blood pressure, blood lipids (fats), obesity, and physical activity."[59]

The effects of loneliness may be even greater than originally thought, as researchers look into a variety of situations. In one fascinating study, researchers decided to find out whether companionship that alleviated loneliness could make a difference in the outcome of labor and delivery. To test their notion, researchers randomly divided first-time moth-ers into two groups. In the first group, each mother went through labor alone, except for occasional checks by the hospital staff; in the second group, each had the companionship of an untrained woman throughout labor. The mothers in the second group had never met their companions; the support provided during labor varied from mere companion-ship to holding hands, talking, or rubbing the mother's back during labor.[60]

The results were striking. Among the mothers who underwent labor alone, 75 percent developed complications during labor or birth, including induced labor, fetal distress, still-births, or caesarean section deliveries. Only 12 percent of the mothers with companions developed complications. When researchers looked at just the uncomplicated labors, there was still a marked difference. The unsupported mothers had an average length of labor of 19.3 hours; the mothers who enjoyed support averaged 8.7 hours—less than half as long.[61] The differences continued even after birth. When physicians and researchers observed the mothers for the first hour after the babies were born, the supported mothers were more awake and alert, talked to their babies more, stroked their babies more, and smiled more at their babies.[62]

In a new study that involved 616 women, research director John Kennell of Case Western Reserve University estimated that emotional support during labor could save the health industry $2 billion a year. In his study, Kennell compared women who went through labor and delivery alone to those who were given emotional support and com-panionship by another woman. Those who were less lonely during labor and delivery required fewer caesarean sections, less anesthesia, and fewer induced deliveries. Those with companionship delivered their babies faster, and the babies required shorter hospi-tal stays than those born to women who went through the experience alone.[63]

Loneliness apparently has profound effects at the other end of life as well. In addi-tion to the variety of other physical illnesses that have been linked to loneliness, recent research indicates that loneliness in old age is linked to Alzheimer's disease. Researchers at Rush University Medical Center in Chicago studied 823 senior citizens who were initially free of any dementia; they tested the seniors for cognitive functioning and for loneliness annually over a period of four years.

Those who were lonely at the beginning of the study were also those who had the lowest levels of cognitive functioning as the study began. Those who were lonely also suffered the most rapid decline over the period of the study, and the top 10 percent of people in terms of loneliness were more than twice as likely to develop Alzheimer's disease as those who were least lonely. The greatest factor was loneliness, not isolation.

Interestingly, the factor of loneliness was not correlated with Alzheimer's-associated damage in the brain. Lead researcher in the study, Dr. Robert Wilson, emphasized that loneliness is a real risk factor for Alzheimer's but that researchers need to look outside the typical disease pathways in the brain. He also maintains that loneliness is a risk factor for—and not a reaction to—the disease.[64]

Loneliness and Longevity

University of Maryland psychologist James J. Lynch says that all the available data from hundreds of in-depth studies point to several factors, including lack of human companionship, chronic loneliness, and social isolation, as "among the leading causes of premature death."[65] And, says Lynch, although the effects of human loneliness are related to "virtually every disease," they are particularly strong in heart disease, the leading cause of death in the United States.

Samuel Silverman, associate clinical professor of psychiatry at Harvard University, claims a person can add up to fifteen years to life simply by reducing two "emotional aging factors," one of which is loneliness.[66]

A study by University of Michigan researchers followed 2,754 men and women to determine which behavioral factors influenced health and longevity. Loneliness turned out to be a substantial health risk—and an apparent cause of premature death. According to researchers, women who were lonely and isolated were 1.5 times more likely to die prematurely than women with close social ties. For men, the risk was double.[67]

Another University of Michigan study—this one involving 37,000 people—found that people who lived alone or who had few friends were twice as likely to die during the 10-year period of the study.[68]

In the study conducted on residents of Alameda County, California (detailed in Chapter 9), researchers followed 7,000 men and women for nine years, looking for clues on what leads to health and long life. Again, loneliness was strongly implicated as being detrimental. In that study, the genders seemed to "switch risk": Lonely women had a nearly three times greater risk and lonely men had a doubled risk of illness and premature death than men and women who had close ties with family and friends.

Loneliness and Immune Function

A host of studies has shown that loneliness has a considerable effect on immune system function. Loneliness itself is actually a stress—just like stressors such as illness, injury, loss, exhaustion, fatigue, fear, pain, and grief—and it causes the same stress reaction in the body, complete with the stress hormones. Solid scientific research has proven that those stress hormones impact immunity and eventually affect every cell in the body. Simply stated, loneliness can make us sick, keep us sick, and interfere with our recovery.[69]

A recent study at Carnegie Mellon University looked at freshmen students who were away from home for the first time. Researchers often use response to the flu vaccine as a measure of how well the immune system is functioning. All the students in the study were healthy when the study began and received their first-ever flu shots on campus. Those students who rated themselves as lonely or who felt isolated had the weakest immune response to the flu vaccine; the weakest responses of all were among those who felt both lonely and isolated.[70]

In another measure of loneliness, researchers at Harvard Medical School studied 111 students—78 men and 33 women. All students in the study were physically healthy, and none was taking drugs that would have suppressed the immune system. Students were given the Minnesota Multiphasic Personality Inventory, a questionnaire-form test that rates, among other things, depression, loneliness, social isolation, and maladjustment. They were also given blood tests that measured the activity of natural killer cells, white blood cells that attack tumors and viruses even without being previously exposed to them. There was a definite correlation in the study: Students who showed high levels of loneliness also had significantly low functioning of the immune system. Researchers found that their natural killer cells were not as active and that they were less able to fight off the Epstein-Barr virus.[71]

A closely related study yielded the same results. Researchers administered a blood test and the UCLA Loneliness Scale—a psychological test measuring loneliness—to a group of first-year medical students and a group of psychiatric inpatients. When researchers measured immune system function, they found that the lonelier medical students and the lonelier psychiatric patients both had significantly lower levels of natural killer cell activity than those who were not lonely.[72]

Apparently there's a medical reason for the reduction in immune system functioning: Lonely people secrete an excessive amount of the hormone cortisol, which suppresses the immune system. When loneliness is coupled with stress, another condition that stimulates cortisol production, the results can be particularly crippling.

A study that measured the effects of loneliness coupled with stress was carried out at Harvard Medical School; researchers measured the levels and activity of natural killer cells in students both before and after they took exams. As expected, the activity of natural killer cells declined under the stress of taking an exam, but the students who were also lonely had the lowest natural killer cell activity.[73]

Researchers at Ohio State University carried the tests a step further by involving a specific disease: herpes.[74] Researchers looked at herpes simplex type 1, which causes common cold sores, and herpes simples type 2, which causes genital, or venereal, herpes. Those who were lonely were not able to fight against herpes viruses of either type. Their immune systems were compromised.

It appears that loneliness may even affect the way people perceive and deal with stress. A pair of University of Chicago psychologists studied middle-aged and elderly people to determine which were lonely and how their loneliness impacted their health. They found that those who were lonely suffered the same number of stress events as everyone else, but they recalled more adversity from their childhood, identified more sources of chronic stress, seemed more threatened and helpless in the face of the stress, and were less likely to seek help in dealing with the stress.[75] Furthermore, the lonely people had more epinephrine—one of the key stress hormones—circulating through their bodies, indicating that lonely people may go through life in the heightened state of arousal that inflicts wear and tear on the body.[76]

Loneliness and Heart Function

Researchers looked for ways in which the mind had an influence over the heart. One of the brain's perceptions—that a person is lonely—apparently has a significant effect on that individual's heart. In the largest study yet attempted of the impact of loneliness on cardiac health, Dr. Kristina Orth-Gomer of the Karolinska Institute in Sweden and Dr. Jeffrey Johnson of the Johns Hopkins School of Public Health studied 17,433 Swedes. Orth-Gomer and Johnson looked at how lonely the Swedes were, as measured by how much they interacted with family, friends, neighbors, and coworkers, and compared the loneliest with those who were not lonely for a period of six years. Then the researchers made allowances for typical heart disease risks, such as age, smoking, physical inactivity, and a family history of heart disease. After making these allowances, they reasoned, they should be able to determine what actual impact loneliness had. They found that those who were lonely had a 40 percent greater risk of dying from cardiovascular disease than the rest of the people in the study.[77]

Orth-Gomer and her colleagues followed up with a second study that zeroed in even more carefully on loneliness and its impact on heart disease. She and her colleagues studied 150 middle-aged men between the ages of 40 and 65, observing them for 10 years beginning in 1976. One-third of the men were healthy, one-third had heart disease, and the last third were at high risk for developing heart disease. The researchers tested the men's physical health in a variety of ways and examined a range of psychosocial factors to determine which factors were most strongly associated with those who eventually died of heart disease. After 10 years, 37 men had died from heart disease. Of those who died, almost all had been initially categorized as socially isolated and lonely. In fact, loneliness was as strong a factor as the strongest physical factor— having an irregular heartbeat—in determining who would eventually die from heart disease.[78]

Another interesting finding stemmed from the study at Karolinska Institute: Researchers found that there is apparently an actual physiological link between loneliness and heart disease. According to the researchers, loneliness creates neuroendocrine changes that lead to atherosclerosis.[79] Some studies indicate that there may be differences between the genders when it comes to the effect of loneliness on the cardiovascular system. In one study of middle-aged working men and women, loneliness was shown to compound the effect of stress on high blood pressure—but only among the women. The authors of the study concluded that loneliness has potentially adverse effects on how well people adjust to and cope with stress.[80]

In still another study of more than 1,700 elderly men and women in Odense, Denmark, a feeling of loneliness was found to be associated with death from cardiovascular disease. That association was especially true for the men.[81]

Apparently loneliness has what one researcher calls a "stunning" impact on blood pressure. In people over the age of fifty, loneliness significantly increases the risk of high blood pressure. In fact, in one study, those who were most lonely had blood pressure readings that were thirty points higher—enough to move a blood pressure from normal to hypertension. Researchers concluded that the effect of loneliness on blood pressure was as significant as that of being overweight or inactive.[82]

One of the most comprehensive retrospective studies of early predictors of disease and premature death involved 50,000 former students from the University of Pennsylvania and Harvard University who attended college between the years of 1921 and 1950. Dr. Ralph Paffenbarger and his colleagues carefully studied the records of the first 590 men who had died of coronary heart disease and compared them with 1,180 randomly selected classmates of equivalent age who were still alive.[83]

Nine factors distinguished the men who died of heart disease: heavy cigarette smoking, high blood pressure, increased body weight, shortness of body height, early parental death, absence of siblings, nonparticipation in sports, a higher emotional index, and scarlet fever in childhood. Researchers said several of those factors, including early parental death, absence of siblings, and nonparticipation in sports, were clear and accurate indicators of which were the loneliest. And, researchers say, those who were loneliest and most socially isolated were the ones most at risk to die of heart disease.[84]

Paffenbarger and his colleagues then did a second study involving 40,000 students. In the years following graduation, 225 of them had committed suicide. When researchers compared the suicides with a large number of randomly selected students, they found that the students who committed suicide were lonely, socially isolated, and came from homes in which the parents had separated early or in which the father had died early. The students who committed suicide tended to have fathers who had a professional status and parents who were college-trained.[85]

All of these factors worked together to bring about loneliness, researchers say. As Paffenbarger commented, "Lack of participation in extracurricular activities seems to acquire meaning in loneliness, fear, hostility, or frustration. Wealth or success of the father may have an adverse influence on the son through paternal absence, deprivation of companionship and counsel, overbearing demand for emulation, possible lack of interest or lack of need for individual success or effort in the son."[86]

An opposite scenario is the case study provided by the city of Seattle, Washington, where an unusually high percentage of its population—over 40 percent—is trained in cardiopulmonary resuscitation (CPR). In Seattle, say observers, it's considered a "civic virtue" to know what to do for possible cardiac arrest; it's considered important to care, to be prepared to save someone else. Seattle has the highest rate in the country for recovery from cardiac arrest, in part because it addresses the question of loneliness.[87]

The Importance of Good Friends

One of the greatest benefits provided by friends is that they avert the distress of loneliness. As Robert Louis Stevenson said, "A friend is a present you give yourself." People without friends are lonelier. Studies involving neurotic people have noted that they have far fewer friends (usually no more than one).[88]

And, even though friends are clearly less important in terms of social support than are spouses, it's also clear that close friendships help buffer stress and help overcome the health effects of loneliness. In the study of 7,000 residents of Alameda County, California, it was concluded that a "larger network size and greater frequency of contact was related to decreased mortality for both men and women at all ages, even when other factors, such as socioeconomic status, initial health status, and health practices," were taken into account.[89]

Researchers stress that although having a few close friends is critical to health, it's also wise to have a large social support network. A larger network gives a greater likelihood of finding someone who can provide the kind of support needed when things get tough.

In some cases, the support of close friends may be even more important than the support of family. One study looked at persons aged 55 and older in three North Carolina communities. The researchers first determined who had the greatest satisfaction with life—who were the happiest, healthiest, and generally most satisfied. Then they searched to determine what kinds of social support seemed to contribute most to that satisfaction. For this elderly population, at least, the frequency of contacts with family and the satisfaction with contacts from family weren't what made people happiest in life. It was contact with close friends that made the biggest difference.[90]

In a study conducted by Ohio State University, researchers reviewed how many visitors nursing home patients had and how strong the patients' immune systems were. Researchers measured the immune systems by taking blood samples and measuring both levels of antibodies and natural killer cell activity. The elderly residents who had visitors three times a week or more had significantly stronger immune systems than did the elderly residents who had fewer visitors.

Friends contribute to health by providing all the functions of the family. In some cases, friends may be closer confidants than family members are. And people who are able to build close relationships with friends have greater health protection against stress.[91]

A study of working-class women in London demonstrates the point. Women who were under severe stress were much more likely to be depressed. The women who had close friendships still suffered stress, but the effects of the stress were four times less severe. In summing up the results of the study, researchers said that the difference was due to the "protective effect of confidants" and that those with fewer close friends were more vulnerable to both psychiatric and physical illness.

Types of Friends

Judith Viorst has categorized friends by the five different functions they fulfill in our lives:[92]

1. Convenience friends. These are the neighbors or the office mates with whom we exchange pleasantries. We engage in "pleasant chitchat" but don't really share our intimate feelings with them. They are important enough to us that we want to keep up a pleasant face with them. We might occasionally ask them for help—such as with a carpool—but don't lean on them for intense support in times of need.

2. Special-interest friends. With these friends we share some interest or activity: members of the bowling team, someone we meet on Saturdays for a game of tennis, the people in a ceramics class. We do things with these people, but we don't share our feelings with them.

3. Historical friends. These are people with whom we have been close at one time or another; but, because of any of a number of reasons, we've drifted apart. We enjoy an occasional telephone call with these friends, perhaps exchange Christmas cards or other infrequent correspondence, and maybe even meet for occasional nostalgic reunions. These friends are important—not because they offer ongoing support but because they help us maintain a link with the past.

4. Cross-generational friends. This type of friendship is between members of different generations. It could be an 18-year-old neighbor who used to babysit your children or an elderly man on the corner who brings you bags of tomatoes and onions from his garden. These friendships can be close, and even intimate, but they don't usually provide intensive support. There's almost always an inequality involved: the older partner usually gives advice, and the younger one is expected to take it.

5. Close friends. These are the gems—the friends we see the most often, the people who are most important to us. They are the ones in whom we confide our deepest feelings, the ones we see and talk with most often, and the ones whose advice and confidence are most important to us. They are the ones who provide the greatest protection from illness and premature death.

Close friendships seem more common among women than among men. Friendship patterns tend to vary a little, too: women have closer friendships with other women and fewer friendships with men, whereas men tend to have closer friendships with women. There could be a variety of reasons, but researchers think it might have to do with the confiding nature of women. A variety of studies has shown that conversations with women tend to do more to relieve loneliness for members of both sexes. Women's conversations are generally more pleasant, are more intimate, tend to involve more self-disclosure, and are likely to be more meaningful than the conversations of men.[93]

Specific Health Benefits of Friends

One loneliness study found that female students visited their physicians less often if they had close contacts with good friends. If the women had friends who were pleasant, intimate, and encouraged them to confide, they had a considerably lower rate of illness than women students with fewer close friends.[94]

Friends can also help buffer the effects of stress—and it's well established that stress can make people sick. Friends help one to weather stress. From the results of two separate studies, researchers believe the harmful consequences of stress can be significantly reduced through an active network of friends and family members. Based on studies, psychologists and other researchers say that people with a number of close friends and confidants, people with a "high capacity for intimacy," and people who can openly discuss their deepest feelings are better able to cope with stress in general. Whereas stress overwhelms and exhausts some, people with friends tend to be challenged and stimulated instead.

Lillian B. Rubin, a psychologist who has studied the health benefits of friends, says that "people who have others with whom they can communicate about the tensions in their lives often find relief for those tensions."[95] Other psychologists agree—and some go so far as to say that a good friend who is willing to listen in confidence is as good as professional counseling when facing a problem.[96]

Friendship protects health because it provides a natural outlet for confiding feelings to others. Researchers have found that openly discussing a traumatic event with someone else—such as a friend—can actually improve physical health even when the traumatic event occurred many years previous.[97] In his research, University of Texas psychologist James Pennebaker found that immune system function is boosted by confiding upsetting events. The health benefits of confiding in a friend are long-lasting: Pennebaker's research shows that immune function improvement lasts as long as six weeks afterward![98]

According to a study conducted by the California Department of Mental Health, close, confiding personal relationships—good friends—have been found to buffer the stress not only from life's major changes (such as death of a loved one), but from life's daily hassles as well. People in crisis—whether from a major life change or from an accumulation of daily hassles—have higher morale, fewer physical symptoms, and less illness if they have support from and contact with close friends.[99]

In addition to the factor of social support, friends may help protect health because they are familiar. They are comforting because we are used to them. What is familiar is often less threatening because it seems more predictable and manageable.

Those who don't have friends or other people who can alleviate loneliness may resort to anthropomorphism—the tendency to develop human-like connections with pets, other animals, gods or other supreme beings, angels, or even gadgets. One of the most well-known examples was the character played by Tom Hanks in *Castaway*, who, when confronted by complete isolation on a deserted island, anthropomorphized a volleyball. Wilson, the name he gave the volleyball, became his confidant and dear friend while he was on the island. Essentially, it's a way for people to alleviate the pain of loneliness; and, say the researchers, it can actually provide many of the same psychological and physical benefits that come from connections with other people.[100]

The Importance of Pets

Research into the health benefits of pet ownership has shown beyond a doubt that comfort does not always have to come only from people.[101] There are an estimated 100 million pets in the United States—pets who are sheltered, groomed, petted, talked to, babied, and showered with toys. More than half of all American homes have one or more pets. Those pets may return a health benefit to the owners who care for them.

According to research,[102] pets fulfill a variety of needs for their human owners. They provide a chance for interaction with another living thing and fulfill the natural craving for companionship and emotional relationships. They provide for our need to care and our desire to be loved. They act as a stimulus for exercise. As anyone who owns a pet knows, they also give love in return.

The discovery that pets benefit health came quite by accident at first and was due to three landmark events. The first occurred in 1959, when New York child psychiatrist Boris Levinson happened to have his dog Jingles with him when a patient paid an unexpected visit. The young patient had been withdrawn and isolated and had failed to respond to the repeated attempts to help. Jingles suddenly ran up to the boy and licked his face. The child broke out of his usual withdrawal and started to play with the dog. Levinson began using pets as a way to break the ice with his young patients.[103]

The second landmark event also occurred quite by accident. In the mid-1970s, Ohio State University psychologist Samuel A. Corson kept a kennel of dogs on the grounds for use in his research. When mental patients in an adjoining hospital heard the dogs barking, they insisted on seeing the dogs. They began to visit, they developed relationships filled with trust and affection, and as a result they were able to trust their physicians and make great progress in their treatment.[104]

The final landmark event in pet studies occurred in 1980 when University of Pennsylvania researchers Aaron Katcher and Erika Friedmann found that people with pets lived longer after experiencing heart attacks than did those without pets[105] and that pet ownership may facilitate both physical and mental fitness. Subsequent research has shown that among people who have heart attacks, pet owners have one-fifth the death rate of those who do not have pets.[106]

The benefits of pet ownership even extend to a population that is traditionally the most prone to health problems: the elderly. A study by Judith M. Siegel and her colleagues at UCLA followed 1,000 Medicare enrollees for one year. The elderly were interviewed at the beginning of the study and then every two months throughout the year of the study. In addition, they were assessed for psychological distress at 6 months and 12 months. Siegel found that more than one-third of the people involved in the study owned pets—cats, dogs, birds, and fish.[107]

She found that pet owners enjoyed better health and had fewer visits to the doctor than did those without pets. Even among those under the most stress during the year of the study, the pet owners had 16 percent fewer physician visits.

Of interest was the finding that the greatest benefit seemed to come from dog ownership—perhaps because those who owned dogs "spent more time outdoors with them, spent more time talking to them, felt more attached to them, and, during the course of the study, had fewer physician contacts than other pet owners."[108] Researchers found that even the most highly stressed dog owners in the study had 21 percent fewer physician contacts than did people without pets.[109]

People who own pets have better health, recover more quickly from all kinds of illness and surgery, and live longer lives than those who don't have pets.

As the title of Shelley Levitt's article says, "Pet Two Poodles and Call Me in the Morning."[110]

Why Pets Benefit Health

Pets, among other things, alleviate loneliness. They provide companionship. They make us feel safe. They help us feel calm. No matter what else may happen around us, they are a constant amid the change. And they can exert an overall good influence. University of California, Davis, researchers found that elderly people with pets not only enjoyed an improvement in their well-being but worked actively to improve their overall living conditions, too.[111]

As mentioned, the first notice of the health benefits of pets on a scientific level was quite by accident. A team of medical researchers from the University of Maryland and the University of Pennsylvania designed and carried out a study to determine how social conditions affect heart disease. They delved into the backgrounds and living conditions of people who had been hospitalized with heart disease. They checked out income, marital status, lifestyle, and a number of other "social" factors. A year after the patients were released from the hospital, researchers followed up to see which ones were still alive. They also did detailed computer analyses to figure out which factors had helped keep those patients alive.

People who owned pets had fared much better than people who didn't. In fact, three times as many of the nonowners had died in the year since they had been released from the hospital![112] One of the reasons may be, simply, that pets enhance social interactions between people, and pet owners are more likely to have strong social interactions—which have been shown in numerous studies to benefit both health and longevity.[113]

The Cardiovascular System

One of the studies almost exactly duplicated the initial, accidental study. At the University of Pennsylvania's Center for Interaction of Animals and Society, researchers studied 92 patients who had been hospitalized for coronary disease. Those with pets had one-third the death rate of the people who did not have pets. In that study, researchers discovered one possible reason for the coronary survivals: Patients actually had lower heart rates when they were with their pets. Friedmann maintains that's an important result because "even small reductions in the heart rate repeated thousands of times per week could provide direct health benefits by decreasing the frequency of arterial damage, and thus slowing the arteriosclerotic process. The results of this research may have important implications for middle-aged and elderly individuals with a variety of stress-related chronic diseases."[114] Subsequent research at Brooklyn College showed that pets do, indeed, slow the heart rate, even among high-stressed, high-intensity, type A personalities.

Studies show that pet owners tend to have lower blood pressure,[115] lower levels of triglycerides in the blood, and lower cholesterol—findings that are especially pronounced in men over the age of 40. Other studies have shown that pet owners have better survival rates after heart attack, and that simply getting a pet is associated with an elevated sense of psychological well-being.[116]

Pets have another important effect on the cardiovascular system: they help reduce blood pressure. In a number of studies, pets of all kinds have been shown to lower blood pressure. Petting a dog decreased blood pressure among healthy college students, hospitalized elderly, and adults with hypertension. The blood pressure of bird owners dropped an average of ten points when they were talking to their birds. Watching fish in an aquarium brought blood pressure to below resting levels.[117]

One of the least sterile and most clinical studies was carried out by researcher James Lynch in the recreation room of his home with the help of his three children. For the study, Lynch and his kids invited neighborhood children to come over and read in the recreation room. Each child's blood pressure was measured both while sitting quietly and while reading aloud—and both while alone and while a dog was in the room. The kids had lower blood pressure while the dog was in the room, whether they were sitting quietly or reading aloud. The dog seemed to be what made the difference.[118] Some researchers think pets help lower blood pressure because of their calming influence and because most people slow down and become more calm and gentle when talking to their pets.

People in hospitals, including mental hospitals, recover more completely and more quickly and are discharged sooner if they have pets waiting for them at home. The patients might feel a responsibility for the pet and want to get home to resume caring for the pet. Some hospitals have started allowing pets to visit patients, a practice that has been found to speed recovery. Swedish-American Hospital in Rockford, Illinois, initiated use of a "pet visiting room," where pets can be brought to visit their hospitalized owners. Researchers in charge of the project have found that visits from pets calm the patient, boost patient morale, and improve and speed postsurgical recovery.[119] Many believe that, for the patients, the pet represents an important source of companionship and love and an alleviation of loneliness. And study results still point to the effect of reducing blood pressure.

Effects of reducing blood pressure have been most profound among elderly people and children, even though it seems to work regardless of age. In one experiment, children at the University of Pennsylvania School of Veterinary Medicine were brought into a room and interviewed by a stranger. The reaction of the children was predictable: they experienced stress, and their blood pressure increased. When a friendly dog was brought into the room, the children relaxed and their blood pressure dropped.[120]

Stress

Pets also help alleviate the effects of stress. To test that notion, researchers at the University of Oklahoma decided to try it against one of life's most stressful situations: the death of a spouse.[121] Researchers compared two groups of recent widows; one group had pets and the other did not. The two groups were studied to see how they responded in terms of physical complaints, lifestyles, interactions with others, and feelings toward self. The widows with pets did significantly better than the widows who did not have pets. Those with pets were healthier, had fewer illnesses and physical complaints, and were able to interact with others better. The widows without pets had more persistent fears, headaches, and feelings of panic—and they tended to take more medications than did the pet owners.

In another study, psychologists Karen M. Allen and James J. Blascovich of the State University of New York at Buffalo gave 45 women a challenge that's often used in the laboratory to create stress: performing mental arithmetic.[122] The women had to rapidly count backwards by threes from a four-digit number. During the test, the researchers measured the women's pulse rate, blood pressure, and electrical skin conductance—all measures that can indicate how stressed someone is feeling.

What happened? The women who had a human friend at their side during the test had poor performance and a lot of stress. The women who had their pet dogs at their side during the test did much better on the arithmetic—and they did it with lower blood pressure and fewer other physical responses to stress.[123]

Pet-Facilitated Therapy

Pets have been shown to have such a benefit on both physical and mental health that they are now being used in a whole new field of therapy called pet-facilitated therapy. They are being used with hospitalized patients, with mental patients, with the elderly in convalescent centers, and even in prisons.

In one of the most successful programs of its kind, social worker David Lee of Lima State Hospital for the Criminally Insane in Ohio introduced small animals—fish, parakeets, and so on—to the prisoners as "mascots." Among the prisoners were murderers, rapists, and others who had committed violent crimes. Allowing the criminals to care for the animals almost completely stopped suicide attempts and fighting among prisoners.[124]

Recent findings in a St. Louis nursing home showed that you may not need the real thing: a sophisticated robotic dog appeared to work equally well as a real dog in alleviating loneliness and allowing nursing home residents to form attachments.[125]

WHAT DID YOU LEARN?

1. What is the difference between loneliness and being alone?
2. How common is loneliness in America?
3. What are the major causes/risk factors for loneliness?
4. What are the major health consequences of loneliness?
5. How may having good friends and pet ownership dispel loneliness?

ENDNOTES

1. Louise Bernikow, *Alone in America* (New York: Harper & Row, 1986).
2. Harry T. Reis, "Relationship Experiences and Emotional Well-Being," in Carol D. Ryff and Burton H. Singer, eds., *Emotion, Social Relationships, and Health* (New York: Oxford University Press, 2001).
3. Susan L. Duncan, "Loneliness: A Health Hazard of Modern Times," *Interactions* 13, no. 1 (1995): 5–9.
4. Joan Borysenko, *Fire in the Soul* (New York: Warner Books, 1993), 83.
5. "Loneliness: A Healthy Approach," *Longevity* (April 1990): 22.
6. Boris Blai, "Health Consequences of Loneliness: A Review of the Literature," *Journal of American College Health* 37 (1989): 163.
7. Blai, "Health Consequences of Loneliness."
8. Ibid., 163.
9. Louise Hawkley and John Cacioppo, "Loneliness and Its Effects on Health," *Current Directions in Psychological Science* (August 2007).

10. Robert Ornstein and David Sobel, *Healthy Pleasures* (Reading, MA: Addison-Wesley, 1989), 222–23.
11. "You're Not Alone When It Comes to Loneliness," *Harvard Health Letter* 24, no. 7 (1999): 4.
12. Bill Harms, "New Research Reveals How Loneliness Can Undermine Health," *The University of Chicago Chronicle* 19, no. 20 (August 17, 2000).
13. Anne Morrow Lindbergh *Gift from the Sea* (New York: Random House, 1997), 122.
14. John Cacioppo, "Biological Costs of Social Stress in the Elderly" (paper delivered at a meeting of the American Psychological Association, Washington, DC, August 6, 2000).
15. "Census: More Americans Living Alone," *USA Today* (September 2, 2005).
16. "Americans Marrying Older, Living Alone More, See Households Shrinking, Census Bureau Reports," *U. S. Census Bureau News* (May 25, 2006).
17. Marc Pilisuk and Susan Hillier Parks, *The Healing Web* (Hanover, NH: University Press of New England, 1986).
18. "Americans Marrying Older, Living Alone More, See Households Shrinking, Census Bureau Reports," *U.S. Census Bureau News* (May 25, 2006).
19. "Domestic Migration Across Regions, Divisions, and States: 1995 to 2000," *Census 2000 Special Reports* (August 2003): 1.
20. Pilisuk and Parks, *The Healing Web.*
21. Carin Rubenstein and Phillip Shaver, "Are You Lonely? How to Find Intimacy, Love, and Happiness," *Shape* (August 1987): 72.
22. Rubenstein and Shaver, "Are You Lonely?" 75.
23. Larry Dossey, *Meaning and Medicine* (New York: Bantam, 1991), 70.
24. Hafen and Frandsen, *People Need People* (Cordillera Press, 1987).
25. S. Lau and C. K. Kong, "The Acceptance of Lonely Others: Effects of Loneliness and Gender of the Target Person and Loneliness of the Perceiver," *Journal of Social Psychology* 139, no. 2 (April 1999): 229–41.
26. Duncan, "Loneliness."
27. "You're Not Alone."
28. "Most Senior Citizens Experience Loneliness, Say Researchers," *SeniorJournal.com,* from www.rotaryclubofsantamonica.org/In%20The%20News/2002-2003/ seniorjournaldotcom.htm, posted November 21, 2005.
29. Pirkko E. Routasalo et al., "Social Contacts and Their Relationship to Loneliness Among Aged People—A Population-Based Study," *Gerontology* 52 (2006): 181–7.
30. Ibid.
31. J. R. Vicary and D. A. Corneal, "A Comparison of Young Women's Psychosocial Status Based on Age of Their First Childbirth," *Family Community Health* 24, no. 2 (July 2001): 73–84.
32. D. B. Hudson, S. M. Elek, and C. Campbell-Gorssman, "Depression, Self-Esteem, Loneliness, and Social Support Among Adolescent Mothers Participating in the New Parents Project," *Adolescence* 35, no. 139 (Autumn 2000): 445–53.
33. Bernikow, 18.
34. Ibid.
35. Hafen and Frandsen, *People Need People* (Cordillera Press, 1987), 32.
36. T. Koropeckyj-Cox, "Loneliness and Depression in Middle and Old Age: Are the Childless More Vulnerable?" *Journals of Gerontology Series B Psychological Sciences and Social Sciences* 53, no. 6 (November 1998): S303–12.
37. Cacioppo, "Biological Costs of Social Stress."

38. A. Steptoe, N. Owen, S. R. Kunz-Ebrecht, and L. Brydon, "Loneliness and Neuroendocrine, Cardiovascular, and Inflammatory Stress Responses in Middle-Aged Men and Women," *Psychoneuroendocrinology* 29, no. 5 (June 2004): 593–611.
39. Reis, "Relationship Experiences and Emotional Well-Being."
40. Ibid., 33.
41. Ibid.
42. Sheldon Cohen, "Social Relationships and Susceptibility to the Common Cold," in Chapter 7, Carol D. Ryff and Burton H. Singer, eds., *Emotion, Social Relationships, and Health* (New York: Oxford University Press, 2001).
43. "You're Not Alone."
44. Ibid.
45. Noreen E. Mahon, Adela Yarcheski, and Thomas J. Yarcheski, "Social Support and Positive Health Practices in Young Adults," *Clinical Nursing Research* 7, no. 3 (1998): 292–308.
46. L. C. Hawkley and J. T. Cacioppo, "Loneliness and Pathways to Disease," *Brain, Behavior, and Immunity* 17, suppl. 1 (February 2003): S98–105.
47. Cacioppo, "Biological Costs of Social Stress."
48. L. C. Hawkley and J. T. Cacioppo, "Loneliness and Pathways to Disease."
49. Cohen, "Social Relationships and Susceptibility."
50. Bernikow, *Alone in America,* 18.
51. "Why Loneliness May Damage Health," *BBC News* (September 12, 2007).
52. Ibid.
53. A. M. Ponizovsky and M. S. Ritsner, "Patterns of Loneliness in an Immigrant Population," *Comprehensive Psychiatry* 45, no. 5 (September–October 2004): 408–14.
54. Hawkley and Cacioppo, "Loneliness and Pathways to Disease, " 98–105.
55. Dossey, *Meaning and Medicine,* 94.
56. Ibid.
57. Pilisuk and Parks, *The Healing Web.*
58. Ibid.
59. "Lack of Social Relationships Increases Risk of Illness and Death," *Wellness Newsletter* (November–December 1988): 4.
60. Robert Ornstein and David Sobel, *The Healing Brain* (New York: Simon & Schuster, 1987), 195–6.
61. Ibid.
62. Ibid.
63. Bruce Bower, "Emotional Aid Delivers Labor-Saving Results," *Science News* 139 (1991): 277.
64. Robert S. Wilson et al., "Loneliness and Risk of Alzheimer Disease," *Archives of General Psychiatry* 64 (February 2, 2007): 234–40.
65. Sharon Faelten, David Diamond, and the editors of *Prevention* magazine, *Take Control of Your Life: A Complete Guide to Stress Relief* (Emmaus, PA: Rodale Press, 1988), 58.
66. Frances Sheridan Goulart, "How to Live a Longer, Healthier Life," (n.p., n.d.).
67. "Lack of Social Relationships," 4.
68. Gyanish Gungaram, "Serious Health Risks of Loneliness: How to Cultivate New Friendships and Live Longer," *Diethack* (March 18, 2008).
69. Duncan, "Loneliness."
70. Miranda Hitti, "Researchers Say Lonely College Freshmen Show Weaker Immune Response," *WebMD Health News,* from http://www.webmd.com/ accessed May 2, 2005.
71. Barbara R. Sarason, Irwin G. Sarason, and Gregory R. Pierce, *Social Support: An Interactional View* (New York: John Wiley & Sons, 1990), 256; and J. Stephen Heisel, Steven E. Locke, Linda J. Kraus, and R. Michael Williams, "Natural Killer Cell Activity and

MMPI Scores of a Cohort of College Students," *American Journal of Psychiatry* 143 (1986): 1382–6.

72. Janice Kiecolt-Glaser and Ronald Glaser, "Q & A," *Medical Aspects of Human Sexuality* 19, no. 12: 56–57.

73. "Depression and Immunity," *Harvard Medical School Mental Health Letter* (n.d.): 8.

74. Ibid., 8.

75. Hawkley and Cacioppo, "Loneliness and Its Effects on Health," 2007.

76. Ibid.

77. Alix Kerr, "Hearts Need Friends," *Physician's Weekly*, (n.d.).

78. "Social Isolation Tied to Heart Attack Deaths," *Deseret News* (May 1, 1988): A10.

79. The editors of *Prevention* magazine, *Positive Living and Health: The Complete Guide to Brain/Body Healing and Mental Empowerment* (Emmaus, PA: Rodale Press, 1990), 154.

80. Ibid.

81. Rolf Bang Olsen, Jorn Olsen, Finn Gunner-Svennsson, and Bodil Waldstrom, "Social Networks and Longevity: A 14-Year Follow-up Study Among Elderly in Denmark," *Social Science Medicine* 33, no. 10 (1999): 1189–95.

82. "Loneliness Linked to High Blood Pressure," *CBS News* (March 28, 2006).

83. Lynch, *The Broken Heart* (New York: Basic Books 1985), 183.

84. Ibid., 183.

85. Ibid., 184.

86. Ibid., 184.

87. Bernikow, *Alone in America*.

88. Michael Argyle, *The Psychology of Happiness* (New York: Methuen and Company, 1987).

89. Sheldon Cohen and S. Leonard Syme, *Social Support and Health* (Orlando, FL: Academic Press, 1985).

90. Cohen and Syme, *Social Support and Health*.

91. Leonard A. Sagan, *The Health of Nations* (New York: Basic Books, 1987).

92. Ibid.

93. Argyle, *The Psychology of Happiness*.

94. Ibid., 182–83.

95. Faelten, Diamond, and the editors of *Prevention* magazine, *Take Control of Your Life*, 272.

96. Ibid.

97. J. W. Pennebaker et al., "Disclosure of Traumas and Health among Holocaust Survivors," *Psychosomatic Medicine* 51 (1989): 577–89.

98. Sarah Hoying, "Confess for Your Health?" *Self* (September 1990): 96.

99. Faelten, Diamond, and the editors of *Prevention* magazine, *Take Control of Your Life*, 273.

100. "Loneliness May Be Alleviated by Animals, Gadgets, Spiritual Beliefs, Not Just People," *Medical News Today* (January 21, 2008, reporting on article in February 2008 *Psychological Science*).

101. Robert Ornstein and Charles Swencionis, *The Healing Brain: A Scientific Reader* (New York: Guilford Press, 1990), 93.

102. Lea B. Jennings, "Potential Benefits of Pet Ownership in Health Promotion," *Journal of Holistic Nursing* 15, no. 4: 358–72.

103. Editors of *Prevention* magazine, *Positive Living and Health*, 298.

104. Ornstein and Sobel, *The Healing Brain*, 229.

105. Jennings, "Potential Benefits of Pet Ownership."

106. Ibid.

107. "Health Benefits of Pet Ownership," *Journal of Personality and Social Psychology* 115, no. 4 (June 1990): 423.

108. "Pet Ownership Reduces Stress and Physician Visits Among Elderly," *Healthline* (October 1990), 8, originally cited by the American Psychological Association.

109. "Health Benefits of Pet Ownership," *Journal of Personality and Social Psychology.*

110. Shelley Levitt, "Pet Two Poodles and Call Me in the Morning," *50 Plus* (July 1988): 56–61.

111. Editors of *Prevention* magazine, *Positive Living and Health,* 157.

112. Lynne Lohmeier, "The Healing Power of Pets," *East/West* (June 1988): 52.

113. June McNicholas and Glyn M. Collis, "Dogs as Catalysts for Social Interactions: Robustness of the Effect," *British Journal of Psychology* 19, no. 1 (February 2000): 61.

114. Leavitt, 57.

115. Duncan, "Loneliness."

116. McNicholas and Collis, "Dogs as Catalysts for Social Interactions."

117. Lohmeier, "The Healing Power of Pets," 58.

118. Ornstein and Sobel, *The Healing Brain,* 166.

119. Editors of *Prevention* magazine, *Positive Living and Health,* 235.

120. Hafen and Frandsen, *People Need People* (Cordillera Press, 1987), 78.

121. Bruce Bower, "Stress Goes to the Dogs," *Science News* 140 (1992): 285.

122. Ibid.

123. Ibid.

124. Karen M. Allen, "The Human-Animal Bond," *Insights* (n.d.): 5.

125. "Doggie Robot Eases Loneliness in Nursing Home Residents as Well as Real Dog, Study Finds," *Science Daily,* February 26, 2008.

CHAPTER 11

Marriage and Health

To be happy at home is the ultimate result of all ambition.

—Samuel Johnson

LEARNING OBJECTIVES

- Understand the health hazards related to divorce for both adults and children.
- Identify how divorce differs from an unhappy marriage in impacting health.
- Understand the health benefits of a happy marriage.

Marriage—a good one, that is—has all kinds of benefits. According to psychologist John Gottman, a pioneer in the field of marriage research and the James Mifflin Professor in the University of Washington Department of Psychology, those benefits include "better physical health, more resistance to infection, fewer infections, and a reduced likelihood of dying from cancer, from heart disease, from all major killers. The other health benefit is longevity: People live longer if they are in marital relationships, particularly if they are good, satisfying relationships. There are physical benefits and mental health benefits. You have less depression, less anxiety disorders, less posttraumatic stress disorders, fewer phobias. You also have fewer injuries due to accidents."

Divorced people and those who are unhappily married don't fare nearly as well in terms of health and long life. A four-year survey conducted by the National Center for Health Statistics showed that married adults are generally healthier than adults with any other marital status,[1] and evidence from more than five dozen articles published in the past decade show that martial functioning has significant consequences on health.[2] And the impact seems to vary, depending on age and gender (the health impact of dissolving a marriage seems to be greatest on men).[3]

According to the latest census figures, marriage demographics have changed dramatically over the last decade. Today, 25 million American adults live alone, and married couples make up the smallest percentage of the nation's households in two centuries. According to the U. S. Census Bureau from the 2000 census (the most recent actual data available), only 59 percent of the nation's households include married couples—down from 62 percent in 1990 and 72 percent in 1970. In fact, in 2005 the Census Bureau said the number of unmarried women would soon surpass the number of married women in the United States. The number of "unmarried couple households" (those people who are living together but who are not married) is increasing steadily: up to 3.7 million in 2000.

The Health Hazards of Divorce

Divorce rates have been on a roller coaster in this country since the end of World War I, when family life was pretty stable and the divorce rate was relatively low. Following World War II, when soldiers started coming back from the war, the divorce rate soared but only temporarily. For a period of time after World War II, the divorce rates fell back to their prewar level. Since the postwar period, divorce rates have steadily increased—from about 10 percent in the early 1950s to a rate that approaches 50 percent today. In one disturbing trend, increasing numbers of couples are ending longtime marriages. The percentage of divorces among people over the age of 65 more than doubled in the past two decades. Research Associate Professor Marjorie A. Pett of the University of Utah pinpointed five basic reasons for divorce among older couples: they had grown apart and no longer shared dreams, they had personal differences, there was an extramarital relationship, the couples had poor communication, and the marriage was plagued by financial difficulty.

Overall, as a country, the United States has the highest divorce rate in the world.[4] According to statistics, the parents of more than 1 million children divorce in the United States every year.[5] Those same statistics tell us that 30 percent of America's white children and 40 percent of black children spend at least part of their formative years in postdivorce, single-parent families. More than 90 percent of all postdivorce children live with their mother—and only one in three children see their noncustodial parent as often as once a month.

Increasingly, children are being subjected to a second divorce during their childhood. The custodial parent of more than 70 percent of all white children involved in divorce remarries within five years, and more than half of those divorce a second time.[6] The median age at the time of a *second* divorce is 34 for men, 32 for women.[7] According to researchers, the children of these "twice-divorced parents are often seriously disturbed."[8]

Effects on Children

The effect of divorce on children is perhaps a good starting point in the discussion of how divorce impacts health because it is often the children who suffer the most profoundly. And the suffering is long-lasting as well as deep, according to a study that followed more than 100 children for 15 years following their parents' divorce.[9]

Researcher Ann S. Masten points out:

> A stressful event rarely occurs in isolation. Divorce is not a single event, but a series of related events embedded in the ongoing lives of people. It often occurs in the context of extreme family conflict and emotional crisis. It can precipitate recurrent financial

problems and separations, custodial conflicts, changes of school, home, and daily routine. Above all, divorce can be so devastating to the parents that the children temporarily lose the most important protective factor in their lives, a healthy, well-functioning caregiver.[10]

The numbers of children affected by divorce and the profile of those caregivers have changed steadily over the past few decades. The number of single-parent families has more than doubled since 1978, and the percentage of children living in single-parent families rose from 9 percent in 1960 to 30 percent in 2005.[11] According to *The State of Our Unions 2005,* a report issued by the National Marriage Project at Rutgers University, only 63 percent of American children grow up with both biological parents—the lowest rate in the Western world. As of 2003, 43.7 percent of custodial mothers and 56.2 percent of custodial fathers were either separated or divorced. Although the largest category of single-parent families is that headed by a divorced mother, the number of children living with the father alone has more than doubled since 1970.[12] Even children living in two-parent families are not immune from the stresses involved in divorce. Many are living with one parent who is not their natural parent. The often hostile relationships that exist between stepparents and stepchildren are well known.

However, parents of conventional two-parent families can't be too smug about their children being protected from the damaging consequences of divorce. With the increasing frequency and visibility of divorce, even children in stable families are anxious about the possibility of it affecting them.

For children, divorce is one of the most disruptive life events possible—and it leads to changes in biological health. Children almost universally experience divorce as a profound personal, familial, and social loss.[13] In addition to health problems, most children involved in divorce suffer emotional and behavioral changes that can also impact health. Adding insult to injury, most divorced families end up with less affluence—forcing children along with the rest of the family to adjust to a whole new spectrum of reduced economic advantages.

There is a wide range of social, academic, and health problems associated with the children of divorce. According to researchers cited in *City Journal,* the nation's premiere urban policy magazine, children who grow up outside of intact marriages are much more likely to "slip into poverty, become victims of child abuse, fail at school and drop out, use illegal drugs, launch into premature sexual activity, become unwed teen mothers, divorce, commit suicide, and experience other signs of mental illness, become physically ill, and commit crimes and go to jail."[14] They visit health clinics and physicians more often; and some childhood cancer and other alterations in physical health as a result of injury have been strongly associated with divorce.[15] On the emotional side, children are prone to become depressed and aggressive and to suffer regression in development; some develop psychosomatic disorders. Many adopt delinquent behavior. Boys especially seem to bear the brunt of divorce. Studies have shown that, following a divorce, boys (more than girls) suffer from poor self-image, loss of self-concept, bedwetting, a sense of sorrow, below-average academic performance, anger, withdrawal, delinquent-like behavior, aggression, and frequent fighting.[16]

Divorce is particularly damaging to a child's emotional and physical health if it involves a move. Moves have been implicated in "a variety of childhood disorders" and, coupled with the stress of a divorce, can be very damaging to a child. "For children especially," researchers say, "stable identification with a place and home seems to represent an important predictor of health."[17]

Effects on Adults

Children aren't the only ones who face health risks following divorce. Every major study agrees that divorced people—and others who are separated from their spouses—experience more physical and mental illness than do those who are married. Divorced people visit physicians significantly more often than do married or single people.[18] Through in-depth studies, divorce has been significantly related to depression,[19] alcoholism, increased traffic accidents, admission to psychiatric facilities, homicides, and death from disease in general.[20] A review found that 70 percent of chronic problem drinkers were either separated or divorced; only 15 percent were married—and single men are more than three times as likely to die of cirrhosis of the liver.[21] According to research, divorce has the same impact on health as smoking a pack of cigarettes a day.[22] Furthermore, most therapists agree that divorced people have higher rates of cancer, heart disease, pneumonia, high blood pressure, and accidental death than do married, single, or widowed persons.[23]

Many theories have been extended to explain why. Perhaps it is because a person who has just been through a divorce all too often loses a major source of protecting social support: the family. The family of origin may not approve of the divorce or may be going through its own crises at the time, unable to spare the considerable emotional strength to be of real support. Access to needed resources may also play a role: Women have low relative income compared to men, and divorce has been solidly shown to increase female poverty.[24] The difficulty of coping with divorce is considerable. According to one prominent researcher, new evidence suggests that divorce may be even more devastating to many people than losing a spouse to death, "since it's harder to accept that the relationship is really over."[25]

Various studies give insight into the specific health hazards of divorce. In one study, divorced Caucasian men under age 70 who live alone have twice the death rate from heart disease, stomach cancer, and cirrhosis of the liver, and three times the incidence of high blood pressure of married men under age 70. James Lynch, who has done extensive research into the phenomenon of divorce and loneliness, says those facts are true for both men and women of all ages.[26]

In another study,[27]British researchers looked at two groups of people in their forties from the MRC National Survey of Health and Development. The people in one group were married and had never been divorced or separated. The people in the second group had been divorced or separated at least once. A total of 2,085 people participated in the study. After all other traditional risk factors were considered, researchers found that divorce and separation were strongly associated with depression and anxiety and increased the risk of alcohol abuse. These risks were true even for those who were remarried or who had reunited with their spouses at the time of the study.

Statistics from a variety of nations reveal a significantly higher death rate among divorced men and women than among the married. The divorced die much more frequently from suicide, homicide, and accidental death. The death rate among the divorced is also significantly higher for alcoholism, diabetes, tuberculosis, and lung cancer.[28]

Research has shown that divorce can actually compromise the immune system, which helps explain why there is an increase in illness and death among the divorced. Immune system compromise is especially apparent the first year following divorce. A study of divorced or separated women during the first year following divorce or separation showed that they had poor cellular immune function, a lower number of natural killer cells, and a deficit in their ability to fight disease with responsive lymphocytes.[29]

Research shows that age at the time of divorce may significantly influence how the divorce impacts health. In one study,[30] researchers from the University of Pennsylvania did two successive five-year studies on a large national sample of women (originally derived from the National Longitudinal Surveys of Young Women). When the study started, all women were between the ages of 24 and 34; researchers compared those who had never been married with those who had been divorced or separated. At the conclusion of the first study, the women who had never married had worse health trends and worse overall health than those who had been divorced or separated. However, at the conclusion of the second study, when the women were older, it was the divorced and separated women who had experienced the more harmful health effects—findings that were exactly reversed when compared to the first study.

For some reason, divorce also seems to have its most deleterious effects on men. Divorced men suffer significantly more disease and die in far greater numbers before the age of 64 than do their married counterparts. The statistics are sobering. Ten times as many die of tuberculosis; seven times as many die of pneumonia and are killed in homicides. More than twice as many die of heart disease, and almost three times as many die of lung cancer. More than twice as many die of complications of strokes, of cancer of the digestive system, and of high blood pressure. More than three times as many commit suicide, and almost eight times as many die of cirrhosis of the liver. Almost four times as many are killed in motor vehicle accidents.[31]

Dr. Robert Seagraves of the University of Chicago Medical School points out:

> It is difficult for happily married individuals to appreciate the extent of disruption caused by divorce. The individual has lost a social network as well as a spouse. Typically, close friends of married couples are themselves married, and many of these friendships are lost following divorce. The divorced individual reenters the world of dating, feeling rusty in middle age, and facing the same insecurities experienced as a teenager.[32]

Studies show that in all psychiatric hospitals, divorced people are overrepresented— and married people are underrepresented. Risks of disease in almost every category soar with divorce. And, apparently, divorce even affects longevity, as clearly evidenced by the fact that the state of Nevada had the second highest death rate from all causes in the United States during the years when it was the divorce center of the country.[33]

Divorce has also been shown to have a particular result on the aging: Those older people who divorce are often forced to live with adult children, get financial assistance from adult children, rely on adult children for informal care, or pay for help from non-related caregivers. The effects are most pronounced for elderly men, and remarriage can often cause even more deleterious effects, especially for stepchildren.[34]

The Divorced Versus the Unhappily Married

New evidence shows that unhappily married people may be the worst off in terms of good health and long life! All social relationships involve some level of stress—and involve both wanted and unwanted demands, gratification, conflict, irritation, and pleasure.[35] The stress this creates is even more intense in an intimate relationship as important as marriage. While the health benefits of a good marriage are well recognized and documented, negative impact on health can occur when the marriage involves things like frequent conflict, anger, jealousy, criticism, moodiness, extreme financial problems, abuse, emotional or physical violence, or sexual assault.[36] According to research, the bad effects of a negative marriage are significantly stronger than the good effects from a positive marriage.[37] In fact, an unhappy marriage can increase the chance of becoming ill by 35 percent and can reduce longevity by four years for both men and women.[38]

Research results from a number of cross-sectional studies are all showing that unhappily married people have poorer health than their single counterparts—even the ones who are divorced. An unhappy marriage is linked not only to lifestyle risk factors and nonadherence to medical regimens, but to more depression, hostility, and anger.[39] Apparently, a major variable in marriage and health is happiness: It isn't just being married that gives you a better chance of being psychologically well-adjusted and physically healthier, but being happily married.[40] According to research, unhappily married people are, healthwise, worse off than anyone else.[41]

Studies now offer preliminary evidence that actual physical changes occur during marital conflict. Couples who handle conflict in a negative way don't heal as well. Studies show that couples in unhappy marriages that handled conflict with sarcasm and put-downs healed 40 percent more slowly than those in happy marriages who handled conflict in a positive way. And the impact was more profound on women. "Biologically, the different reactions women have . . . are enormous. Women just have a more intense physiological reaction to hostility in relationships than men do," said Janice Kiecolt-Glaser, Director of Health Psychology at Ohio State University's College of Medicine.[42] A different study, however, showed that men and women in bad relationships face equal health risks.[43]

According to researchers at Stanford University, blood pressure is strongly correlated to positive and negative interactions: During positive interactions, blood pressure is lower, but during negative interactions—fights—it can skyrocket.[44] Similar research at the University of Washington and the University of California, Berkeley, shows that marital conflict affects the heart rate, pulse, and skin resistance.[45] Critical to maintaining health is to eliminate criticism, contempt, defensiveness, and "stonewalling" (refusing to respond) from conflict: Research shows it's not the conflict itself that causes the problems, but the way people generally respond to conflict.[46]

New studies show that marital fights actually weaken the immune system (especially in women), raise blood pressure, and speed up heart rate. A host of studies shows that marital stress plays a significant role in overall health, increasing the risk for everything from chronic pain to heart attack. Research, in fact, has shown that the risk of a bad marriage is as strong as other medical risks.[47] For women, simply discussing their angry feelings leads to these stressed-out body reactions. For men, the stress seems to accompany the act of talking louder and faster.

In one study, researchers brought 90 newlywed couples into the laboratory, those you would normally expect to have the least amount of conflict. The researchers gave each couple a role-play and asked them to resolve the disagreement involved. Interestingly, researchers noted a number of hostile behaviors—including criticizing, denying responsibility, interrupting, disagreeing, making excuses, and trying to coerce each other into accepting their point of view—even among what researchers considered to be mild disputes.[48]

Scientists monitored the couples' blood continuously for the next 24 hours to determine immune response, including measures of natural killer cells, which fight off infection.

"There was a far stronger effect on the immune system than we ever anticipated," said psychologist Janice Kiecolt-Glaser and immunologist Ronald Glaser, both of Ohio State University. "Those couples who expressed the most hostility during the discussions showed a drop of eight measures [of immunity] for the next 24 hours."[49]

The effects of an unhappy marriage apparently differ when it comes to gender. Another study of newlyweds conducted at Ohio State University showed that among those in unhappy marriages, the impact was greater on the women. Women who talked about the negative aspects of their marriages produced more cortisol, a hormone characteristically produced during stress, than the men who discussed the negative aspects of their marriages. Interestingly, the amount of cortisol produced by the men didn't have any correlation to their marital status 8 to 10 years later—but the women who produced more cortisol as they talked about their marriages were more than twice as likely to be divorced a decade later.[50]

The gender difference seems to persist throughout life. When researchers studied older couples who had been married an average of 42 years, they found that stress hormones increased during conflict—but only among women.[51]

In reporting on a large study conducted by the Human Population Laboratory of the California Department of Public Health, researchers believe that, in terms of health and longevity, it's better to be single than unhappily married. Unhappy marriage has been implicated in a number of specific health problems by teams of researchers who have studied large groups of people. Coronary disease is among the most prevalent among the unhappily married. In one revealing study, researchers screened 10,000 Israeli men before any symptoms of coronary heart disease had appeared. They then observed this population for five years. The men who later had a myocardial infarction reported far more dissatisfaction with their marital life than did those men who remained healthy.[52]

Separate studies seem to confirm these findings. Patients with coronary heart disease reported far more frequent dissatisfaction in their marriages than did those without heart disease—and they reported far more marital problems. A series of recent reports has revealed a trend: The occurrence of marital dissatisfaction and a sense of personal rejection stemming from unhappy marriage is the apparent trigger for a surprising number of acute myocardial infarctions.

A study of more than 9,000 couples showed that those with the worst marriages were 34 percent more likely to have heart attacks or other cardiac problems over a twelve-year period than were those who had good relationships, even if the good relationships were with partners, close relatives, and friends. Lead researcher Roberto de Vogli said that the quality of the marriage matters significantly.[53]

Psychologist Vicki Helgeson of Carnegie-Mellon University found in a recent study that male cardiac patients were far less prone to follow-up heart attacks if they were able to discuss matters easily with their wives. Married men in the study who reported poor communication with their wives fared even worse than those who were not married. According to Helgeson, "The strong influence of good marriages has caused a general misappraisal of marriage's role in preserving health. A poor marriage may be worse than none at all."[54]

Marital problems apparently can also drive up blood pressure. Recent research done at Brigham Young University shows that a happy marriage is good for blood pressure, but an unhappy marriage has greater negative impact on blood pressure than does being single. The more marital satisfaction, the lower the average blood pressure, but those in unhappy marriages had higher average blood pressure than did single people. "I think this study is worth some attention," responded Karen Matthews, a professor of psychiatry, psychology, and epidemiology at the University of Pittsburgh.[55]

Researchers at the Department of Psychology at the University of Michigan and at the university's School of Public Health studied almost 700 men and women for 12 years.[56] They found that people with unhappy marriages, especially those who can't easily express their anger, are at twice the risk of death. One key appears to be the way they deal with anger and conflict. Those who suppress anger suffer the greatest consequence of all among the unhappily married. The risks of high blood pressure are greatest for women between the ages of 45 and 69, who are the most likely to suppress their anger, and for unhappily married women between the ages of 30 and 44, who are apt to feel guilty about expressing anger toward their husbands.

Those who are unhappily married are at a much higher risk for all kinds of illness. A reason could be reduced functioning in the immune system.[57]

Interestingly, preliminary data show that women may bear the greatest health brunt of unhappy marriages. Psychologist Robert W. Levenson of the University of California, Berkeley, studied married couples to determine the health effects of unhappiness in marriage.[58] In Levenson's study, there was no correlation between unhappiness in marriage and the well-being of the husbands. On the other hand, the wives in those unhappy marriages suffered from anxiety, depression, and other stress-related illnesses.

In commenting on the study, psychologist Lynn Fainsilber Katz said that our culture makes emotional work "more of a woman's job. Women take on more of the responsibility for regulating the marriage, and in a distressed marriage, this takes a toll."[59]

In a study done by researchers from San Diego State University and the University of Pittsburgh, women in happy marriages were compared to women in unhappy marriages and to women who were not married. Those in happy marriages had lower risk of cardiovascular disease as well as lower psychological cardiovascular risk factors, such as depression, anxiety, and anger.[60]

Finally, marital satisfaction has a real bearing on not just physical, but also mental, health. Researchers have found a definite relationship between depression and dissatisfaction with one's marriage; the marriage relationship has such an impact on mental health because it is such an important and valued social tie.[61] In a study on depression conducted by the National Institute of Mental Health, 15,000 adults were given personality surveys and other tests that helped determine their level of depression. Only 2.4 percent of single men and 3.9 percent of single women reported major episodes of depression. However, the figures changed drastically when researchers looked at those who were unhappily married: almost one-fifth of all unhappily married men and nearly half of all unhappily married women had major episodes of depression.[62]

In a survey conducted several years ago by researchers at Vanderbilt University, sociologists quizzed 1,100 people nationwide about their feelings and followed up by giving these people personality tests. Those who said they were "not too happy" or "not at all happy" with their marriages were in poorer mental health than were people who were single, divorced, or widowed.[63]

Results of a separate study were the same: In the more than 5,000 people who were extensively studied, people who were unhappy or dissatisfied with their marriages were in poorer mental health than any of the people who were single—whether they had never married, had divorced, or had been widowed. Results of a recent study on marital stress indicate that unhappy marriages have an even greater impact on mental health than on physical well-being, and the researchers from Rutgers University who authored the study call for further studies examining how marriage affects mental health.[64]

The Health Benefits of a Happy Marriage

While the relationship between marriage and health is more complex that was originally believed, the greatest benefits regarding health and long life come to those who are happily married. Studies generally have found that married people are healthier than unmarried people—whether the unmarried are never married, divorced, separated, or widowed. Those who are happily married seem healthier overall than any other group, according to government researchers with the National Center for Health Statistics. The Center, which recently completed a survey of 122,859 people in 47,240 families nationwide, found that married people have fewer health problems than do unmarried people.[65] According to the Centers for Disease Control, which co-sponsored the study, "Married persons were healthier for nearly every measure of health,"[66] something that was true for all ages, ethnicities, and levels of income and education. Charlotte Schoenborn, who was instrumental in conducting the study for the government, said that the results "demonstrate that in spite of the recent changes in American marital patterns, there is still a clear association between being well and being married."[67]

Researchers with the Framingham Heart Study, which tracked the health of more than 5,000 people for more than three decades, reported that getting—and staying—married was a predictor for a long, healthy life.[68] According to one researcher, "Studies consistently find that the married are in better mental and physical health than the unmarried. On the whole, married people live longer than the unmarried, and they make fewer demands on health care services."[69]

Why would being married help people be healthier and live longer? There are probably a number of factors at work; social, emotional, and economic, to name a few. There are two general theories. One, *marriage protection,* is the theory that married people have more advantages in terms of economic resources, social and psychological support, and support for healthy lifestyles (for example, rates of cigarette smoking are lowest among married adults). The other, *marriage selection,* is the theory that healthier people get married and stay married, whereas less healthy people either do not marry or are more likely to become separated, divorced, or widowed.[70]

In addition, there are probably other indirect factors at work. One is social support—by its very nature, marriage protects against social isolation. Generally, married people tend to eat better, take better care of themselves, and live a more stable and secure lifestyle. In addition, a spouse is more likely to influence health-promoting behaviors and to discourage risks or unhealthy behaviors. Marriage has been shown to contribute to elevated feelings of overall happiness, improve sexual fulfillment, and increase individual earnings, which leads to the fact that married people are more likely to have socioeconomic resources that enable them to obtain quality health care.[71]

Obviously, there are some differences that occur as a result of aging itself. Middle-aged adults are most likely to be married, while adults aged 65 and older are most likely to be widowed. Older adults are more likely to be in fair or poor health or to have some sort of health limitation, a situation that is compounded by widowhood: Fair or poor health is highest among widowed adults and lowest among married adults. Among the adults aged 65 and older, widows are 50 percent more likely to have some limitation in daily living activities when compared to those who are married. Those who are widowed are also the most likely to be physically inactive, which is a factor in health problems.[72]

The only area in which marriage was not correlated to health was in obesity. Married men especially are more likely to be overweight or obese, and the problem is greatest among middle-aged men: Three out of four married men between the ages of 45 and 64 are overweight or obese. Men and women who have never married are the slimmest.[73]

Social Support

Married couples are usually better integrated into the community than are single people. Although single people, especially in large cities, struggle to make friends and meet new people, married couples generally have a much easier time developing a strong social network. It may not be only the marriage, then, but also the entire spectrum of social networking that is enhanced or made easier by marriage.

One researcher believes that the health benefits of married life might be because married people seem to follow through better—maybe because each partner has someone to remind him or her. Married couples, she says, have a tendency "to eat more balanced, regular meals or to be more willing to see a doctor when they suspect something's wrong. Maybe it's having someone around to nag them, but married couples also seem to follow through more completely on taking medicines than do singles."[74]

The health benefits of marriage also might be due to economic factors, as previously mentioned. Many married couples have the benefit of double incomes, and married couples are less likely than singles or single-parent families to be living at or below poverty levels. In addition, statistics have established that the more money you make and the more educated you are, the more healthy you will generally be.[75]

The health benefits of marriage seem to be even greater for men than for women, as previously discussed. (Some studies, in fact, indicate that single women who have never married may fare almost as well as married women in terms of health and longevity.)

One reason may be the nature of the friendships outside the marriage. A man's friendships are traditionally "situational"—men have friends at work, friends they fish with, sports buddies, and so on. Women's friendships, on the other hand, are traditionally much longer and more permanent, serving as a source of great emotional strength. Women, unlike men, tend to maintain close confidants with whom they stay in regular contact after marriage. Friendships are important, even in marriage. Research shows that single people with strong networks of friends run fewer risks healthwise than do married people who are relatively isolated.

Social support and the socialization aspects of marriage may indeed play a strong role in health, and some researchers are trying to duplicate it or create a stronger social network for high-risk people, those who have separated or divorced. Results are lending credence to the belief that the social support of marriage is at least partially what helps keep married individuals healthy.

Injuries and Medical Insurance

According to a National Health Interview Survey, married people report fewer injuries per year than single and divorced people (but, interestingly, more than widowed people). The survey, which studied 122,859 Americans, showed that divorced people had "by far" the highest rate of injuries, with divorced women having more than twice as many as married women.[76]

The same survey showed an interesting trend about insurance: married people are more likely to be insured than are single people, probably—according to a National Center for Health Statistics researcher—because spouses "share each other's employment benefits."[77] According to the Center, about 84.5 percent of married women had private health insurance, compared with 66.9 percent of divorced women, 66.5 percent of widows, and 46.5 percent of those who were separated. According to government statisticians, women who are separated are the most likely to be uninsured; even though about 23 percent have public coverage, almost one-third are completely uninsured.

Marital status of parents also affects the health coverage of children. Approximately 80 percent of children who live with both parents are covered by private health insurance. Contrast that with children in single-parent families: Close to two-thirds of children living with their father only are covered by private health insurance, and fewer than one-half of children living with their mother only are covered. Even with public coverage taken into consideration, approximately 29 percent of the children living with fathers and 19.5 percent of the children living with mothers are completely uninsured.

Coronary Heart Disease and High Blood Pressure

Detailed studies conducted by several researchers have carefully compared deaths from coronary heart disease between people who are married and those who are single, widowed, and divorced. Marriage seems to be a definite protecting factor. Coronary heart disease deaths in the United States per 100,000 individuals in the general population are 176 among the married and 362 among the divorced. Death rates for single, divorced, and widowed individuals are significantly higher than the rates for married individuals; this holds true for coronary heart disease deaths among both men and women and for both whites and nonwhites. Marriage seems to provide an even greater protection for some groups: Divorced white men between the ages of 25 and 34 have 2.83 times higher death rate from coronary heart disease than do married men of the same age.[78] And those in a happy marriage are much better off than those in an unhappy one—people who are not married or who are in an unhappy marriage have greater metabolic risk factors and suffer a more acute stress response, both of which contribute to cardiovascular disease and death from heart disease. The result is cumulative: by middle age, say researchers, the cumulative impact of being unmarried or of being in an unhappy marriage has already occurred.[79]

One researcher who has specialized in the study of heart disease says that "the magnitudes of some of the increases in death rates in the nonmarried groups are most impressive, sometimes exceeding the married death rates by as much as five times. The differences are greatest at younger ages and tend to diminish somewhat with age. However, the death rates of the unmarried groups never fall below those for married individuals."[80]

Furthermore, the researcher adds, differences are sometimes even more pronounced. "The excess risk in the widowed under age 35, compared to the married, was greater than tenfold for at least one of the specific age-sex groups, involving several leading causes of death, including arteriosclerotic heart diseases," a degenerative disease that can begin in childhood and that generally progresses very slowly throughout life.[81] Bereavement and other emotions connected with the breakup of a marriage, the researcher says, can hasten the progress of arteriosclerotic heart disease, a disease that generally develops at an "imperceptibly slow pace" over the course of decades.[82]

Data from the Israel Ischemic Heart Disease Project[83] indicate another benefit of marriage in relationship to heart disease. Among men with angina, a wife's love and support appear to protect against the disease, particularly in men who also suffer from high levels of anxiety. University of Rochester School of Medicine researcher Thomas Campbell, in fact, believes that angina is an "illness behavior" rather than a sign of underlying coronary heart disease—and he says that statistics show it is much more common in unhappy marriages.[84]

As far as high blood pressure goes, married men and women are 20 percent less likely to have high blood pressure than are people who are single, separated, divorced, or widowed.[85] Married men and women are also more likely to be aware of high blood pressure and to get help when they do develop it, according to researchers who studied a group of more than 4,000 people. In summing up the study, a University of Texas epidemiologist said, "Married people with high blood pressure were 59 percent more likely to be receiving treatment for it, and 78 percent more likely to have it under control."[86]

Cancer

Earlier research has shown that married people statistically have a lower incidence of cancer at many sites. Only recently, however, has careful study shown that marriage itself actually has an influence on survival rates from cancer.

In one energetic study, researchers collected data on 27,779 cases of cancer on file at the New Mexico Tumor Registry, part of the National Cancer Institute's surveillance program. All the cancer patients in the study were older than 20 years. Researchers did not consider cancers that were diagnosed only from a death certificate or autopsy, cancers on which there was incomplete information, or cancer patients with unknown marital status. Researchers wanted to find out how marital status affected the diagnosis, treatment, and survival of people who had been diagnosed with cancer.[87]

Marital status at the time of diagnosis was used in the study. Patients were coded as single (never married), currently married, divorced, separated, or widowed. Follow-up information and updated files were obtained from the patients' private physicians. At the time of the study, more than one-half of the patients had died; almost two-thirds of the patients who were still alive had been diagnosed more than five years earlier.

In analyzing the results, being unmarried was associated with decreased survival for patients diagnosed with cancer. The percentage of persons surviving at least five years was greater for married persons than for unmarried persons in almost every category of age, gender, and stage of cancer. Being unmarried was associated with poorer survival at all stages of cancer. All three categories of unmarried people—single (never married), divorced/separated, and widowed—were more likely to develop cancers that had spread beyond a local site, were less likely to receive definitive treatment, and had poorer survival after the diagnosis of cancer.

Researchers point out that the improved survival rate of married persons might be because married people have better health habits—and they are prone to seek medical help at an earlier stage. As stated earlier, marriage also provides important social support, which is widely accepted as buffering the effects of many diseases. And, finally, researchers note that survival from cancer increases as socioeconomic status increases, probably because cancer victims with more money can seek earlier and better medical care and are not apt to delay treatment. As discussed earlier, married people tend to be in higher socioeconomic classes and are more likely to have health insurance coverage, which would promote earlier medical care.

The most controversial finding of the study was this: even when the disease was diagnosed at a more advanced stage, the best odds for survival seemed to lie with those who were married. James Goodwin, director of the study, summed it up by saying that "the protective impact of being married affected every stage of cancer care."[88]

"Treatment for cancer often involves frequent trips to the hospital for chemotherapy or radiation. If you're married, you're twice as likely to have help getting there, and to have support when your motivation is waning," said Dr. Goodwin. "Sometimes health care is complex, and if there's no one there to say, 'Hey, wait a minute—that doesn't make sense,' you may ignore information you don't quite understand."[89]

A separate study that had similar results involved researchers who combed through information at the M. D. Anderson Hospital and Tumor Institute in Houston, Texas. Researchers studied 910 married white women with breast cancer and 351 widowed white women with breast cancer. They considered a number of factors, such as how old the women were, what their socioeconomic status was, what stage the disease was in at the time of diagnosis, and whether the women delayed in seeking medical treatment. Again, marriage came out a winner: Widowed patients were less likely to survive than married patients with similar histories. According to the researchers, marital status was "the strongest predictor" of survival among the breast cancer patients.[90]

In still another study, Medical College of Wisconsin researcher James Goodwin showed that the married have much better cancer survival rates. The difference, he says, is probably due to social support and/or better financial conditions among the married, both of which can enable a married person to seek a higher quality of medical care.[91]

Immune System Function

A number of tests and several careful studies have shown that marriage helps keep the immune system strong—one possible reason why married people enjoy better health than their single, divorced, or widowed counterparts. According to measures of the immune system function (as determined by blood tests that measure the level of immune cells in the bloodstream), married people fare the best. Next are singles—those who have never been married. Singles are followed by those who have been widowed. The group of people with the lowest immune system function is those who are divorced or separated.

Researchers at Ohio State University compared the immune function of thirty-eight separated or divorced women with that of thirty-eight married women.[92] Their findings confirm the belief that a happy, stable marriage provides health benefits. Researchers found the following:

- Women within the first year of separation had significantly poorer immune function than very well-matched counterparts in the community who were married.

- Among the married women, those who described their marriage as better had better immune function.

- The longer that separated or divorced women had been separated or divorced (that is, the less they were still attached to their ex-husbands), the better their immune systems were working.

A separate group of researchers at Ohio State University's College of Medicine decided to take a look at men with herpes, an infection that tends to directly mirror the strength of the immune system.[93] (When the immune system is compromised, the herpes infection flares up; when the immune system is strong, the infection is kept in check.) All the men in the study had active herpes infection. All were given psychological and immunological tests, and researchers compared the married men with the ones who were separated or divorced. Again, strong marriages were demonstrated to be the best protection as far as a boost in immune function. The researchers found that:

- The separated or divorced men were more anxious, depressed, and lonely than were their married counterparts—and, not surprisingly, their immune systems were significantly weaker.

- Among the married men, the ones who were happy with their marriages had the strongest immune functioning.

- Those who had unhappy or unsatisfying relationships with their wives had higher levels of active herpes antibodies as well as lower ratios of T helper cells to suppressor cells.

In another study, researchers studied women, comparing married women to divorced women. In tests measuring the strength of the immune system, the married women came out on top. Those who had been separated or divorced for less than a year—and were still attached to their ex-husbands—fared the worst.[94]

Mental Health

People who are married have, on average, better levels of psychological well-being—as measured by lower rates of depression, substance abuse, and alcoholism—than do people who have never married or are divorced, widowed, or separated.[95] One of the most consistent findings is that the highest rates of mental disorder are among the divorced and separated, and the lowest is among the married.[96] And it's not simply that mentally healthy people are the ones who get married: researchers followed a group of adults over a period of years and watched as they married, got divorced, or remained single. When people got married, their mental health improved—substantially and consistently. The people who divorced suffered a substantial deterioration in both emotional and mental well-being, including increased rates of depression.[97]

Research shows that marriage has a significant impact on happiness: married adults at any income level are more likely to report being happy than even the wealthiest unmarried adults. Approximately 64 percent of married people say they are very satisfied with the way their personal life is going, compared to only 43 percent of those who are not married.[98]

Hosts of studies show that married people are less likely to have all kinds of mental disorders than the never married, separated, divorced, and widowed. Research dating back as far as 1936 shows that the first-time psychiatric admissions for men suffering from schizophrenia are more than five times higher for unmarried men than for married men. Study author Dr. Benjamin Malzberg says that "the evidence seems clear that the married population had, in general, much lower rates of mental disease than any of the other marital groups."[99]

Interestingly, studies show that the protective factor of marriage does not apply equally across ethnic lines. A study conducted by researchers in Hawaii compared four ethnic groups—white Americans, Japanese Americans, Filipino Americans, and native Hawaiians—to determine whether single people suffered more psychiatric symptoms than do married people.[100]

The researchers concluded that marriage definitely seemed to provide protection from psychiatric symptoms among white Americans and native Hawaiians but not among Japanese Americans and Filipino Americans. Marriage simply did not seem to be as important to mental health among these two groups. There could be many reasons why, said the researchers, but a main, likely reason is that people in those cultures derive a great deal of good social support from sources outside of marriage.

The impact of marriage and relationships on mental health also seems to vary based on gender. The mental health of women has been shown to be better in marriage, but getting back into a relationship after a marriage fails is good for men's mental health but bad for the mental health of the woman involved. Women who stay single after a divorce actually tend to have better mental health than women who remarry; studies show that women's mental health deteriorate progressively the more relationships they experience and the more times they move on to other relationships.[101]

A great deal of marriage's protection probably has to do with the fact that it provides "instant" social support: People with a supportive spouse are much less likely to become depressed following stressful incidents in their lives. Among women with stress, almost half who get little or no support from their husbands become deeply depressed. When married women have a high level of support from their husbands, only about 10 percent become depressed.[102]

Marriage and Life Expectancy

As study results poured in, researchers reached the same conclusion: Happy marriage dramatically increases life expectancy. Statisticians Bernard Cohen and I-Sing Lee, after compiling a catalog of relative mortality risks, said that "being unmarried is one of the greatest risks that people voluntarily subject themselves to."[103] In fact, a man who marries can expect to automatically add about nine years and seven months to his life.[104] In one large-scale study of Swedish men, married men had a mortality rate of only 9 percent during the three years of the study; their divorced counterparts had a rate of 20 percent.[105]

The health risks of the unmarried tend to escalate as they age; by the time a divorced man reaches the age of 50, for example, his health will deteriorate much more rapidly than a man his age who is married.[106] One recent study of unmarried middle-aged men and women showed that they faced twice the risk of dying within 10 years as did those still living with their spouses.[107] The study, which involved more than 7,600 people nationwide, was conducted by researchers at the University of California, San Francisco. They found a significant gap between the married and the unmarried—and divorce is a key factor in putting people at risk.

Marriage itself, they concluded, seems to be the key factor. "Of particular interest is that both men who live alone and those who live with someone other than a spouse are equally disadvantaged for survival," said epidemiologist Maradee Davis, who led the study. "The critical factor seems to be the presence of a spouse."[108]

Researcher Robert Coombs said that "virtually every study of mortality and marital status shows the unmarried of both sexes have higher death rates, whether by accident, disease, or self-inflicted wounds, and this is found in every country that maintains accurate health statistics."[109]

One study showed that there was no association between unhappy marriages and early death. However, the same study found that over a 10-year period, wives who kept silent during marital arguments had a greater risk of dying than those wives who expressed their feelings. For men, the greatest factor is simply being married: Married men in studies are less likely to die than single men.[110]

Researchers agree: The unmarried have higher death rates from all causes of death. The differences are greatest at younger ages, and the differences are the most apparent among men. Mortality rates in the United States for all causes of death are consistently higher for divorced, single, and widowed individuals of both sexes and all races.[111] In fact, according to one researcher who has specialized in the study of heart disease and other causes of death, some of the increased death rates in unmarried individuals are "astounding," rising as high as 10 times the rates for married individuals of comparable ages.[112] The researcher sums up:

> The overall death rate for divorced individuals in the United States is almost double that of married individuals. For every major cause of death, rates for divorced males range anywhere from two to six times higher than those of their married counterparts. Single and widowed males show similarly high death rates when compared to those who were married.[113]

WHAT DID YOU LEARN?

1. In what direction are marriage demographics going?
2. What are the specific health hazards of divorce on adults and children?
3. Is it harder on health to be divorced or remain in an unhappy marriage?
4. What are the health benefits of a happy marriage?
5. How does marriage affect life expectancy?

ENDNOTES

1. Charlotte A. Schoenborn, "Marital Status and Health: United States, 1999–2002," *Advance Data* 351 (December 15, 2004): 351.
2. J. K. Keicolt-Glaser and T. L. Newton, "Marriage and Health: His and Hers," *Psychology Bulletin* 127, no. 4 (2001): 472–503.
3. K. Williams and D. Umberson, "Marital Status, Marital Transitions, and Health: A Gendered Life Course Perspective," *Journal of Health and Social Behavior* 45, no. 1 (March 2004): 81–98.
4. Leonard A. Sagan, *The Health of Nations* (New York: Basic Books, 1987).
5. Neil Kalter, "Effects of Divorce on Boys Versus Girls," *Medical Aspects of Human Sexuality* (November 1989): 26–34.
6. Ibid.
7. National Center for Health Statistics and U.S. Census Bureau reports.
8. Sagan, *The Health of Nations*.
9. Judith Wallerstein and Sandra Blakeslee, "A Family Divided: Time Bombs of Divorce," *American Health* (June 1989): 49–59.
10. Ann S. Masten, "Stress, Coping, and Children's Health," *Pediatric Annals* 14, no. 8: 544–7.
11. Statistics from the U.S. Census Bureau.
12. Sagan, *The Health of Nations*.
13. Sheldon Cohen and S. Leonard Syme, eds., *Social Support and Health* (London: Academic Press, 1985).
14. Maggie Gallagher, "Why Marriage Is Good for You," *City Journal* (Autumn 2000).
15. Cohen and Syme, *Social Support and Health*.
16. Kalter, "Effects of Divorce."
17. Cohen and Syme, *Social Support and Health*.
18. Barbara R. Sarason, Irwin G. Sarason, and Gregory R. Pierce, *Social Support: An Interactional View* (New York: John Wiley & Sons, 1990), 257.

19. Ibid.

20. Marc Pilisuk and Susan Hillier Parks, *The Healing Web* (Hanover, NH: University Press of New England, 1986).

21. Glenn T. Stanton, "Only a Piece of Paper? How Marriage Improves Adult Health," *Divorce Statistics Collection—Smart Marriages Archive,* http://www.palmettofamily.org/viewarticle. asp?ID=10, accessed May 27, 2008.

22. H. Morowitz, "Hiding in the Hammond Report," *Hospital Practice* (August 1975): 35–9.

23. Bernie S. Siegel, *Love, Medicine, and Miracles* (New York: Harper & Row, 1986).

24. C. A. Heath and D. H. Ciscel, "Patriarchy, Family Structure and the Exploitation of Women's Labor," *Journal of Economic Issues* 22, no. 3 (September 1988): 781–94.

25. Siegel, *Love, Medicine, and Miracles.*

26. Brent Q. Hafen and Kathryn J. Frandsen, *People Need People: The Importance of Relationships to Health and Wellness* (Evergreen, CO: Cordillera Press, 1987), 33–4.

27. M. Richards, R. Hardy, and M. Wadsworth, "The Effects of Divorce and Separation on Mental Health in a National UK Birth Cohort," *Psychological Medicine* 72 (1997): 1121–8.

28. R. Taylor Segraves, "Divorce and Health Problems," *Medical Aspects of Human Sexuality* 19 (June 1989): 106.

29. Sarason et al., *Social Support.*

30. Ingrid Waldron, Christopher C. Weiss, and Mary Elizabeth Hughes, "Marital Status Effects on Health: Are There Differences Between Never Married Women and Divorced and Separated Women?" *Social Sciences and Medicine* 45, no. 9 (November 1997): 1387–97.

31. Hafen and Frandsen, *People Need People,* 35.

32. Ibid.

33. Barbara Powell, *Alone, Alive, and Well* (Emmaus, PA: Rodale Press, 1985).

34. L. E. Pezzin and B. S. Schone, "Parental Marital Disruption and Intergenerational Transfers: An Analysis of Lone Elderly Parents and Their Children," *Demography* 36, no. 3 (August 1999): 287–97.

35. Allan V. Horwitz, Julie McLaughlin, and Helen Raskin White, "How the Negative and Positive Aspects of Partner Relationships Affect the Mental Health of Young Married People," *Journal of Health and Social Behavior* 39, no. 2 (1973): 124–36; and George Homans, *Social Behavior,* 2nd ed. (New York: Harcourt Brace Jovanovich, 1974).

36. Horwitz et al., "How the Negative"; and Paul R. Amato and Stacey J. Rogers, "A Longitudinal Study of Marital Problems and Subsequent Divorce," *Journal of Marriage and the Family* 59 (1997): 612–24.

37. Tracy A. Revenson, Kathleen M. Schiaffino, S. Deborah Majerovitz, and Allan Giborsky, "Social Support as a Double-Edged Sword: The Relation of Positive and Problematic Support to Depression Among Rheumatoid Arthritis Patients," *Social Science and Medicine* 33 (1991): 807–13; Heather A. Turner, "Gender and Social Support: Taking the Bad with the Good?" *Sex Roles* 30 (1994): 521–41; and Debra Umberson et al., "The Effect of Social Relationships on Psychological Well-Being: Are Men and Women Really So Different?" *American Sociological Review* 61 (1996): 837–57.

38. Poonam Sharma, "Marriage and Health," http://1stholistic.com/Reading/health/health-marriage-and-health.htm, accessed May 27, 2008.

39. Linda C. Gallo, Wendy M. Troxel, Karen A. Matthews, and Lewis H. Kuller, "Marital Status and Quality in Middle-Aged Women: Associations with Levels and Trajectories of Cardiovascular Risk Factors," *Health Psychology* 22, no. 5 (September 2003): 719–30.

40. Sarason et al., *Social Support,* 258.

41. Powell, *Alone, Alive, and Well.*

42. Sarah Mahoney, "The High Price of a Bad Relationship," *Prevention* (February 2006): 167.

43. Study reported in *Archives of Internal Medicine* (October 8, 2007).

44. Bonnie Burman and Gayla Margolin, "Marriage and Health," *Advances* 6, no. 4 (1994): 51–8.

45. Ibid.

46. Sharma, "Marriage and Health."

47. Tara Parker-Pope, "When Your Spouse Makes You Sick: Research Probes Toll of Marital Stress," *Wall Street Journal* (May 4, 2004): D1.

48. Victoria E. Burns, Douglas Carroll, Christopher Ring, and Mark Drayson "Antibody Response to Vaccination and Psychosocial Stress in Humans: Relationships and Mechanisms," *Psychosomatic Medicine* 55 (1993): 395–409.

49. Linda Murray, "Mad Marriages: Arguing Your Way to Better Health," *Longevity* (October 1993): 30.

50. Janice K. Kiecolt-Glaser, "Marriage Has Different Health Costs for Men and Women," *SelfhelpMagazine,* http://www.selfhelpmagazine.com/articles/health/marriage.html, accessed May 27, 2008.

51. Mahoney, "The High Price of a Bad Relationship."

52. James J. Lynch, *The Broken Heart: The Medical Consequences of Loneliness* (New York: Basic Books, 1977).

53. Study reported in Archives of Internal Medicine, October 8, 2007.

54. "Communication with Spouse Reduces Cardiac Risk," *Brain/Mind and Common Sense* 17, no. 12 (2001): 1.

55. Julianne Holt-Lunstad, "Can Hostility Interfere with the Health Benefits of Giving and Receiving Social" as reported in the *Annals of Behavioral Medicine* 35, no. 3 (March 20, 2008): 319–30.

56. Sharon Faelten, David Diamond, and the editors of *Prevention* Magazine, *Take Control of Your Life: A Complete Guide to Stress Relief* (Emmaus, PA: Rodale Press, 1988), 143–44.

57. Sarason et al., *Social Support.*

58. Linda Murray, "Love and Longevity," *Longevity* (January 1993): 56.

59. Ibid.,56.

60. Gallo et al., "Marital Status and Quality."

61. Horwitz et al., "How the Negative."

62. Catherine Houck, "Uncovering the Secrets of Happiness," *Cosmopolitan,* n.d., 236–40.

63. Powell, *Alone, Alive, and Well.*

64. Horwitz et al., "How the Negative."

65. Schoenborn, "Marital Status and Health."

66. Miranda Hitti, "The Health Perks of Marriage," *WebMD Medical News,* http://www.webmd.com/balance/news/20041215/health-perks-of-marriage, accessed May 27, 2008.

67. Charlotte A. Schoenborn, "Marital Status and Health." United States 1999–2002, Centers for Disease Control, *Advance Data from Vital and Health Statistics* 351 (Dec. 15, 2004): 73.

68. Carol Turkington, "Have You Hugged Your Immune System Today?" *Self* (October 1988): 184.

69. Powell, *Alone, Alive and Well,* 159.

70. Robert G. Wood, Brian Goesling, and Sarah Avellar, *The Effects of Marriage on Health: A Synthesis of Recent Research Evidence,* U.S. Department of Health and Human Services, June 2007.

71. Ibid.

72. Schoenborn, "Marital Status and Health."

73. Hitti, "The Health Perks of Marriage."

74. Turkington, "Have You Hugged Your Immune System," 184.

75. Ibid.

76. Emily Friedman, "Marriage May Promote Health," *Medical World News* (December 26, 1988): 34.

77. Ibid.

78. Lynch, *The Broken Heart.*

79. Gallo et al., "Marital Status and Quality."

80. Ibid.

81. Ibid.

82. Ibid.

83. J. H. Medalie and U. Goldbourt, "Angina Pectoris Among 10,000: II. Psychosocial and Other Risk Factors as Evidenced by a Multivariate Analysis of a Five-Year Incidence Study," *American Journal of Medicine* 60 (1976): 10–21.

84. Burman and Margolin, "Marriage and Health."

85. Sally Squires, "Marriage—Good for the Heart," *American Health* (July 1987): 111.

86. Ibid.

87. James S. Goodwin, William C. Hunt, Charles R. Key, and Jonathan M. Samet, "The Effect of Marital Status on Stage, Treatment, and Survival of Cancer Patients," *Journal of the American Medical Association* 258, no. 21 (1987): 3125–30.

88. Turkington, "Have You Hugged Your Immune System," 184.

89. Ibid., 184.

90. A. V. Neale, B. C. Tilley, and S. W. Vernon, "Marital Status, Delay in Seeking Treatment, and Survival from Breast Cancer," *Social Science and Medicine* 23, no. 3 (1986): 305–12.

91. The editors of *Prevention* magazine and the Center for Positive Living, *Positive Living and Health: The Complete Guide to Brain/Body Healing and Mental Empowerment* (Emmaus, PA: Rodale Press, 1990), 337.

92. "Is Marriage Good for Your Health? An Interview with Janice Kiecolt-Glaser," *Mind/Body/Health Digest* 1, no. 2: 1.

93. Rick Weiss, "Worried Sick: Hassles and Herpes," *Science News* 132 (1987): 360.

94. J. K. Kiecolt-Glaser et al., "Marital Quality, Marital Disruption, and Immune Function," *Psychosomatic Medicine* 49 (1987): 13–34.

95. Adrianne Frech and Kristi Williams, "Depression and the Psychological Benefits of Entering Marriage," Journal *of Health and Social Behavior* 48, no. 7 (2007): 149.

96. Stanton, "Only a Piece of Paper?"

97. Gallagher, "Why Marriage Is Good for You."

98. Jennifer Warner, "Marriage Beats Money for Happiness," *eMedicineHealth,* http://www.emedicinehealth.com/script.main/art.asp?articlekey=78837, accessed May 27, 2008.

99. Glen T. Stanton, "Only a Piece of Paper. The Unquestionable Benefits of Lifelong Marriage," Colorado Springs, CO. Focus on the Family August 1995.

100. From D. T. Takeuchi and K. N. Speechley, "Ethnic Differences in the Marital Status and Psychosocial Relationship," *Social Psychiatry and Psychiatric Epidemiology* 24 (1989): 288–94.

101. "Cohabiting Better for Men's Mental Health; Marriage Better for Women's," *Mental Health About.com,* http://mentalhealth.about.com/cs/mindandbody/a/cohab0104.htm, accessed May 27, 2008.

102. Michael Argyle, *The Psychology of Happiness*, (Methuen, 1987), 27.
103. Gallagher, "Why Marriage Is Good for You."
104. Jo Ann Tooley and Lynn Y. Anderson, "Living Is Risky," *U.S. News and World Report* (January 25, 1988): 77.
105. Rosengren et al., "Marital Status."
106. Lee A. Lillard and Constantijn W.A. Panis, "Marital Status and Mortality: The Roles of Health," *Demography* 33, no. 3 (1996): 313–27.
107. Morton Hunt, "Long-Life Insurance: For Men, It's Marriage," *Longevity* (February 1991): 10.
108. Ibid., 10.
109. Stanton, "Only a Piece of Paper?"
110. "Toxic Marriage May (Literally) Hurt Your Heart," Associated Press, reporting on studies cited in *Archives of Internal Medicine*, October 8, 2007.
111. Lynch, *The Broken Heart*.
112. Ibid.
113. Ibid.

CHAPTER 12

Families and Health

The happiest moments of my life have been the few which I have passed at home in the bosom of my family.

—Thomas Jefferson

- Define the concept of family.
- Explain how the early influence of parents impacts the health and longevity of their children.
- Discuss the traits of weak or stressed families and their negative impact on health.
- Understand the traits of strong families and know how those families contribute to the health and longevity of their members.
- Explain the importance of family reunions and other traditions that keep families close.

In an October 1965 speech delivered at New York's Abbott House, the Reverend Martin Luther King, Jr., summarized the role of the family this way:

> Family life not only educates in general, but its quality ultimately determines the individual's capacity to love. The institution of the family is decisive in determining not only if a person has the capacity to love another individual, but, in the larger sense, whether he is capable of loving his fellow men collectively. The whole of society rests on this foundation for stability, understanding, and social peace.[1]

What Is a Family?

It used to be relatively easy to define the term *family*—it was a father, mother, and children, living together in a relationship defined by love, marriage, procreation, and mutual dependence.[2] But today, Americans have virtually remade society—and, along with it, the family. Essentially, there is no longer a universal definition of *the family;* instead, definitions depend on situation, generation, race, perception, and purpose. The beliefs of any one person can radically bias the perception of what a family is or should be.

There is a movement across the nation to change narrow legal definitions of *family* so that people who are living together, but who are not married, can enjoy the same legal benefits as those who are legally married. (As one example, a partner doesn't have the same rights as a spouse when it comes to hospital visitation, making health care decisions, or suing over the wrongful death of a partner.) In California, the Supreme Court ruled that all needy children living in the same household under the care of a relative constitute a "family" for purposes of welfare grants.[3]

In other cities across the nation, municipalities are grappling with the issue of just what defines a family—and, according to one columnist, the result is "mini culture wars" as planning commissions, zoning boards, and city councils try to decide who may, and may not, live in a residential area designated for "single-family occupancy." A zoning law in Manassas, Virginia, restricts households to immediate relatives;[4] in Provo, Utah, planners made a similar change, saying that only people related by blood, marriage, or adoption could live in a single-family structure.[5] On the other hand, courts in California and New Jersey ruled that groups of people could live together as long as they *function* as a family—even if they weren't related by blood, marriage, or adoption.[6]

Advocates of these types of rulings say that *family* should be defined by function, not by structure. The statistics tell at least part of the story of what has happened to bring us to this point: according to a special issue of *Newsweek*,[7] today's American family is likely to be very different from Ozzie and Harriet or the Cosbys.

The divorce rate is maintaining at an all-time high, and demographers project that half of all first marriages will end in divorce. Six out of ten second marriages will probably also collapse. One out of every three children today is being raised by a single parent; and, while some certainly flourish, on average they are at greater risk of living in poverty, suffering academic problems, and developing behavioral problems.[8]

Trends in America today have resulted in a variety of "family units"—and the only thing in common among them is that their members live under one roof. The following types of families have resulted from the complex industrial, technological, and social changes that have occurred in the last few decades:[9]

- **Married nuclear families.** This is the "traditional" family unit: a married man and woman are both the biological parents of the children. There are several different iterations of this family: the father may work outside the home while the mother cares for the children, the mother may work outside the home while the father cares for the children, or both parents may work outside the home.

- **Single-parent families.** There is only one parent in the home due to divorce, the death of a spouse, or an adult who chose not to marry. This is the fastest-growing type of family in America, and 88 percent of them are headed by women.

- **Stepfamilies.** There is a married man and woman, but they are not both the biological parents of the children in the home. Most commonly, these families are created by divorce and remarriage. Nine thousand new stepfamilies are created each week in this country.

- **Cohabitation families.** Two unmarried adults are committed to each other and live in a long-term relationship. They may have children together or may bring children from previous relationships into the family.

- **Cross-generational families.** Two or more adults from different generations of a family intend to share a household for the foreseeable future. This type of family may include children; for example, a grandparent may be raising grandchildren.

- **Joint/shared-custody families.** The biological parents of the children are not living together as a result of divorce. Depending on the legal arrangement between the parents, the children generally move back and forth between the residences of each parent.

- **Foster families (or group home families).** Children are cared for by foster parents or institutional child-care workers, who become a child's "substitute family."

Despite the chaos that surrounds the family, the image of Ozzie and Harriet is still with us, say researchers who are studying the family—and it still has a great deal of impact on today's family unit, regardless of how many changes take place. According to Yale historian John Demos, "In a time when parents seem to feel a great deal of change in family experience, that image is comfortingly solid and secure, a counterpoint to what we think is threatening for the future."[10]

Whatever the family unit, a family is a group that shares common goals and values, and they work together to achieve those goals. And we know that what goes on in a family—the network of relationships between its members—can have a profound influence on the health and longevity of its members. In fact, the health of each member of the family can be influenced by many factors: how big the family is, how many fights the family engages in, whether one or both parents work, whether family members can effectively communicate with each other, and more. A family member's health can even be affected by whether the family holds regular family reunions!

The Early Influence of Parents

Parents have an incredible impact on the health, development, and behavior of children.

The way parents treat their children determines in large part the way the children will feel about themselves, both while they are children and when they become adults. Parents can endow them with a healthy self-image or engender feelings of low self-esteem. Children react to parents' emotions, moods, and behavior. If the parents are stressed, they can rear children who are stressed—and, therefore, are prone to disease.

Relationships in early childhood seem to play a huge role in the development and health of family members, and the impact of the mother appears to be especially important. For example, monkeys who are raised by their peers instead of by their mothers have reduced function of serotonin in the central nervous system, a condition that has been linked in humans to violence, alienation, social isolation, and suicide.[11] There seems to be another impact on the brain as well: Adult rats that were handled and nurtured as infants experience slower aging of the hippocampus, the center in the brain that shows the earlier degeneration in Alzheimer's disease.[12] Those rats that were raised in a toy-filled "complex" with other rats had 30 percent more nerve cell connections in their brains, which are associated with better performance on difficult learning and problem-solving tasks.[13]

The impact of early relationships also seems to have an effect on how well we respond to stress. In one study, researchers subjected adult rats from nine litters to 20 minutes of restraint; the rats that were licked and groomed more as pups showed much lower response to the stress of being restrained.[14] And infants who lived for at least eight months amid the emotional and physical deprivation of Romanian orphanages were still producing much higher levels of stress hormones six years later when compared to children who had not lived in the orphanages.[15]

Experiments with Monkeys

Other experiments have shown the importance of a parent's presence and touch. Dr. Harry F. Harlow at the University of Wisconsin noticed that baby monkeys that had cloth pads on the floor of their wire cages were stronger and huskier than the baby monkeys with no cloth pad. The babies treated the cloth pad much as a child treats a teddy bear; they cuddled it, caressed it, and played with it. That observation prompted Harlow to construct a kind of surrogate "mother" for the monkeys—a wire monkey covered with terry cloth that had a light bulb inside (to radiate heat) and a rubber nipple (to dispense milk). The baby monkeys were enthusiastic in their acceptance.

His success with the surrogate "mother" prompted him to examine whether the babies really needed a mother that was so touchable. He constructed a second "mother," this time of wire alone. There was no terry cloth and no light bulb to provide warmth. There was a rubber nipple and a supply of milk, but that was all. Of the eight baby monkeys, four were allowed to nurse from the terry cloth mother while the other four were allowed to nurse only from the wire mother. All eight of the monkeys spent most of their time cuddling the terry cloth mother. At feeding time, the four would go to the wire mother for their milk, but they would instantly return to the terrycloth mother as soon as they were finished eating. Whenever they were frightened, all eight would climb onto the terrycloth mother for solace.

In still other experiments, monkeys were placed in cages with nothing but a wire mother. Although they took their nourishment from her, many of them did not survive. Those who did had poor coping mechanisms. When placed under stress, they cowered in a corner, hid their faces under their arms, or screamed. Their deprived development occurred even though they could see, hear, and smell other baby monkeys.

Results of the study and its implications about early attachment between mothers and infants "reflects [sic] millions of years of evolutionary history," says Dr. Stephen Suomi, chief of the Laboratory of Comparative Ethology at the National Institute of Child Health and Human Development in Bethesda, Maryland, who worked with Harlow on the monkey experiments. "The mother buffers the child from the big, scary world. How she does that can have profound impact on her youngster's ability to function socially, as well as on their basic biology."[16]

Studies with Human Babies

The same thing seems to apply to human beings. Twenty-five years ago Dr. Rene Spitz, now at the University of Colorado Medical Center, first described "marasmus" (a physical wasting away from malnutrition) in infants who had suddenly lost their mothers. Some infants who suddenly lost their mothers refused to eat and, even when force-fed, would eventually die.[17]

In studies conducted by Dr. Spitz and Katherine Wolf, 91 infants in foundling homes throughout the United States and Canada were carefully observed. Even though all of the babies were well cared for physically, they didn't grow as rapidly as normal babies; none gained the weight they should have, and some even lost weight. There were effects other than the physical ones, too; the babies seemed depressed and anxious. A little more than one-third of the babies in the foundling hospitals—34 of the babies—died despite what researchers said was "good food and meticulous medical care."[18]

In one study of orphaned infants, half of the orphans were placed in foster homes and half were placed in institutions. After one year, researchers studied both sets of babies. The children who had been placed in foster homes did better in every way, both mentally and physically. At that point, when all the children were one year old, those who had been originally placed in institutions were placed in foster homes. Researchers then took another look when the children were five. Although the institutionalized children had improved in both behavior and performance, they were, five years later, still behind in development when compared with the children who had been placed in foster homes at birth. The researchers concluded that the psychic trauma "of the first year of neglect was never overcome."[19]

The Effects of Neglect

Other experiments had similar results. Researchers studied a group of one-year-old children who had been born to mothers with an average IQ (intelligence quotient) of 70 and who were unable to care for their children. Half of the children were routinely placed in institutions. The other half, who had been randomly selected from the group, were placed in a hospital ward of mentally retarded adults where each was assigned a one-to-one relationship with an individual woman who assumed a motherly role. Three years later researchers took a look at the children. Those in the routine institutional care hadn't fared very well: They had deteriorated and were significantly retarded. As a group, they had lost an average of 26 IQ points each. The group of children who had been cared for by the retarded women had gained an average of 29 IQ points each.[20]

Researchers didn't stop there. Thirty years later, they followed up on each child who had been part of the study. Again, the institutionalized children presented a bleak picture. All were still institutionalized; a number were dead. The most advanced among them had completed the third grade. In sharp contrast, the children who had been cared for by a "mother" in the hospital had made impressive gains. Most had completed high school. A few had even completed a year of college. All were self-supporting. The children in the study clearly illustrated "the debilitating effect of neglect during childhood, and of the benefit to intellectual development of affectionate care even by retarded mothers."[21]

Apparently the importance of a parent's influence is present at the moment of birth. The animal world presents many examples. Researchers at Cornell Animal Behavior Farm noted that when mother sheep were prevented from licking their newborn after birth, the lambs were unable to stand on their legs—and subsequently died. Almost the opposite occurs when mother animals are allowed "gentling" of their young; the baby animals show an increased immune response when they are experimentally exposed to vaccinations later in life. In one experiment, in fact, the enhanced immune response proved true in every animal tested![22]

Again, similar results have been obtained with human babies. In one study, mothers who had extra contact with a child during the first hours after birth demonstrated significantly more fondling, soothing, and eye contact with the child one month later. Two years later, these same mothers spoke to their children with more questions, fewer commands, and more words per proposition.[23]

In a separate study, 301 new mothers were randomly assigned to different postpartum nursing schedules: 134 of the infants were roomed with their mothers; the other 143 were roomed in the nursery and given routine visits to their mothers. Researchers kept track of the infants' progress during the next 21 months. Of the 143 babies roomed in the nursery, away from their mothers, 9 were hospitalized because of "parenting disturbances"—for abuse, neglect, abandonment, or failure to thrive. Of the 134 babies who had been roomed with their mothers, only 1 required hospitalization during the subsequent 21 months. The study should not only have an impact in setting hospital policy but should also "demonstrate the extreme sensitivity of the infant to the care given in the first hours of life."[24]

Dr. Mary D. Salter Ainsworth, recognized as one of the top researchers in infant-mother attachment, believes that a parent's influence is significant from the moment of birth, and she's conducted studies to prove her point. In one study, she examined groups of babies who had been treated differently during their first year of life. Some had been virtually ignored, having little physical contact with their mothers; these mothers typically felt that by not "coddling" their babies, they were allowing their babies to develop a sense of independence and were avoiding what they felt to be an unhealthy "attachment." The second group of babies had been occasionally cuddled and held by their mothers; but, for the most part, they had been encouraged to be independent. The third group had mothers who consistently responded to their signals, especially their crying, by picking them up and comforting them.

At one year of age, the most secure, well-adjusted babies were the ones in the third group—the ones whose mothers had comforted them consistently. The babies in the second group (the ones whose mothers had occasionally responded to them) had a form of "anxious attachment." They seemed anxious and worried when separated from their mothers and yet were not able to relate normally to their mothers, either. The worst of the babies were those in the first group, the ones whose mothers gave them little physical contact during the first year and who did not respond to their signals, such as crying. These babies were anxious and resistant. When researchers first separated them from their mothers by placing them in a strange room and then returning them to their mothers, the babies avoided contact with their mothers and resisted being held.

Ainsworth's conclusion speaks strongly about the influence of parents in a child's early life: "Babies under a year need a certain kind of tender, responsive holding when they're upset. If they don't get it, they learn to count on not having their needs met,"[25] a situation that makes them hostile, angry, and rejecting. The influence of parents and the quality of relationship that a child has with the parents apparently continues to be a strong factor in both physical and mental health—even beyond the first few critical years.

Parental Styles

The influence is great, too, for parental style when it comes to disciplining children. University of California psychologist Diana Baumrind reported findings to the American Psychological Association that were surprising even to her after she studied teenagers, their parents, and their health. Baumrind and her colleagues were looking for evidence that would validate one parenting style over another in terms of producing children who were healthy both physically and emotionally. "We expected that at puberty, some imbalance in favor of freedom over control would have become desirable, but that did not happen," she reports.[26] In fact, the healthiest children came from families in which the parents were authoritative, placing restrictions and demands on children but providing good support as well. These children did better academically, used fewer drugs and less alcohol, and showed the most social competence, maturity, and optimism.

In discussing the study results, Baumrind stressed the importance of support. Authoritative parents, she explains, "are not bossy. They make it their business to know their children, how they're doing in school, and who their friends are. Their control reflects a high level of commitment to the child, and they are not afraid to confront the child."[27]

Educators trying to reverse the trend of adolescent involvement with drugs, alcohol, tobacco, sexual relationships, and gang violence, which are happening at progressively earlier ages, focused on awareness. However, studies found that the greatest effect in keeping children away from these risks was the direction of their parents—who, despite adverse publicity to the contrary, continue to be the strongest role models and to have the strongest indirect influence on their children throughout adolescence.[28]

Another long-range study of medical school graduates followed more than 900 of them from 1948 through 1964. At various intervals these graduates were given personality tests—tests that measured, among other things, how close they felt to their parents. By the middle of 1973, 26 of the graduates had developed malignant tumors. Researchers were curious about what those graduates might have had in common, so they poured over the personality tests the graduates had taken when they were healthy. Twenty of the cancer victims had scored extremely low on questions determining closeness to their parents.

The affection style of parents also seems to have an impact on the health and development of the children in the family, especially on their emotional development. Those from families in which both parents were affectionate show less neuroticism as well as significantly less anxiety and depression. Here again, the mother may have the greatest influence. Those who had affectionate fathers but not affectionate mothers suffered greater emotional problems—and those families were marked by greater conflict, separation/divorce of the parents, emotional problems in the parents, and mistreatment by the parents.[29]

Even the willingness of parents to take certain risks can impact their children. Researchers in the United States have found a strong link between teenage sex and risky behavior by parents—parents who smoke or who don't wear seatbelts in cars, for example. An analysis of the National Longitudinal Study of Adolescent Health, a study that includes information on the sexual behavior of 19,000 adolescents between the ages of 12 and 18, found that:

- Teenagers were more likely to have sex before the age of 16 if their parents smoked.

- Teenagers were more likely to have sex early in adolescence if their parents drank heavily.

- Boys were more likely to have sex during high school if their parents drove without wearing a seatbelt.

The same study found a link between parents who smoked and drank and children who became involved with drugs and the police. Adolescents whose parents engage in risky behavior, "especially smoking, are especially likely to be sexually active. They are also more likely to smoke, drink, associate with substance-abusing peers, and participate in delinquent behavior."[30]

Parental Loss

Even more devastating is the loss of a parent, especially during childhood. Early parental loss is directly related to a wide variety of physical, emotional, and intellectual problems in the child—and children deprived of one parent during childhood have a greatly increased risk of many individual diseases, as well as suicide and alcoholism.

A research group at Rochester Medical School decided to look into the backgrounds of the patients at the hospital. They found that a significant number of the adult patients hospitalized with physical disease had lost one or both parents when they were children. Similarly, data from two prominent heart studies showed that a significant number of coronary patients had lost their father to death, usually between ages 5 and 17.

Traits of Weak or Stressed Families

Health problems can be traced to weak or stressed families, and many of those families share certain characteristics that help us identify them. Many of those families are also a product of the times. America is no longer a nation of extended families. Fifty years ago almost three-fourths of all households in the United States included at least one grandparent as an active, full-time member of the household. Today, fewer than 2 percent have a grandparent as a resource. Families have lost that important outlet, a person to lean on in times of stress.

In 1930, children spent an estimated four hours a day in close personal contact with members of the extended family: parents, grandparents, aunts, uncles, and cousins who lived nearby. Today, in a mobile society, chances are great that a child's grandparents, aunts, uncles, and cousins are spread across the state, if not across the nation. Few live in the same neighborhood. Extended families are not living under the same roof anymore.

Americans have been reduced to what is called the "nuclear" family, consisting of parents and children.

Interaction within the nuclear family does not approach the three or four hours of intensive daily interaction in families earlier in the last century. Experts estimate that interaction in most nuclear families is limited to a few *minutes* a day—and those aren't necessarily positive. "Of those few minutes, more than half are used in one-way, negatively toned communications of parents issuing warnings or reproaching children for things done wrong."[31]

Then there's the trend toward two-career families. In 1940, more than 90 percent of all households in the United States had a full-time homemaker who spent approximately thirty-nine hours a week doing domestic chores. Even with time-saving appliances and methods, it still takes about thirty-seven hours a week to successfully run a household. Today, nearly 88 percent of all children who return home from school in the United States enter a household where every living member has been gone the best 10 hours of the day. The scenario is vastly different: everyone comes home at the end of an exhausting day, still faced with the routine business of the household. Little wonder that no one has lots of spare time for meaningful family interaction![32]

Now team up those trends with the ten top stresses for today's families:

1. Economics, finances, and budgeting
2. Children's behavior, discipline, and sibling fighting
3. Insufficient couple time for adults
4. Lack of shared responsibility in the family
5. Communicating with children
6. Insufficient "me" time
7. Guilt for not accomplishing more
8. Poor spousal relationships
9. Insufficient family play time
10. An overscheduled family calendar[33]

No wonder families experience breakdown!

A number of traits signify tension and distress in a family:

1. **Physical symptoms.** Children may bite their nails, stutter, or have other nervous habits usually associated with tension. Those over age six may still wet the bed. When children are placed under stress, they may react by throwing violent tantrums. Parents and children alike may have frequent and unexplainable illnesses, often hallmarked by a collection of vague symptoms that persist for months (such as chronic headache, indigestion, or fatigue).

2. **Signs of stress.** In problem families, molehills often do become mountains. Small disagreements or conflicts often escalate into major battlefields. There are far too many quarrels and misunderstandings, not to mention conflicts between husband and wife. Nobody seems able to relax. There never seems to be enough

time to accomplish even basic goals. As a consequence, family members try to escape from each other—to the office, a room with a locked door, anywhere they don't have to deal with the pressures of the family.

3. **Burnout.** Instead of being a joy, family life becomes a burden. Parents get to the point at which they no longer enjoy their children; they feel as though they are standing by helplessly while the children dominate the family. This is the same kind of burnout that renders executives and medical personnel helpless.

4. **Lack of communication.** Children in troubled families don't feel free to approach their parents about difficult subjects, such as drug or alcohol use or premarital sex. Instead of depending on their parents for help, they try to cope with things on their own. These problem families have trouble talking about simple things as well. Too much of the time, confusion reigns; and, in the meantime, nobody explores ideas, talks about feelings, or reaches solutions. Nobody really listens to anybody else.

5. **"Controlled" arguments.** A few good shouting matches between family members are okay. In fact, this is desirable—if family members use good communication skills to patch things up afterward. That's what happens in healthy families. In troubled families, arguments are quite different. Troubled families often have an unwritten or unspoken rule that all anger must be controlled. Disagreements are buried in silence. Instead of getting things out in the open, these families let disagreements smolder beneath the surface for weeks. When somebody finally gets around to talking about what's happened, no one seems to care (or hear) what is being said. Instead of negotiating and compromising, family members become absorbed with who is in control and who is right.

6. **Interaction with others.** In healthy families, members have a deep sense of loyalty and concern for members of the family, but they also have rich and rewarding relationships outside the family. No one in the family is threatened by these. Troubled families seem to be at one of two extremes. At one end of the spectrum, family members belong to a tight-knit group; parents insist that children have no outside friends, interests, or activities. All family members are forced into doing things only with other members of the family. At the other end of the spectrum, the families are extremely loosely constructed; each family member has his or her own interests and activities and very little interaction occurs between family members.

7. **Lack of affection.** Even if family members were able to share affection when children were young, they stop at some point, and in most troubled families, parents stay a "safe" distance from their children. Little, if any, hugging and kissing go on—which the children come to interpret as a lack of concern.

8. **Infidelity.** Many troubled families are characterized by sexual infidelity—but there is other infidelity, too. Some spouses become "unfaithful" by having an "affair" with their work, a hobby, an outside interest, or another relationship so that no time or effort is invested in the marriage.

Clinical psychologist Harriet B. Braiker defines the seven deadly sins of toxic relationships as anxiety, helplessness, hostility, frustration, depression, cynicism, and low self-worth.[34]

Health Problems in Weak or Stressed Families

Results of studies gathered over many years demonstrate soundly that a healthy family and supportive family members have a great deal to do with the health of individuals in the family unit. On the other side of the coin, marital stress and tension, troubled family life, and other problems in the family unit can contribute to illness and stress in individual family members. Research has even shown that problems in the family unit can lead to greater chronic anger among family members.[35]

Family stress occurs when the demands on the family exceed the family's abilities to meet those demands, and an imbalance results.[36] That imbalance can be real or perceived. Remember that stressors, those things that create demands, can be both positive and negative, ranging from the birth of a child or the promotion and relocation of the primary wage-earner to the divorce of parents, unexpected medical expenses following an accident, or the death of a family member. Each of these things causes the family's coping pattern to change and results in stress. If the family sees the stressor (the "demand") as an uncontrollable event that could ruin the family—instead of a challenge to be met with a sense of adventure—the stress can escalate until the family unit, like the individual, becomes exhausted.

Criticism from family members can be especially detrimental on both physical and mental health. While a great deal of research has focused on the mental and emotional impact of criticism in the family, several recent studies have shown the impact of criticism on the physical health of family members as well. In one study, conducted at a primary medical care facility in upstate New York, almost 900 patients answered questionnaires about the amount of criticism in their families. Two scientifically accepted measurement tools were then used to assess the results. Researchers found that those who had the highest amount of criticism from family members also had the most harmful health behaviors, including smoking, lack of exercise, and high-fat diets. Those who were criticized the most not only had the most negative outlook but also had the poorest physical health.[37]

Learned Pain

Something as basic as pain, for example, may be learned from the family you grow up in. Psychologist Patrick Edwards of North Dakota State University believes that pain can be something children learn, something parents help them "rehearse." In a survey of 288 college students, he asked them to catalog the length, intensity, and frequency of their own pain experiences—pain from things like backache, toothache, headache, muscle ache, abdominal pain, and neck soreness. Then he asked the college students to recall how much and what types of pain their families suffered. He found that children who grew up in pain-plagued households were more likely to experience pain themselves. Girls seemed to be more influenced by the way other family members felt than were boys. Some of the college students who grew up in families with lots of physical pain developed an attitude of helplessness; they believed that pain was beyond their control and would happen no matter what.[38]

Edwards followed up with another study, which again showed the profound influence of families on pain. He asked 224 college students to describe their own pains and the pains of their families—and to describe how much time their parents took off from work because of pain. The findings showed that the students who felt the most pain, and whose parents apparently were in the most pain, were also the ones whose parents missed quite a bit of work. Children interpreted pain as a way to gain; the "gains of pain" became special attention, sympathy, or a way out of difficult tasks. These children had learned to use pain as a way to miss school, a way to get out of doing chores, or a way to escape other things they wanted to get out of. An additional result was that these children tended to focus on pain more than was necessary. In some cases, they were conditioned to look for pain when it scarcely existed.[39]

Other researchers agree with Edwards that families can encourage or discourage physical distress and suffering. Some believe a family's response to a family member's complaints will influence how sick he or she feels, the way he or she feels about the symptoms, and, in the end, even how disabled he or she becomes.

A few researchers think family reaction can cause a sick person to "use" an illness to gain power and position in the family. At first glance, a sick person may seem to be "the weakest and most defenseless member of the family," one researcher says. But, in reality, "He is often the most powerful member, because his illness entitles him to special consideration, and his needs now have top priority: A sick family member can cause routine family life to grind to a halt and center on him."[40] Because illness confers this kind of power, it sometimes becomes a solution to family problems. In families that are rigid, enmeshed, and unable to openly acknowledge their difficulties, a family member's suffering may temporarily stabilize the family.

Strep Infections

Aside from the issue of learned pain or illness used to gain power or attention, stress or weakness in the family unit can actually lead to illness. Two Harvard Medical School researchers decided to test that theory by doing extensive examinations of 16 families—consisting of 100 people—for a year. Every three weeks, these two pediatricians performed throat cultures on each family member in addition to other clinical tests to determine whether the family members had any signs of streptococcal illness. Because of their situations, each of the families had about the same chance as the others to pick up a streptococcal infection: They all had a similar number of school-aged children, lived in similar degrees of neighborhood crowding, and had fathers with similar occupations.[41]

A number of the family members did acquire strep infections during the study period; but, most of the time, the acquisition of strep bacteria did not result in illness. Families with high levels of chronic stress not only got infected more often, but their infections developed into illness four times more frequently than in families without chronic stress.[42]

Cancer

At Jefferson Medical College in Philadelphia, many cancer patients described their parents as "aloof, cold people." Their own emotional rigidity, which may lead to cancer, seemed a product of their strict upbringing.[43] When cancer patients were asked about childhood traumas, they tended to gloss over the death of a parent or sibling; some had to be prodded to even remember that a parent had died when they were very young. Perhaps they repressed the death, or perhaps they were not really emotionally attached to the person who died—but the researchers agreed that cancer patients tended to "bottle up" their emotions.

In a number of studies, cancer patients described themselves as "emotionally detached" from their parents—and they described their parents as having been disagreeable to each other. In the study involving Johns Hopkins graduates, more negative attitudes about the family prevailed among the cancer patients than among any other group in the study.[44]

Asthma

Problems in the family may contribute to asthma. Studies of people with asthma reveal that many consider their parents to be rejecting or overbearing. In one study, researchers sent the parents of asthmatic children on paid vacations and left trained observers to care for the children. Without any other treatment, about half of the children improved.[45]

A similar experiment also pointed a finger at the family. In research done nearly 30 years ago, a physician studied a group of children who were genuinely allergic to house dust; inhaling the dust in their homes brought on violent asthma attacks. Then the doctor hospitalized each of the children. Next, he secretly took dust from each child's home and sprayed it into each child's hospital room. Only one of the twenty children had an asthma attack. Away from home and family, the rest of the children were healthy.[46]

Diabetes

Almost 20 years ago, a psychiatrist from Albert Einstein College of Medicine in New York wondered why diabetes strikes certain people at certain times in their lives. He decided to do some investigating at a local clinic where he had been counseling adolescents with diabetes. The clinic had kept detailed records of the age at which each adolescent became ill, as well as personal information about the family: deaths, divorces, family disturbances, and the like.[47]

In carefully studying these records, the doctor found that well over two-thirds of the diabetes patients had experienced the loss of a parent or a disturbed family life (characterized by serious illness of a parent, parental fighting, chaotic atmosphere, and so on). Only about one-fifth of a diabetes-free control group had experienced similar family problems. In about half of the diabetic teens, the parental loss had occurred before the onset of diabetes, suggesting a possible connection between the two.[48]

Apparently the health of the family has a great deal to do with the way children adapt to and cope with the stress of their own chronic illness. Researchers at Case Western Reserve University School of Medicine compiled the results of 57 studies of children with chronic illness.[49] Those studies clearly show that children who come from weak, stressed families characterized by conflict and psychological distress in the mother were consistently less capable of adjusting to and coping with their illness. Those children who came from strong, healthy families were significantly better able to adjust to and cope with chronic illness, such as asthma and diabetes.

Anorexia Nervosa

The same pattern seems to hold true for victims of anorexia nervosa. Some professionals think the development of anorexia nervosa is closely related to abnormal patterns of interaction between the patient and her family (anorexia nervosa usually occurs in girls), mostly involving overly restrictive or suffocating relationships. A leading family therapist who has worked extensively with anorexic victims claims that "the boundaries that keep family members over-involved with each other and separated from the world are well defined and strong. The boundaries within the family, however, are diffuse and weak."[50]

A study conducted at Duke University Medical Center indicated that people from weak families also tended to have weak health. The study showed that families weak in structure and support produced people with more symptoms, impaired physical health, and weakened emotional health.[51]

Traits of Strong Families

Just as weak or stressed families can contribute to illness, strong families can contribute to good health and long lives. Children reared in a healthy, happy family have a better than average chance of enjoying a healthy, long life—in part because strong families encourage exercise, eat balanced diets, know how to cope with stress, encourage friendship and support, and emphasize pride and loyalty.

What are the hallmarks of a healthy family? Different researchers have different answers and different ways of arriving at an opinion, but there is more unity of opinion than we might think among America's families. Researchers at the University of Nebraska–Lincoln wanted to know whether the perceptions of a strong family differed between ethnic groups, so they asked more than 500 people from five ethnic groups—Native Americans, Hmong refugees, blacks, Hispanics, and Caucasians—what they thought made a strong family. The responses were remarkably similar: the traits were trust, support, and effective communication, with encouragement of individuality, teaching of moral principles, and working together for the welfare of the family.[52]

Hamilton McCubbin, a family stress researcher at the University of Wisconsin, emphasized that strong families do things together, build esteem in each other (and themselves), develop social support within the community (as opposed to becoming isolated from the community), enjoy the lifestyle they have adopted, and use a variety of things to reduce tension—such as exercise, relaxation, a positive outlook, and staying involved in activities.[53]

Years of research show that strong families cultivate six characteristics: they have commitment, express appreciation, spend time together, develop spiritually, deal effectively with stress and crisis, and have "rhythm"—the rituals and traditions that give structure and meaning to everyday life.[54]

One researcher who wanted to define the traits of healthy families sent out questionnaires to more than 500 family professionals: teachers, pastors, pediatricians, social workers, counselors, and leaders of volunteer organizations. In the end the lists look much the same. Number one, according to all the experts, is the family's ability to communicate. The lists have the following traits in common.[55]

Commitment

Members of the family know that the family comes first—which means they find time to spend together, do things together, create a good balance between family and the other demands in life, and recognize the family unit as something special. Family members are willing to compromise and make changes in their own activities occasionally to accommodate the interests of the whole. They support each other and lend a hand in times of difficulty. Because of their commitment to the family, stresses, either those that affect an individual or the family as a whole, don't destroy that commitment.

Communication and Listening

Strong families gather around the table at mealtime and talk about what happened during the day and also about feelings. A lot of listening goes on, too. Parents listen in a way that encourages more communication. Instead of jumping to conclusions and reacting based on scanty information, they listen attentively and draw out more information. They know each family member well enough that they can read nonverbal messages. They know when a child feels inadequate, ugly, clumsy, stupid, unloved, or just plain worthless. Family members use positive words and phrases, and they stay away from sensitive subjects (like a brother's carrot-red hair or a sister's orthodontic braces).

There's a proper perspective on television watching. Family members enjoy it, but it doesn't take the place of fun family activities. Parents use what is on television to stimulate family discussions on subjects such as ethics, politics, sportsmanship, fidelity, or sexuality.

When parents communicate, there is clearly an equality. No one communicates in a way that indicates power or submission. Healthy families resist the urge to use silence as a "weapon" or punishment. When arguments take place, as they inevitably do, there's a reconciliation soon afterward. Things are talked out, and feelings are explored.

Affirmation and Support

Everyone hungers after love and support—and members of healthy families give it freely to other family members. In a healthy family, members develop good self-esteem; they feel good about themselves, and they genuinely like the other members of the family. The parents are positive, confident, and secure; they have the esteem and courage to face the world, knowing that a defeat may be disappointing but not devastating. The family's basic outlook is positive, too: Family members help each other, support each other, and forget their own interests temporarily if someone in the family needs a hand. Each family member takes an active interest in every other family member.

Findings of a variety of studies show that *being connected to their families* helped protect teens against every health risk behavior—including violence and drug abuse—except pregnancy. The researchers determined that the role of parents and family in shaping the health of adolescents is critical. And even though the physical presence of a parent in the home at key times obviously reduces risk (especially of drug abuse), the factor of greatest significance, say the researchers, is a sense of connectedness with parents—feelings of warmth, love, and caring from parents.[56]

Respect

Children in healthy families are taught self-respect, both verbally and by example. Children are taught to respect each other—and, since individuality is valued, the family teaches respect for individual differences (the two children who love to get up early on Saturday morning, for example, have learned to be relatively quiet so they don't disturb the child who likes to sleep in). Respect isn't a "special occasion–only" quality, either; it's a universal value meant for all people of all persuasions. Children are encouraged to associate with a broad spectrum of people—people of all religions, races, and philosophies. Because a child has learned self-respect, his or her parents need not fear losing their own sense of values.

Parents in healthy families respect a child's individual decisions (a father who always hoped his daughter would attend college gave her his full support when she enrolled instead in a nursing program at a local technical college). Children in healthy families, too, are taught to respect others and the property of others (a seven-year-old who shoplifts a candy bar is accompanied back to the store by his mother, who stands by him while he returns the candy bar and apologizes to the store manager).

Trust

Members of healthy families trust each other because they have earned that trust. Children are gradually given opportunities to earn trust—and if a trust is broken, family members realize that it can be mended. Having trust is so important that members of healthy families constantly work to help all family members develop it. Family confidences are kept confidential. Nobody breaks a trust by betraying another family member. Trust isn't just for the children. In healthy families, the parents demonstrate that they can be trusted, too. They follow through on commitments and keep promises.

Enjoyment

Healthy families enjoy each other—and they work together to get enjoyment out of life. They get away from the problems and pressures of everyday life. You might find them relaxing on the porch, sipping a glass of icy lemonade, and watching the fireflies dance. They work hard, but they know how to play, too. They get together for a Trivial Pursuit tournament, followed up by some homemade ice cream, or they pack a picnic lunch and ride their bicycles to the park.

Members of healthy families recognize their "breaking point"—the point at which stress has become too much. At that point they step back, cancel their scheduled activities, and get together for some good, spirited fun. They diffuse stress with laughter and play, and the members of healthy families share a great sense of humor.

Positive and Equal Interaction

In healthy families, the family is important; it's a priority to each of the members. Family members take time from work and other activities and give it to each other; and, if one member of the family has an emergency or deadline pressure, other members rally around in support. They try hard not to bring work home at night or on the weekends, and they plan carefully so there is plenty of time for family activities. Those family times reflect equality and sharing between family members. No one member dominates; there are no cliques or coalitions. Family members perform sometimes-complicated juggling acts to give a fair share to each other.

Leisure Time

Healthy families have a balanced amount of leisure time, spending some of it in pursuit of their own activities and some of it together as a family. Healthy families usually say that the most enjoyed activities are the ones that are the least structured: playing touch football in the leaves on the front lawn, shopping for a new television set, deciding to sleep outside on a warm summer night. And, although it's important to spend leisure time together as a family, members of healthy families usually spend time, too, with just one other family member: A husband and wife get away together for the evening, two sisters go horseback riding together, or a father takes his six-year-old daughter out to lunch. The leisure time that families spend together isn't just "leftover" time; it's a priority that is definitely planned.

Shared Responsibility

Parents in healthy families delight in the chance to give their children responsibility—and then they follow through by helping their children fulfill their responsibility. Family members realize that they need each other, and everyone pitches in to make sure the family keeps running smoothly. Everyone shares in the running of the household; one person does not exist to "serve" the others. Members of healthy families share responsibility for more than just chores; they also take responsibility for creating a great home atmosphere, for boosting each other up, and for providing support. Children who take responsibility are praised, recognized, and commended for their efforts.

A Sense of Right and Wrong

Although values are a very personal thing and vary from family to family, values in healthy families clearly include the differences between right and wrong. Those differences are taught to all family members. The husband and wife agree on basic values and give their children clear, specific guidelines about what is right and wrong.

Traditions

Healthy families share traditions. Some involve special occasions (the kids always put out a plate of cookies for Santa Claus, and there's always a big Easter egg hunt the morning before Easter), but some "traditions" are part of the everyday fabric of life, too (every Sunday afternoon Grandma comes over for dinner, and Mom makes the rounds every night to tuck everyone in bed).

Healthy families treasure their stories and the things family members have left behind—a yellowed diary kept by an early farmer, a collection of letters from a young immigrant to his parents in the homeland, a patchwork quilt pieced from a thousand tiny scraps of fabric and stitched by hand in front of a stone fireplace.

Rituals are an important part of healthy families; some are very simple (a child gets to choose the dinner menu on her birthday). Families are eager to accept all their members, new babies and elderly grandparents alike, and the door is always open for visits, even when no invitation has been extended.

Religion

Healthy families seem to share a strong religious core that brings them faith, a set of moral values, and a system of beliefs as a guideline. Parents make it a priority to pass religious faith on to their children by example and to help their children understand various tenets of the faith. Even when parents are not of the same religious faith, they tend to take the strong aspects of each religion and use them as strengths in the family. Healthy parents do not force a child to accept a religion but encourage it by example.

Respect for Privacy

Although healthy families enjoy each other and do plenty of things as a group, they also recognize the need to nurture each person as an individual. In a healthy family, parents recognize that each person is a private being who has the right to be alone—physically or emotionally—sometimes. The right to be private is the right to be different, the right to change gradually over the years, the right to mature, and the right to eventually leave home as a mature, functioning adult.

Respecting privacy means knocking on a child's closed door before entering the room; it also means allowing a child to make some of his or her own decisions and respecting confidences.

Service

Healthy families stress the importance of service to others, not only within the family circle but outside it as well. Parents encourage their children to participate in volunteer activities, and they set an example by doing it themselves. In addition, family members are hospitable and make others feel comfortable in their home.

Solving Problems

The healthy family is not a problem-free family, but it is a family that works toward solving problems. Members admit problems, face them head-on, and do whatever is needed to solve the problems. If necessary, they seek outside help. They expect problems because they know that problems are a part of everyday life, so they develop their own problem-solving abilities to work things out. When problems do occur, such as illness, job loss, devastating property or income loss, or even death, they do not destroy the family because the family has consciously developed mechanisms to help them surmount the challenges that could occur.

The Health Benefits of Strong Families

The family is our refuge and springboard;
nourished on it, we can advance
to new horizons. In every
conceivable manner, the family is
the link to our past, bridge to our future.
—Alex Haley

As with all basic relationships, the family determines to a large extent how healthy its members are. Those who belong to a healthy family find that their stress levels are lower, they suffer significantly less illness, and they recover from illness and disease much more rapidly. Their coping mechanisms are better, and they are able to function at a higher level. Those from healthy families, overall, are healthier people.

In a special Gallup Poll commissioned by *American Health* magazine, Americans credit much of their health—and most of their positive health changes—to the influence of the family. In the poll, 87 percent of those surveyed reported making positive health changes during the past few years; they included quitting smoking, drinking less alcohol, controlling job stress, exercising more, losing weight, and eating healthier foods.

The family, not the physician, was responsible for those changes, poll results show. The editor of the magazine reported the poll results with the comment: "Family and loved ones shape our health habits more than doctors do. . . . The computer showed that marriage and family played an even deeper role than we realized."

Social support has been demonstrated to be an important factor in protecting good health and long life. If you belong to a strong, healthy family, you've got "an unconditional charter membership in an emotional support group wherever you roam."[57] No one is in a better position to help than your family; no one knows you better. Members of your family can be counted on to provide practical and concrete aid in times of crisis. One family counselor summed it up this way: "The person from a really supportive family doesn't have to go it alone. That person is part of something bigger—a family that cares enough to let him or her know he or she is okay."[58]

The strongest social ties we have are our family: our parents, spouse, siblings, and children. Research has shown that of all the different kinds of social support available, that provided by the family is the most critical and the strongest.[59] The family unit itself is a source of the joy that brings good health. In a variety of studies, parents have expressed that children provide love and companionship, give a sense of self-fulfillment, and bring joy and pleasure as parents watch them develop and grow.

If it is true that stress causes disease, which has been demonstrated beyond doubt through years of scientific studies, it is also true that a strong family helps an individual cope better with stress, thus reducing the risk of illness and disease. As one researcher put it, "During periods of crisis, as doubts arise and confidence flags, families offer reassurance and bolster the individual in his resolution. This is particularly important during periods of loss, desertion, or other crises."[60] Studies of people during particularly stressful periods—such as the Great Depression and World War II—showed that family integration, family adaptability, and marital adjustment were the factors most enabling people to adjust to crisis.

Studies of other stressful situations illustrate the buffering effect of strong families. The American farm crisis provides an example.[61] During the 1970s, farmers faced incredible odds: The cost of production skyrocketed, but they couldn't command a high enough price for farm commodities. Many farmers faced staggering debt; some underwent foreclosure. A number of family farms were destroyed in the process.

As many as half the farmers in some states were bankrupted. Those who weren't teetered on the edge, not knowing from one month to the next whether they would survive financially—or whether it would be their farm on the next auction block. In one small Iowa community of only 8,000, three farmers committed suicide in an 18-month period because of the prospect of losing their farms.

Consider the stress created by this kind of scenario. The family faced not only economic distress but also a feeling of personal failure. Some of the farms had been run by families for many generations; the failure or loss of a farm was an embarrassment and disgrace not only for the farmer, but also for dozens of members of the extended family. The economic and emotional load for the head of the family would be unbearable; and the children, who had nothing to do with the source of the problem and little control over its solution, undoubtedly stood to pay much of the price in the form of stress.

Some of these farm families undoubtedly suffered tremendously, but many, according to research, rallied. They fought off the effects of stress. They did not fall prey to illness or disease as a result. They were families. The strength of the family—its interactions, communication patterns, and problem-solving abilities—enabled them to weather the storm.

The unique social support provided by families comes from several different functions in the family. A family endows a person with the feeling that he or she is loved and cared for. It gives a person a sense of being valued and esteemed. It gives a person a sense of belonging to a group, a group in which he or she has responsibilities and obligations. All of that translates into a buffer for the stress we all experience in daily living—and it helps prevent disease and illness.

Evidence of that buffering effect abounds.[62] Children experience less stress from hospital procedures when parents are present, so many hospitals are now allowing parents to stay in the room with sick infants and children. People with strong families recover more quickly from surgery, tend to follow medical instructions, maintain treatment recommendations, take prescribed medications, and get better more quickly and with fewer complications.

People with strong families also tend to manage chronic illness better. Wendy Auslander, a medical social worker at Washington University, studied children with diabetes; she found that the most significant factor influencing children's metabolic stability was family stress. Her findings are important nationally: diabetes affects more than 1 million children in the United States. Auslander and her colleagues discovered that children with the healthiest families were best able to control their disease. It's not just diabetes, either, says Auslander. The strength or weakness of the family and the findings of her study can be generalized "to other diseases, like cystic fibrosis, asthma, renal disease, and leukemia."[63]

People with strong families are more likely to survive a heart attack. And people with strong families are less likely to develop heart disease, even when standard risk factors are present.

People with strong families are able to weather the storm of unemployment; and, in a situation that often causes illness, they are often buffered from getting sick. People with strong families do better after the death of a loved one. They do better, in fact, in almost any stressful situation.

Research shows that a strong family can even mitigate the stresses usually experienced by single-parent families. Generally, single-parent families are seen as problematic, and the experience of losing a parent through separation, divorce, or death has been shown to lead to health problems in children. However, the strength of the remaining parent and his or her ability to create a cohesive family unit helps overcome some of those problems, thereby indicating that it is the strength of the family, not the number of parents, that has the greatest impact. In one Canadian study of 138 two-parent families and single-parent families headed by women, researchers looked at how the health of the children was impacted by family cohesiveness.[64] They especially looked at family cohesion, family pride, general self-efficiency, network support, community support, family income, the mother's educational level, internal locus of control, and the mother's nontraditional sex role orientation. They found that strong families—even those headed by a single parent—promote the health of their members because of their ability to focus on healthy behavior and to make and act upon informed choices about healthy living.

Finally, people in strong families tend to live longer than people in weak families or people without children. People who are married do best; compared to married people, those who were previously married have higher death rates regardless of whether they live alone, live with their older children, or live with others. In fact, previously married people who live with relatives other than their parents or their children are more than 50 percent more likely to die.[65] Researchers believe that part of the protective power of strong families comes from the quality of social support felt by their members.

People with strong families are twice as likely to be alive at any given age, and studies have shown that members of strong families even expect to live longer.[66] Family therapists and researchers Nick Stinnett and John DeFrain summed it up this way:

> Strong families are pleasant, positive places to live because members have learned some beneficial ways of treating each other. Family members can count on each other for support, love, and loyalty. They can talk to each other, and they enjoy each other.
>
> Members of strong families feel good about themselves as a family unit or team; they have a sense of belonging with each other—a sense of "we." At the same time, no individual gets lost or smothered; each family member is encouraged to develop his or her potential.
>
> Finally, strong families can best be defined as places where we enter for comfort, development, and regeneration and places from which we go forth renewed and charged with power for positive living.[67]

Family Reunions: More than a Good Time

Family reunions are more than just fun. They apparently provide some health benefits, too. Researchers were first prompted to study the health benefits of family reunions after watching what happens in the wild: elephants have a practice of gathering around a sick beast, offering help and support. Also, the oldest healing form in tribal medicine involved bringing the whole family—the entire clan—together and working things through for a few days.

Harold Wise, MD, who has studied family reunions, believes that they can have tremendous healing power, even for conditions as serious as cancer. As a result of the research of Wise and others, some physicians have begun encouraging "therapeutic" family reunions. Extended families are brought together to rally around a sick member. Family members are encouraged to tune in to each other. One person is encouraged to speak for the others. Wise says it's "a very primal feeling, a sense that you have stepped out of time. And once the family is into that level, no one will leave."

Wise says that, although he doesn't understand exactly how the reunions work, he does know that they work. He has experienced only one reunion in which the family member did not improve in health. "It's a very moving event," he says. "And to my astonishment, there have been some remissions of the disease in the dying person."

Wise believes that the reunions—in which family members are urged to bring up problems, discuss feelings, and forgive each other—help people feel more "connected," which brings tremendous health benefits. According to Wise:

> I have a lot of notions about what's happening, but I don't have a theory that satisfies me. All I know is that the reunions are very healthful for the family. And as the ill person is a part of the family, it's also critical to that person.
>
> You can clear out everything that prevents families from getting together, the unresolved grief, the unexpressed anger, and get to what lies underneath—a tremendous amount of love. If people feel supported and loved, they seem to heal better. The immune system seems to work better. But whether there's a remission of the disease or not, I know that this work is important for the healing of the family itself.[68]

Having a family reunion is only one way to boost the strength of your family. Try developing other family traditions or customs that have special meaning for every member of your family. You might come up with certain rituals you always remember on birthdays, anniversaries, or other holidays. Or your customs might be as simple as gathering the family for prayer before everyone leaves in the morning, reading a few pages of a classic novel together at bedtime, or going on a family walk around the block just before dinner. You might try a "penny parade": Each time you reach a corner, flip a penny. Heads, you go left—tails, you go right.

Another good idea is to take on a volunteer effort as a family. Involve the entire family from the beginning. Work together to decide on a project, plan for what each family member will do, and carry out all your plans. If you're creative, you'll be able to find ways to involve even young children.

Alternatively, try working together on a project that benefits everyone in the family. Try a family garden—work together to plan what you'll plant, read up on how to plant, prepare the soil, place the seeds, and stake off the area. Take turns watering and weeding, and work together to harvest. You might even set up a family "assembly line" to preserve your harvest by freezing, canning, or drying it.

Finally, you might consider setting aside a regular, structured block of time for "family night" or family councils. Use a certain night each week or each month to make plans, compare schedules, discuss problems, set goals, or work on a special project. Make sure you add some fun time—a romp in the leaves, a swim at the local pool, or a round of banana splits for everyone!

WHAT DID YOU LEARN?

1. How does early influence of parents affect the health of their children?
2. What are the traits of distressed families and how does that affect family health?
3. What are the traits or characteristics of strong families and how does that affect family health?
4. What part do family reunions play in fostering good health?

ENDNOTES

1. Leonard A. Sagan, *The Health of Nations* (New York: Basic Books, 1987).
2. Phillip L. Rice, *Stress and Health: Principles and Practice for Coping and Wellness* (Monterey, CA: Brooks/Cole Publishing Company, 1987), 122.
3. Linda Greenhouse, "Ruling on Definition of 'Family,' Justices Back a Welfare Curb," *The New York Times* (March 23, 1995).
4. Stephanie McCrummen, "Manassas Changes Definition of Family," *Washington Post* (December 28, 2006): A01.
5. Thomas F. Coleman, "More Cities Grapple with Definition of 'Family,'" *Eye on Unmarried America* (March 27, 2006).
6. Ibid.
7. Jerrold K. Footlick, "What Happened to the Family?" *Newsweek* (Special Issue; Winter/Spring 1990): 16.
8. "Building Strong Families: Can Well-Designed Interventions Help?" *Mathematica Policy Research, Inc.*, http://www.buildingstrongfamilies.info/About/index.htm, accessed May 28, 2008.
9. Saralee Jamieson and Lisa Wallace, "Family Strengths," University of Missouri, http://extension.missouri.edu/bsf/strengths/index.htm, accessed May 28, 2008.
10. Footlick, "What Happened to the Family?" 17.
11. J. Higley et al., "A Nonhuman Primate Model of Excessive Alcohol Intake: Personality and Neurobiological Parallels of Type I- and Type II-Like Alcoholism," in M. Galanter, ed., *Recent Developments in Alcoholism, vol. 13: Alcoholism and Violence* (New York: Plenum Press, 1997); and J. Higley, et al., "Low Central Nervous System Serotonergic Activity Is Traitlike and Correlates with Impulsive Behavior," *Annals of the New York Academy of Sciences* 836 (December 29, 1997): 39–56.
12. B. McEwen et al., "Corticosteroids, the Aging Brain and Cognition," *Trends in Endrocrinology and Metabolism* 10, no. 3 (1999): 92–6.
13. T. Comery et al., "Rapid Communication: Differential Rearing Alters Spine Density on Medium-Sized Spiny Neurons in the Rat Corpus Striatum: Evidence for Association of Morphological Plasticity with Early Response Gene Expression," *Neurobiology of Learning and Memory* 63 (1995): 217–9.

14. D. Liu et al., "Maternal Care, Hippocampal Glucocorticoid Receptors, and Hypothalamic-Pituitary-Adrenal Activity," *Science* 277 (September 12, 1997): 1659–62.

15. M. Gunnar, "Early Adversity and the Development of Stress Reactivity and Regulation," in C. A. Nelson, ed., *The Effects of Adversity on Neurobehavioral Development: The Minnesota Symposia on Child Psychology* 31 (New Jersey: Lawrence Erlbaum Associates, 2000).

16. Stephen Suomi, "Attachment in Rhesus Monkeys," in J. Cassidy and P. Shaver, eds., *Handbook of Attachment: Theory, Research, and Clinical Applications* (New York: Guilford Press, 1999): 181–96.

17. James J. Lynch, *The Broken Heart: The Medical Consequences of Loneliness* (New York: Basic Books, 1977).

18. Ibid.

19. Ibid.

20. Ibid.

21. Ibid., 81.

22. Ibid.

23. Ibid.

24. Ibid., 82.

25. Mary D. Salter Ainsworth, *Patterns of Attachment* (with M. Blehar, E. Waters, and S. Wall, Hillsdale, NJ: Erlbaum, 1978), 28–43.

26. B. Bower, "Teenagers Reap Broad Benefits from 'Authoritative' Parents," *Science News* 136 (1989): 117–8.

27. Ibid.

28. Brent V. Nelson, Troy H. Patience, and David C. MacDonald, "Adolescent Risk Behavior and the Influence of Parents and Education," *Journal of the American Board of Family Practice* 12, no. 6 (1999): 436–43.

29. A. E. Jorm, K. B. G. Dear, B. Rodgers, and H. Christensen, "Interaction Between Mother's and Father's Affection as a Risk Factor for Anxiety and Depressive Symptoms: Evidence for Increased Risk in Adults Who Rate Their Father as Having Been More Affectionate Than Their Mother," *Social Psychiatry and Psychiatric Epidemiology* 38 (2003): 173–9.

30. "Parents Influence Age of Teenage Sex," *BBC News* (August 30, 2002).

31. H. Stephen Glenn and Jane Nelsen, *Raising Children for Success* (Fair Oaks, CA: Sunrise Press, 1987).

32. Ibid.

33. Dolores Curran, *Stress and the Healthy Family* (Minneapolis, MN: Winston Press, 1985).

34. Harriet B. Braiker, *Lethal Lovers and Poisonous People* (New York: Pocket Books, 1992).

35. N. E. Mahon, A. Yarcheski, and T. J. Yarcheski, "Anger, Anxiety, and Depression in Early Adolescents from Intact and Divorced Families," *Journal of Pediatric Nursing* 18, no. 4 (2003): 267–73.

36. Clemson University Extension, "From Family Stress to Family Strengths," *Stress* (February 1997).

37. Kevin Fiscella and Thomas L. Campbell, "Association of Perceived Family Criticism with Health Behaviors," *Journal of Family Practice* 48, no. 2 (2005): 128–34.

38. "Pain: Is It All in Your Family?" *Executive Fitness* (May 1987): 7.

39. Ibid.

40. Arthur J. Barsky, *Worried Sick: Our Troubled Quest for Wellness* (Boston: Little, Brown, 1988).

41. Blair Justice, *Who Gets Sick: Thinking and Health* (Houston, TX: Peak Press, 1987), 37–8.

42. Ibid.

43. Steven Locke and Douglas Colligan, *The Healer Within: The New Medicine of Mind and Body* (New York: E. P. Dutton, 1986), 141.

44. Ibid.

45. S. I. McMillen, *None of These Diseases,* rev. ed. (Old Tappan, NJ: Fleming H. Revell Company, 1984).

46. Locke and Colligan, *The Healer Within,* 118–9.

47. Ibid.

48. Ibid.

49. Dennis Drotar, "Relating Parent and Family Functioning to the Psychological Adjustment of Children with Chronic Health Conditions: What Have We Learned? What Do We Need to Know?" *Journal of Pediatric Psychology* 22, no. 2 (1997): 149–65.

50. Barbara Powell, *Good Relationships Are Good Medicine* (Emmaus, PA: Rodale Press, 1987).

51. G. R. Parkerson et al., "Associations Among Family Support, Family Stress, and Personal Functional Health Status," *Journal of Clinical Epidemiology* 42, no. 3 (1989): 217–29.

52. Douglas A. Abbott and William H. Meredith, "Characteristics of Strong Families: Perceptions of Ethnic Parents," *Family and Consumer Sciences Research Journal* 17, no. 2 (1988): 140–7.

53. Clemson University Extension, "From Family Stress to Family Strengths."

54. "The Family Journey: Characteristics of Strong Families," University of Arkansas, http://www.arfamilies.org/family_life/family/characteristics_strong_families.htm, accessed May 28, 2008.

55. "Influence of Parents and Family on Children's Drug Use and Other Problem Behaviors: Review of the Literature," Office of National Drug Control Policy, 1998.

56. From Dolores Curran, *Traits of a Healthy Family* (Minneapolis, MN: Winston Press, 1983).

57. Sharon Faelten, David Diamond, and the editors of *Prevention* magazine, *Take Control of Your Life: A Complete Guide to Stress Relief* (Emmaus, PA: Rodale Press, 1988), 273.

58. Ibid.

59. C. E. Ross and J. Mirowsky, "Family Relationships, Social Support and Subjective Life Expectancy," *Journal of Health and Social Behavior* 43, no. 4 (December 2002): 469–89.

60. Sagan, *The Health of Nations.*

61. Rice, *Stress and Health,* 140.

62. Nick Stinnett and John DeFrain, *Secrets of Strong Families* (New York: Berkley Books, 1985).

63. "Cutting Family Stress Aids in Controlling Child's Illness," *Deseret News* (July 16, 1989): 11A.

64. Marilyn Ford-Gilboe, "Family Strengths, Motivation, and Resources as Predictors of Health Promotion Behavior in Single-Parent and Two-Parent Families," *Research in Nursing & Health* 20, no. 3 (1997): 205–17.

65. Richard G. Rogers, "The Effects of Family Composition, Health, and Social Support Linkages on Mortality," *Journal of Health and Social Behavior* 37, no. 4 (1997): 326–38.

66. Ross and Mirowsky, "Family Relationships."

67. Stinnett and DeFrain, *Secrets of Strong Families.*

68. Harold Wise, MD, "Netletter" 4, no. 1 (May 1989).

CHAPTER 13

Grief, Bereavement, and Health

Every man has his secret sorrows which the world knows not; and oftentimes we call a man cold when he is only sad.

—Henry Wadsworth Longfellow

LEARNING OBJECTIVES

- Understand the relationship between loss and grief.
- Define *grief* and *bereavement*.
- Explain the health consequences of bereavement.
- Explain how grief and bereavement impact mortality.
- Consider ways of helping to reduce the risk of grief on health.

For more than 2,000 years, people have recognized that grief—the overwhelming sorrow that follows a loss—can make people sick; even longer ago, philosophers and physicians knew that grief alone could kill. An early epitaph by Sir Henry Wootton crisply summarizes the effect that grief and bereavement can have on those who mourn:

> He first deceased; she for a little tried
> To live without him; liked it not, and died.[1]

Clearly, we've made considerable advancements in medical technology during the past 2,000 years. But something else is just as clear: Grief still makes people sick—and, unfortunately, it even kills them. Although some come through the experience of loss and the grief that follows it with relative ease, many are not so fortunate. Grief-related disorders can range all the way from mild distress and depression to major illness and death.

Our understanding of the grief and bereavement process is made all the more important by several emerging trends:[2]

- Most deaths in the United States occur in health care settings, such as hospitals and long-term care facilities; an estimated 60 percent happen in hospitals or medical clinics; and an additional 16 percent occur in nursing homes or hospice facilities. Staff in these health care settings have an increased role in caring for survivors and helping through the initial grief process.

- Research on grief and study of the care that is given to survivors has increased dramatically in the last 20 years.

- Biomedical research advances made during the past 20 years have the potential of substantially improving our understanding of the biological changes that occur as part of the grief and bereavement process.

- There are likely to be greater demands on the nation's health care systems—including the demand for end-of-life services—as the sizable "baby boomer" generation ages and faces death.

The Loss That Leads to Grief

Researchers and physicians have long recognized a specific pattern relating to human loss: loss is often followed by depression and disease. Early physicians recognized it. Some chronicled that entire kingdoms and villages in England were "daunted" by the death of a national hero.[3]

Today loss is still recognized as a precursor to distress, depression, and disease. Loss has even been implicated as a factor in premature death. Dr. Arthur Schmale studied 42 consecutive patients admitted to the Rochester Memorial Hospital; their medical problems ranged from cardiovascular problems to respiratory, digestive, and skin diseases. Hoping to find some common thread among them, he interviewed patients and their families regarding the events that led up to the illness. Schmale did indeed find a common thread: loss. Thirty-one of the patients—approximately 75 percent—developed their disease within one week of the loss of a loved one. The loss led to feelings of helplessness or hopelessness, and illness followed.[4] Researchers believe that the illness and death that so often follow loss is no coincidence: Researcher Steven Schleifer of New York's Mount Sinai Hospital estimates that 20 percent of all people who die within a year of losing a spouse die as a direct result of the loss.[5]

Loss has been shown to be a factor in a variety of illnesses, but it seems to have particular influence in some—notably, cancer. Renowned surgeon Bernie Siegel, who has become well known for his work with cancer patients, said, "One of the most common precursors of cancer is a traumatic loss or a feeling of emptiness in one's life. When a salamander loses a limb, it grows a new one. In an analogous way, when a human being suffers an emotional loss that is not properly dealt with, the body often responds by developing a new growth. It appears that if we can react to loss with personal growth, we can prevent growth gone wrong within us."[6]

The loss that precedes illness doesn't always have to be the loss of a person or a relationship. Illness might also follow the loss of a job, the loss of self-respect, the loss of feelings of usefulness, the loss of security, or the loss of an important possession. In fact, grief and illness do not always necessarily follow a loss that involves death or separation from a loved one. One study yielded the "unexpected finding" that other losses had greater impact on health than did bereavement.[7]

Possessions may be especially important to elderly people, and the loss of a cherished possession may place them at particular risk for illness. According to researchers, possessions for the elderly seem to explain where they fit in and how they are related to the bigger scheme of things. When the elderly "see their possessions as extensions of themselves or as a personal record of their memories and experiences, then depriving older people of objects they care about may be the equivalent of destroying their identity."[8] This can be particularly true of having to leave one's home.

For children, another kind of loss—the loss of a parent—can be particularly devastating. Dr. Rene Spitz described how infants who suddenly lost their mothers physically wasted away, dying of marasmus, a severe protein deficiency disease usually seen only in poor countries. These infants refused to eat and eventually died, even when they were force-fed.[9]

In an attempt to determine the impact of parental loss on children, in a classic set of studies, Spitz and Katherine Wolf carefully observed 91 infants who were reared in foundling homes in the United States and Canada. All of the infants were physically well cared for, but they didn't gain weight or grow as rapidly as other infants. In fact, some of them even lost weight. Despite excellent physical care, the infants seemed anxious and depressed. Of the 91 infants in the study, 34—or more than one-third—died despite what researchers say was "good food and meticulous medical care."[10] Even among those who survived, almost all showed varying signs of emotional and physical retardation. The last trimester of an infant's first year of life seems to be of particular significance. Most of the deaths in the study occurred during this period.

Parental loss—the loss of a parent through death, separation, or divorce—has been shown in a wide variety of studies to lead to later health problems. Unfortunately, the likelihood of losing a parent has remained almost constant since 1900. Even though mortality rates have dipped—making it less likely that a parent will die—the divorce rates have increased, making it more likely that divorce or separation will create the parental loss.[11]

From what researchers can determine, early loss of a parent leads to both physical and psychological illness. In an expansion of his earlier study, Schmale and other members of the Rochester Medical School research group studied adult patients who had been admitted to the hospital with physical complaints. A significant number of the men and women had lost one or both parents early in life. Now, as adults, they had suffered some new loss—or had merely been threatened with such a loss—and they reacted with physical illness, including cardiac disorders.[12] A new loss can be more devastating when it reignites the trauma of an old loss.

The psychological problems that follow the loss of a parent can be devastating, too. Delinquency, accidents, psychosis, and suicide are all more pronounced among children who lost a parent early in life. The risk of suicide is seven times greater among children who have lost both parents than for those raised in an intact family.[13]

Eager to find out how much influence parental loss had over thoughts of suicide, researchers decided to study college students. They examined students who had come from intact families and students who had been separated from at least one parent during childhood. The differences between the two groups of students were vast: Only 10 percent of the students from intact families had ever had serious thoughts about suicide. In sharp contrast, almost half of the students who had lost a parent had seriously contemplated ending their own lives.[14]

Grief: The Natural Effect of Loss

According to one psychologist, grief is the natural and predictable process of healing from the pain of loss. Grief has been called the "quintessential mind-body problem," providing rich evidence of how an emotional experience translates into very real biological consequences. Psychiatrist Paul Pearsall calls grief a completely natural emotion—as natural, in fact, as joy—and concludes that his patients who grieve the most intensely are also those who experience the greatest joy.

Because it is a process of healing, grief is necessary. Those who don't grieve, says professor of psychiatry Glen Davidson, become chronically disoriented. An entire array of studies shows that incomplete or abnormal grief can cause serious physical and psychological problems.

For grief to progress "normally," most experts agree, a person often passes through the stages of grief made famous by Dr. Elisabeth Kübler-Ross:

- Denial—a disbelief that the loss has actually occurred

- Anger over the loss

- Bargaining—a person typically "bargains" with him or herself or with God, desperately attempting to reverse the loss by offering something in exchange

- Depression—feeling intense sorrow over the loss

- Acceptance of the loss

- Hope for the future

Even though grief is normal, natural, and necessary, it can cause illness because it involves intense emotions and because it is so inseparably connected to loss. The best health protection against the consequences of grief is to allow enough time to grieve—enough time for the healing process to take place—and to affirm and acknowledge feelings about the loss. Psychiatrist Glen Davidson, chief of thanatology at Southern Illinois University School of Medicine, emphasizes that a wide range of emotions is apt to accompany grief. In his in-depth work with mourners, he has found that emotions like sorrow, guilt, anger, depression, fear, shame, anxiety, and loneliness are all normal.[15]

As the old saying goes, "Time heals all wounds." Nothing could be more appropriate in describing what's needed to heal grief. Research now shows that trying to stifle grief, trying to "keep a stiff upper lip," is actually more stressful on the body than allowing yourself to grieve. Formal psychiatry has sometimes suggested that "uncomplicated bereavement" should be completed in two months—a notion that Gerald Koocher, an expert on grief and chief psychologist at Children's Hospital in Boston, calls "... ridiculous. A person can grieve continuously for a loved one for as long as two years, and intermittently for many years after"—something that should not be considered wrong or unhealthy.[16]

Other researchers in the area of grief agree with Koocher's assessment. Stephen Goldston, a psychologist who has done comprehensive research on grief, says we have adopted a cultural attitude that

> A person who isn't "back to normal" four to six weeks after a loss is somehow sick or wallowing in self-pity. This places a burden on grieving people, who then think they should "snap out of it" after a few weeks. But people just can't recover from a major loss that quickly. And when they don't, they are made to feel abnormal or guilty about experiencing normal, understandable emotions. In fact, it takes most people a full year to resume life after bereavement, and it can take as long as three. They find ways to cope with a loss themselves, at their own pace. In fact, that is really the only way to handle grief.[17]

Although Davidson's research shows that the average recovery time from a major loss is between 18 and 24 months, that time can vary greatly—and can even be much longer under some circumstances—without being considered prolonged or abnormal. A full-fledged clinical depression evolving from the grief might be considered abnormal, however. Such depression can be difficult to distinguish from normal grief. A cardinal symptom of clinical depression that is considered unlikely after two or three months of grief is *anhedonia,* the inability to experience pleasure. If a person is distracted from the loss and is unable to enjoy things that normally would be very enjoyable, there is a possibility that the grief has triggered clinical depression. This is a particular possibility if there is a past history or family history of such depression or if the sad feelings become so pronounced that they interfere with the ability to function—the inability to shop or socialize, the tendency to miss work, the creation of unnecessary conflicts, or feelings of giving up.

In a two-year study of more than 300 mourners, Dr. Holly Prigerson—director of the Center for Psycho-Oncology and Palliative Care Research at the Dana-Farber Cancer Institute in Boston—found that, while nearly all went through a rough time of crying, longing, and having trouble concentrating, 85 percent return to feeling normal after six months of the loss.[18] Complicated grief that requires treatment is apparent if, after that point, the mourning is prolonged and if several of the following problems have ensued: trouble accepting the reality of the loss, excessive bitterness, detachment from others, the feeling that life is meaningless and hopeless, or agitation that causes difficulty.[19] There are a number of innovative ways of treating this complication, such as online intervention[20] or desensitization methods. Dr. Katherine Shear of Columbia University studied an innovative treatment for 95 people with complicated grief. She recorded the mourners describing their loved one's death. Then she had the mourners take the recording home and listen to it regularly. "Some people told us that when they listened to the tape, they finally believed their loved one was truly gone." That is, they came to some acceptance. The results showed 51 percent using the tape had a good result compared to 28 percent who had a good result with traditional psychotherapy.[21]

A number of things can help ease the grieving process and can thereby reduce the risk of ensuing illness. Among them are regular exercise, a balanced diet, a healthy fluid intake, and plenty of rest. Also critical to the eventual healthy outcome is a nurturing social network. Mourners who have good support from family and friends (even if it's just a few close friends) do better than those who don't have such support. Talking a lot about one's feelings, memories, and how to reorganize life helps a lot to move the grieving process along. In contrast, bottling up those feelings and memories prolongs the grieving process. A good listener is a great asset to one who is grieving. And, researchers say, as important as all the other factors is attitude—the courage to face the loss and the willingness to fully rejoin life.

The Health Consequences of Bereavement

Bereavement, the loss of a loved one through death, leads to a special kind of grief. A universal experience, it has been described as the process of disbanding from someone who played an important role in one's life—someone who is now gone. Bereavement has been defined by some researchers as a "broad term that encompasses the entire experience of family members and friends in the anticipation, death, and subsequent adjustment to living following the death of a loved one."[22] That definition would include external circumstances and changes (such as a change in living conditions) as well as internal, physiological changes and the expressions and experiences of grief.

Grief, on the other hand, has been defined as "a complex set of cognitive, emotional and social difficulties that follow the death of a loved one."[23] Researchers who use that definition point out that people vary enormously in the kind of grief they experience, its duration and intensity, and their way of expressing it.

Because much of the research does not differentiate between grief and bereavement, the studies cited throughout the rest of this chapter may use either or both terms to describe the same general phenomenon.

The intense and prolonged grief involved in bereavement has been shown to have significant health risks, ranging all the way from immune system disorders to suicides, sudden deaths, and increased death rates from all causes. According to some research, how you grieve determines to a large extent how healthy you stay.[24]

According to the National Institute of Mental Health, the likelihood of suffering through bereavement at some time in your life is great. Each year, more than 2.5 million people die in the United States, and an estimated 8 million Americans suffer the death of an immediate family member. There are approximately 12.5 million widows and widowers in this country. Suicide occurs in at least 33,500 families each year (and probably in many more, since suicide is heavily underreported). Approximately 100,000 children and young adults under the age of 25 die each year in the United States.[25]

Because of the tremendous increase in grief research over recent decades, we know much more about bereavement and its effects on the body:

- Everyone experiences loss, but not everyone reacts to that experience in the same way—and there is no one clearly defined way to grieve. There are many factors that can influence the way a person grieves; among them are gender, age, stage of development, familial relationships, religion, culture, existing social networks, history of loss, previous trauma, the type of loss (anticipated, violent, or traumatic), the quality of the relationship with the deceased person, and the presence of any depressive or other psychiatric disorder. Most people cope well with loss, but, because we haven't fully identified all the "normal" responses to loss, it's sometimes difficult to determine when someone has a problematic reaction to grief.[26]

- We have made progress in distinguishing "normal" reactions to grief from complicated grief and in determining the risks that complicated grief entails. A small but significant percentage of the population experiences complicated (sometimes called "pathological") grief. We have made progress in defining what that means, and we also know that those are the people who are most likely to suffer adverse physical reactions to their grief.[27]

- Maintaining continuing emotional or psychological bonds with the deceased is not necessarily a sign of pathological grief. We used to think that "breaking bonds" with the deceased was a critical part of normal, healthy grief.[28] Recent research,[29] however, indicates that people who maintain emotional and psychological ties to the deceased can often have a very positive adaptation to bereavement.

- Positive emotions are possible following loss.[30] In fact, the loss of a loved one might change a person in very positive ways. Researchers have found numerous accounts of people who have been transformed for the better as a result of struggling with the loss of a loved one.[31]

- Some people do not experience what we understand as distress or grief following the loss of a loved one.[32] In the past, we considered someone who didn't experience distress or grief as having an abnormal or pathological reaction, both of which indicated problems. However, researchers now realize that the death of a loved one may actually signal the end of a very difficult situation, relief from a terminal illness, or even the end of an abusive relationship,[33] which would obviously not cause distress. Even when negative circumstances did not exist, the loss of a loved one may result in important personal growth.[34]

- Research shows that grief counseling may not help people who are going through "normal" grief—and, in fact, it might even be detrimental.[35]

- Significant advancements have been made in identifying, measuring, and understanding the biological effects of grief.[36] These advances can help us more clearly understand how pathological grief may lead to negative health effects and will help us determine how to help those who are grieving.

- The bereaved are susceptible to serious illness and even death. At a minimum, bereaved people may report pain; gastrointestinal problems, sleep and appetite disturbances; and other vegetative symptoms that may signal the onset of a depression.

A special type of bereavement occurs when a woman involuntarily loses her baby during pregnancy. Research shows that women tend to experience greater symptoms of grief than do their male partners. In one study involving 109 Australian women who lost their babies either during pregnancy or at birth,[37] 91 percent of the women saw the death as the worst thing that had ever happened to them, and 77 percent said the death of the baby led to a marked decline in their ability to function. Most reported that their social environment did not give them "permission" to grieve. However, 68 percent said they were eventually able to attribute something positive to the experience.

In another study of 74 African American women,[38] almost all the women said they considered the loss to be of the baby, not the pregnancy. Contemplating memories of the baby helped these women, as did reliance on spiritual and religious practices and beliefs and the effort to connect with other people.

Another special type of bereavement occurs in parents who lose a child—a type of loss that is regarded as more intense than the loss of a spouse or parent.[39] Parents who lose a child are more likely to suffer from increased anxiety and other types of distress;[40] conflict and anger, breakdown in communication, differences in grief intensity, lowered expression of intimacy between parents;[41] and complicated grief.[42] In one study of 204 families who lost a child by accident, homicide, or suicide, parents indicated it took three or four years to put the child's death into perspective; those whose children died by homicide suffered the highest rate of posttraumatic stress disorder, and marital satisfaction decreased over time for all parents, regardless of how the child died.[43]

One prominent psychologist maintained that every death has at least two victims—and that it is the surviving "victim" who hurts the most deeply. The one who is left behind is at significantly increased risk for a number of health problems.

A survivor's health is at least partly dependent on how much he or she thinks about or talks about the death. To study that effect, researchers obtained coroner's records of everyone who had died in a large metropolitan area within a single year and singled out the people who had committed suicide or died in a car accident.[44] To further narrow the study, any deaths used as part of the study had to meet three criteria. The deceased person had to have (a) been married, (b) been between the ages of 25 and 45, and (c) died within 24 hours of the suicide attempt or accident.

Researchers then sent questionnaires to the surviving spouses approximately one year after the death; 62 percent of those who received them returned the questionnaires. The questionnaires tried to determine three things:

1. What kind of illnesses the survivors had in the year following the death.

2. How much the survivors had talked to others about their spouse's death.

3. How much they thought about their spouse's death.

Three interesting findings emerged. First, the more people talked about a spouse's death, the fewer health problems they had during the year following the death. Second, the more they talked about the death, the less they thought about it. Finally, the more they thought about the death, the more health problems they had.

The spouses of car accident victims had more health problems than the spouses of suicide victims. Those whose spouses died in car accidents tended to talk about the accident less and think about it more; those whose spouses died as a result of suicide seemed more eager to seek out a "listening ear" and to talk about the death.

Apparently the health effects of widowhood depend in part on how old the person is when he or she is widowed. Although divorce takes a greater toll at older ages, the harmful health effects of widowhood are greater at younger ages. The younger a person is when a spouse dies, the greater the likelihood that health problems or premature death will follow.[45]

The health effects of widowhood also depend on how swiftly the spouse dies; and, even then, there are differences in the ways men and women react. A study led by researchers from Yale looked at whether bereavement led to different health outcomes in men and women, depending on gender.[46] The study involved almost 100 women and more than 50 men, who were first interviewed when their terminally ill spouses were admitted to the hospital and who were followed for more than two years. The study looked for all kinds of physical and behavioral problems known to be associated with grief and bereavement, including heart attack, heart disease, stroke, smoking, alcohol abuse, sleep problems, and depression. They noted any hospitalization and also recorded how the men and women rated their own health at periodic follow-up intervals.

The researchers found that both men and women suffered three distinct symptom "clusters"—traumatic grief, depression, and anxiety. Both men and women experienced easing of these symptoms over a similar period of time; neither the men nor the women were able to ease their emotional stress more rapidly than the other group. However, the way these symptoms impacted health was different for men and women, depending on gender.

At approximately the one-year anniversary of their wives' death, the men in the study who suffered a high level of grief had an increased rate of accidents, hospitalization, and "physical events" (being told by a physician that they had cancer, stroke, or heart attack). The women in the study who had significant grief had a high rate of sleep changes. Men who suffered depression had higher rates of hospitalization and accidents; women who were depressed had higher rates of arthritis, thoughts of suicide, and poor self-rated health. High levels of anxiety tended to produce poor self-rated health among both men and women.[47]

At approximately two years after the spouse's death, high levels of grief caused high blood pressure among the men; it caused heart problems, "physical events," and changes in eating habits among the women. Significant depression caused high blood pressure, poor self-rated health, and changes in sleep habits for men; high depression caused higher levels of traumatic grief among the women. High levels of anxiety caused thoughts of suicide among the men but heart attack and stomach problems among the women.[48]

Research conducted at the University of Utah in Salt Lake City and sponsored by the National Institute on Aging led to findings that women fare better than men when a spouse dies suddenly and that men do better than women after a spouse dies of a chronic illness.[49] According to the research, men whose wives die suddenly are at 52 percent greater risk of dying soon than are men of similar age and background whose wives are still alive. If the wife dies of chronic illness, her husband's risk of premature death drops to 13 percent—still elevated above normal but one-fourth the risk of those whose wives die suddenly.

The risks appear to be reversed for women. Sociologist Ken R. Smith, who spearheaded the study, says that a woman whose husband dies of a chronic illness faces 49 percent higher risk of premature death than other women her age whose husbands are still alive. If the husband dies suddenly, her risk of premature death plummets to 1 percent.

Smith speculates that the difference between men and women has to do with the woman's role as caregiver. Men whose wives died suddenly aren't prepared for the loss of the one who nurtured them; if the wife dies of a chronic illness, the man has probably had a chance to "prepare" by finding someone to take care of his needs. A woman, on the other hand, faces the burden of giving care to a chronically ill husband and the financial loss that follows his death.[50]

Those who are caregivers—especially the elderly—may suffer particular effects of grief once the patient dies,[51] depending on how much strain was involved in the caregiving. In a study of 129 people between the ages of 66 and 96 (75 percent women, and 90 percent Caucasian), researchers divided the group into caregivers who were strained, caregivers who were not strained, and people who were not caregivers.

The strained caregivers suffered greater symptoms of depression and had worse health practices; they didn't take time to go to the physician when they were sick, didn't get enough rest, had trouble slowing down, didn't take time to exercise, and forgot to take medications. However, researchers indicate that the death of a spouse may not necessarily increase the levels of distress for strained caregivers, who may interpret the death as the relief of a significant burden. The people who were not caregivers had higher levels of depression, increased use of antidepressants, and suffered weight loss. The nonstrained caregivers fell somewhere in the middle, experiencing only minor increases in depression.

Widowhood seems to have a profound effect especially on the well-being of men.[52]

Contrary to theories that women may be more sensitive to bereavement,[53] research shows that men may be even harder hit than women. The effects of bereavement become greater with age: The older the man, the more his health is affected by the loss of a spouse, adult child, parent, sibling, or friend.[54]

Dr. Anne Peplau, a psychologist at the University of California, Los Angeles, says:

> One of the myths we have been debunking is that the people you really need to worry about are lonely old ladies, that men somehow do better. The evidence comes out overwhelmingly opposite—women seem to be better able to adjust to old age and widowhood than men do, especially if the men are not married. Through most of men's lives, marriage seems to provide a social buffer for them. If their wives die before they do, men are in trouble in terms of their physical health and their mental health.[55]

Studies bear out Peplau's contention that men are less able to make full adjustments. In one large-scale study, researchers observed bereaved men and women beginning in the second year after the spouse's death and continued the study through the tenth year. They found a slight but significant increase in illness and death among the men when compared with the rates of illness and premature death among the women, especially among men who did not remarry.[56]

Adjustment following the death of a spouse depends on a number of factors, including age, the quality of the relationship, self-blame, and self-assessment of initial grief symptoms[57]. In general, an entire host of symptoms and illnesses strike with greater frequency among the bereaved. One mail survey evaluated the health of a group of widows in the Boston area; all were under the age of 60, and each had been widowed 13 months earlier. Researchers then found a group of 199 other women who were used as a matched control group; they were extremely similar to the widows in age, profession, and other circumstances, except that members of the control group were married.[58] Researchers looked at (a) what kinds of physical symptoms each of the groups had, (b) which group had the most physical symptoms, and (c) which group had the greatest "deterioration in health" during the previous 13 months.

Findings of the study confirmed the health problems associated with bereavement. Members of the widowed group had a significantly higher number of physical symptoms, ranging from sleeplessness to serious disease conditions, such as asthma. The most common symptoms generally associated with bereavement were headaches, dizziness, fainting spells, skin rashes, excessive sweating, indigestion, difficulty in swallowing, and chest pain.[59]

The second part of the study confirmed that the bereaved continued to have more loss of health in the subsequent year: 28 percent of the bereaved reported that they had experienced a significant deterioration in health, whereas only about 4.5 percent of the control group had experienced such a decline.[60]

A study of the survivors of more than 200 deaths showed that if the death occurs as a result of chronic illness, the survivors will have an increase in minor illnesses, but if the death is sudden, the survivors will have an increased risk for serious illnesses.[61]

The ability of a person to make sense of a death may depend in large part on religious faith. In one study,[62] researchers studied 205 adults who had suffered the loss of a spouse/partner, parent, child, sibling, other relative, or friend; they asked participants whether they had been able to make sense of the death or had been able to find anything positive in the experience. The researchers found that those with fewer problems were the ones who had religious or spiritual beliefs about death that helped them make sense of the situation.

Those who were able to make sense of the death within the first six months were much less likely to suffer emotional distress—and those who couldn't make sense of the death within the first six months were also unlikely to be able to make sense of it later. Most reported that they had perceived something positive from the experience, most often growth in character, strengthening of relationships, and changes in perspective. Importantly, making sense of the death and finding something positive in the death are not related.

A study of relatives and friends of dying patients in a London care center[63] found that those with strong spiritual beliefs had the strongest pattern of recovery over the nine months following the death. Those with low levels of spiritual belief showed little change by nine months following the death but tended to recover quickly from then on. Those with no spiritual beliefs actually showed a decline at nine months that intensified at fourteen months following the death. Authors of the study suggest that the strength of spiritual beliefs may play a role in the timing and resolution of grief following the death of a loved one.

Heart Disease

We've all heard about people who "died of a broken heart." According to research, there may be much more fact than fiction to that notion. As an example, the heart attack rate of widows between the ages of 25 and 34 is five times that of married women in the same age group. The greatest risk is in the first week after loss of one's spouse, when the death risk is two fold.[64] In an attempt to determine the rate of premature death among widowed people, British researchers studied 4,486 people (over age 55) for 9 years. During the first six months after a spouse's death, the rate of premature death was startling: 40 percent above the expected rate for married men of the same age. The mortality rates gradually decreased over the next few years until it had become the same as control groups by the end of five years. Almost half of all the deaths during the first six months were due to heart problems.

As a result, researchers dubbed it the "broken heart" study—and announced that the bereaved can, indeed, die of a broken heart.[65] Subsequent studies have confirmed the findings, although the exact percentages vary slightly. Widowers are significantly more likely to die than men the same age who have not lost their wives; the increased risk for the men persists for at least six years unless the man remarries. The duration of risk for women who are widowed appears to be shorter, usually recovering by the third year.[66]

A handful of critics have eyed bereavement studies with suspicion, saying that marriage and remarriage may not have that great an influence. Critics believe that the people involved in these studies were probably too sick to get remarried—and that's not only why they failed to remarry, but it's probably why they died, too. However, the results of a number of studies directly refute that line of thinking. The most persuasive was a study in which a high number of surviving spouses died during the first six months of bereavement. The study finding "clearly implies that the increase in mortality in widows and widowers is not due to the fact that these individual are simply too sick to remarry. Most of the increase in sudden deaths occurs before there would have been sufficient time to remarry in any event."[67] The "broken heart" syndrome might again have influence: Three-fourths of the bereaved people who died fell prey to either arteriosclerosis or coronary thrombosis. The mechanisms of how stress and depression cause coronary events (more vessel plaque, spasms, and clots) as well as heart rhythm abnormalities are likely similar in bereavement (see Chapters 2, 4, and 6).

In another study, the "broken heart" notion held true, but those who died had a different kind of bereavement. Dr. William Greene and his colleagues carefully studied the circumstances surrounding 26 Eastman Kodak Company employees who died of sudden coronary deaths. To gather their information, they studied medical records and also interviewed the next of kin, usually the wife. Most of the 26 men who had died suddenly from coronary heart problems were grieving—not the loss of a spouse but a child. More than half were depressed over "the departure of the last or only child in the family for college or marriage." Greene and his colleagues also noticed during the course of the study that a large number of patients who had a heart attack but who survived to reach the hospital mentioned that a child had recently left home.[68] This may counter the popular notion that "an empty nest is a happy nest" (at least for the first few months).

Immune System Function

Researchers say there's a logical reason why the bereaved have greater health problems than usual: The process of bereavement compromises the immune system. This link was first discovered in a 1977 study. Four Australian researchers decided to study immune system response in 26 people who had lost their spouses. The researchers conducted blood tests two weeks after the spouses died and again six weeks later. They then compared the test results with people whose spouses were still living. The results demonstrated for the first time that bereavement had real, physical effects. In both sets of blood tests—the test two weeks after the deaths and the test six weeks later—there were significant abnormalities in both T and B cell activity.[69]

Numerous follow-up studies have shown the same result. Physicians from Florida's Veterans Administration Medical Center and the University of Miami School of Medicine studied a group of 60 men; the average age was 54. Each man had experienced serious illness or death of a close family member during the previous six months. In each case, the men had a reduced activity level of lymphocytes, cells vital to the functioning of the immune system.[70]

Researchers working in the laboratory with animals have had similar results. University of Colorado psychiatrist Martin Reite and his colleagues created depression in monkeys by separating them from their mothers at the age of six months. The baby monkeys, who were put into cages separate from their mothers, showed all the classic signs of depression. To test immune response, Reite took blood samples from the baby monkeys both before and after the separation; as part of the tests he ran, he checked the ability of white blood cells to proliferate. Following separation from their mothers, the baby monkeys showed a "significant reduction" in white blood cell activity.[71]

A team of researchers at Mount Sinai Hospital in New York City headed by psychiatrists Steven Schleifer and Marvin Stein and immunologist Steven Keller studied a group of men whose wives had died from breast cancer. To test how well the widowers' immune systems were functioning, researchers injected the men with a mitogen, a chemical that kicks the immune system into gear and triggers lymphocyte activity. For two months following the wives' deaths, the widowers' immune activity (measured by the response of T cells and B cells) was "significantly suppressed." For a year longer, the men's immune systems didn't completely bound back; throughout the year, the immune system lymphocytes showed only an "intermediate level" of activity. In assessing the results of the study, Schleifer and his colleagues summarized that the increased death rate among bereaved widowers is due (at least in part) to the changes in the immune system.[72]

Test results are similar for women who are bereaved. Dr. Michael Irwin and his colleagues at the University of California, San Diego measured natural killer–cell activity in women whose husbands had recently died. The role of natural killer cells is a vital one: They appear to protect the body against viral disease and against tumor growth; natural killer cells become immediately activated against virus and tumor cells, even when they have never been exposed to those cells previously. The researchers compared natural killer–cell activity among widows to natural killer–cell activity among women whose husbands were healthy.

The results showed that the women whose husbands were healthy had normal levels of natural killer–cell activity. Those who were bereaved—whose husbands had died—had "significantly reduced" natural killer–cell activity.[73] This often contributes to increased and prolonged infections. Similar abnormalities in natural killer–cell function (and white blood cell counts) were found in people who sustained losses after devastating Hurricane Andrew slammed into Florida in 1992. In that study, the immune changes seemed mediated by the new sleep loss associated with the devastating personal losses.[74] One might wonder if close attention to sleep in such circumstances would lessen the impact of grief on immunity.

It is not only the event of bereavement that causes these problems; more important may be perception and attitude—how we think and, specifically, our thoughts regarding the loss. That theory is supported by a study conducted at Norway's University of Bergen. Thirty-nine Norwegian women were studied approximately one month after the death of their husbands and again a year later. Researchers found that immunity was strongest among women who had good "coping"—defined as a positive expectation about their longer-term outcome of the experience.[75]

That theory may also receive credence from a study involving women who had undergone abortion. Research scientists from Israel's Weizmann Institute of Science and Jerusalem's Kaplan Hospital studied women who had lost their unborn children.[76] Some of the women had experienced spontaneous abortion (miscarriage); others had requested medically induced abortions. Researchers were interested in finding out which factor influenced the immune system. Was it the type of abortion, or was it how the women perceived the abortions?

To test the women, psychiatrists divided them into two groups. In the first group were those who did not accept the abortion, regardless of the way it happened. In the second group were the women who were more accepting, less anxious, and less upset. Blood samples were then taken and compared with each other as well as with samples from women of similar ages who had not suffered the loss of an unborn child. The women who were having trouble coping and adjusting to the loss of the child suffered "a definite shift" in immune system activity; they had "more feeble T cell strength" than the women who had adjusted better to the loss. The woman's thinking seemed to be the critical factor; whether the abortion was accidental and unplanned or medically requested didn't seem to make a difference.[77] As one researcher said, "The heart cannot decide that a loved one's death in a train wreck is too much to bear; the liver does not feel the shame of embarrassment; the immune system does not know whether its client is employed or not, divorced or happily married. It is the brain that knows and feels."[78] Thus changes in the thinking brain create changes in immune responses. Stress-vulnerable thinking leads to greater vulnerability of the immune system to its challenges. (Reasons for this were taken up in the discussion of psychoneuroimmunology in Chapter 1.)

After the devastating 1994 Northridge earthquake in California, a study of the psychological and immune response effects showed much less immune disruption among those with a more "appropriate" and "realistic" response to the losses.[79] The degree of immune impact correlates with the perception of loss of control.[80] After natural catastrophes, perceived loss has greater immune and health impact than actual damage from the catastrophe. After expressing one's grief, dealing well with the hopeless or intrusive thoughts and creating a realistic response plan may be important keys to diminishing the health effects of loss.[81]

Timing after a loss also has an effect on what kind of impact on the immune system occurs. Similar to the differences in health effects of acute stress versus chronic stress, immunity may actually become acutely overresponsive (as with hives or asthma) and then may diminish as one begins to give up. Thus, complex immune reactions may be seen, depending on how soon after the loss the effects are measured.[82] Neither too much nor too little immune response is desirable. Research at Norway's University of Bergen shows that immune system function usually recovers improved function after one year of bereavement.[83]

Sudden Deaths

Those who are mourning a loss have a higher than expected rate of sudden death. We already discussed the sudden deaths among Eastman Kodak employees in Rochester; at least half of the sudden deaths were preceded by "the departure of the last or only child in the family for college or marriage."[84] Throughout most of medical history, physicians have documented cases in which a person died suddenly and unexpectedly following a loss; in fact, "grief" used to be listed as a cause of death on death certificates.[85] As medicine became more sophisticated and technology became more advanced, however, physicians began searching instead for signs of disease or illness; the factor of "grief" as a cause of death became mere speculation among friends and family members.

In any event, a number of researchers have shown that loss, grief, mourning, and bereavement can and do result in sudden death. One of the most notable pioneering researchers in the mind-body field, Dr. George Engle, studied 170 sudden deaths in 1971. Engle, who is affiliated with the University of Rochester Medical School in New York, studied 170 newspaper reports (many from the Rochester press) of sudden death during a six-year period. Engle used the 170 deaths in his study because he could rule out suicide as a factor and because he could reconstruct the circumstances surrounding the deaths. The following are examples of the cases:

- During a physical examination, a 52-year-old man passed an electrocardiogram with "flying colors"; the test showed no evidence of coronary disease. Six months later, his wife died of lung cancer. The day after her funeral, the man died suddenly of a massive myocardial infarction (heart attack).

- When an 88-year-old man was told of the sudden death of his daughter, he began wringing his hands and asking, "Why has this happened to me?" Even though he had no known heart disease, he developed acute pulmonary edema while talking on the phone to his son; he died just as a physician reached his house.

- A 71-year-old woman rode in the ambulance with her 61-year-old sister, who was pronounced dead on arrival at the hospital. The instant she received the news that her sister was dead, the older woman "collapsed." Physicians did an electrocardiogram, which showed she had sustained damage to her heart; within a few minutes, she developed ventricular fibrillation (disruption of the heart's rhythm) and died.

- A 14-year-old girl suddenly "dropped dead" when told that her 17-year-old brother had died unexpectedly.

- An 18-year-old girl died suddenly and unexpectedly when told that her grandfather, who had helped raise her, was dead.[86]

In more than half of the sudden deaths he investigated, Engle was able to document that the death was immediately preceded by some kind of interpersonal loss. In both men and women, most of the deaths occurred after the collapse or death of a loved one, during acute grief (within 16 days of the loss), or during the threat of loss of a loved one.[87]

As in the last two cases (the young girls), the kinds of sudden death that occur as a result of grief or bereavement don't just happen to the elderly or to people who are already ill. Engle points out that they often occur in young, apparently healthy people. When they suddenly and unexpectedly lose someone close, they apparently become convinced that life is "unbearable." In many ways, says Engle, they simply "will their own death."

A more physiological explanation involves the effects of stress hormones on the heart. Most sudden deaths are caused by a sudden arrhythmia, when the heart develops an irritable site of new electrical discharges affecting the usual normal beating pattern. The ventricular fibrillation described in one of the cases above (the 71-year-old woman) is a classical example. Instead of the usual pacemaker controlling the rhythm, a site down on the lower heart ventricle takes over so it beats out of control, and effective blood flow stops. It is well known that a flood of catecholamines in response to stress can trigger such an event. Such a flood of stress hormones also at times can cause severe coronary spasm and pressure loads that cause sudden myocardial necrosis, or death of the heart muscle. This damage often also triggers an arrhythmia and heart pumping failure, causing the pulmonary edema (fluid backing up in the lungs) described in one of the above cases (the 88-year-old man).

Researchers Ian Wilson and John Reece reported on the case of inseparable twin sisters in North Carolina. Neither married or stayed away from the other for any prolonged period. When they were 21, both of the young women started showing signs of schizophrenia; within 10 years, both had to be hospitalized. During the next year, they were in and out of the hospital several times; with each readmission they became worse, until finally they both refused to eat. Hospital authorities theorized that they reinforced each other's behavior and refusal to accept food, so the twins were separated and placed on separate floors of the hospital. Early one morning, one of the twins was found dead. Within minutes her twin sister went to the window, looked up at her sister's room a floor above, and—without even knowing that her sister was dead—slumped to the floor. She, too, was dead.[88]

The phenomenon isn't isolated to people. Based on his years of research, Engle says that animals, too, seem to give up and die suddenly if a lifelong companion dies. Based on his studies, he tells the following story of Charlie and Josephine, who had been inseparable for 13 years:

> In a senseless act of violence, Charlie, in full view of Josephine, was shot and killed in a melee with the police. Josephine first stood motionless, then slowly approached his prostrate form, sank to her knees, and silently rested her head on the dead and bloody body. Concerned persons attempted to help her away, but she refused to move. Hoping she would soon surmount her overwhelming grief, they let her be. But she never rose again; in fifteen minutes, she was dead.
>
>   The remarkable part of the story is that Charlie and Josephine were llamas in the zoo! They had escaped from their pen during a snowstorm and Charlie, a mean animal to begin with, was shot when he proved unmanageable. I was able to establish from the zookeeper that to all intents and purposes Josephine had been normally frisky and healthy right up to the moment of the tragic event.[89]

Another phenomenon related to the sudden death among the bereaved has been dubbed the "anniversary" death: A bereaved person may die suddenly and unexpectedly on the anniversary of a loved one's death. Sometimes these deaths occur on actual anniversaries; at other times, they occur as the result of a powerful reminder of the dead person. For example, the widow of Louis "Satchmo" Armstrong suffered a fatal heart attack as she played the final chord of *St. Louis Blues* at a memorial concert for her husband.[90]

Bereavement's Effect on General Mortality Rates

Many studies show that people who are widowed are more likely to die early than people of the same age whose spouses are living. In the study conducted in Finland, the rate of death from all causes was 6.5 percent higher than expected for their age and gender.

The increase was sharpest during the first months; during the first week alone, mortality rates doubled for both men and women. Women seemed to recover more rapidly than men to the emotional rigors of being widowed: Their death rates from natural causes returned to average by the end of the first month. In men older than 65, the death rates returned to average by the end of six months. Men younger than 65 fared the worst; after being widowed, their death rates were still 50 percent higher than expected after three years.[91]

Studies done in England confirmed that men are affected more gravely. In the British research called "The Broken Heart Study"[92] described above, the high initial mortality rates started to gradually decline after six months, until, by five years, they reached the death rates for married men of the same age.[93] According to one researcher, among the widowers the death rate from cardiovascular disease was 67 percent higher than would have been expected.[94]

Widows are affected as well. They die at rates 3 to 13 times as high as those of married women for every known major cause of death.[95] Both men and women who lose their mates are among the highest-risk groups for premature death. As mentioned earlier, studies conducted at New York's Mount Sinai School of Medicine indicate that about 35,000 bereaved partners die each year—and that one in five can be directly attributed to the loss of their mate.[96]

However, a National Institute on Aging study shows that widowed persons who survive for two years after their loss resume the likelihood of living a normal life expectancy. The study, which involved 14,000 adults in the United States and West Germany, half of whom were widowed, was conducted from 1970 to 1981. During the first two years after the death of their spouses, the widowed had a "consistently higher death rate" than those of the same age who were married. The newly widowed were more likely to die as a result of disease or accidents and also more likely to commit suicide. However, data reveal, "after the two-year mark, the mortality rate slowed significantly, and the researchers could see no differences in the health and well-being of the long-term widowed and married people of the same age."[97] This two year transition back toward normalization in women was also confirmed in the large Women's Health Initiative study.[98]

In a rural community in Wales, researchers studied 903 close relatives of almost 400 residents who died during a five-year period. Nearly 5 percent of the relatives died within the first year after being bereaved; only 0.7 percent of the nonbereaved people of the same age who lived in the same community died during the year.[99] This is a sevenfold increase in the death rate for surviving close relatives—spouses, children, parents, or siblings. The place of death was also significant: If the person died in the hospital, the relative's risk of death during the first year was two times higher. If the person died elsewhere, the relative's risk jumped to five times higher.

What bereaved people die of may differ between men and women and even somewhat with age. According to statistics, bereaved women tend to die more often than expected from cancer, heart disease, tuberculosis, cirrhosis, and alcoholism. Bereaved men have a higher risk of dying from heart disease, tuberculosis, influenza, pneumonia, cirrhosis, alcoholism, accidents, and suicide.[100] Yale researchers, however, urge caution in separating the genders when considering the impact of bereavement. While it makes sense that the emotion of losing a spouse may differ between men and women, they indicate that further studies are needed, regarding differences in the physical impact.[101]

One researcher, who did an extensive review of the literature,[102] cautions that a number of issues complicate the interpretation of published findings about the relationship of bereavement and increased mortality. He argues that these findings should be considered tentative and that the prospective data on grief, depression, immune function, and neuroendocrine function are needed before it will be possible for researchers to substantiate claims that bereavement either weakens the immune system or causes premature death.

Cutting the Risk

The best thing bereaved people can do to protect themselves, researchers say, is to surround themselves with people who are supportive. If they perceive that their social support is strong, health improves.

Researchers studied a group of women 13 months after the death of their husbands. The group was divided into those who perceived their social support to be adequate and those who did not. Only about 1 in 5 of those who felt their social support was good had poor health; in stark contrast, almost 9 of 10 of the women with inadequate social support had poor health.[103]

Researchers then took the women who felt their support was inadequate and put them in a program of supportive counseling; the women were able to gain much social support from the counselors and the group. As a result, the percentage with poor health went from a staggering 86 percent to only 13 percent. In summing up the findings, researchers said that "adverse health effects associated with bereavement are absent or at least reduced when the individual maintains close supportive relationships."[104]

Similarly, 200 widows were assessed during the first few weeks following the husband's death. Researchers judged that 64 of them were at high risk for developing disease because of weak support from family and friends, an ambiguous relationship with the husband, and additional life crises at the time of the study. Researchers took the 64 widows considered to be at high risk and divided the group in half. Half of the group received no support; the other half received support and counseling. At 13 months following the bereavement, the group that had received social support and counseling did the best; only about a third showed increased health problems. By contrast, more than half of the unsupported group had worsening mental and physical symptoms.[105]

In the final analysis, support and an opportunity to talk to an understanding person may be the most crucial factors. Itzhak Levav of the University of Hebrew and Hadassah School of Public Health and Community Medicine studied the effect of support on bereavement. His researchers examined 3,600 Israeli parents who had lost adult sons either in the Yom Kippur War of 1973 or through accidents occurring between 1971 and 1975. The bereaved parents were compared with the general populace, and researchers compared not only illness and disease but death rates as well. The widowed and divorced mothers of the deceased sons did have increased mortality, but the married parents demonstrated "no consistent evidence of an elevated risk of death." Researchers conducting the study concluded that marriage—and the social support it provides—protects against the potential health and mortality dangers of bereavement.[106]

How can you best help the bereaved? According to research, traits that help protect a person in the event of loss, in addition to social support, include strong religious belief, rituals, and belief that one can feel some control in the bereavement.[107] One writer suggests the following:

- Be there.
- Listen.
- Avoid clichés.
- Keep in touch.
- Send a note.
- Be patient.
- Accentuate the positive.

And, the writer says, don't forget to touch—a hug or a squeeze of the hand can do wonders.[108]

Coping with Grief

A person experiencing grief might consider these suggestions from the Counseling and Mental Health Center at the University of Texas, Austin[109]:

Talk to family or friends	Seek counseling
Read poetry or books	Engage in social activities
Exercise	Eat healthy foods
Seek spiritual support	Take time to relax
Join a support group	Listen to music
Be patient with yourself	Let yourself feel grief

In addition, various studies show the following to be very helpful:

- When reminiscing about the relationship with the person you have lost, focus on the good things you are grateful to have had instead of focusing on the loss.
- Avoid alcohol.
- Tell funny stories involving the deceased, and laugh about good times with that person.
- Develop a new, ongoing relationship with the deceased: mentally express gratitude to him or her and sense the deceased person's counsel and love.
- Rediscover your sense of purpose in life, and throw yourself into it.

Also, helpful resources and insights can be found from good guidebooks,[110] or on reliable websites.[111]

WHAT DID YOU LEARN?

1. Define both *grief* and *bereavement*.
2. How might you tell if normal grief has evolved into clinical depression?
3. Describe how grief might cause sudden death.
4. What is probably the single most important factor in dealing well with grief?

ENDNOTES

1. Wolfgang Stroebe and Margaret S. Stroebe, *Bereavement and Health* (Cambridge, MA: Cambridge University Press, 1987), 1.
2. Center for the Advancement of Health, *Report on Bereavement and Grief Research* (New York: Brunner-Routledge, 2004), 495.
3. Stroebe and Stroebe, *Bereavement and Health,* 2.
4. James J. Lynch, *The Broken Heart: The Medical Consequences of Loneliness* (New York: Basic Books, 1977).
5. Larry Dossey, *Meaning and Medicine: A Doctor's Tales of Breakthrough and Healing* (New York: Bantam Books, 1991), 90.
6. Bemie S. Siegel, *Love, Medicine, and Miracles* (New York: Harper & Row, 1986).
7. S. A. Murreil, S. Himmelfarb, and J. F. Phifer, "Effects of Bereavement/Loss and Pre-Event Status on Subsequent Physical Health in Older Adults," *International Journal of Aging/Human Development* 27, no. 2 (1988): 89–107.
8. Ann McCracken, "Emotional Impact of Possession Loss," *Journal of Gerontological Nursing* 13, no. 2 (1987): 14–9.
9. Lynch, *The Broken Heart.*
10. R. A. Spitz and K. M. Wolf, "Anaclitic Depression: An Inquiry into the Genesis of Psychiatric Conditions in Early Childhood, II," *Psychoanalytic Study of the Child* 2 (1946): 313–42.
11. Leonard A. Sagan, *The Health of Nations* (New York: Basic Books, 1987).
12. Lynch, *The Broken Heart.*
13. Sagan, *The Health of Nations.*
14. Ibid.
15. Brent Q. Hafen and Kathryn J. Frandsen, *People Who Need People: The Importance of Relationships to Health and Wellness* (Evergreen, CO: Cordillera Press, 1987), 37.
16. Sharon Faelten, David Diamond, and the editors of *Prevention* magazine, *Take Control of Your Life: A Complete Guide to Stress Relief* (Emmaus, PA: Rodale Press, 1988), 134.
17. Ibid.
18. H.G. Prigerson et al., "Traumatic Grief as a Risk Factor for Mental and Physical Morbidity," *American Journal of Psychiatry* 154 (1997): 616–23.
19. K. Hawton, "Complicated Grief After Bereavement," *British Medical Journal* 334 (2007): 962–3.
20. B. Wagner, C. Knaelvelsrud, and A. Maerker, "Internet Based Cognitive Behavioral Therapy for Complicated Grief: A Randomized, Controlled Trial," *Death Studies* 30 (2006): 429–53.
21. K. Shear et al., "Treatment of Complicated Grief: A Randomized, Controlled Trial," *Journal of the American Medical Association* 292 (2005): 2601–8.

22. G. Christ, G. Bonanno, R. Malkinson, and S. Rubin, "Bereavement Experiences After the Death of a Child," in Institute of Medicine, M. Field, and R. Behrman, eds., *When Children Die: Improving Palliative and End-of-Life Care for Children and Their Families* (Washington, DC: National Academy Press, 2003), 554.
23. Ibid., 555.
24. J. Amold, "Rethinking Grief: Nursing Implications for Health Promotion," *Home Health Nurse* 14, no. 10 (September 1997): 777–83.
25. Figures are from the U.S. Census Bureau and the Centers for Disease Control for 2005 and 2006.
26. Center for Advancement of Health, *Report on Phase I of the Grief Research Gaps, Needs, and Action Project* (Washington, DC: Center for Advancement of Health, 2003).
27. H. Prigerson and S. Jacobs, "Traumatic Grief as a Distinct Disorder: A Rationale, Consensus Criteria, and a Preliminary Empirical Test," in M. Stroebe et al., eds., *Handbook of Bereavement: Consequences, Coping, and Care* (Washington, DC: American Psychological Association, 2001), Part V, Chapter 27.
28. M. Stroebe, "Bereavement Research and Theory: Retrospective and Prospective," *American Behavioral Scientist* 44 (2001): 854–65.
29. D. Klass, and T. Walter, "Process of Grieving: How Bonds Are Continued," in M. Stroebe et al., eds., *Handbook of Bereavement*, Part IV, Chapter 19.
30. G. Bonanno, "Introduction: New Directions in Bereavement Research and Theory," *American Behavioral Scientist* 44 (2001): 718–25.
31. L. Calhoun and R. Tedeschi, "The Positive Lessons of Loss," pp. 157–72 in R. Neimeyer, ed., *Meaning Reconstruction and the Experience of Loss* (Washington, DC: American Psychological Association, 2001).
32. G. Bonanno, "Grief and Emotion: A Social-Functional Perspective," in M. Stroebe et al., eds., *Handbook of Bereavement*, Part V, Chapter 22.
33. C. B. Wortman and R. C. Silver, "The Myths of Coping with Loss Revisited," in M. Stroebe et al., eds., *Handbook of Bereavement*, Part IV, Chapter 18.
34. Calhoun and Tedeschi, "The Positive Lessons of Loss."
35. J. Jordan and R. Neimeyer, "Does Grief Counseling Work?" *Death Studies* 27 (2003): 765–86; and H. Schut, M. Stroebe, J. Van den Bout, and M. Terheggen, "The Efficacy of Bereavement Interventions: Determining Who Benefits," in M. Stroebe et al., eds., *Handbook of Bereavement*, Part VI, Chapter 30.
36. K. Goodkin et al., "Physiological Effects of Bereavement and Bereavement Support Group Intervention," in M. Stroebe et al., eds., *Handbook of Bereavement,* Part VI, Chapter 26; and M. Hall and M. Irwin, "Physiological Indices of Functioning in Bereavement," in M. Stroebe et al., eds., *Handbook of Bereavement*, Part V, Chapter 21.
37. T. Uren and C. Wastell, "Attachment and Meaning Making in Perinatal Bereavement," I 26 (2002): 279–306.
38. P. Van and A. Meleis, "Coping with Grief after Involuntary Pregnancy Loss: Perspective of African American Women," I 32, no. 1 (2003): 28–39.
39. Christ et al., "Bereavement Experiences," 554.
40. S. S. Rubin and R. Malkinson, "Parental Response to Child Loss Across the Life Cycle: Clinical and Research Perspectives," in M. Stroebe et al., eds., *Handbook of Bereavement*, Part II, Chapter 10.
41. Christ et al., "Bereavement Experiences."
42. Ibid.
43. S. Murphy et al., "Bereaved Parents' Outcomes 1 to 60 Months After Their Children's Deaths by Accident, Suicide, or Homicide: A Comparative Study Demonstrating Differences," *Death Studies* 27, no. 1 (2003): 39–61.

44. J. H. Chen et al., "Gender Differences in the Effects of Bereavement-Related Psychological Distress in Health Outcomes," *Psychological Medicine* 29, no. 2 (1999): 367–80.

45. Ibid.

46. Ibid.

47. James J. Pennebaker and Joan R. Susman, "Disclosure of Traumas and Psychosomatic Processes," *Social Science Medicine* 26, no. 3 (1988): 327–32.

48. Sheldon Cohen and S. Leonard Syme, *Social Support and Health* (Orlando, FL: Academic Press, 1985).

49. "Swiftness of Spouse's Death Affects Mate's Mortality Risk," *Medical World News* (September 11, 1989): 27.

50. "When Death Does Us Part: The Difference Between Widows and Widowers," *Psychology Today* (November 1989): 14.

51. R. Schulz et al., "Involvement in Caregiving and Adjustment to Death of a Spouse: Findings from the Caregiver Health Effects Study," *Journal of the American Medical Association* 285 (2001): 3123–9.

52. Cohen and Syme, *Social Support and Health*.

53. Genevieve Davis Ginsburg, "Coping with Widowhood: 'Who Am I Without My Mate'?" *50 Plus* (June 1987): 44–53.

54. T. R. Fitzpatrick, "Bereaved Events among Elderly Men: The Effects of Stress and Health," *Journal of Applied Gerontology* 17, no. 2 (October 1996): 204–28.

55. Louise Bemikow, *Alone in America* (New York: Harper & Row, 1986).

56. "On the Health Consequences of Bereavement," *New England Journal of Medicine* 319, no. 8 (1988): 510–1.

57. Stroebe and Stroebe, *Bereavement and Health*, 143.

58. Ibid.

59. Ibid., 145.

60. J. Van Eijk, A. Smits, F. Huygen, and H. van der Hoogen, "Effect of Bereavement on the Health of the Remaining Family Members," *Family Practitioner* 5, no. 4 (1988): 278–82.

61. C. Davis and S. Nolen-Hoeksema, "Loss and Meaning: How Do People Make Sense of Loss?" *American Behavioral Scientist* 44 (2001): 726–41.

62. K. Walsh, M. King, et al., "Spiritual Beliefs May Affect Outcome of Bereavement: Prospective Study," *British Medical Journal* 324 (2002): 1–5.

63. Lynch, *The Broken Heart*.

64. J. Kaprio, M. Koskenvuo, and H. Rita, "Mortality after Bereavement, a Prospective Study of 95,647 Widowed Persons," *American Journal of Public Health* 77 (1987): 283–7.

65. C. Murray Parkes, B. Benjamin, and R. G. Fitzgerald. "Broken Heart: A Statistical Study among Widowers," *British Medical Journal* 1(56 46) (1969): 740–743.

66. S. Wilcox, et al., "The Effects of Widowhood on Physical and Mental Health, Health Behaviors, and Health Outcomes: The Woman's Health Initiative," *Health Psychology* 22 (2003): 513–22. Also see B. Bower, "Widows Show Third Year Rebound," *Science News* 164, no. 12 (Sept. 20, 2003): 189.

67. Lynch, *The Broken Heart*.

68. Ibid.

69. V. E. Bartrop et al., "Depressed Lymphocyte Function After Bereavement," *Lancet* 1, no. 8016 (1977): 834–6.

70. B. S. Linn, M. W. Linn, and M. D. Jensen, "Degree of Depression and Immune Responsiveness," *Psychosomatic Medicine* 44 (1982): 128–9.

71. Steven Locke and Douglas Colligan, *The Healer Within: The New Medicine of Mind and Body* (New York: E. P. Dutton, 1986), 68.

72. Signe Hammer, "The Mind as Healer," *Science Digest* (April 1984): 47–9, 100.
73. "Bereavement: An Immune Reaction," *Mind/Body Health Digest* 1, no. 2 (1987): 2.
74. G. Ironsen et al., "Posttraumatic Stress Symptoms, Intrusive Thoughts, Loss and Immune Function After Hurricane Andrew," *Psychosomatic Medicine* 59 (1997): 128–41.
75. Torill Christine Lindstrom, "Immunity and Health After Bereavement in Relation to Coping," *Scandinavian Journal of Psychology* 38, no. 3 (September 1997): 253–9.
76. Locke and Colligan, *The Healer Within*, 72.
77. Locke and Colligan, *The Healer Within*.
78. Robert Ornstein and David Sobel, "The Healing Brain," *Psychology Today* (March 1987): 48–52.
79. G. F. Solomon et al., "Shaking Up Immunity: Psychological and Immunological Changes After a Natural Disaster," *Psychosomatic Medicine* 59 (1997): 142–3.
80. A. Galinowski, "Stress and Panic. Immunologic Aspects," *Encephale* 19, spec. no.1 (1993):147–51.
81. Ironsen et al., p. 139.
82. A. Sabioncello et al., "Immune, Endocrine and Psychological Responses in Civilians Displaced by War," *Psychosomatic Medicine* 62 (2000): 502–8.
83. Torill Christine Lindstrom, "Immunity and Somatic Health in Bereavement: A Prospective Study of 39 Norwegian Widows," *Omega: Journal of Death and Dying* 35, no. 2 (1997): 231–41.
84. Lynch, *The Broken Heart*.
85. Ibid.
86. G. I. Engle, "Sudden and Rapid Death During Psychological Stress," *Annals of Internal Medicine* 74 (1971): 771–82.
87. Lynch, *The Broken Heart*.
88. I. C. Wilson and J. C. Reece, "Simultaneous Death in Schizophrenic Twins," *Archives of General Psychiatry* 11 (1964): 377–84.
89. G. I. Engle, "A Life Setting Conducive to Illness: The Giving Up-Given Up Complex," *Bulletin of the Menninger Clinic* 32 (1968): 358.
90. Blair Justice, *Who Gets Sick: Thinking and Health* (Houston, TX: Peak Press 1987), 196.
91. Jaakko Kaprio, Markku Koskenvuo, and Heli Rita, "Mortality After Bereavement: A Prospective Study of 95,647 Widowed Persons," *American Journal of Public Health* 77 (1987): 283–7.
92. Lynch, *The Broken Heart*.
93. C. Murray Parkes, et al., "Broken Heart".
94. Peter Reich, "How Much Does Stress Contribute to Cardiovascular Disease?" *Journal of Cardiological Medicine* (July 1983): 825–31.
95. Claudia Wallis, "Stress: Can We Cope?" *Time* (June 6, 1983): 48–54.
96. Brent Q. Hafen and Kathryn J. Frandsen, *People Who Need People* (Provo, UT: Behavioral Health Associates).
97. M. S. Stroebe, W. Stroebe, and R. O. Hansson, *Handbook of Bereavement: Theory and Research* (Cambridge University Press, 1997), 196–203.
98. S. Wilcox, "The Effects of Widowhood on Physical and Mental Health, Health Behaviors, and Health Outcomes."
99. Lynch, *The Broken Heart*.
100. Hafen and Frandsen, *People Who Need People*.
101. Chen et al., "Gender Differences."
102. P. R. Duberstein, "Death Cannot Keep Us Apart: Mortality Following Bereavement," pp. 250–331, in P. R. Duberstein and J. M. Musling, eds., *Psychodynamic Perspectives on Sickness and Health* (Washington, DC: American Psychological Association, 2000).

103. M. Pilusuk and S. H. Parks, *The Healing Web: Social Networks and Human Survival* (Hanover, NH: University Press of New England, 1986).

104. Ibid.

105. Robert Ornstein and David Sobel, *The Healing Brain: Breakthrough Discoveries About How the Brain Keeps Us Healthy* (New York: Simon & Schuster: 1987), 195.

106. I. Levav, et al., "An Epidemiology Study of Mortality among Bereaved Parents," *New England Journal of Medicine* 319 (1988): 457–61.

107. K. A. Gass, "The Health of Conjugally Bereaved Older Widows: The Role of Appraisal, Coping, and Resources," *Research in Nursing and Health* 10 (1987): 39–47.

108. Victor M. Parachin, "Eight Ways to Say I Care," *Complete Woman* (April 1991).

109. University of Texas Counseling and Mental Health Center, Grief and Loss; accessed online at: http://www.utexas.edu/student/cmhc/booklets/Grief/grief.html#anchor20291050).

110. P. Kelley, *Companion to Grief* (New York: Simon & Schuster, 1997); Alan Wolfelt, *The Journey Through Grief* (Fort Collins, CO: Companion Press, 1997); and *The Road to Recovery,* accessed online at www.GriefHelp.org.

111. HELPGUIDE.org, *Coping with Grief and Loss*, accessed at http://helpguide.org/mental/grief_loss.htm.

CHAPTER 14

The Healing Power of Faith, Spirituality, and Religion

It is difficult to make a man miserable while he feels he is worthy of himself and claims kindred to the great God who made him.

—Abraham Lincoln

LEARNING OBJECTIVES

- Be able to define *spirituality, religion,* and *healing.*
- Describe how faith and placebos affect health.
- Create awareness of the difference between the two minds involved in spiritual transformation and of practices that facilitate this transformation.
- Describe the effects of spiritual and religious practices on health.
- Clarify the essential principles of spiritual well-being, particularly as defined by health outcomes.

"[One] who is seriously involved in the pursuit of science becomes convinced that a Spirit is manifest in the Laws of the Universe," reflected Albert Einstein—"a Spirit vastly superior to that of man, and one in the face of which we, with our modest powers, must feel humble."

In a Harris Poll, 1,254 people were asked about their aches and pains. The results were rather surprising. First of all, what age group do you think has the most pain? Young adults! (Maybe that is not so surprising when you realize that some of the most common pains—headaches, menstrual cramps, abdominal pains, and the like—tend to subside with age.) The pains reported in the poll were highly associated with the "hassles of life." (See Chapter 5 for a discussion of how anxiety impacts pain.) The next surprise was where people get their best pain relief. Respondents said that physicians provided relief 73 percent of the time. Other practitioners provided pain relief 65 to 70 percent of the time. Most helpful of all were *spiritual counselors*—at 85 percent. How could spiritual counseling relieve physical pain? Could it be by reducing the stress of life's hassles?

Here's another example: Most people with a common, chronic muscle pain condition called fibromyalgia seek "alternative care"—in other words, help beyond the conventional medical system. A survey of these chronic pain patients asked what had been helpful to them and, on a scale of 1 to 10, how helpful each had been. The results are shown in Table 14.1.

Table 14.1   Therapies Used by Fibromyalgia Patients in the Treatment of Muscle Pain

Therapy	Percentage of Patients Using Therapy	How satisfying? (0–10)
■ Over-the-counter items	70	5
■ Dietary modifications	26	5
■ Practitioners	40	8
■ Spiritual Practices	48	**9**
■ Prayers	41	
■ Meditation	38	
■ Relaxation	10	
■ Self-help	6	
■ Spiritual healing	5	

Source: M. Pioro-Boisset, J. M. Esdaille, and M. A. Fitzcharles, "Alternative Medicine Use in the Fibromyalgia Syndrome," *Arthritis Care Research* 9 (1996): 13–7.

Note that the spiritual practices listed were regarded as even more helpful (9 out of 10 in satisfaction) than other methods or practitioners. How would spiritual practices improve pain management?

History of Religious Belief and Medicine

Before we assign any definition to spiritual health, consider history: Spirituality and medicine were intertwined from the beginning of time. The earliest doctors of which we have record were the religious figures in tribes and groups—the priests and the medicine men and women. Cardiologist Bruno Cortis points out that disease was originally considered to be supernatural, and those who dealt with disease were the ones considered to have power over the bad spirits thought to be causing it. Not until Hippocrates, says Cortis, was medicine separated from religion.[1]

For millennia before the late 1800s, medicine, hospitals, and beliefs about health were intimately tied to religion and the need for divine help in healing. After the scientific revolution, medicine went in the opposite direction (perhaps to an extreme), thinking of healing processes along purely biological and psychological lines. The prevailing belief was that "germs" and other offenders caused disease, and the way to treat or prevent disease was to kill or avoid the causative agent.

As we became more aware, it was obvious that some people exposed to disease-causing agents got sick, and some didn't. The concept of "host resistance" evolved. As described through many chapters in this book, many factors play into that resistance: not only organic problems but also social factors and such things as coping ability. All of these modulate the homeostasis and immune responses that make up the disease-resistant person (see Chapter 8). So now the pendulum is swinging back toward rediscovering the role that spiritual issues play in the well-being (health) equation.

Almost three-quarters of Americans say that their coping and overall approach to the stresses of life are centrally grounded in their religious beliefs.[2] In a Gallup Poll conducted in May 2007, 86 percent of Americans believe in God, and 82 percent consider spirituality to be important in their daily lives. A separate survey indicated that 61 percent believe that spirituality or religion can answer most of life's perplexing problems. Surveys suggest that a very large majority (86 percent) believe that God, prayer, and spiritual practices are very important to them in healing at a time of serious illness.[3] Several reviews of medical literature (involving hundreds of studies) show that both spiritual and religious factors play a significant role in both the prevention of illness and in health outcomes when people are recovering from physical or mental illness.[4] The scientific studies are quite consistent in demonstrating a significant beneficial effect of spiritual issues on health outcomes. These benefits cross different religions, nationalities, ages, genders, and types of medical practice.[5]

It seems that the ancients knew something important about spirituality—and today, that connection is being rediscovered. Evidence suggests that increasing numbers of physicians are taking the spirituality of their patients into account as part of patient care.[6] These physicians are forming a "therapeutic alliance" with their patients that affirms the importance of their spirituality. Indeed, says one writer, "As physicians respectfully explore patient spirituality, a reciprocal enhancement in patient regard for physicians and a deepening of the alliance between patients and their physicians becomes possible, potentially resulting in more effective treatment."[7]

The same type of spiritual involvement is being incorporated into mental health treatment and has been recognized as "a crucially important dimension" in acute mental care.[8] Unfortunately, the current medical system is not well designed to deal well with this exceptionally important factor. Many organizations are taking steps toward recognizing the importance of spirituality in mental health treatment; in the United Kingdom, for example, the Code of Professional Conduct requires that mental health nurses "recognize and respect the uniqueness and dignity of each patient, including their religious beliefs."[9]

As physicians have sought support and training in dealing with their patients on a spiritual level, rapidly increasing numbers of medical schools and other training programs have responded favorably. Funds have also been dedicated to the spiritual education of physicians. For example, the John Templeton Foundation recently established start-up grants for medical schools to initiate courses in spirituality and medicine as a regular part of physician education. In the past decade, such efforts and studies have led to more than half of medical schools starting courses on dealing well with spirituality in medical care.

Research shows that patients, too, are supportive of a patient-physician relationship that takes spirituality into account. A number of studies show that patients long for their physicians to be more involved with them on a spiritual level. In a survey of the American public, 74 percent of sick patients feel a physician should do at least one of the following:

- Introduce a discussion about an ill patient's spiritual needs
- Refer a patient to a spiritual advisor (rabbi, priest, minister, or chaplain)
- Suggest prayer

At the end of life, the number hoping for their physician to include spiritual considerations increases to 90 percent—but this is done only 24 percent of the time. A Gallup Poll indicates that 60 percent of patients would like their physicians to pray with them.[10] In the current health system, however, such a practice would often be awkward. At the very least, new guidelines suggest that physicians should ask patients about their spiritual beliefs, practices, and values as a routine part of assessment and should incorporate those into the patient's ongoing care.[11] When the local culture of a community is taken into consideration, activities such as prayer, anointing, testimonials, and other worship practices can be explored as potential health resources.[12] When this is done, sick people often feel the comfort and hope for which they are yearning.

Sometimes illness has the potential to motivate spiritual transformation, a process that invites greater love and forgiveness. And this healing transformation has at times been associated with surprising medical improvements, even "spontaneous cures." Bernie Siegel, cancer surgeon, comments, "When a doctor reports amazing improvements in a patient's condition, he or she almost never mentions that person's beliefs or lifestyle, but when I inquire, I find the patient *always* has made some drastic change toward a more loving and accepting outlook."[13] And beyond such healing, spiritual well-being may also have a role in preventing illness in the first place.

Faith and Health: The Placebo Effect

To understand how powerfully faith and belief can impact health, it's important to understand how powerful the placebo effect can be. One of the most striking demonstrations of faith in action (and one of the most scientifically proven) is the *placebo effect*: the physical change that occurs as a result of what we believe a pill or a procedure will do. Giving a placebo is nearly always more effective than doing nothing. Because generally about a third of sick people respond well to a placebo, all reliable treatment studies require a placebo control to be compared to the "active" treatment. Simply, the placebo is a tangible way to elicit faith and hope.

If a person deeply believes that a pill is going to work in a certain way, chances are it will—even if the pill is fashioned of nothing more than table sugar, distilled water, or saline solution.[14] The healer is actually faith, not pharmacology. Interestingly enough, however, such faith creates some of the same physiological changes as an active pharmacological treatment. This is demonstrated in some historically classical examples. (Many of these following studies could not be done under ethical guidelines today, for which complete disclosure to patients is now required.)

One dramatic example of the placebo effect occurred in a New York hospital in 1950. In the experiment, Dr. Stewart Wolf treated women who were suffering severe nausea and vomiting from pregnancy. Wolf told the women he was going to give them a drug known to effectively alleviate nausea and vomiting. In reality, however, Wolf gave the women syrup of ipecac—a drug used to induce vomiting.

What happened? The patients' nausea and vomiting disappeared after taking the syrup of ipecac. According to researchers, the women's belief in the drug's powers was so potent that it actually counteracted the pharmacologic actions of the drug.[15]

The power of the placebo also extends to surgery. Some of the most convincing evidence regarding the placebo effect stems from surgical procedures in which incisions are made while the patient is under anesthesia, but no operation is performed.[16] One of the most classic examples of this hails from the mid-1950s. At that time, a new surgical procedure was introduced to help relieve chest pains resulting from coronary heart disease. The surgery called an "internal mammary artery ligation," involved tying off an artery in the chest wall, the internal mammary artery, and sometimes implanting it into the heart, in an attempt to get more blood to the heart.

Initial response to the surgery was overwhelming. Almost half of the patients reported an improvement in chest pain—and two-thirds of them said that the improvement was considerable. Surgeons who pioneered the operation said that the patients also did better on an electrocardiogram after the surgery, and their exercise tolerance also improved. Thousands of patients requested the surgery, and the operation gained in popularity.[17]

However, not all of the surgeons who looked into the operation were equally enthusiastic about it. In fact, two groups of surgeons were extremely skeptical and decided to test the procedure against a placebo. (Remember that this kind of test would not be allowed under today's rules of medical ethics.) For their test, the skeptical surgeons randomly divided patients slotted for surgery into one of two groups. The first group would receive the internal mammary artery ligation, as planned. The second group, without knowing it, would be put under general anesthesia, an incision would be made in the chest, the incision would be closed, yet no surgical procedure would be performed on any artery.

The results were almost identical, regardless of whether the patients had arteries tied. Many of the patients in both groups experienced less chest pain, increased tolerance for exercise, improvements on the electrocardiogram, and a reduced need for nitroglycerin. The studies demonstrated that surgery on "the internal mammary artery was no better than a skin incision, and that such an incision could lead to a dramatic, sustained placebo effect."[18]

After more than 10,000 patients underwent an internal mammary artery ligation, the surgery was abandoned.

According to Yale oncologist and surgeon Bernie Siegel, "What the placebo suggests to us is that we may be able to change what takes place in our bodies by changing our state of mind."[19]

Researcher Daniel Goleman maintains that belief "is the hidden ingredient in Western medicine and every traditional system of 'healing' I know about. In the West, doctors have long been aware of its curative power. A large number of illnesses can be treated more successfully if the patient believes in a particular cure."[20]

Psychiatrist Jerome Frank ascribes even greater powers to faith. He says faith is a key element, even in modern medicine, that brings about a recovery. "The physician's main function is to use his medical skills to stimulate the patient's mechanisms of repair," Frank explains. "Nonmedical healers, whether African witch doctors or religious faith healers in Western countries, intuitively understand this. Their rituals and laying on of hands are designed to release or strengthen the patient's inner healing powers."[21]

"Faith" is not the property of a certain religion nor does it owe its effectiveness to a certain shrine or ritual. All religions have members who have experienced seemingly magical, spontaneous cures from life-threatening or incurable diseases. Miracles have occurred at shrines scattered throughout the world, and patients who seemed stripped of any possibility of a cure have responded to a broad spectrum of rituals (such as laying on of hands for "faith healing").

"There is no denying that religious shrines unleash powerful healing emotions of hope in the pilgrim," maintains Frank. "One cannot attribute this to any particular religious faith or object of worship, since all religions can cite instances of these seemingly magical cures. The more likely explanation is that the cure results from the individual's state of mind—his expectant faith."[22]

The growing appreciation of the healing power of faith among members of the medical community is characterized in the comments of Dr. Joan Borysenko, a former instructor at Harvard Medical School:

> Two thousand years ago a woman who had suffered prolonged uterine bleeding approached Jesus of Nazareth. Coming up to him in a crowd, she touched the hem of his garment and was instantly healed. Jesus turned to her and explained that it was her faith that had made her whole. After centuries of slow progress toward rational explanations of the physical world, even scientists can at least begin to appreciate the truth of His assessment. We are entering a new level in the scientific understanding of mechanisms by which faith, belief, and imagination can actually unlock the mysteries of healing.[23]

Thus belief strongly impacts health outcomes. And the belief of a large majority of Americans is connected to their religious commitments. For example:[24]

- Ninety-five percent of all Americans believe in God or a higher power.
- Seventy-five percent of Americans say that their religious faith forms the foundation for their approach to life.
- Seventy-three percent of Americans say that prayer is an important part of their daily life, and 33 percent of all Americans use prayer to heal their medical conditions.
- Seventy-four percent of all Americans associate the word *spirituality* with positive feelings.
- Sixty-five percent of Americans connect religion with positive associations.
- More than 40 percent of Americans attend weekly religious services.

Religious belief provides power for an individual. With such beliefs so prevalent, it is no surprise that religious faith plays a significant role in healing.

Healing and the Religious Shrine

One obvious example is probably the best-known healing shrine in Lourdes, France. Since the visions of Marie Bernarde Soubirous and the mid–nineteenth century discovery of the healing spring, there have been countless documented cases of people who went to the spring with faith and who were cured of severe illness. Lame people have left Lourdes with the ability to walk; the deaf have been blessed with the gift of sound, and sight has been restored to the blind. Many of the cures have been dramatic.

Today, more than 2 million people visit Lourdes each year from all corners of the world in hope of being healed. Many have been told there is no cure for their condition; for most, Lourdes is a last resort. Many make the pilgrimage only after years of drugs and therapies that have not yielded results.

The reputation of Lourdes as a "healing" shrine is well deserved. People are healed, sometimes of lifelong conditions. Are those healings due to some magical property of the springs themselves? Or to a special healing power possessed by the priests, nurses, and orderlies? Probably the major component of the healing is due to the expectant faith of the pilgrim who comes to Lourdes to be healed. As one eyewitness describes the scene at the shrine each afternoon, "The sick line up in two rows. . . . Every few feet, in front of them, kneeling priests with arms outstretched praying earnestly, leading the responses. Nurses and orderlies on their knees, praying too. . . . The Sacred Host is raised above each sick one. The great crowd falls to its knees. All arms are outstretched in one vast cry to Heaven. As far as one can see in any direction, people are on their knees, praying."

The stirring services, the sense of support, and the outpouring of emotion at Lourdes and shrines like it "can only serve to reinforce the expectant faith that pilgrims bring with them," explains Frank. This faith, he adds, explains "the spontaneous remissions of disease and improved bodily functions experienced by some, as well as the increased sense of hope and improved morale that even the uncured take home with them."[25]

Other Examples of Faith and Healing

Lourdes is only one example of how faith works to heal the sick. There are many other examples, and a number of scientific studies have even been able to document the healing power of faith. In one study, researchers studied a group of patients who were about to undergo surgery for a detached retina.[26] The researchers gave each patient a "score" that reflected his or her expectations about the surgery. After the surgery, the surgeon—who did not know the patient's "score"—gauged the speed of recovery and noted any complications. Those who had faith in the surgeon and faith in their own ability to cope with the surgery did the best. The researchers concluded that the body's own healing ability is actually stimulated "by a patient's faith in the healer and his methods, an optimistic outlook toward the treatment, and other psychological variables that, taken together, may be called an attitude of expectant faith."

A separate study provides a graphic description of how powerful faith can be in the healing process—even when the faith is not justified.[27] A hospital-based physician was frustrated with three patients who, despite his best efforts, had not been helped by medical treatment. All three were women in their sixties. One suffered from chronic inflammation of the gall bladder. One was wasting away after failing to recuperate from surgery for pancreatitis. The third had inoperable cancer of the uterus; to complicate matters, she also had tremendous swelling of the legs and anemia.

The doctor called in a faith healer but did not tell any of the women about him. He practiced his rituals on an absentee basis, without any of the three patients being aware of his efforts. After twelve healing sessions, there was no change in any of the patients' conditions. The physician dismissed the faith healer.

Then the physician went to the three patients, described the faith healer in enthusiastic and glowing terms, and told the women that they were extremely lucky: The faith healer would be working on their behalf each morning for three days. Of course, this wasn't true; the doctor had dismissed the faith healer. As far as the women were concerned, however, they believed that the faith healer was working for them.

What the doctor saw was both dramatic and almost unbelievable: All three patients were relieved of their symptoms. All three were able to leave the hospital within a week. The patient with pancreatitis, who had been literally wasting away, got out of bed after what she believed to be the first "healing session." She rapidly gained 30 pounds—a feat medical approaches had been unable to help her accomplish—and she remained well, without any relapse of her condition. Most amazing was the cancer patient. The swelling in her legs disappeared. Her red blood cell level rose, reversing her anemia. Five days after the "healing sessions" began, she returned home, where she was able to function normally until her death several months later.

One of the most striking and profound examples of how faith influences even the course of medication is the well-known story of a patient treated by Dr. Bruno Klopfer in the late 1950s.[28] The patient was suffering from a widespread lymphoma, a serious cancer of the immune system, that was in its late stages. At the time, a supplement called Krebiozen was being touted in the alternative medicine community as a cure for cancer, though its effectiveness had not been proven. The patient demanded that Klopfer administer Krebiozen, and the doctor agreed. Within two days of receiving the Krebiozen, the patient experienced a remarkable turnaround. As one account described it, the large tumors that covered his body began "melting like snowballs." After ten days of treatment with Krebiozen, the patient was released from the hospital, apparently free of disease. Klopfer believed that a medical miracle had occurred.

A medical miracle *had* occurred—but it was due to the patient's faith in the Krebiozen, not due to the drug itself. As fate would have it, that faith was short-lived. A few months after the patient was released from the hospital, newspapers around the country announced that Krebiozen had been proven worthless, and the news was brought to the patient's attention. His tumors promptly reappeared.

Klopfer was fascinated by this turn of events. Based on what happened, he strongly suspected that the patient's belief had cured him and that the drug had nothing to do with the cure. Klopfer became convinced that he could once again harness the man's faith if the conditions were right. He called his patient in, reassured him, and told him the newspaper accounts were inaccurate and an extra-strength, improved, refined form of the drug had just been released to physicians. Klopfer offered this "refined" form of the drug to his eager patient. But Klopfer didn't actually have any improved Krebiozen. He gave his patient distilled water. (Again, this would not be ethically allowed today.)

With distilled water coursing through his veins, the patient who believed that he had a new super Krebiozen staged another remarkable recovery. Within days, his tumors again disappeared. He was released from the hospital a second time, again apparently disease-free.

Unfortunately, it didn't last. Three months after his recovery, the patient read a newspaper report published by the American Medical Association. Definitive tests had proven beyond a doubt, the report said, that Krebiozen was worthless. Top-ranking officials in the American Medical Association proclaimed the drug as useless in the fight against cancer. The patient, who had left the hospital three months earlier free of tumors, read the report. His faith was shattered. His tumors ballooned. Days after he read the newspaper report, he literally laid down and died.

How Do Placebos Work?

All of these examples demonstrate the ability of the mind to elicit the anticipated response clear down to cellular levels by creating an expectant, usually mentally pictured outcome. At a purely physiological level, all of this is not so mysterious when one considers the mechanisms of psychoneuroimmunology (see Chapter 1), the effect of belief on neurotransmitters, and the impact of these neurotransmitters on other body systems (see Chapters 2, 5, and 6). The hope engendered by taking a placebo has been shown to have significant impact on the neurotransmitters dopamine and endorphins[29], as well as turning on the brain function that suppresses pain—similar to taking an opiate.[30] On functional MRI brain scans, a placebo elicits the same neurofunctional and neurochemical brain effects as an active drug.[31]

Some, eager to dismiss the phenomenon of faith healing, overlook the impact of faith on health. By doing so, say many researchers, they risk overlooking a potentially powerful source of healing for many patients. Responding to criticism in his field about the prospect of faith healing, one professor of nursing wrote:

> It may be that some force is activated that we do not yet understand (although [scientists] offer us perfectly rational explanations), but . . . we risk putting an incredibly useful idea outside scientific and rational enquiry, thereby keeping it out of the mainstream of health care—exactly where it is needed. A bit of humility, clear thinking, and free speech in the face of the awesome mystery of healing would not come amiss from very many of our "healers."[32]

One of the most diligent physicians of all time recognized the power and value of our faith and our beliefs. When he was asked to explain the secret of African witch doctors, humanitarian Albert Schweitzer replied with a simplicity that carries a message for all of us:

> The witch doctor succeeds for the same reason all the rest of us succeed. Each patient carries his own doctor inside him. We are at our best when we give the doctor within each patient a chance to go to work.[33]

What Is Spirituality and Spiritual Health?

Before discussing spiritual health, let's look at the terms *religion, spirituality,* and *healing.* The word *religion* derives from the Latin root *religio,* which signifies a bond between humanity and some greater-than-human power. In ancient times, the experience of interacting with that power, and the rituals involved, were central to religion. More recently, religion has seemed to become less a personal experience with that power and, in some cases, more identified with a fixed doctrinal and ecclesiastical system (such as what is seen with denominations, theologies, and organizational practices). Religion and the beliefs associated with it provide ways to interpret the deeper purposes of life, to give life and its events meaning and structure, and to organize one's actions in keeping with those precepts. Religious communities provide a means to explore and share spiritual ideals and experience and to potentially receive caring support. At times, however, there is also potential for being judged and excluded for violating the society's norms.

Motivations used in religious groups to encourage "proper" behavior can vary: either using unconditional love and support or else motivating with conditional guilt, shame, and fear. The health and well-being effects of religion can thus vary, depending on which approach is taken. In some of the studies cited below,[34] intrinsic religious experience improved health, but extrinsic religious commitment showed little benefit.[35] Intrinsic religion refers to being motivated by core, internalized beliefs that reflect deeply who a person is and that for which he or she most hopes. Intrinsic religion is deeply God-centered and is not subject as much to social pressures and conformity. Extrinsic religious commitment, on the other hand, usually involves using religion for other ends, such as security, social acceptance, or self-justification. Extrinsic religion is often driven by social pressures and conformity and tends to be more self-centered. Extrinsic religion is often driven by ego issues, and intrinsic religion by deep felt purpose and authenticity to one's larger core self (more on this difference later). As you'll see from the studies below, intrinsic religion is healthy, but extrinsic religiosity is usually not.

The word *spirituality* derives from the Latin *spiritus*, meaning "breath" or "life." In the Jewish and Christian traditions, biblical words translated as "spirit" (Hebrew *ruach* and Greek *pneuma*) also mean breath (and the source of life). Much like Eastern religions today, ancient biblical people used breathing meditative techniques to "breathe in" and thus experience spiritual power. Shamanic healing ceremonies among Native Americans and Polynesians invoke similar rituals of drawing healing spiritual power within one who needs it. The experience of oneness with the sources of spiritual power and life seems central to spirituality. Those same energies are sensed as sources of healing. In recent years, the rise of secularism together with the yearning for such experience with the transcendent has led to many nonreligious approaches to seeking spirituality, such as the New Age movement and nonreligious meditation.

Comparing Spirituality and Religion

Spirituality involves an integrative energy that "encompasses all aspects of a human being and is a means of experiencing life."[36] It is often based on feeling and experience, not intellect, and can be manifested in experiences of interconnectedness—not only with a divine being but also with the larger self, the earth, the environment, the cosmos, nature, animals, or others. Thus full spirituality often consists of a mystical quality coupled with real day-to-day application.

Religion is generally recognized as the way in which people practice, expand, or express their spirituality; simply stated, it is the organized practice of a person's beliefs. While spirituality and religion are similar in many ways, they do have some important distinctions:[37]

- Spirituality focuses on individual and integrated growth, while religion focuses on creating a community.

- Religion is much more formal in worship, systematic in doctrine, and authoritarian in direction, and it involves more formally prescribed behaviors than does spirituality.

- Spirituality is much more difficult to identify and objectively measure than is religion.

- Spirituality is feeling-based and focuses on inner experiences; religion is behavior-based and focuses on outward, observable practices.

- Spirituality is universal and emphasizes unity with others; religion is particular and sometimes segregates one group from another.

- Spirituality creates vision and power for possibilities; religion gives practical form to that vision.

Religiosity (behavior) is easier to measure than spirituality and is thus more studied, often with the hope that religiosity is a surrogate marker for a developing spirituality. Health research demonstrates that religion is usually associated with institutional and ritual-practice elements, while spirituality is more associated with personal experience with the transcendent.

But what exactly is spiritual well-being? Interestingly, we may be able to help define the answer to that important question by scientific analysis of which spiritual elements powerfully affect mental and physical well-being (health). When we determine that, it becomes increasingly clear that the mind-body connection is more accurately a mind-body-spirit triad.

As we try to define healing, we find some fascinating overlap between medical and spiritual terminology. Drawing once again on ancient wisdom, the words *heal* and *health* originally referred to being made whole—and both are associated with the concept of "holy." The biblical Greek word *sozo* is translated as both "to heal" and also "to save." The biblical Greek word *soteria* is translated as either "health" (total well-being) or "salvation." Thus, to ancient people, salvation—the end goal of religious and spiritual practice—meant total well-being (health): spiritual, mental, physical, and social. That ancient insight is very worthy of our consideration today.

To heal also has to do with bringing separated things back together: that concept applies both to skin that has been cut or a relationship that has been damaged. It thus has to do with creating oneness; not only reestablishing the interactive homeostasis of physical systems but also mentally and socially becoming "at one"—no longer feeling internally torn apart nor alienated from oneself, from others, or from the sources of one's spiritual strength. As we'll see, when people heal social and spiritual relationships, they tend to heal physically as well. We usually artificially separate these things, but the larger and wiser brain, mind, and soul do not.

Healing of any kind tends to make people feel more fully alive and more grateful for life. Indeed, deep-felt gratitude for all that life offers may be one of the best markers for spiritual well-being. This healing usually means more than simply a return to the former condition. More often, it involves enlarging the circle of our being to include more that is loved and understood.

Dr. Bernie Siegel tells the story of a woman who had been reared in an alcoholic family where everyone committed suicide. She wrote that she felt she "didn't have a choice" regarding the family she was born into and that she felt like she was a prisoner. However, she wrote to Siegel, "When I let love into my prison, it healed all the things in my life." She still has her illness, but she is at peace. "We don't have choices about who our parents are and how they treated us," Siegel says, "but we have a choice about whether we forgive our parents and heal ourselves."[38] Love is the great healer.

Although spirituality is not the same as organized religion, spiritual experience is the cornerstone of religion. Religion is a means to an end (often a very powerful means). What is that end? Might it be spiritual well-being? Thus defining the core components of spiritual well-being might best guide how one "does" his or her religion.

Spiritual health is not the same thing as physical health: a person can enjoy optimum spiritual health while battling the ravages of terminal cancer. Indeed, healing does not always "result in a physical cure," points out *Psychology Today* editor Marc Barasch. "But the quest for wholeness is never in vain, no matter what the outcome. To find it, we may have to forsake, once and for all, that misapprehension that sees Good in what aggrandizes us, Beauty in what is unblemished, Wholeness only in what is intact. For those who can summon the courage to tread a path with heart, illness's dark passage may provide a glimpse not only of what it is like to become whole, but what it means to be fully human."[39]

"I believe that the power of the mind goes far beyond what I first imagined," wrote renowned radiation oncologist O. Carl Simonton, following years of research on the connection between the mind and the body. "In addition, I believe that, beyond the body and mind, there is another aspect of healing that needs to be addressed: the spiritual aspect. . . . The dictionary defines spirit as the life principle, especially in humans, and the feelings and motivating part of our lives. . . . Our work with patients has demonstrated that health involves body, mind, and spirit. And while the mind alone can be used to influence the physical state, it is used most effectively when it is aware of spirit."[40]

One researcher attempted to arrive at a definition of spirituality by questioning health professionals, health educators, health students, and others who worked in the health and medical fields. Her characterization eventually merged many of the ideas of people involved in health. Her resulting definition of the spiritual dimension involved eight different ideas. She determined that the spiritual dimension is:[41]

1. Something that gives meaning or purpose to life

2. A set of principles or ethics to live by

3. The sense of selflessness and an altruistic feeling for others; a willingness to give of yourself

4. Commitment to God, which includes an ultimate concern

5. Perception of what causes the universe to work the way it does

6. Something for which there is not yet any rational explanation; recognition of powers beyond the known natural and rational

7. Something perceived as being intuitively known; something for which there is no easy explanation, and so it becomes a matter of faith

8. The most pleasure-producing quality of humans

Combining all of these ideas and others she collected, this researcher identified what she believed to be the four aspects of spiritual health:

1. The spiritual dimension of health acts as a *unifying force* that integrates the other dimensions of health: physical, mental, emotional, and social. The spiritual dimension brings all these into a single whole.

2. The spiritual dimension of health creates or brings into focus *meaning in life*. The exact components of that meaning vary from one individual to another. For one, it may be centered on family relationships, whereas for another it may be focused on humanitarian efforts or the result of professional effort. Regardless of the source of the meaning, it can serve as a powerful inner drive for personal accomplishment and contribution. Regardless of its source, it is vital. Without some meaning in life, the will to live is lost.

3. Because the spiritual dimension of health transcends the individual, it has the capacity to be a common bond between individuals. It rises above the individual and *goes beyond the limits of the individual*. With this common bond, we are enabled to share *love, warmth, and compassion* with other people—and we are able to do unselfish and compassionate things for others, things that go beyond ourselves. We are able to put someone else's life, safety, security, and interest before our own. This common bond also enables us to follow a set of ethical principles and to make a commitment to God (or the source of one's spiritual power).

4. The spiritual dimension of health is based on individual perceptions and faith. We acknowledge that there is some higher power at work and perceive that such a power is the cause behind the natural workings of the universe. Our perceptions and our faith bring us pleasure and convince us of our ability to survive.[42]

Medical evaluations for indications of spirituality have included prayer, meaningful contemplation, coming to a sense of purpose and meaning in life, a sense of closeness to a higher being and to others, and other experiences that reflect spiritual awareness.[43] The scope of decisions influenced by spirituality is vast; the wide range of decisions that have spiritual overtones include the degree of sexual intimacy engaged in, the decision to donate organs, the movies seen, the literature read, the music sung or listened to, smoking, drinking alcohol, taking drugs, and many more.[44]

Transformation: Moving from the Little Self to the Large Self

In *The Path of Transformation*, Shakti Gawain writes that "contact with our spiritual self gives us an expanded perspective on our lives, both as individuals and as part of humanity. Rather than just being caught up in the daily frustrations and struggles of our personality, we are able to see things from the perspective of the soul. We're able to look at the bigger picture of life on earth, which helps us to understand a lot more about why we're here and what we're doing. It helps to make our daily problems seem not quite so huge, and makes our lives feel more meaningful."[45]

One researcher developed a slightly different definition of spiritual health. Optimum spiritual health, he says, is the ability to develop our spiritual nature to its fullest potential. Part and parcel of that is the ability to discover and articulate our own basic purpose in life. It's the ability to learn how to experience love, joy, peace, and fulfillment. And it's the experience of helping ourselves and others achieve full potential.[46] This conceptualization assumes that within each of us there is a core spiritual nature (the large "I am") that, like a flower from a seed, is yearning to blossom.

Nearly all great spiritual traditions explore the importance of this transforming movement from "the little I" (or ego mind) toward the "large I am" (or core, wise, big mind). Some traditions do this more explicitly and some with more subtlety than others.[47] We all seem to have these two "selves" within us. Contemplating human suffering suggests that responding to life through the little I or ego mind causes most of our difficulties. Responding through the large, wise I am seems to heal those difficulties. Coming from the little I, you are on your own. Coming from the big I am draws on the power of connectedness. Awareness of the difference between these two selves, and sensing the ability to choose which to come from, are powerful in creating desired change. So what is the difference between them? Study carefully these differences (as described by the spiritual traditions) summarized in Table 14.2. Do you recognize both aspects of yourself?

Moving from the little I to the big I am is sometimes called the process of spiritual transformation. Methods and practices shown to greatly facilitate this transformation are summarized in Table 14.3.[48]

The Connectedness of Spirituality

One of the keys to spirituality and spiritual health lies in our relationship with others and the experiences we share. Those experiences are of prime importance. According to several researchers who spoke at Harvard Medical School's Mind/Body Institute Symposium: "Spirituality and Healing in Medicine,"[49] the greatest health benefits of spirituality are rooted in experience, not just belief. Apparently, those who "believe" but do not experience miss out on the psychological and physical benefits of spirituality. (Speakers were quick to point out that many people probably have spiritual experiences all the time but do not recognize them as such.) Those experiences are the moments of love and compassion, of feeling part of something much larger, of really seeing beauty, of resonating with what feels deeply true, and of experiencing joy. Simply getting caught up in a magnificent sunset, feeling the awe and gratitude for such beauty (and feeling one with it), might be one of those spiritually joyful moments.

The notion of spirituality itself implies that we are able to give as well as to receive[50]—that we can receive love and joy and peace and fulfillment, but that, through our experiences, we can give those things as well—and that in the giving of such things, we receive. Notice the circular and reciprocal flow of this. Dr. Deepak Chopra describes what is flowing back and forth as spiritual energy, the same energy that gives life.[51] We can give peace to another by offering words of encouragement or forgiveness (and in so doing we feel more encouraged and forgivable ourselves). We can give joy by giving someone else a deeply desired gift. We can share love by countless acts of kindness, by compassionately considering someone else's needs. Spirituality can be manifested by listening to a friend's heartaches, by walking with a child, by leaving a box of groceries

Table 14.2 The Two Selves

The little I (ego mind)	The large "I AM" (wise mind)
Fear and self driven	**Love motivated**
– What's in it for me?	– What's best for all?
– Protecting ego	– Safe
– Social mask	– Authentic
– The world's a dangerous place	– The world's a beautiful place
– Cynical, doubtful	– Trusting, hopeful
Separate	**Connected, at one**
– Competitive, comparisons	– Enjoys others' success
– Power over	– Power with
– Isolated	– Closeness to the source of love & strength
Proving self	**Acceptance & liking self**
– Externally justified	– Internally OK
"I'm only OK if . . ."	"It's OK to be in process"
– Pride	– Humility with intrinsic power
– Easily offended	– Can't be offended
– Defensive	– Takes criticism as valuable feedback
Controlled by externals	**Internal locus of control**
– Victim	– Accepts responsibility for response
– Controlling behavior	– Trusts the process
Internal turbulence	**Inner peace**
Scarcity mentality	**Abundance mentality**
– Grasping, clinging	– Generous
– Feeling deprived	– Feeling deeply grateful
Insecure	**Intrinsically secure**
– Attachment (to ego issues)	– No need for attachment (letting go)
– Externally rewarded	– Actions are intrinsically rewarding
– Transience	– Permanence
Lacking meaning ("empty")	**Filled with purpose**
Much unrealized potential	**Realizing "fullness" of potential**
Joy elusive	**Joy experienced**

on the porch of a young family whose husband lost his job. Nearly all of the spiritual traditions suggest that in such unconditional giving, good gifts tend to naturally flow back. Spirituality can be enhanced by sitting at the edge of a meadow studded with wildflowers, befriending someone who is lonely, listening to a symphony, or watching a child find a safe home for a bug they've found.

Table 14.3 Principles and Practices Facilitating Transformation

1. **Awareness** of the difference in the two selves (or minds)
   - **a.** Identify and label the ego thoughts as "My smaller ego is thinking . . ." (It's the larger mind that does this)
   - **b.** Smile at the devices used by the ego to seem important
   - **c.** Feelings (distressed or empowered) will tell you which self you are coming from
   - **d.** Choose which mind to which you give **attention** (and thus power)
2. **Stillness**:
   - **a.** Creating newness occurs in the gaps between ego thoughts
   - **b.** "Come to your senses": Breathing, listening, touching, *see* nature
   - **c.** Daily practice of being nonjudgmental (experiment with this)
   - – Being at peace with what arises
   - **d.** *Meditation, mindfulness*
3. Embrace **the present**: this is what is real
   - **a.** Accept that what is there, is there
   - **b.** Take responsibility to creatively respond
   - – How do I choose to be here and now?
4. Take the path of **least resistance**
   - **a.** Drop the burdens of defensiveness, resentment, hurtfulness, offense
   - **b.** Open to all points of view: relinquish the need to prove you are right
   - **c.** Refuse to take offense
   - **d.** Assume the positive intentions of others, and seek to identify and honor them
   - **e.** Effort motivated by love is easy
5. Assume **abundance**
   - **a.** Trust the principle that what you sow (give) is what you reap
   - **b.** Give of your talent and care freely
   - **c.** Constantly look for and receive the gifts of life gratefully
6. Your heart-felt **intention** is key to transformation and what you create
   - **a.** What do you want to bring and give to each encounter?
   - **b.** **Attention** to this then gives it power
7. **Visualize** responding as you would love to be
8. **Trust** the power of the "I am"
   - – Let go of ego requirements and attachments

Through the spiritual dimension, we emphasize our "connectedness" to other members of the human family and often to other creatures as well. Because of that connectedness, say some, we have a responsibility to help others experience spiritual growth—to help others find joy, peace, fulfillment, and a purpose in life. When we do so, we find that the experience is reciprocated; as we affect the spirituality of others, we receive help and support as well.[52]

An important distinction has to be made: In this results-oriented society in which we live, we need to realize that spirituality and spiritual health are a process or a journey, not an end point. It is a lifestyle, not a prescribed set of activities to accomplish once. There is no standard recipe to follow to achieve spirituality or spiritual health; spirituality and spiritual health involve intentional choices made over an entire lifetime. They involve living a series of experiences that define and fulfill our purpose in life and lead us eventually to feelings of joy, peace, and love in most of life's moments.

Joan Borysenko was formerly the Director of the Harvard Mind-Body Clinic. Her experiences there led her to observe:

> Wholeness has to do with the acceptance of both darkness and light, so that the work of healing and transformation can begin. Healing is a state of authenticity that allows freedom of creativity and is marked by peace, joy, compassion, and acceptance of the wide range of emotions that carry the information required to continue learning. It is a splendid coincidence that healing is often associated with better physical functioning, but the person who is truly evolving toward healing realizes that illness is a part of a Sacred Mystery that can never be reduced solely to the physical, emotional, behavioral, or spiritual (in the limited perspective we have as human beings).[53]

Influences of Spirituality on Health

We have suggested that the cultivation of spiritual health can have an influence on physical, mental, and emotional health—sometimes in very dramatic ways. What is the evidence for this connection, and how does it work? The impact of spirituality on health may be due in part to the fact that ". . . attitudes, of faith, hope, and commitment imply an internal locus of control, and following an ethical path that involves fulfillment, purpose, and meaning may lead to enhanced self-esteem and a sense of connectedness with self and others."[54] You may notice in this description of key spiritual elements the four mental principles well-proven to be highly associated with better health: hope, internal control, purpose and meaning, and connectedness (see Chapter 8).

How could such things as a sense of control or purpose, of love or hope, cause better physical health? Let's take the example of pain, or of depression, with its damage to health. We have already described the neurochemistry of how depression or anxiety cause more disease and pain (through deficiencies of neurotransmitters such as serotonin, noradrenaline, gamma-aminobutyric acid [GABA], or dopamine), and how enhancing the function of these neurotransmitters reduces pain or depression and enhances mental function. Earlier we cited examples of how spiritual practices reduce pain. Interestingly, in studies at the University of California Los Angeles, a personal sense of control was shown to significantly increase serotonin function (much like an antidepressant medication would). Deeply loving relationships and vivid spiritual experience raise dopamine levels. That's not all: getting "turned on" with purpose to a project you believe in can raise central noradrenaline levels. Meditation can raise GABA function, a neurotransmitter that calms the overresponsive nervous system characteristic of many common illnesses such as headache, irritable bowel, anxiety, or chronic pain. Each of these neurochemical effects improves nervous system suppression of pain. So all this may explain somewhat how a person with pain who falls in love and experiences joy will at times find his or her pain subsiding. It may also explain how interventions that quiet hostility and improve relationships can reduce heart attacks.[55] Spiritual well-being greatly impacts the experience of life stressors, turning distress (the bad kind for health) into eustress (the good kind).

Cardiologist Bruno Cortis asks, "How can health be without spirituality? . . . The spiritual powers within . . . lift all of humanity."[56] Experienced clinician and educator Paul Pearsall, who founded and directs the Problems of Daily Living Clinic in the Department of Psychiatry at Sinai Hospital in Detroit, Michigan, remembers a woman who exemplified spiritual health:

> I will never forget her. As she laughed, her hand went to her forehead to brush her hair from her eyes. Purple numbers were tattooed on her wrist. She called them her death marks but said that they had strangely protected and renewed her life during her suffering. She had been tortured, seen her own parents and almost all of her relatives killed, and had lived in the agony, squalor, and starvation of a prison camp for most of the young years of her life. She had every reason to be weak, bitter, sick, and depressed. Instead, she was one of the most joyful, hardy women I have ever met.[57]

Pearsall attributes her health, strength, and resilience to a deep sense of spiritual strength. She was a person whose spirituality enabled her to find meaning and purpose in life—even in the midst of crisis.

Similarly, Viktor Frankl, himself a Jewish survivor of a Nazi prison camp and an astute observer of what allowed some to bear it well, eloquently describes the key to such resilience as a sense of purpose and meaning. In his classic book, *Man's Search for Meaning*,[58] Frankl describes how resilient people find meaning in all the vicissitudes of life, even in the worst of stress, such as the tragedy of the camp.

Researchers are beginning to view spirituality with new interest, especially as it relates to physical health. One pioneer of such research is Kenneth Pelletier—who, with his colleagues at the Corporate Health Promotion Project at the University of California–San Francisco, investigated the link between spirituality and health. Pelletier started his research by exploring the lives of top business executives and other prominent people who have achieved what most consider to be "success."

He found first that most of the professionally successful men and women participating in the study had strong spiritual values and beliefs. Further, most of them had suffered a major psychological or physical trauma early in life. Despite these traumas—or maybe because of them, Pelletier surmises—these people now have a more effective style of coping with life crises.[59] (As discussed in a Harvard Medical School conference, spiritual people weather crises better—partially because they are able to find purpose and meaning in life despite the crisis and even from the crisis.)

Preliminary findings from the study found the correlation between good spiritual health and good physical health to be "striking." People with a deep sense of spirituality reported less use of medical services, fewer minor illnesses, and more complete recovery from minor illness than the national average. Similar findings were reported from a study of 300 terminally ill and non–terminally ill hospitalized adults. Even if their illnesses were terminal, those with the greatest spirituality showed resilient emotional health. Spirituality was significantly related to "low death fear, low discomfort, decreased loneliness, emotional adjustment, and positive death perspectives among terminal cancer and other seriously ill patients."[60]

In another study of more than 100 geriatric patients at a clinic, researchers measured each patient's "religious activity" by determining the amount of each one's religious community activity, private devotional activity (such as prayer), and intrinsic religious orientation. They found that those who had little religious activity had much higher rates of cancer, chronic anxiety, depression, cigarette smoking, and alcohol use. On the other hand, patients with high levels of religious activity enjoyed better overall physical and mental health.[61]

Some of the improvement in overall health may well relate to the benefits of spiritual practice on mental health and reduction of feeling distressed. One researcher concluded that the evidence showed that spirituality can reduce anxiety, foster better intimacy, enhance a sense of purpose and meaning for life, and foster personal growth and control.[62] A panel of experts carefully reviewed many studies in the medical literature;[63] their conclusions are summarized in Table 14.4.

Table 14.4 Correlates of Spirituality and Religiousness

Spirituality and Religiousness are associated with greater levels of:	Spirituality and Religiousness are associated with lower levels of:
Subjective well-being	Depression symptoms
Life satisfaction	Delinquency
Marital satisfaction	Drug and alcohol abuse

When dealing with stressful events, some aspects of religious coping—such as seeking reassurance from God and seeking support within one's religious community—were more helpful than others (including praying for a miracle). On the other hand, some forms of religiousness had deleterious mental effects; these included beliefs in a punitive God, extrinsic religiosity, conflict with or feeling judged by clergy, and hyper-rigid religiousness). Flexibility appears to be important in healing.

Mindful meditative practice reduces anxiety in the long term.[64] This has been shown to reduce physical problems considerably, as do other treatments for anxiety.[65] For example, by reducing stress hormones, transcendental meditation can lead to regression of carotid artery thickening[66] (compared to progressive thickening in control groups) and improved coronary disease outcomes.[67]

One message from all this is that the ultimate healer is not so much the doctor but rather ourselves. Paul Pearsall states, "Determination on the part of the patient, not the physician, is what makes healing and joy possible."[68] Or, as Buddha summarized, "It is you who must make the effort. The masters only point the way." Pearsall remarks that contemporary psychologists call this combination of faith and determination a "sense of trust"—"a trust in the spirit of God within each of us as the source of all joy."

Relationships are an essential part of spiritual well-being. Those in truly great relationships know the joy that comes in desiring the good of the beloved. In this, a person comes to feel more fully alive, and, in fact, the person is more fully alive. Such empowering relationships have a powerful effect to enhance health in all its dimensions (see Chapter 9).

Pearsall emphasizes that choosing to care well for oneself is another aspect of spirituality. This requires a good sense of self-acceptance:

> We seem to be alienated from our own affection for ourselves. We believe that once we lose weight, make more money, or learn some new skill, we will then become more acceptable to ourselves. This sequence is backward. We must begin with a celebration of self, not a diagnosis of our flaws. If you can't say something good about yourself, maybe you shouldn't be saying anything at all until you look a little closer at just how special you really are. . . . To love oneself is only possible by first learning to love others and by developing a tolerance, acceptance, and empathy that are necessary if we are ever going to get closer to one another than we have been until now.[69]

Crisis as a Growth Experience

People with a deep sense of spirituality see life differently. They have a purpose, they enjoy a sense of meaning in life, and they have a broader perspective. Spirituality buffers stress; people with a deep sense of spirituality are not defeated by crisis. They are able to relax their minds, elicit the relaxation response, and heal more quickly and completely. Deep spirituality brings inner peace and hope in the face of whatever arises.

At a deep level, how important is growth to you—that is, how important to you is it to be better today than you were five years ago and to be wiser and stronger tomorrow than you are today? To most of us, that seems very important. Yet we often try to avoid the very parts of life that best bring that maturation. Much of what life is about seems to be related to that growing process: becoming wiser and more loving. Praying for no difficulties is probably a prayer that is unlikely to be answered. It is those who acknowledge life's purposes, and even enjoy rising to the challenge, who become more resilient.[70]

Spirituality helps people interpret crisis in a growth-producing way. Even when a disease takes a life, spirituality can make the experience one of creating resilience. In talking about how spirituality can influence attitude, Yale cancer surgeon Dr. Bernie Siegel remarks, "I simply try to heal the life. I hate to have somebody die with an unhealed life. I hate to have somebody die who says, 'I have never lived; I have never experienced love; I have always felt worthless.' Through the disease, I try to bring something to their lives, so the disease can be a gift."[71]

In the effort to "heal a life," Siegel says, we need to figure out "what is the self trying to get me as a patient to learn about myself?" . . . "If you turn toward what threatens you and say, 'Why are you here? Why do you want to kill me? What can I learn from you?' then you help heal your life and find out who you are."[72] He further says that when "you take on life's afflictions and challenges, you are a winner." He adds that he hopes people can

> understand that there can be a gift in the disease and you can help heal everyone around you. Hemingway said that the world breaks everyone and some of us are strong at the broken places. I am talking about people who are strong at the broken places: the quadriplegics can have healed lives; people who aren't cured of cancer can be incredibly inspiring and teach all of us; people with multiple sclerosis can teach us.[73]

Not everyone will be cured. At some time or another, everyone dies. But people who are busy living, who are trying to make changes in their lives, experience great growth even in the face of serious illness. People who face disease with that attitude, Siegel says,

> define their disease as a gift, a challenge, a wake-up call, a new beginning, and a beauty mark. And they are not necessarily saying, "I am cured." The exceptional people accept their mortality. They have heard they're going to die, but they don't take it as a sentence. So they don't go home and die. They take it as an opportunity to live until they die.[74]

In discussing the entire issue of spirituality and the growth that can come from illness or other adversity, Siegel talks about what he calls "a spiritual flat tire":

> I simply say that sometimes adversity and affliction direct you into the proper place so that when you have a flat tire that makes you miss a plane that later crashes, you embrace the tire, bronze it, and hang it over your fireplace as the spiritual flat tire that saved your life. But while you are fixing the tire you are screaming and yelling and getting dirty and mad that you are going to miss your plane. There are many things in life that redirect our lives. So I don't judge things as good, bad, right or wrong. Just sit back and say, "We'll see."[75]

In viewing illness or crisis as a positive redirection in life, perhaps most important, says Siegel, is to infuse your situation with spirituality and love:

> The only way you can live forever is to love somebody: then you can really leave a gift behind. And when you live that way, as I have seen happen with people who have physical illnesses, it is even possible to decide when you die. You can say, "Thank you, I've used my body to its limit. I have loved as much as I possibly can, and I'm leaving at two o'clock today." And you go. Then maybe you spend half an hour dying and the rest of your day living. But when these things are not done, you may spend a lot of your life dying, and only a little living.[76]

Spiritual healing, says one researcher, "is not a complicated system of diagnoses and remedies but seems to work on the level of unselfish love and compassion. Not an emotional love, that is bound up with one's own needs, but a caring, unconditional, detached love with no beginning and no end."[77]

The Power of Prayer on Health

A 76-year-old Spanish-speaking man who lives in a small village north of Santa Fe, New Mexico, described the essential rhythms of his life in this way:

> For us the day begins with a prayer of thanks to God, for giving us another day here. And in the evening, when we go to bed, we stop and say thank you, dear Lord, for the gift of another day with our children and grandchildren. It is only a few moments any of us is here, we know—because life goes on and on and on, and we're but one stalk of corn, and many stalks are planted and grow and are harvested, season after season. But the one who puts us here and then gathers us up—He is the one who should hear from us with a please, a thank you, a wave, a smile. If we cry, He'd like to know why. If we're happy, He'd like to know why. It's not right to think you're the lord and master of this place. He is the one who has His eyes on us and wants the best for us.

True, we have to build our lives for ourselves; He has let us do that. But He's not beyond giving us a boost now and then—if we ask! When we get sick, we don't go right down to Santa Fe or Albuquerque right away. No sir, we stop and try to figure out what has happened; and we call the priest; and we get down on our hands and knees and call Him to us, the Lord, and tell Him what's up. When we do that—well, you hear what you've said, and believe me, there are times when just listening to your own prayers makes you feel better![78]

The elderly villager describes what many have felt: Your prayers can make you feel better, particularly those prayers that are filled with gratitude and hope. Prayer is often the mediator of our spirituality and is at the core of most spiritual experiences. According to a recent Gallup Poll, 87 percent of all Americans pray to God. When we pray, we are in a state of relaxed alertness, peace, joy, contentment, and emotional release. During prayer, we empty the mind, yet we receive some inner direction. Part of the magnetism of prayer comes from our own belief, our own faith—the powerful suggestion that prayer will work, that something will happen.[79]

A study of nearly 4,000 mostly Christian people over age 65 found that those who never or rarely prayed ran about a 50 percent greater risk of dying over a period of six years.[80] The authors postulate that the relaxation and meditative effects of prayer may play a role in the protection it provides. From a naturalistic perspective, one might also think that the 64 percent of people who pray for their health[81] and trust in prayer's efficacy tap into the power of hope and optimistic expectation that improves outcomes (see Chapter 16).

It's the subtle peace-and-quiet effect of prayer that may be the most effective. In one study of spontaneous remission of cancer conducted at Kyushu University School of Medicine in Japan, researchers found that prayer preceded the cure in every case. However, say the researchers, it wasn't "robust, aggressive prayer for specific outcomes, including eradication of the cancer" that did the trick but "a prayerful, prayerlike attitude of devotion and acceptance."[82]

Dr. Larry Dossey, an internist who has pioneered prayer research, writes, "I would describe prayer as any psychological activity—conscious or unconscious—that places us in closer contact with the transcendent. This can involve words, but it can also be subconscious or unconscious. Prayer can even occur during sleep. The state of mind that I call prayerfulness seems to involve certain fairly specific qualities, in particular, empathy. The most successful prayer experiments have always linked outcome to the empathy, love, and sense of involvement felt by the people doing the praying."[83] One concept going on here is that the powerful ingredient of prayer is not so much the words said as it is a feeling of hope and gratitude, of being thankful for the answer to prayer, and of all involved being blessed by the prayer.[84]

The Relaxation Response

Prayer can have powerful physiological effects on the body as well. Of 131 controlled experiments on prayer-based healing, more than half showed statistically significant benefits.[85] Dr. Herbert Benson, Associate Professor of Medicine at the Harvard Medical School and chief of the Section on Behavioral Medicine at the New England Deaconess Hospital, has focused the last two decades of his clinical work on what he has come to call the "relaxation response." The relaxation response is the body's ability to enter a "scientifically definable state" of relaxation. During the relaxation response, changes occur in the body. Metabolism slows down, blood pressure drops, breathing slows, heart rate lowers, and even the brain waves are less active.[86] During the relaxation response, the distress response is reversed.

According to Benson, the relaxation response, "with all its physiological benefits, has most often and effectively been elicited through forms of prayer."[87] In his own practice, as he has struggled to teach patients the relaxation response, he has watched the significant physical results of prayer. He has written extensively of those results; in one woman, crippling angina was resolved. In another, life-threatening high blood pressure was dropped.

The relaxation response gives us one clue as to why prayer improves health: it helps us meditate, relieving stress. Prayer may be the most common kind of meditation in the Western world. When patients pray, they're usually focusing on their deepest values, contemplating ways to operate within those values, and drawing on powers to fulfill those values (thus increasing an internal locus of control). In prayer, they draw on spiritual support that develops both a sense of connectedness and hope. Once again, recall that a sense of control, connectedness, and hope all have been known to positively affect medical outcomes. The mind has the ability to heal when those elements are elicited.

Apparently, most of the benefits from prayer come from what researchers call "meditative" prayer—being still, knowing that God is God. In moments of stillness, between ego thoughts and fears, inspiration comes. According to University of Akron sociologist Margaret Poloma, research suggests that people who use only active, petitionary prayer but don't get into meditative prayer "aren't as likely to find peace and serenity" through their prayers.[88]

Poloma and her colleague, Brian Pendleton, found that different types of prayers affected people in different ways. Happiness, they say, seems to be predicted not by the frequency of prayer but by its quality. In a study of 560 Akron-area residents, Poloma and Pendleton identified four main types of prayer that are performed away from church:

1. Meditative (feeling or quietly thinking about God)

2. Colloquial (asking for guidance or forgiveness)

3. Petitional (asking for explicit favors)

4. Ritual (reading specific prayers)[89]

According to Poloma and Pendleton, meditative prayer was closely associated with "existential well-being" and religious satisfaction, whereas colloquial prayer was related to overall happiness.

In summary, when we pray, we reap much physical, emotional, and spiritual benefit.

The Healing Power of Forgiveness

Essential to a spiritual nature is forgiveness—the ability to release from the mind all the past hurts and failures, all sense of guilt and loss. Counselor Suzanne Simon defines forgiveness as a "process of healing." What some have also called "the first step on the pathway to healing," forgiveness enables one to banish resentment. It is, as Dr. Joan Borysenko put it, "accepting the core of every human being as the same as yourself and giving them the gift of not judging them."[90]

According to psychotherapist Robin Casarjian, founder and director of the Lionheart Foundation, forgiveness is "a relationship with life that frees the forgiver from the psychological bondage of chronic fear, hostility, anger, and unhealthy guilt."[91] Forgiveness, she says, is an attitude that implies that you are willing to accept responsibility for your perceptions, realizing that "your perceptions are a choice and not an objective fact."

We forgive others, and we must forgive ourselves. According to one researcher, forgiveness "removes whatever has blocked your creative mind from operating positively for you and for your good."[92]

Forgiveness isn't easy; in fact, most people who responded to one poll said they had great difficulty in forgiving others. Apparently, forgiveness is the most difficult when we are called upon to forgive ourselves. Psychologists estimate that at least 7 of every 10 people carry throughout life a sense of guilt—a feeling of having committed a sin or mistake for which they have never been forgiven.[93]

Forgiveness is not condoning negative, inappropriate behavior, whether your own or someone else's, says Casarjian. It is also not "pretending everything is just fine when you feel it isn't, or assuming an attitude of superiority or self-righteousness." Instead, she says, it is a "decision to see beyond the limits of another's personality . . . and to gradually transform yourself from being a helpless victim of your circumstances to being a powerful and loving co-creator of your reality."[94]

Our own chosen thoughts about what the offender has done are far more powerful in creating our reaction than is their act itself. For example, when Ingrid saw her physician for abdominal pains and headaches, she spoke very angrily and in condemning terms about her teenage daughter's sassy, rebellious attitude the day before. "Cally makes me so angry! I hate her when she acts that way!" To Ingrid, Cally's acts seemed to reach inside her to make Ingrid bitterly angry and hateful, causing her to lash out at Cally with putdowns in retaliation.

Afterward, however, Ingrid felt some remorse, even guilt, about the way she had put her daughter down. "I don't want to be that kind of mother," Ingrid admitted. "Cally is going through a lot, and trying to let go of being dependent and controlled by me. I don't deserve to be treated that way, but neither does she. When I try to put myself in her shoes, and see the world through her eyes, I can feel my heart softening and the anger melts away."

Ingrid was beginning to understand an essential key to reclaiming one's life, to feeling the sense of personal control that has been so consistently linked to better health and medical outcomes. That key is called forgiveness. Forgiveness can at first seem difficult, like giving a magnanimous gift to some jerk who doesn't deserve it or letting them off the hook of deserved consequences and retribution. However, with a bit of reflection, the real meaning of forgiveness begins to emerge. Forgiveness is refusing any longer to blame someone else, or circumstances, for making one feel or act in ways they would not want. Forgiveness is taking back control of one's life, behavior, and personal actions. This recovery of a sense of personal control is essential to wholeness and well-being (health). A low sense of personal control leads to all the negative emotions: anger, guilt, fear, anxiety, and frustration (with all of their adverse health implications). On the other hand, a high sense of personal control (of one's self, not of the world out there) leads to all the positive emotions: confidence, inner peace, hope, and loving kindness (even for a rebellious daughter).

The foremost way to get a high personal sense of control is to fully accept personal responsibility for how one chooses to think about and respond to the acts of others (or of fate). Blaming makes it feel like the other has taken control of you, making you act and feel ways you would not want. The fact is they don't have that kind of control over you. Only you do. So call your control back by refusing to blame any longer what they have done for making you be other than what you want to be—by forgiving. Such a choice may well require help beyond your own. Forgiveness is taking back control of your life and, if possible, as Ingrid did, seeing the pain or insecurity that drives the other's behavior. This may even lead to compassion.

To determine the physical effects of forgiveness, it is first necessary to determine what happens to us physically when we don't forgive. The resulting hatred drives all the mechanisms causing poor health described in the chapters on stress (Chapter 2) and anger (Chapter 4). With forgiveness, the anger and resentment dissolve. The body stops pouring high-voltage chemicals into the bloodstream. The healing begins.

One of the greatest examples of the healing power of forgiveness can be found in nature. As one author put it:

> Nature always forgives. Nature is the great giver and the great forgiver. Should you cut your hand with a sharp knife, the forces of nature set about immediately to repair the damage. It was a mistake to cut your hand, but nature does not withhold the repairing of the wound. Nature immediately forgives and starts at once to make repairs. If you eat food that does not agree with you and you have indigestion, nature immediately starts to repair the damage. Although it was a mistake to eat the wrong food, you do not need to go through the rest of your life with indigestion. Nature even repairs the ravages of the battlefield by covering it with grass and flowers. [No one] can go forward if he is tied to the past. No one can think straight and efficiently if his mind is cluttered up with thoughts of hate or memories of hurts and mistakes; hence the necessity of forgiving so that we can love ourselves, our neighbor, and God.[95]

To bring a greater sense of forgiveness into your own life, try following what Dwight Wolter presented as the "tools of forgiveness."[96]

- Begin by letting go of your unforgiving stance.
- Admit that the events and feelings you are struggling with really happened.
- Admit that the past cannot be undone. After all, there is really no hope for a better yesterday.
- Recognize that you no longer need to depend on others, including your parents, for approval. When you realize your independence, you assume your rightful power, and you learn to be who you want to be regardless of the actions of others.
- Don't expect others to respond to your efforts to forgive.
- Release any unrealistic expectations of yourself.
- Accept others for who they are rather than who you want them to be.
- Be flexible about rules of conduct for yourself and others.
- Talk about issues as they come up.

Overall forgiveness means to refuse any longer to blame.

In addition to those suggestions, Robin Casarjian suggests fostering a forgiving attitude by praying, meditating, expressing gratitude (to people or to a higher power), spending time in nature and allowing yourself to experience its wonder, serving others selflessly, and creating through any art form.[97]

Church Affiliation and Health

Many studies have demonstrated that people with active religious faith and people who are strongly affiliated with a church or other religious community generally enjoy better health. For example, those who attend religious services one or more times a week have dramatically lower death rates—especially from coronary artery disease (50 percent less), emphysema (56 percent less), cirrhosis of the liver (74 percent less), and suicide (53 percent less).[98] Generally, in the here and now, religion is a means to the end of spiritual well-being and sometimes provides the opportunity to create a sense of community with common ideals. From the health standpoint, focusing one's religion on the principles of spiritual well-being has very positive effects. Using religion for other purposes has less of a health benefit.

There are two basic orientations of religion:

1. **Personal.** Personal religion involves a person's values, beliefs, and attitudes. Spiritual experience is the cornerstone of this religion and becomes an important way to discover and know God. The personal orientation of religion can be either intrinsic or extrinsic. Those with an intrinsic sense of religion participate in their chosen religion for spiritual reasons, "because that's who they are"; to them, their religion is often loved and becomes a powerful force in their lives. Those with an extrinsic sense of religion do not share the "zeal" or commitment of those with an intrinsic orientation; religion for them is secondary and does not represent a primary need. They "belong," often for the benefits that the religion provides or to avoid problems, but they do not always "live" their religion. Studies show intrinsic religion has far more health benefit than extrinsic religion.[99]

2. **Institutional.** Individuals adopt a church or religion because of group-related benefits: They enjoy attending church, participating in group activities or rituals, and receiving community support.

Studies indicate that religion may enhance well-being in at least four ways:[100] (1) through social integration and support; (2) through the establishment of a personal relationship with a divine other; (3) through the provision of systems of meaning and existential coherence; and (4) through the promotion of specific patterns of a more healthy personal lifestyle. Globally, but at a somewhat simplified level, it is understandable how each of these may improve dealing with the distress that impacts health. Many spiritual traditions suggest the ability to tap into the healing spiritual powers that connect all people.

Regardless of how it works, evidence exists that religion does enhance health. Numerous studies provide evidence that, on average, high levels of religious involvement are associated with better health. These studies have involved both men and women, numerous racial and ethnic groups, people from diverse social and economic backgrounds, people of all ages, and members of a wide variety of different churches. While some studies focus on particular religions (such as the healthy lifestyle of

Mormons or Adventists – such as less smoking or meat, emphasis on family life, etc.), others show that factors such as frequency of attendance, some specific religious practices, and certain types of religious belief are also important in protecting health.[101]

Studies that examined several specific medical problems (including the rate of heart disease, high blood pressure, stroke, cancer, digestive disease, physical disability, self-rated health, and self-reported symptoms) showed a strong relationship between religious participation and good health.[102] A study by the National Institute on Aging found that elderly people living at home who attended church regularly were less depressed and physically healthier than those who did not attend church.[103] This association, of course, doesn't prove a causal relationship. Healthier people may be more likely to attend church. Attendance is used as an easily measured marker for religiosity. However, many studies show similar results. For example:

- Those patients who undergo open-heart surgery have a much greater chance of surviving if they gain comfort and strength from religious faith.[104]

- The greater longevity of those who enjoy regular religious affiliation is probably due in part to better social support.[105]

- The elderly who regularly attend church have significantly better physical and mental health and lower death rates.[106] (One study, in fact, showed that some elderly people in New Haven, Connecticut, actually postponed the timing of their death until the conclusion of major religious holidays, such as Easter or Christmas.[107])

In one study of 850 hospitalized men, researchers at a North Carolina Veterans' Administration hospital found that religion was an important coping factor for the men. One in five said religion is "the most important thing that keeps me going." Nearly half of the patients rated religion as very helpful to them in coping with the situation of being hospitalized. According to the men in the study, they derived a feeling of peace and comfort from prayer, Bible study, faith in God, and the emotional support of a pastor or other church members. Those who were religious had high levels of social support, low levels of alcohol use, and significantly less clinical depression (each of which improves health outcomes).

A detailed review of all such studies[108] revealed that high religious commitment and participation is associated with the following:

Better physical health outcomes

- 212 studies: 75 percent positive; 17 percent mixed; and 7 percent negative (primarily including heart disease, cancer, survival, hypertension, general health, and overall functioning)

Better mental health outcomes

- in 18 of 19 studies: better adjustment and coping

- in 15 of 15 studies: less drug abuse

- in 20 of 24 studies: less alcohol abuse

- in 15 of 18 studies: less psychiatric illness

- in 13 of 19 studies: less depression

Better quality of life

- in 18 of 19 studies: better life satisfaction
- in 10 of 10 studies: better marriage adjustment
- in 20 of 22 studies: better overall well-being
- in 14 of 21 studies: less anxiety about death

Let's discuss some specifics of these studies. For example, Harold Koenig and David Larson studied 542 people aged over 60, finding that over a year, those who attended church at least weekly were hospitalized 56 percent less (43 percent less after controlling for illness, age, and depression) than were those who attended less frequently. Also, when hospitalized, those affiliated with any religion stayed less than half as long as those who claimed no religion.

"Many people—especially those with fewer health, social, and financial resources—turn to religion for solace in the face of situations over which they have no control," said the researchers, commenting on the study. "Their religious beliefs and involvement may counteract feelings of helplessness, provide meaning and order to challenging life experiences, and restore a sense of control."[109]

Researchers at Duke University, confirming these positive effects of religion on health, theorized that the relationship had to do with the comfort religion provides in time of difficulty or crisis. Dr. Harold G. Koenig, co-director of the Center for Spirituality, Theology, and Health at Duke University Medical Center, summarized studies in this area thus:

> If you have nothing stressing you, if you're wealthy and you're well educated, you've got plenty of friends, you're probably going to be pretty happy—[religious or not]. But if you're studying instead a group of people who are undergoing stress—they're physically ill, they're disabled, maybe they are in bereavement, or they've lost a job—then if you look at religious people compared to those who are less religious, you're going to find the religious people are coping better . . .
>
> So these [religious] rules and regulations and laws—love your neighbor and help your neighbor and forgive your neighbor—are good for us, they're good for our mental and our physical health.[110]

Patients themselves tend to confirm those theories. An Internet study recruited 157 people to describe their "alternative" practices in mental health. Very similar patterns were found in a much larger study of 5827 older adults with need for mental health treatment.[111] Most of those surveyed had bipolar mood disorders, depression, or schizophrenia. The methods most commonly used were:

- Spiritual/religious practices: 50 percent
- Meditation: 43 percent
- Massage: 31 percent
- Yoga: 20 percent
- Imagery: 17 percent
- Herbs: 16 percent
- Dietary supplements: 13 percent

Eighty-six percent were also taking medication. Adding the above practices provided the following enhanced benefits (each reported by more than 20 percent of the group):

- Increased calmness and stability
- Better cognitive function
- Improved relationships
- Greater sense of purpose
- Feelings of being spiritually nurtured
- Improved general functioning

In a study of elderly people who were depressed, Bosworth found that the significantly better improvement in those who were religious came from much more than simply social support.[112]

Attendance and Affiliation

However, while almost 90 percent of all Americans report some religious affiliation, despite their belief in God and the Bible, many American Christians are not active in church affiliations. While 85 percent of Americans consider religion "very important or fairly important" in their lives,[113] their church attendance does not always reflect that attitude. According to a Gallup Poll, only about 40 percent of all Americans attend a place of worship weekly, and about 60 percent attend monthly.[114]

Even churchgoers have a growing dissatisfaction with organized religion. Of those surveyed, 59 percent think churches spend too much time on organization issues; 32 percent believe organized religion is too restrictive in its moral teachings. Almost one in four of the respondents to the Gallup Poll say they turned away from their church in search of "deeper spiritual meaning."[115]

Even so, extensive research indicates that all across the age spectrum, active participation in a church or synagogue boosts health,[116] acts as a buffer against stress, and may even prolong life. A case can be made that the social support of active religious community has an advantage over isolated spirituality. Researchers at Southern California College found that elderly people who are religiously active tend to be more optimistic and better able to cope with illness than people who are less religious. Psychologists from Yale and Rutgers Universities, studying nearly 3000 retirees from New Haven, Connecticut, similarly showed that religion gave a significant sense of well being and comfort to the seniors.[117]

At the other end of the age spectrum, similar effects are seen in youth. A study of 19,000 high school seniors conducted at the University of Michigan explains one reason why religious affiliation appears to protect the health of adolescents: Those who have a strong religious affiliation are less likely to behave in ways that compromise their health, such as getting into fights, carrying weapons, smoking cigarettes, using marijuana, and driving under the influence of alcohol. They are also more likely to behave in ways that enhance their health, such as eating well, getting proper nutrition, getting regular exercise, and getting plenty of rest.[118] Research shows that religious beliefs and behaviors are fairly widespread among American teens. Among those aged 13 to 17, 95 percent report being affiliated with a religious group or denomination, and 40 percent say they try very hard to follow the teachings of their religion. Of youth in that age group:[119]

- 95 percent believe in God or a universal spirit.
- 93 percent believe that God loves them.
- 91 percent believe in heaven.

Interestingly, an adolescent's health may even be protected by the fact that his or her mother regularly attends church. A study of 143 teenagers in the Baltimore area looked at the significant risks for psychiatric disorders and examined adolescents who were considered at high risk. Researchers found that those whose mothers attended religious services at least once a week had greater overall satisfaction with their lives, had more involvement with their families, felt greater support from friends, and had better skills in solving health-related problems. The only factor that had a greater influence in the study was family income.[120]

What specific areas of health are impacted by religion? One review of 200 epidemiological studies found that religion particularly improved health in eight areas: cancer of the uterus and cervix, all other cancers, colitis and enteritis, cardiovascular disease, hypertension and stroke, general health, general longevity, and disease and death among the clergy.[121]

Relationship to Church Teachings

An obvious way that some religions improve health is by actively promoting healthier lifestyles, such as eating healthy, nutritious foods and less meat, drinking less alcohol, avoiding caffeine-containing foods and drinks, and not smoking.[122] They may also encourage family and social patterns of helping and caring, proper rest, life balance, and exercise.

Religious teachings often encourage support in times of need— a belief in life after death, for example, makes it much less stressful to face the terminal illness of a loved one. Many religions also discourage behavior that is harmful to health, often counseling against harmful drugs, immoral activities (including promiscuous sex with its elevated risks of contracting sexually transmitted diseases), and activities that have a high probability of injuring the body.[123]

Researchers point out, however, that not all religions act to preserve life and promote health. Some religions include the use of contaminated substances in rituals, burials, and other practices; placing the dead in rivers; ritual suicide; religious wars; tortures and executions in the name of religion; and endogamous marriage customs that may engender and perpetuate genetic disorders. Some, too, prohibit members from seeking modern medical treatment or from practicing modern health principles—although churches with these policies are in the distinct minority.[124]

Still another way that churches protect health may lie in teachings regarding attitude. According to researcher Ellen Idler at Rutgers University, the religious teachings of many churches help foster a more positive approach to finding resilience and meaning in illness, pain, or disability.[125]

A prominent theory regarding how religious communities protect the health of their members rests with the well-known fact that social support boosts and protects health. People who are active in a church are not as likely to be lonely. Members of a church affiliation are much like members of an extended family: they provide comfort, companionship, and even material assistance when needed. Ministers and other church leaders visit the ill, marry couples, provide comfort when a family member dies, speak at the funeral, and give counsel in difficult circumstances. Churches offer tradition and social support that are lacking in many communities.[126]

What is the effect of religious life on mental and emotional health? Famed psychotherapist Carl Jung commented:

> During the past thirty years, people from all the civilized countries of the earth have consulted me. I have treated many hundreds of patients. . . . Among all my patients in the second half of life—that is to say, over thirty-five—there has not been one whose problem in the last resort was not that of finding a religious outlook on life. . . . It seems to me that, side by side with the decline of religious life, the neuroses grow noticeably more frequent.[127]

Maryland psychologist John Gartner reviewed 200 studies on religious commitment and mental health. Those studies showed that the religiously faithful have lower suicide rates, lower drug use and abuse, less juvenile delinquency, lower divorce rates, higher marital happiness, better overall well-being, and better recovery from mental illness.

"Religious belief gives life a context and restrains many self-destructive impulses," explains Gartner. "For many people it appears to be a solid floor for mental health."[128]

Regardless of why religion works to boost health, abundant evidence shows that regular participation seems to be a key, even after controlling for age, sex, and various other risk factors.[129]

In summary, spiritual practices and attitudes that have been proven to be associated with enhanced physical health include the following:

- Hope
- Forgiveness
- Giving up hostility
- Altruism
- Loving, supportive relationships—community
- Prayer
- Meditation
- Feeling close to God

The Essence of Spirituality and Spiritual Well-Being

What, then, is the essence of spiritual well-being, the state toward which spiritual and religious practices are best directed? Perhaps, from a scientific perspective, we might discover the answer in those spiritual elements that most powerfully impact mental and physical well-being.

Health has been defined by the World Health Organization as total well-being (physical, mental, social, and spiritual), not just the absence of disease. Others have defined health as the quality of existence in which one is at peace within oneself (physically, mentally, and spiritually) and in good concord with the environment. Health science requires the measurements of studies. We can measure physical health very well and mental health quite well, but how do we measure spiritual health?

As one looks at the hundreds of studies in this book for the mental (mind) elements that most powerfully affect physical health (body), at least four principles become very obvious:

1. A sense of empowerment and personal control—not necessarily over the environment but rather over one's self and responses in that environment. This involves being and acting in accord with one's deepest values in any situation, a type of spiritual integrity to deep wisdom.

2. A sense of connectedness—to one's deeper self, to others, to the sources of one's empowerment, and even to the earth and universe, and all regarded as good.

3. A sense of purpose and meaning—giving of oneself for a purpose of value and something believed in, thus having an altruistic sense of mission about one's life. Also sensing purpose in the present here-and-now circumstances (whether difficult or joyful) honoring growth and having a vision of one's potential.

4. Hope—not necessarily for a specific outcome but for the wisdom and capability to deal well with whatever comes and for something of value to come of it.

Notice that these "mental" elements (proven to improve physical and mental health) are at their core also very spiritual elements. We propose that they thus define some of the most important principles of spiritual well-being.[130] These principles thus are the connectors between the triad of body-mind-spirit health. Directing one's spiritual practices and religious motivations toward these principles has been shown to improve total health. Violating these principles, even with the best of intentions, is likely to cause problems.

For example, a parent or religious leader who has very good intentions for a person may use guilt or shame to motivate better behavior. Does that empower the person—or is it more likely to make him or her feel less capable? Does throwing guilt connect us or disconnect us? Does shaming create hope, or imply that one is unworthy? On the other hand, motivating improvement instead with love that accepts people right where they are in their process, conveying a belief and trust in them to rise to their own greater wisdom, might enhance each of the above four principles of spiritual well-being. Thus, knowing what we are going toward might guide one's approach to both religion and spirituality. It seems important not to confuse means and ends. Done well, religion can be a very powerful means to the end of spiritual well-being. Losing sight of those end principles, religion not done so well could cause difficulty.

Physician Rachel Naomi Remen, medical director of the Commonweal Cancer Help Program and a member of the Scientific Advisory Board for the Inner Mechanisms of the Healing Response Program for the Institute of Noetic Sciences, says it may be easiest to define the spiritual by defining what it isn't. The spiritual, she says, is not the moral. Nor is it the ethical. The spiritual is also not the psychic, nor is it the religious.

The spiritual, she says, "is inclusive. It is the deepest sense of belonging and participation. We all participate in the spiritual at all times, whether we know it or not. There's no place to go to be separated from the spiritual. . . . The most important thing in defining spirit is the recognition that spirit is an essential need of human nature. There is something in all of us that seeks the spiritual. This yearning varies in strength from person to person, but it is always there in everyone. And so healing becomes possible."[131]

WHAT DID YOU LEARN?

1. Name four spiritual principles that have been well demonstrated to be associated with good mental and physical health.

2. Describe the difference between *spirituality* and *religion*. In terms of studies, which is more easily measured?

3. Describe at least two ways that religious involvement might improve health.

4. Discuss four or more differences between the "little I" (ego mind) and the "big I am"

5. Describe at least three methods or practices that create transformation to the larger mind.

ENDNOTES

1. Bruno Cortis, *Heart and Soul: A Psychological and Spiritual Guide to Preventing and Healing Heart Disease* (Pocket Books;1997)

2. A. E. Bergin and J. P. Jensen, "Religiosity of Psychotherapists: A National Survey," *Psychotherapy* 27 (1990): 3–7.

3. CBS News Poll 1998 and Yankelovich Partners U.S. Survey. Reported in C. Wallis, "Faith and Healing," *Time* (June 24, 1996): 62.

4. D. B. Larson, *The Faith Factor, Volume II: An Annotated Bibliography of Systematic Review and Clinical Research on Spiritual Subjects* (Rockville, MD: National Institute for Healthcare Research, 1993); D. B. Larson and S. S. Larsen, *The Forgotten Factor in Physical and Mental Health, What Does the Research Show?* (Rockville, MD: National Institute for Healthcare Research, 1994); D. A. Matthews and D. B. Larson, *The Faith Factor, Volume III: Enhancing Life Satisfaction* (Rockville, MD: National Institute for Healthcare Research, 1995); A. E. Bergin, "Psychotherapy and Religious Values," *Journal of Consulting and Clinical Psychotherapy* 48(1980): 95–105; and I. R. Payne et al., "Review of Religion and Mental Health: Prevention and Enhancement of Psychosocial Functioning," *Prevention in Human Services* 9 (1991): 11–40.

5. J. S. Levin, "How Religion Influences Morbidity and Health: Reflections on Natural History, Salutogenesis and Host Resistance," Social Science and Medicine 43 (1996): 849–64.

6. "MDs Discover Prayer Is Good Medicine," *Alternative Therapies in Clinical Practice* 4, no. 2 (1997): 59.

7. David G. Hamilton, "Believing in Patients' Beliefs: Physician Attunement to the Spiritual Dimension as a Positive Factor in Patient Healing and Health," *American Journal of Hospice and Palliative Care* 15, no. 5 (September/October 1998): 276–9.

8. P. J. Charters, "The Religious and Spiritual Needs of Mental Health Clients," *Nursing Standard* 13, no. 26 (October 1999): 34–6.

9. United Kingdom Central Council for Nursing, Midwifery, and Health Visiting (UKCC), *Code of Professional Conduct* (London: UKCC, 1992).

10. George Gallup, quoted at the Harvard Mind/Body Institute Symposium: *Spirituality and Healing in Medicine II*, (Boston, MA, December 1996).

11. Hamilton, W. L. Larimore, M. Parker, and M. Crowther, "Should Clinicians Incorporate Positive Spirituality into Their Practices? What Does the Evidence Say?" *Annals of Behavioral Medicine* 24 (2002): 69–73; and P. S. Mueller, D. J. Plevac, and T. A. Rummans, "Religious Involvement, Spirituality, and Medicine: Implications for Clinical Practice," *Mayo Clinic Proceedings* 76 (2001): 1225–35.

12. Mary Rado Simpson and Marilyn Givens King, "'God Brought All These Churches Together': Issues in Developing Religion-Health Partnerships in an Appalachian Community," *Public Health Nursing* 16, no. 1 (February 1999): 41–9.

13. Bernie Siegel, *Love, Medicine and Miracles,* (New York: Harper and Row: 1986), 41.

14. Tamar Nordenberg, "The Healing Power of Placebos," *FDA Consumer* (January/February 2000): 14–7.

15. Stewart Wolf, "The Pharmacology of Placebos," *Pharmacological Reviews* II (1959): 689–704.

16. Herbert Benson and D. P. McCallie, "Angina Pectoris and the Placebo Effect," *New England Journal of Medicine* 300, no. 25 (1979): 1424–9.

17. E. G. Diamond, C. F. Kittle, and J. E. Crockett, "Evaluation of Internal Mammary Artery Ligation and Sham Procedure in Angina Pectoris," *Circulation* 18 (1958): 712–3.

18. L. A. Cobb et al., "An Evaluation of Internal-Mammary-Artery Ligation by a Double-Blind Technique," *New England Journal of Medicine* 260, no. 2 (1959): 1115–8.

19. Bernie Siegel, *Peace, Love, and Healing* (New York: Harper & Row, 1989), 21.

20. Daniel Goleman, "The Faith Factor," *American Health* (May 1984): 48–53.

21. Jerome D. Frank, "Emotional Reactions of American Soldiers to an Unfamiliar Disease," *American Journal of Psychiatry* 102 (1946): 631–40.

22. Ibid.

23. Joan Borysenko, *Minding the Body, Mending the Mind* (Reading, MA: Addison-Wesley Publishing Company, 1987), 10.

24. D. B. Larsen and H. G. Koenig, "Is God Good for Your Health? The Role of Spirituality in Medical Care," *Cleveland Clinic Journal of Medicine* 67, no. 2 (2000): 80–4; D. A. Matthews, "Prayer and Spirituality," *Rheumatic Diseases Clinics of North America* 26, no. 1 (2000): 177–87; and R. O. Scott, "A Look in the Mirror: Finding Our Way in This New Spiritual Landscape," *Spirituality and Aging* 4, no. 1 (2001): 26.

25. Frank, "Emotional Reactions of American Soldiers."

26. Larry Dossey, *Meaning and Medicine: A Doctor's Tales of Breakthrough and Healing* (New York: Bantam Books, 1991), 158–9.

27. B. S. Oken, "Placebo Effects: Clinical Aspects and Neurobiology," *Brain* 131(Pt 11) (2008): 2812-23.

28. Andrew B. Newberg, Mark Robert Waldman, *Why We Believe What We Believe: Uncovering Our Biological Need for Meaning, Spirituality, and Truth (*Free Press: 2006), pp 3–4; Klopfer's original report can be found in the *Journal of Projective Techniques* (Volume 16, No. 3, September 1952).

29. J. Kong et al., Placebo Analgesia: Findings from Brain Imaging Studies and Emerging Hypotheses. *Reviews in Neuroscience* 18, no. 3/4 (2007): 173–90. Also, K. Wiech, M. Ploner, and I. Tracey, "Neurocognitive Aspects of Pain Perception," *Trends in Cognitive Science* 12, no. 8 (August 2008): 306–13.

30. V. Faria, M. Fredrikson, and T. Furmark, "Imaging the Placebo Response: A Neurofunctional Review," *European Neuropsychopharmacology* 18, np. 7 (July 2008): 473–85.

31. Steve Wright, "Speaking Out," *Nursing Times* 95, no. 10 (March 10–16, 1999), 19.

32. D. B. Larson, J. P. Swyers, and M. E. McCullough, eds., *Scientific Research on Spirituality and Health: A Consensus Report* (Rockville, MD: National Institute for Healthcare Research, 1998).

33. Albert Schweitzer, quoted by F. Charatan, "The Doctor Within," *British Medical Journal* 328(2004): 1426

34. Matthews and Larson, *The Faith Factor, Volume III.*

35. M. J. Donahue, "Intrinsic and Extrinsic Religiousness: Review and Meta-Analysis," *Journal of Personality and Social Psychology* 48 (1985): 400–19.

36. N. Goddard, "A Response to Dawson's Critical Analysis of 'Spirituality as Integrative Energy,'" *Journal of Advanced Nursing* 31, no. 4 (2000): 968–79.

37. Caroline Young and Cyndie Koopsen, *Spirituality, Health, and Healing* (Thorofare, NJ: Slack Incorporated, 2005), 59–60.

38. Bernie Siegel, *How to Live Between Office Visits* (New York: HarperCollins Publisher, 1993) 13.

39. Marc I. Barasch, "The Healing Path: A Soul Approach to Illness," *The Psychology of Health, Immunity, and Disease,* vol. B, 10, in *Proceedings of the Sixth International Conference of the National Institute for the Clinical Application of Behavioral Medicine,* held at Hilton Head Island, SC, December 1994 (Mansfield Center, CT: National Institute for the Clinical Application of Behavioral Medicine:1994).

40. O. Carl Simonton and Reid Henson, *The Healing Journey* (New York: Bantam Books, 1992), 13.

41. R. Banks, "Health and the Spiritual Dimensions: Relationships and Implications for Professional Preparation Programs," *Journal of School Health* 50 (1980): 195–202.

42. Banks, *Health and the Spiritual Dimensions.*

43. Pamela G. Reed, "Spirituality and Well-Being in Terminally Ill Hospitalized Adults," *Research in Nursing and Health* 10 (1987): 335–44.

44. Glenn E. Richardson and Melody Powers Noland, "Treating the Spiritual Dimension Through Educational Imagery," *Health Values* 8, no. 6 (1984): 28.

45. Shakti Gawain, *The Path of Transformation* (Mill Valley, CA: Nataraj Publishing, 1993), 77.

46. Larry S. Chapman, "Developing a Useful Perspective on Spiritual Health: Love, Joy, Peace, and Fulfillment," *American Journal of Health Promotion* (Fall 1987): 12.

47. Ken Wilber, *A Brief History of Everything* (Shambhala: 2nd edition 2001); Eckhart Tolle: *The New Earth: Awakening to Your Life's Purpose* (New York: Plume: 2006).

48. Some useful books that explore this transformation process include: Don Miguel Ruiz, *The Four Agreements: A Practical Guide to Personal Freedom* (A Toltec Wisdom Book) (Amber-Allen Publishing: 1997); Wayne Dyer: *The Power of Intention* (Hay House: 2004); Stanley H. Block: *Come to Your Senses: Demystifying the Mind-Body Connection* (Hillsboro, OR: Beyond Words Publishing:2005); Deepak Chopra: *The Seven Spiritual Laws of Success: A Practical Guide to the Fulfillment of Your Dreams* (New World Library / Amber-Allen Publishing: 1994).

49. Harvard Mind/Body Institute Symposium: "Spirituality and Healing in Medicine," Salt Lake City, May 2002.

50. Ibid., 13.

51. Chopra. *The Seven Spiritual Laws of Success.*

52. Ibid., 13.

53. Joan Borysenko, "Exploring the Heart of Healing: New Findings on Body, Mind and Soul," *The Psychology of Health, Immunity, and Disease,* vol. B, 33, in *Proceedings of the Sixth International Conference of the National Institute for the Clinical Application of Behavioral Medicine,* held at Hilton Head Island, SC, December 1994 (Mansfield Center,CT: National Institute for the Clinical Application of Behavioral Medicine:1994).

54. Phillip J. Waite, Steven R. Hawks, and Julie A. Gast, "The Correlation Between Spiritual Well-Being and Health Behaviors," *American Journal of Health Promotion* 13, no. 3 (January/February 1999): 159–62.

55. J. A. Blumenthal et al., "Stress Management and Exercise Training in Cardiac Patients with Myocardial Ischemia: Effects on prognosis and evaluation of mechanisms." *Archives of Internal Medicine* 157 (1997): 2213–23.

56. Dr. Bruno Cortis, "Spirituality and Medicine," in *Proceedings of the Fourth National Conference on the Psychology of Health, Immunity, and Disease,* held at Hilton Head Island, SC, December 1992. (Mansfield Center, CT: The National Institute for the Clinical Application of Behavioral Medicine:1992).

57. Paul Pearsall, *Super Joy* (New York: Doubleday, 1988), 1.

58. Viktor E. Frankl, *Man's Search for Meaning* (Pocket: 1997) (First published 1946).

59. K. Pelletier, "The Spirit of Health," *Advances: Journal of the Institute for the Advancement of Health* 5, no. 4 (1988): 4.

60. Reed, "Spirituality and Well-Being."

61. H. G. Koenig, D. O. Moberg, and J. N. Kvale, "Religious Activity and Attitudes of Older Adults in a Geriatric Assessment Clinic," *Journal of the American Geriatric Society* 36, no. 4 (1988): 362–74.

62. K. I. Pargament, *The Psychology of Religion and Coping: Theory, Research and Practice* (New York: Guilford Press, 1997).

63. Larson, Swyers, and McCullough, *Scientific Research on Spirituality and Health*, 59–61.

64. J. Kabat-Zinn et al., "Effectiveness of a Meditation-Based Stress Reduction Program in the Treatment of Anxiety Disorders," *American Journal of Psychiatry* 149 (1992): 936–43.

65. J. J. Miller, K. Fletcher, and J. Kabat-Zinn, "Three-Year Follow-Up and Clinical Implications of a Mindfulness-Based Stress Reduction Intervention in the Treatment of Anxiety Disorders," *General Hospital Psychiatry* 17 (1995): 192–200.

66. A. Castillo-Richmond, "Effects of Stress Reduction on Carotid Atherosclerosis in Hypertensive African Americans," *Stroke* 31, no. 3 (2000): 568–73.

67. J. W. Zamarra et al., "Usefulness of the Transcendental Meditation Program in the Treatment of Patients with Coronary Artery Disease," *American Journal of Cardiology* 77 (1996): 867–70.

68. Pearsall, *Super Joy*, 215.

69. Pearsall, *Super Joy*, 54.

70. S. O. Kobasa, "How Much Stress Can You Survive?" *American Health* (September 1984): 67.

71. Siegel, *Peace, Love, and Healing*;130.

72. Ibid.

73. Ibid.

74. Ibid.

75. Ibid.

76. Rick Fields, Rex Weyler, Rick Ingrasci, and Peggy Taylor, *Chop Wood, Carry Water* (Los Angeles, CA: Jeremy P. Tarcher, 1984).

77. A. Taylor, *I Fly Out with Bright Feathers: The Quest of a Novice Healer* (London: Fontana/Collins, 1987).

78. Robert Coles, "The Power of Prayer," *50 Plus* (December 1987): 44.

79. Blair Justice, *Who Gets Sick: Thinking and Health* (Houston, TX: Peak Press, 1987), 275.

80. M. Hughes, et al, "Does Private Religious Activity Prolong Survival? A Six-Year Follow-up Study of 3,851 Older Adults," *Journal of Gerontology A Biological Sciences and Medical Sciences* 55 (2000): M400–M405.

81. CBS News Poll [transcript]. "CBS News." CBS television. April 20–22, 1998.

82. Larry Dossey, *Healing Words* (San Francisco: HarperSanFrancisco, 1993), 31. Also, Anon., "The Power of Prayer: The Spiritual Dimension of Healing," *Medical Tribune,* April 16, 2003/No. 16.

83. Larry Dossey; "Evidence of Prayer's Healing Power," *Brain/Mind* (December 1993): 4–5.

84. Gregg Braden, *Secrets of the Lost Mode of Prayer* (Carlsbad, CA: Hay House, 2006).

85. Rupert Sheldrake, "Prayer: A Challenge for Science," *Noetic Sciences Review* (Summer 1994): 5.

86. Herbert Benson, *Your Maximum Mind* (New York: Times Books/Random House, 1987), 6.

87. Ibid., 46.

88. Gurney Williams III, "Holy-istic Healing," *Longevity* (March 1994): 28.

89. B. F. Pendleton, M. M. Poloma, "The Effects of Prayer and Pprayer Experiences on Measures of General Well-Being." *Journal of Psychology and Theology* 19 (1991): 71–73.

90. Joan Borysenko, *Minding the Body, Mending the Mind* (Reading, MA: Addison-Wesley Publishing Company, 1987), 176.

91. Robin Casarjian, "Forgiveness: An Essential Component in Health and Healing," in *Proceedings of the Fourth National Conference on the Psychology of Health, Immunity, and Disease,* held at Hilton Head Island, SC, December 1992. (Mansfield Center, CT: The National Institute for the Clinical Application of Behavioral Medicine:1992)

92. Dan Custer, *The Miracle of Mind Power* (Englewood Cliffs, NJ: Prentice Hall, 1991).

93. Ibid.

94. Casarjian, "Forgiveness."

95. Custer, *The Miracle of Mind Power.*

96. Dwight Lee Wolter, *Lotus* (Spring 1994): 53.

97. Robin Casarjian, *Forgiveness: A Bold Choice for a Peaceful Heart* (New York: Bantam Books, 1992), 232–3.

98. Caroline Young and Cyndie Koopsen, *Spirituality, Health, and Healing* (Thorofare, NJ: Slack Incorporated, 2005), 61.

99. Matthews and Larson, *The Faith Factor, Volume III.*

100. Christopher G. Ellison, "Religious Involvement and Subjective Well-Being," *Journal of Health and Social Behavior* 32 (1991): 80–99.

101. Christopher G. Ellison and Jeffrey S. Levin, "The Religion-Health Connection: Evidence, Theory, and Future Directions," *Health Education and Behavior* 25, no. 6 (December 1998): 700–20.

102. J. S. Levin and P. L. Schiller, "Is There a Religious Factor in Health?" *Journal of Religion and Health* 26 (1987): 9–36.

103. William W. Parmley, "Separation of Church and State (of Health)," *Journal of American College of Cardiology* 28, no. 4 (October 1996): 1047–8.

104. Ibid.

105. W. J. Strawbridge, R. D. Cohen, S. J. Shema, and G. A. Kaplan, "Frequent Attendance at Religious Services and Mortality over 28 Years," *American Journal of Public Health* 87 (1997): 957–61.

106. Neal Krause, "Religion, Aging, and Health: Current Status and Future Prospects," *Journal of Gerontology* 52B, no. 6 (1997): S291–3.

107. E. L. Idler and S. V. Kasl, "Religion, Disability, Depression, and the Timing of Death," *American Journal of Sociology* 97 (1992): 1052–79.

108. H. G. Koenig and D. B. Larson, "Use of Hospital Services, Religious Attendance and Religious Affiliation." *Southern Medical Journal* 91 (1998): 925–932.

109. Ibid.

110. Harold G. Koenig interview by Lisa Schneider, "What Religion Can Do for Your Health," accessed 2008 at http://www.beliefnet.com/Health/2006/05/What-Religion-Can-Do-For-Your-Health.aspx?p=1.

111. J. G. Jrzywacz JG, et al, "Older Adults' Use of Complementary and Alternative Medicine for Mental Health: Findings from the 2002 National Health Interview Survey." *Journal of Alternative and Complementary Medicine* 12 (2006): 467–73.

112. H. B. Bosworth et al., "The Impact of Religious Practice and Religious Coping on Geriatric Depression," *International Journal of Geriatric Psychiatry* 18 (2003): 905–14

113. Andrew J. Weaver et al., "An Analysis of Research on Religious and Spiritual Variables in Three Major Mental Health Nursing Journals, 1991–1995," *Issues in Mental Health Nursing* 19, no. 3 (May/June 1998): 263–76.

114. G. H. Gallup, *Religion in America: 1992–1993* (Princeton, NJ: Gallup Organization, 1993).

115. Ibid.

116. Leonard A. Sagan, *The Health of Nations* (New York: Basic Books, 1987), 137.

117. E. L. Idler and S. V. Kasl, "Religion, Disability, Depression, and the Timing of Death," *American Journal of Sociology* 97(1992): 1052–79.

118. John M. Wallace, Jr., and Tyrone A. Forman, "Religion's Role in Promoting Health and Reducing Risk Among American Youth," *Health Education and Behavior* 25, no. 6 (December 1998): 721–41.

119. G. H. Gallup, Jr., and R. Bezilla, *The Religious Life of Young Americans* (Princeton, NJ: George H. Gallup International Institute, 1992).

120. Stuart R. Varon and Anne W. Riley, "Relationship Between Maternal Church Attendance and Adolescent Mental Health and Social Functioning," *Psychiatric Services* 50 (1999): 799–805.

121. Laurel Arthur Burton and Jarad D. Kass, "How to Make the Best Use of a Patient's Spirituality," in *Proceedings of the Fourth National Conference on the Psychology of Health, Immunity, and Disease,* held at Hilton Head Island, SC, December 1992. (Mansfield Center, CT: The National Institute for the Clinical Application of Behavioral Medicine:1992).

122. Mark Bricklin, Mark Golin, Deborah Grandinetti, and Alexis Lieberman, *Positive Living and Health* (Emmaus, PA: Rodale Press, 1990).

123. George K. Jarvis and Herbert C. Northcott, "Religion and Differences in Morbidity and Mortality," *Social Science Medicine* 25, no. 7 (1987): 813–24.

124. Ibid.

125. Bricklin et al., *Positive Living and Health.*

126. Brent Q. Hafen and Kathryn J. Frandsen, *People Need People: The Importance of Relationships to Health and Wellness* (Evergreen, CO: Cordillera Press, 1987) 25.

127. S. I. McMillen, *None of These Diseases* (Old Tappan, NJ: Fleming H. Revell Company, 1984), 208.

128. John Gartner, Dave Larson, and George Allen, "Religious Commitment and Mental Health-A Review of the Empirical Literature," *Journal of Psychology and Theology,* 19(1991): 6–25.

129. Jeffrey S. Levin and Preston L. Schiller, "Is There a Religious Factor in Health?" *Journal of Religion and Health* 26, no. 1 (1987): 9-36. Also, Jeffrey S. Levin and Harold Y. Vanderpool, "Is Frequent Religious Attendance Really Conducive to Better Health?: Toward an Epidemiology of Religion," *Social Science and Medicine* 24, no. 7 (1987): 589–600.

130. N. L. Smith, "Healing as the Masters Healed," *Journal of Collegium Aesculapium* 1988 (Winter): 17–27; presented at the Harvard Conference on Spirituality in Medicine (Salt Lake City, UT March 14, 2002), and also at the Psychiatry Grand Rounds (University of Maine, Portland MA September 23, 2003, and University of Utah, Salt Lake City November 6, 2002).

131. Rachel Naomi Remen, "On Defining Spirit," *Noetic Sciences Review* (Autumn 1988): 7.

CHAPTER 15

The Healing Power of Altruism

I don't know what your destiny will be, but one thing I know: the only ones among you who will be truly happy are those who will have sought and found how to serve.

—Albert Schweitzer

- Define *altruism*, and identify the aspect of altruism that may help protect health.
- Discuss how altruism boosts health.
- Identify the characteristics of the altruistic personality.
- Discuss the health benefits of volunteerism and the characteristics of volunteer work that are most beneficial to health.
- Understand how love contributes to well-being and longevity.

Physician and philosopher Albert Schweitzer proclaimed during a selfless career what he believed to be the prescription for happiness. True happiness, he said, is to be found only by serving others. New clinical research has verified that service not only is a prescription for happiness but is a prescription for improved health as well. As German-born physicist and Nobel Prize winner Albert Einstein said, "Only a life lived for others is worth living."

Altruism—the act of giving of oneself out of a genuine concern for other people—has been called one of the healthiest of human attributes. While altruism is a secular impulse, it is a hallmark of virtually every one of the world's religions and great spiritual traditions, and it is practiced by people in all walks of life. Altruism has been defined as "unselfish benevolent love"[1] and gives people the ability to effect meaningful change, even in situations in which they would otherwise feel powerless.[2] It comes from the French word *autrui*, which means "other people," and it involves building a bridge of deep caring to others.[3] Albert Einstein said, "Many times a day I realize how much my own outer and inner life is built upon the labors of my fellow men, both living and dead, and how earnestly I must exert myself in order to give in return as much as I have received."

Recent statistics show that Americans contribute more than $295 billion per year to good causes—and that $223 billion of that comes from individuals.[4] According to one government study, 61.2 million Americans volunteered in 2006, donating an average of 52 hours on their volunteer projects. When you figure that charities use the industry standard of $18.77 per hour to determine the monetary value of their volunteers, those 61.2 million Americans each gave $976 to charity in 2006 through donating their time— a whopping total of more than $59.7 billion.

It's not just the monetary value of giving that counts. The ability to "connect" by regarding another's needs as above one's own appears to contribute to a longer and healthier life. Scientists are beginning to conclude that doing good for others is good for a person, especially for the nervous system and the immune system. In essence, research conducted over decades concludes that people who are generous and giving and who demonstrate their love of others through altruistic service live longer, healthier, and happier lives.[5]

Altruism may actually be one of our earliest skills. Bowling Green State University psychologist Jaak Panksepp believes that helping had an integral part in our biological evolution because it's necessary for reproduction and the survival of certain species. In the evolution of the human species, cooperative efforts may have been not only helpful to survival but also, says Panksepp, a key factor in the development and expansion of the human brain. "Intrinsic helping tendencies may thus, like dominance urges, be embedded in the human brain structure," he theorizes, or "may even be part of what we think of as human nature itself."[6] A landmark new work[7] finds that altruistic behavior is not only related to aspects of human nature such as love but is also closely related to apology, forgiveness, and reconciliation.

Exciting new research by Duke University Medical Center neuroscientists found that activation of a particular region of the brain predicts whether people tend to be selfish or altruistic. A section located at the top and back of the brain—the posterior superior temporal sulcus—showed strikingly increased activity in people who tended to be altruistic. An interesting part of the research that demonstrates the complex nature of altruism found that altruistic behavior may actually originate from how people view the world rather than how they act in it.[8]

How Altruism Boosts Health

Harvard psychologists who wanted to find out how altruistic thoughts impact us conducted a precise experiment on a group of volunteers; the precise measure was the quantity of germ-fighting substance in the saliva of the volunteers. The amount of the substance provides a clear indication of how well the immune system is working. Psychologists measured the saliva of the volunteers both before and after they watched each of three films. The first was a gentle film on gardening, the second was a Nazi war documentary, and the third was a documentary about Mother Teresa, the Nobel Prize–winning nun who has dedicated charitable works to the poor, the lepers, and the orphans in India's most poverty-stricken regions.

Measurements of saliva showed no change during the first two films. After reviewing the third film, the amount of immune agent in the volunteers' saliva rose sharply, even among those who said they dislike Mother Teresa. Volunteers who merely watched altruistic service experienced an actual physical change—one that could possibly help them to stay healthier.[9]

While researchers know that altruism promotes health, they are just beginning to find out how and why. In addition to the direct link to the immune system, it may counteract stress. The American Psychological Association has long asserted that stress impacts the body's ability to fight infection,[10] and altruistic love apparently aids in the healing process by decreasing or eliminating the effects of stress.[11] World-renowned stress expert Dr. Kathleen Hall, a founder of The Stress Institute, says that "altruism creates a physiological response that makes people feel stronger and more energetic and that counters harmful effects of stress."[12] In addition to blocking harmful aspects of the stress response, researchers believe that altruistic love might also activate certain aspects of the relaxation response—the opposing response to stress that helps heart rate, blood pressure, digestion, and hormone levels to return to normal.[13] Canadian physician Hans Selye, one of the world's authorities on the physiological effects of stress, concluded that altruism can help combat the effects of stress by preventing nervous system "overload." By doing good deeds for others, Selye believed, a person wins their affection and gratitude—and the resulting "warmth" helps protect the person from stress.[14]

There may even be a physiological reason for that "warmth": Varied research has shown that altruistic action stimulates the brain to release endorphins, powerful natural painkillers that literally make us feel better. That warmth and those good feelings are so powerful that they often return when people simply remember acts of helping or altruism.[15] Those same endorphins may also be a key to relieving the effects of stress.

Allan Luks, executive director of the Institute for the Advancement of Health in New York City, shares the view that altruistic deeds help relieve stress and lead to the production of powerful pain-killing endorphins. He says that "people who help others frequently report better health than people who don't help. They relate an improved sense of well-being, and decreased problems with stress-related health conditions."[16] Luks added that altruism and the act of helping was especially linked to pain relief in stress-related disorders, including headaches.[17]

We know that the cumulative effects of stress are negative. Kenneth R. Pelletier, associate clinical professor at the University of California School of Medicine, says, "Under conditions of extreme stress, the immune system is depressed. The number and activity of white cells falls. The activity of the natural killer cells is reduced. There are changes in the ratio of helper cells to suppressor cells of the immune system."[18]

The effects of altruism in stabilizing the immune system against the normal immunosuppressing effects of stress may go so far, Pelletier believes, that altruism may even help slow down the inevitable deterioration of the immune system as a person ages.[19] Because of the social contact and sense of purpose associated with altruism, good deeds may help prevent some stress from even beginning.

Some specialists believe that altruism actually helps to preserve life—and a few believe that it is even part of the survival instinct. When University of California–Los Angeles sociologist Linda Nilson studied data from more than 100 disasters, she found that those who survived and did the best were those who reached out to help others. The "tribal cohesiveness" that stemmed from the helping process, says Nilson, is what enabled many to survive even tremendous odds.

Epidemiologist James House and his colleagues at the University of Michigan's Survey Research Center carried out a landmark study of 2,700 people in Tecumseh, Michigan. The study period spanned more than a decade as House and his coworkers followed the volunteers carefully to determine what impact their social relationships had on their health. What House discovered was a powerful testimony for altruism. Among the people studied in Michigan, those who did regular volunteer work had better health and longer lives. Men who volunteered in their community were two and a half times less likely to die during the period of the study than were men who did not volunteer at least once a week.[20] House concluded that doing volunteer work, more than any other activity, dramatically increased life expectancy—and probably health as well.[21]

Other studies confirm House's findings. University of Michigan psychologist Stephanie Brown studied a group of more than four hundred elderly couples over a period of five years. Those who provided no help or service (either practical or emotional) were more than twice as likely to die during the studies as were those who were altruistic. Those who *received* help, incidentally, did not enjoy longer life—but the ones who *provided* help definitely did.[22]

Psychiatrist George Vaillant followed Harvard graduates for four decades. He found that altruism was one of the major qualities that helped the graduates cope with the stresses of life. The absence of altruism apparently has the opposite effect. After an in-depth study, social psychologist Larry Scherwitz of San Francisco's Medical Research Institute concluded that people who are self-centered are more likely to develop coronary heart disease, even when other risk factors are taken into account.[23]

The factor of self-centered thoughts and behavior can in itself contribute to the stress that may lead to disease. Dean Ornish, director of California's Preventive Medicine Research Institute, says, "When a person has a sense of isolation, often what comes with that are feelings of not having enough or not being enough. The person says, 'if only I had more'—more power, more money, more love, whatever—'then I'd be happy.' Once that view of the world is set up, it's ultimately self-defeating because if people don't get more of it, whatever it is, they feel stress. And even when they do, it's never enough."[24]

Altruism and its associated good deeds, says Ornish, help free us from "the stress cycle" by turning our focus away from self-involvement and toward those we are helping.[25] Once our involvement is focused on others, we begin to show the qualities consistent with altruism: a high degree of optimism, a strong sense of purpose and spirituality, and a continued involvement with other people.

Conquering that sense of isolation is another reason why altruism boosts health: some of the strongest findings in the field of mind-body health relate to the importance of social support in protecting health and contributing to longevity. The very essence of altruism requires that people connect to other people, promoting social connectedness with all its health benefits. G. Donald Gale said, "A giving person sees a glass of water and starts looking for someone who might be thirsty." And Abraham Lincoln said, "As you grow older you will discover that you have two hands—one for helping yourself, the other for helping others." As researcher Allan Luks put it, "By helping others—focusing intently on these people and getting good feelings back—the good feelings literally replace your negative feelings. You hold that person's hand, they smile at you, they hug you—these good feelings are buffering and reducing the negative stress in your life. What an incredible antidote to loneliness and isolation."[26]

A group of studies done on altruism found that people who care for others are physically, emotionally, and mentally healthier than are those who concentrate more on their own needs. The positive feelings and energy that result from altruism have been shown to contribute to overall mental health. A study conducted by researchers at the University of Massachusetts Medical School found that churchgoers who provided loving and caring service to others had better mental health than the people who simply received service.[27] Lead researcher Carolyn Schwartz explained, "The act of giving to someone else may have mental health benefits because the very nature of focusing outside the self counters the self-focused nature of anxiety or depression."[28] That shift in focus leads to a change in the way people perceive their health and their quality of life, which also leads to a decrease in stress.[29] (Additional studies have also found that those who receive service don't receive the same benefit as those who give it—underscoring the importance of giving.[30])

Altruism can even boost the ability to learn. College students who volunteered in a Head Start–based Family Literacy Project in Connecticut were studied to determine the impact of their volunteerism. Researchers found that those students who engaged in regular volunteer work had greater self-knowledge, had greater social awareness, and performed better in academics. They also did better in the areas of personal growth, self-esteem, and personal efficacy. The students themselves reported finding more meaning in what was learned in the classroom, increased awareness of important social issues, greater appreciation for diversity, and decreased negative stereotypes.[31]

People who care for others also tend to have an important health-preserving quality: optimism. Psychologist Martin Seligman, author of *Learned Optimism,* says that altruism is an activity "that presupposes a belief that things can change for the better." Optimists, he maintains, "have better health, better immune systems, and so live longer. Indirect evidence would then indicate that altruists might live longer."[32] (For more on optimism and health, see Chapter 16.)

Altruism has also been found to have benefits for all ages; research has shown that it provides increased physical health, better mental health, and improved longevity for youth, adults, and the elderly.[33] A national sample of teens recruited through the Presbyterian Church found that altruistic behavior gives the same kinds of health benefits and sense of well-being to adolescents as it does to adults. The researchers found that altruistic service boosted a sense of well-being in both young men and young women but was most strongly associated with significant health benefits in the young women.[34]

One of the most profound examples of the health and longevity benefits of altruism comes from the life of philanthropist John D. Rockefeller, Sr.[35] Rockefeller entered the business world with gusto and drove himself so hard that by age 33 he had earned his first million dollars. Ten years later he owned and controlled the world's largest business. By the time he was 53, he was the world's first billionaire.

Meanwhile, the people he had crushed in this pursuit of wealth hated him; workers in Pennsylvania's oil fields hanged him in effigy, and he was guarded day and night by bodyguards pledged to protect his life. He had developed alopecia, a condition in which hair falls out; his digestion was so poor that all he could eat was crackers and milk. He was plagued by insomnia. The doctors who struggled to help him agreed that he wouldn't live another year.

Then something happened to John D. Rockefeller. He began to think of—and care about—others more than he did himself. He decided to use his billions of dollars for the benefit of others. Hospitals, universities, missions, and private citizens were the beneficiaries of the hundreds of millions of dollars he gave through the Rockefeller Foundation. His generosity aided in the discovery of penicillin. His contributions to medicine enabled researchers to find cures for tuberculosis, malaria, diphtheria, and many other diseases that had robbed so many of life. His contributions helped rid the U. S. South of its greatest physical and economic plague, the hookworm.

When Rockefeller began using his riches to help other people, he helped himself. For the first time in years, he was able to eat normally. He felt renewed. He slept soundly. He defied the odds and lived to see his 54th birthday—and many birthdays after that. He kept on giving and caring for others, in fact, until he died at the age of 98.

The Altruistic Personality

What makes a person altruistic? Some believe it's instinct, stemming from the time when people lived in small groups of hunters and gatherers. According to Stanford anthropologist John Tooby, those early hunters/gatherers depended highly on each other, not only for food and shelter, but also for survival.[36]

In a supporting point of view, New York psychologist Linda R. Caporall cites a series of experiments conducted over 10 years and reported in *Behavioral and Brain Sciences*. The studies show that human nature is basically social, not selfish—and she agrees that altruism probably stems back to hunter/gatherer times.[37]

A growing number of researchers believe that altruism is a capacity shared by everyone to some extent or another. One large-scale survey showed that women are more likely than men to feel empathy, a quality essential to altruism. The same survey showed that empathy and altruism are unrelated to financial status: people of all socioeconomic levels routinely demonstrate altruistic qualities.[38] Altruism can be learned, say the researchers, depending on social and cultural background, the stage of moral or self-development, previous opportunities to learn altruism, the sense of responsibility and empathy, and the particular situation in which one is called upon to help.[39]

Other researchers believe in a certain "personality"—that altruistic people seem to have, a set of personality traits enabling them to reach out to others. In a classic study of altruism, Samuel P. Oliner and Pearl M. Oliner studied the "rescuers" who provided help to the Jews during Hitler's reign of terror. These rescuers were altruistic—so much so that they often risked their own lives and safety to help others. According to Oliner, altruism is fueled by "empathy, allegiance to their group or institutional norms, or commitment to principle."[40] University of California, Irvine, Professor Kristen Monroe says that research shows altruists tend to view themselves as one with all of humanity rather than acting only in their own behalf.[41]

The Oliners say altruistic people never regard others as inferiors; they have a firm conviction that all people have universal similarities.[42] One rescuer summarized the attitude by remarking that "Jews were just people. We neither looked down on them nor did we look up to them. We never felt they were any different."

The altruistic people the Oliners studied valued human relationships more than money and focused on others rather than on themselves. They believed that ethical values were to be applied universally—that people are worthy of tolerance and respect regardless of their race, religion, or class. They emphasized the values of helpfulness, hospitality, concern, and love, and they sensed a universal obligation to be of help to others. Their commitment to caring for others extended well beyond their friends and loved ones.

The "rescuers" believed in the right of innocent people to be free from persecution—and most were moved by the pain of others. They also had a tendency to believe in a victim's innocence, to believe that people are victimized by external circumstances and not by inherent character flaws. With deep empathy for the sadness and helplessness of others, these rescuers felt a personal responsibility for helping to relieve others' pain and sadness.

That empathy may have been one of their most important emotions. Considerable evidence, both anecdotal and that based on scientific experiments, suggests that empathy somehow connects people. It forms a literal bond, acting almost as a "glue" between living things. We know it works between people and even between people and animals. Now researchers at Princeton University's Engineering Anomalies Research Laboratory have demonstrated that it even works to connect people and machines. According to Larry Dossey, studies show that "the effects of empathic bonding transcend space and time."[43]

These altruistic people had a healthy perspective about themselves. They did not suffer from self-interest or self-preoccupation, both of which reduce the ability to care for others. They did not think too highly of themselves (people with too much self-esteem believe they should be the recipients, not the bestowers, of attention and care). Nor did they think too poorly of themselves (people with too little self-esteem become so absorbed by their own distress that they can't worry about other people's needs). Most were highly independent of the opinions and evaluations of others; they tended to act on their own and did not seek or need external reinforcement for their activities. Actually, most were embarrassed by the thanks or appreciation they received.

The altruistic people the Oliners studied were very "connected" to others, especially to diverse people and groups. They enjoyed close family relationships and had a strong sense of belonging to the community. Their attachment to others began early in life and extended beyond family to embrace friends, acquaintances, and even strangers. The rescuers had a tendency to befriend people who were different from themselves. They perceived their relationships with their family of origin as being very close.[44]

Their commitment to caring was profound—and their internal compulsion was so strong that they often made the decision to help almost instantaneously. They felt a strong sense of inner control, but did not feel the need to control others; although they believed they could control events and shape their own destiny, they were also willing to risk failure. When something didn't go as planned, they spent little time mourning those failures. Most important, they believed they could succeed when others were convinced of failure.

To these rescuers, caring was not a spectator sport—it compelled action. They assumed personal responsibility, not because others required it but because they would have been unhappy if they had failed to act. Although they placed a value on hard work and economic prudence, they never expected a monetary reward for their altruistic actions. They performed those deeds without ulterior motives. The Oliners summed up the rescuers in their study as "not saints, but ordinary people who nonetheless were capable of overcoming their human frailties by virtue of their caring capacities."

The personality traits the Oliners observed among the rescuers are not peculiar to that group of people; the traits, researchers believe, are common among most altruistic people. Nor does altruism necessarily stem from a church or a religious belief; repeated research shows that church members are no more altruistic as a group than are other people.[45] University of Massachusetts psychologist Ervin Staub believes that altruistic people share three general traits:

1. They have a positive view of people in general.
2. They are concerned about others' welfare.
3. They take personal responsibility for how other people are doing.[46]

The tendency toward altruism is a trait that is established early in life, according to a number of researchers. Psychologist Alfie Kohn noted that altruism may be as dramatic as donating a kidney or as "mundane as letting another shopper ahead of you in line. But most of us do it frequently and started doing it very early in life. . . . Caring about others is as much a part of human nature as caring about ourselves."[47]

In studying outstanding altruists, researcher Christie Kiefer found that background and family values help determine the altruistic personality. The altruists she studied "came from families that were warm and nurturing. The emotional self-acceptance they developed in that environment liberated them to be generative, creative, playful, and relaxed." In addition, says Kiefer, they learned a sense of social responsibility from their parents or from another prominent person in their early lives—a sense that "committed them to action on behalf of others or their community."[48]

In their book, *The Altruistic Personality*, the Oliners cited the important lesson all of us can learn from the "rescuers":

> Rescuers point the way. They were and are "ordinary" people. They were farmers and teachers, entrepreneurs and factory workers, rich and poor, parents and single people, Protestants and Catholics. Most had done nothing extraordinary before the war nor have they done much that is extraordinary since. Most were marked neither by exceptional leadership qualities nor by unconventional behavior. They were not heroes cast in larger-than-life molds. What most distinguished them were their connections with others in relationships of commitment and care. It is out of such relationships that they became aware of what was occurring around them and mustered their human and material sources to relieve the pain. Their involvements with Jews grew out of the ways in which they ordinarily related to other people. . . .
>
> They remind us that such courage is not the providence of the independent and the intellectually superior thinkers but that it is available to all through the virtues of connectedness, commitment, and the quality of relationships developed in ordinary human interactions.[49]

The Health Benefits of Volunteerism

Many of the Americans involved in volunteer work do it without organizational support. On their own, they figure out ways to help those who need it or those who are less fortunate. When asked why, two-thirds say it is because they want to "help people."

That instinct to help occurs early in life; as early as the second year of life, a child will respond to someone in distress by reaching out with a comforting touch, offering a favorite toy, or bringing a parent to help.

The acts of volunteering, helping, and serving appear to bring important health benefits to the volunteer. Examples abound. Consider the Retired Senior Volunteer Program, which places a quarter of a million elderly people in community volunteer jobs each year. National Director Alfred N. Larson recognizes the health benefits those seniors have, saying, "Doctors tell us that elderly people who engage in volunteer work are a lot better off, visit the doctor less often, and have fewer complaints."[50] One elderly volunteer in Baltimore explained, "Involvement makes you keep well so you can keep giving. It makes you take care of your health. It's a blessing to ward off old age."

The health benefits aren't restricted to consciously taking better care of health, however. Yale University Professor of Public Health Lowell Levin points out that "when you're a helper, your self-concept improves. You are somebody. You are worthwhile. And there's nothing more exhilarating than that. That can influence your health." Consider these examples:

- Kay Arnold joined SENSE, a group of Connecticut entertainers who perform for the elderly and disabled. Her audiences benefit—and Kay herself says her volunteer work gives her "a sense of worth I never had before." And when she performs, her arthritis pain disappears.

- Vince Ward is the advertising and public relations director for one of the nation's largest telecommunications firms. His job is considered one of the highest-stress positions imaginable, yet he does not have high blood pressure. How has he been able to overcome one of the most common physiological effects of stress? The key could lie in the way he spends his spare time. Vince Ward is busy away from the office, too, raising money for a children's home, working with parolees from Kansas State Penitentiary, and donating blood to the Community Blood Bank of Greater Kansas City.

- In one study, the experiences of more than 1,700 women who regularly volunteered to help others were analyzed at the Institute for the Advancement of Health in New York City. The women who helped experienced relief of actual physical ailments, including headaches, loss of voice, pain due to lupus and multiple sclerosis, and depression. Approximately 90 percent of the women in the survey rated their health as better than or as good as others their age.[51]

Women in two major studies about volunteerism described a "helper's high," similar in nature to the "runner's high" experienced during exercising.[52] Research at Carnegie Mellon University shows that volunteerism helps improve mood and gives a "high." Scientists studying the phenomenon believe the act of volunteering, of serving and helping others, may cause the release of endorphins. One researcher who has been studying the effects of altruism in animal studies concludes that it is "just about proven that it is our own natural opiates, the endorphins, that produce the good feelings" associated with reaching out to help others.[53]

Deeper insight about the "high" experienced by volunteers stemmed in part from a study conducted by Allan Luks, then at the Institute for the Advancement of Health, and psychologist Howard Andrews, a senior research scientist with the New York State Psychiatric Institute. What did they learn? After collecting surveys from more than 3,000 volunteers, they found twofold health benefits from volunteer work. The "healthy-helper syndrome," as they call it, starts with a physical high—a "rush" of good feeling that is characterized by increased energy, sudden warmth, and a sense of euphoria. The physical sensations associated with the "helper's high," which 95 percent of the people surveyed experienced, suggest that the brain releases endorphins in response to the act of helping.

The second stage of the healthy-helper syndrome—which more than half of the volunteers reported—is a longer lasting sense of calm and heightened emotional well-being. Together, say Luks and Andrews, the "high" associated with volunteering is a powerful antidote to stress, a key to happiness and optimism (see Chapter 16), and a way to combat feelings of helplessness and depression.[54]

A national survey that led to the definition of the healthy-helper syndrome definitely delineated the two distinct phases—one an "immediate physical feel-good sensation," the second a sense of calmness and relaxation. According to Luks, the survey showed that those who volunteer have better perceived health and that the more often they volunteer, the greater the health benefits. Luks says those who volunteered once a week reported ten times better health and had specific improvements in health that ranged from less pain and fewer colds to overall well-being.[55]

Famed Harvard cardiologist Herbert Benson, well-known for his research on the effects of relaxation, feels that helping others works much the same way as yoga, spirituality, and meditation to help people "forget oneself, to experience decreased metabolic rates and blood pressure, heart rate, and other health benefits."[56] Volunteer service can result in a condition sometimes described as "helper's calm" or helper's high. Under stress, the heart pumps faster, the adrenal glands release corticosteroids (the "stress hormones"), organ functions are disrupted, and breathing speeds up. As a result, the person is more sensitive to pain, and the stress hormones that start coursing through the veins raise the level of blood cholesterol, elevate blood sugar, and reduce functioning of the immune system. Apparently volunteer service works in the opposite way, reducing the effects of stress.[57] It works so well, in fact, that people in various studies have reported "treating" their stress-induced illnesses by engaging in altruistic volunteer work.

According to Luks and Howard, the volunteers who experienced the healthy-helper syndrome noticed an improvement in their own physical ills, including fewer arthritis pains, lupus symptoms, asthma attacks, migraine headaches, colds, and bouts of flu. The researchers believe that volunteerism, or altruism, can also alleviate the stress and other physiological conditions that lead to heart attacks.

Luks and Howard credit a combination of factors for the improved health of volunteers: "the strengthening of immune system activity; the diminishing of both the intensity and awareness of physical pain; the activation of emotions vital to the maintenance of good health; the reduction of the incidence of attitudes, such as chronic hostility, that negatively arouse and damage the body; and the multiple benefits to the body's systems provided by stress relief."[58]

One-on-One Contact

The benefits of volunteer work depend on several factors. According to Allan Luks and Peggy Payne, the most health benefits from volunteering occur when you make personal contact, do it frequently (two or more hours a week), help a stranger, find a shared problem, work with an organization, use your skills, and "let go" of results.[59]

Of those, one of the most important is one-on-one contact—that the helper actually connects with people. The health benefits of volunteer work don't seem as pronounced when the volunteer simply donates money (no matter how important the cause) or spends volunteer time doing things isolated from close physical contact.[60] The physical contact seems to be a key. It is vital to good health and longevity.

The direct contact involved in volunteer work seems to provide some of its value, but the direct contact apparently doesn't have to be physical, as long as it's one-on-one contact. In various studies, people who have done one-on-one crisis counseling or intervention by telephone have experienced and reported helper's high, whereas those doing nonpeople tasks, such as stuffing envelopes, don't experience the "high."

Furthermore, helper's high results most from helping people we don't know: the greatest chance of experiencing helper's high in several experiments was correlated with giving service to strangers.[61]

Desire to Volunteer

In addition to actual contact with the people one is helping, another important factor in achieving the health benefits of volunteer work seems to hinge on the word *volunteer*: A person has to want to do it. Forcing a person to be of help doesn't reap the health benefits of the helping service. In fact, some researchers now believe that one reason why altruism benefits health is that it gives one a sense of control—but only by being able to choose the circumstances of the altruistic deeds.

That sense of control may even be crucial. A number of studies have shown that a lack of control can undermine health (as discussed elsewhere in this book). One landmark project carried out in a housing project for the elderly in San Francisco underscores the health benefits that follow the sense of control that volunteer work brings.

Liking the Work

Another factor in reaping health benefits from volunteer work is to choose work a person likes to do—something that is suitable, brings pleasure, and is a joy to do. If volunteer work does not bring happiness or even make a person feel slightly exhilarated, he or she should probably consider switching to another project or type of work.

Consistency

Consistency seems important, too. Although an occasional good deed is certainly appreciated by the recipient, it doesn't seem to carry the same health benefits to the bestower as do regular altruistic acts or consistent volunteer work. In studies of altruism and volunteerism, the greatest health benefits have been reaped by those who do consistent, regular volunteer work—at least once a week.[62]

Motive

Will you get the good-health benefits of volunteer work if you embark on a project out of selfish motives to improve your own health? Some say you can. Luks, who has been involved in studying the benefits of altruism, points out that "people help for all sorts of reasons: empathy for the homeless; peer pressure from a neighbor; guilt over some problem; or pressure from church or community. But it doesn't seem to matter. If they continue with the helping, most likely, they'll get the feel-good sensation."[63]

Research shows that people may not fare as well if they expect repayment for their altruism or if they expect something in return. If repayment is expected but withheld, the helper does not gain the emotional benefits from helping, says Carnegie Mellon University researcher Gail Williamson.[64] The "repayment" expected by some volunteers varies tremendously, too; some expect monetary reward, whereas others hope for payment in terms of increased status.[65]

Volunteer work has several unique aspects that could make the health benefits even greater. First, good feelings—and, almost certainly, health benefits—last far beyond the altruistic act itself. People in one study described more than one positive benefit associated with helping; 95 percent felt good while helping, and almost 80 percent said that the good feelings kept recurring long after the helping activity had ended.[66]

Participants in studies say they can recapture the helper's high, although sometimes not as intensely, by merely remembering or thinking about their charitable acts. For those participants, the health benefits of helping—fewer aches and pains, relief of depression, strength, energy, and increased self-worth—kept returning when they remembered the altruistic deeds. In fact, more than 80 percent could recapture the physical benefits just by thinking about their volunteer work.[67]

For the best health benefits from volunteering, researchers advise avoiding "unhelpful helping"—a style of volunteerism that causes the person being helped to actually become progressively more helpless and to eventually lose skills. To avoid that kind of helping, David Sobel offers these suggestions:

- Try to empower the person you're helping; you need to help that person gain as much control over his or her own life as possible.
- Encourage independence.
- As much as you can, allow the other person to make decisions.
- Give the other person clear responsibilities whenever possible—even for things you know you could do better or faster.
- Break down complicated tasks into small, easy steps.
- Allow mistakes and reward efforts, even if the results fall short of what you expected or what you know is possible.
- Limit your availability; the person you are helping should be increasingly independent. If you are always there, you stifle independence instead.

- Don't shield the person from all bad news or all problems; allow the person to appropriately express disappointment, anger, or sadness.[68]

And, because volunteering can become very demanding, Sobel advises that you avoid burnout by doing the following:

- First, monitor yourself and watch for the signs of burnout. You're probably getting burned out if you feel overwhelmed, helpless, out of control, resentful, guilty, or stressed.

- Pay attention to your own needs; if your own bucket is empty, you won't have anything to share with someone else.

- Recognize your limits. It would be nice to help at the homeless shelter every night, but that's just not realistic for most people. Or you might have a difficult time volunteering at a center for abused children if you were abused and have not dealt with those issues in your own life.

- Get help if you need it.

- Pace yourself; go only as fast as you comfortably can. Take what you can handle, and pass on what will overwhelm you.

- Don't get discouraged; if things don't work out with a certain situation, find another helping situation that's better for you. You might feel overwhelmed in a situation where you're expected to help a gang member rehabilitate—try helping an elderly person learn to read instead.

- Cancel any guilt trips you're considering.

- Finally, give yourself a pat on the back. You deserve it![69]

Love: The Emotion Behind It

In essence, the health benefits of altruism and volunteer service may depend on the driving emotion behind it all—love, a projection of one's own good feelings onto other people. True love for others is a reflection of love of oneself,[70] a willingness to project warmth and affectionate concern. The love that brings health benefits goes beyond romantic love and kinship ties to include feelings of friendship, compassion, respect, admiration, and gratitude for others. True love, too, is a verb—an action word that calls on us to demonstrate and apply our good feelings through specific actions or deeds.

After a careful analysis of thousands of his patients, psychiatrist Alfred Adler wrote, "The most important task imposed by religion has always been, 'Love thy neighbor. . . .' It is the individual who is not interested in his fellow man who has the greatest difficulties in life and provides the greatest injury to others. It is from such individuals that all human failures spring."[71]

According to researchers who have studied the effects of love, a truly loving relationship—one of acceptance and safety—is earmarked by freedom from expectations and demands. And when that kind of relationship exists, they say, love and health go hand in hand.

An important kind of love is something called *altruistic love,* prizing someone else's happiness and well-being above your own. A survey conducted by the University of Chicago's National Opinion Research Center found that married people who had a high degree of altruistic love for their spouse had happier marriages. That kind of love, says the survey director, creates a positive cycle in relationships: one spouse puts the other's interest first, and in turn, the spouse reciprocates. The survey also found that people (regardless of marital status) who felt altruistic love for at least one other person were happier in general than those who did not.[72]

Some even believe that love is an important key in the healing process. People who become more loving and less fearful, who replace negative thoughts with the emotion of love, are often able to achieve physical healing.

Most of us are familiar with the emotional effects of love, the way love makes us feel inside. But it doesn't stop there. True love—a love that is patient, trusting, protecting, optimistic, and kind—has actual physical effects on the body, too.

Bernie S. Siegel, prominent Yale surgeon and oncologist, claims that love and support, whether from an individual or a group, is an important facet of all healing. Its importance is so marked that even outsiders who observe the loving process can see clear evidence of its healing effects. Based on his own observations over the years, Siegel says, support and love from a physician can even result in noticeable improvement in a patient's condition.[73] Reflecting on his own practice, which has spanned more than three decades, Siegel concludes, "Someday we will understand the physiological and psychological workings of love well enough to turn on its full force more reliably. Once it is scientific, it will be accepted."[74]

Although we are not yet at that ideal level of understanding, there is much we do know and understand about the physiological effects of love. One of the most important effects of love is a boost of immune system function. Based on his studies, Harvard psychologist David McClelland concludes that love aids lymphocytes and improves immune functions—even though he is not sure how.[75]

Tests conducted at the Menninger Clinic in Topeka, Kansas, seem to confirm the effect of love on the immune system. At the clinic, it was found that people who were romantically in love had white cells that were significantly more active in fighting infection. As a result, they suffered fewer colds. They also had lower levels of lactic acid in their blood, which means they were less likely to get tired, and they had higher levels of endorphins in their blood, which may contribute to a sense of euphoria and may help reduce pain.[76]

People with personality traits that enable them to love others and to enjoy intimate relationships tend to fare better overall in immune system function. In a group of studies, those who loved and cared most for others had the best immune system balance: a high ratio of helper-suppressor T cells and low levels of the stress hormone norepinephrine.[77] Those who scored highest on the ability to have an intimate relationship also had the highest levels of immunoglobulin A (Ig-A), an important immune agent that enables people to resist disease.[78]

Love and Animals

The power of love has even been profoundly demonstrated in experiments with animals. Love and the handling that goes along with it have been shown to influence a baby animal's weight gain, emotional reactions, ability to respond to stress, and learning behaviors.[79]

Studies have shown that animals raised without love (and the handling that goes along with it) have weakened immune systems.

Animals deprived of love also have a greater tendency to develop disease, whereas those exposed to love and handling seem better able to resist disease. In one experiment, two groups of laboratory rabbits were each fed a diet high in fat. One group of rabbits was treated routinely in the laboratory. The other group was shown "love"; these rabbits were talked to, handled gently, and petted often. The rabbits that were shown affection developed significantly less atherosclerosis than the rabbits treated routinely.[80]

Love and Children

In the book *Vulnerable but Invincible,* the effects of an early loving relationship become apparent. To determine in part what helps us resist stress, researchers studied 650 children reared in poverty on the island of Kauai in the Hawaiian Islands. Their families had a multitude of problems. Many of the children were reared by single-parent mothers who were themselves troubled by depression and schizophrenia in addition to the rigors of extreme poverty.[81]

Researchers first did an extensive follow-up on the children when they turned 10 years old. Half of them were already in serious trouble. Many had serious physical problems and problems in school, among other difficulties. Eight years later, researchers did another follow-up on the children, now 18 years old. One-fourth of them had developed "very serious" physical and psychological problems. By the time they became adults, more than three-fourths showed the effects of their impoverished environment. Many had profound psychological and behavioral problems; even more were in poor physical health.

Of greatest interest to researchers, however, were the 15 to 20 percent who remained resilient. Despite their impoverished and difficult existence, these children were able to successfully resist the stress of that environment. Study findings give us a powerful insight into the effect of love. The children who remained resilient and healthy had a warm and loving relationship with another person during their first year of life. The children who developed serious psychological and physical problems did not.

Psychotherapist Harmon Bro, a former professor at Syracuse University, emphasizes the importance of early, affirming love. People who have "never developed the capacity for loving find lovelessness reflected in their bodies"—in poor health, muscular tension, shallow breathing, and other physical "ills" that reflect in a very real way an illness of the spirit.

WHAT DID YOU LEARN?

1. How does altruism boost health?
2. What characteristics are found in the altruistic personality?
3. What are the health benefits of volunteerism?

ENDNOTES

1. "Compassion RX: The Many Health Benefits of Altruism," Earthpages.org, http://epages.wordpress.com/2007/10/26/compassion-rx-the-many-health-benefits-of-altruism/, accessed October 26, 2007.

2. Carolyn Schwartz, Janice Bell Meisenhelder, Yunsheng Ma, and George Reed, "Altruistic Social Interest Behaviors Are Associated With Better Mental Health," *Psychosomatic Medicine,* 65 (2003): 778–85.

3. Edith L. B. Turner, "Discussion: Altruism, Spiritually Merging with a Fellow Human Being's Suffering," *Zygon,* 41, no. 4 (December 2006): 933–9.

4. Benevon, AAFRC Trust for Philanthropy, *Giving USA 2007: The Annual Report on Philanthropy.*

5. Stephen Post and Jill Neimark, *Why Good Things Happen to Good People* (New York: Broadway Books, 2008).

6. Allan Luks and Peggy Payne, *The Healing Power of Doing Good* (New York: Fawcett Columbine, 1992).

7. Samuel Oliner and Piotr Olaf Zylicz, *Altruism, Intergroup Apology, Forgiveness, and Reconciliation* (St. Paul, MN: Paragon House, 2008).

8. "Activation of Brain Region Predicts Altruism," *Health News Today* (St. Paul, MN, January 21, 2007).

9. Eileen Rockefeller Growald and Allan Luks, "Beyond Self," *American Health* (March 1988): 51–3.

10. American Psychological Association, "Stress Affects Immunity in Ways Related to Stress Type and Duration, As Shown by Nearly 300 Studies," http://www.apa.org/releases/stress_immune.html, July 4, 2004 (revised 2007).

11. "Compassion RX."

12. Kathleen Hall, "Stress Reducing Tips," The Stress Institute, 2005.

13. Esther M. Sternberg, "Approaches to Defining Mechanisms by Which Altruistic Love Affects Health," The Institute for Research on Unlimited Love, http://www.unlimitedloveinstitute.org/publications/pdf/whitepapers/Mechanisms_Altruistic.pdf, accessed June 3, 2008.

14. Growald and Luks, "Beyond Self."

15. "Compassion RX."

16. Sarah Lang, "Extend Your Hand, Extend Your Life," *Longevity* (March 1989): 18.

17. Allan Luks, "Helper's High: Volunteering Makes People Feel Good, Physically and Emotionally," *Psychology Today* (October 1988), cited in "Compassion RX."

18. Lang, "Extend Your Hand," 19.

19. Ibid.

20. Gregg D. Jacobs, "Clinical Applications of the Relaxation Response and Mind-Body Interventions," *Journal of Alternative and Complementary Medicine,* 7, no. 1 (December 2001): 93–101.

21. Growald and Luks, "Beyond Self," 51–3.

22. Diane Swanbrow, "People Who Give Live Longer, IRS Study Shows," *The University Record Online,* http://www.umich.edu/~urecord/0102/Nov18_02/15.shtml, November 18, 2002 (accessed June 3, 2008).

23. George E. Vaillant, MD, *Aging Well* (New York: Little, Brown Book Group, 2002), 62–81.

24. Lang, "Extend Your Hand," 19.

25. Ibid., 19.

26. Allan Luke, *The Healing Power of Doing Good* (New York: Fawcett, 1992), 80-81.

27. Ibid.
28. Schwartz et al., "Altruistic Social Interest Behaviors Are Associated With Better Mental Health," *Psychosomatic Medicine* 65 (2003): 778–5.
29. Ibid.
30. William Michael Brown, Nathan S. Consedine, and Carol Magai, "Altruism Relates to Health in an Ethnically Diverse Sample of Older Adults," *Journal of Gerontology* 60B, no. 3 (2005): P143–52.
31. J. Primavera, "The Unintended Consequences of Volunteerism: Positive Outcomes for Those Who Serve," *Journal of Prevention and Intervention in the Community* 18 (1999): 1–2.
32. Lang, "Extend Your Hand."
33. Stephen G. Post, ed., *Altruism and Health: Perspectives from Empirical Research* (London: Oxford University Press, 2007).
34. Carolyn E. Schwartz, Penelope M. Keyl, John P. Marcum, and Rita Bode, "Helping Others Shows Differential Benefits on Health and Well-Being for Male and Female Teens," *Journal of Happiness Studies* No 2 (April 2008).
35. S. I. McMillen, *None of These Diseases,* rev. ed. (Old Tappan, NJ: Fleming H. Revell, 1984), 188–9.
36. Geoffrey Cowley, "A Disaster Brings Out the Best in People. Why?" *Newsweek* (November 6, 1989): 40, 44.
37. Bruce Bower, "Getting Out from Number One," *Science News* 137 (1990): 266–7.
38. Robert Preidt, "Love for Others May Bring Rewards," 2004 *ScoutNews,* from Fairness.com, updated 2007.
39. Tom Hurley, "Another Look at Altruism: Notes on an International Conference," Noetic Sciences Building, August/September 1989, 3.
40. Samuel P. Oliner and Pearl M. Oliner, *The Altruistic Personality: Rescuers of Jews in Nazi Europe* (New York: Macmillan/Free Press, 1988).
41. "Dr. Frederick Franck: An Artist, Physician, and Author Searches for What It Means to Be Human," *Your Personal Best* (November 1989): 14–5.
42. Oliner and Oliner, *The Altruistic Personality.*
43. Larry Dossey, *Healing Words* (San Francisco: Harper San Francisco, 1993), 110–3.
44. Oliner and Oliner, *The Altruistic Personality.*
45. Alfie Kohn, "Do Religious People Help More?" *Psychology Today,* December 1989.
46. Alfie Kohn, "Beyond Selfishness," *Psychology Today* (October 1988): 38.
47. "Research: Altruism and Transformation," *Noetic Sciences Review* (Autumn 1990): 33.
48. Ibid.
49. Oliner and Oliner, *The Altruistic Personality,* 419.
50. Allan Luks with Peggy Payne, "Helper's High," *New Age Journal* (September/October 1991): 49, 121; from Allan Luks with Peggy Payne, *The Healing Power of Doing Good: The Health and Spiritual Benefits of Helping Others* (New York: Ballantine Books, 1991).
51. Allan Luks, "Helper's High," *Psychology Today* (October 1988): 39–42.
52. Luks, "Helper's High," 39.
53. "The Return of Generosity," *Health* (August 1989): 13.
54. Luks and Payne, "Helper's High."
55. Ibid.
56. Luks, "Helper's High," 42.
57. Ibid.
58. Luks and Payne, "Helper's High," 121.
59. Ibid.
60. Luks, "Helper's High."

61. Luks and Payne, "Helper's High."

62. Ibid.

63. Ibid.

64. "The Return of Generosity," *Health* (August 1989): 13.

65. Cowley, "A Disaster Brings Out the Best."

66. Howard F. Andrews, "Helping and Health: The Relationship Between Volunteer Activity and Health-Related Outcomes," *Advances* 7, no. 1 (1990): 25–34.

67. Luks, "Helper's High," 42.

68. David Sobel, "Rx: Helping Others."

69. Ibid.75.

70. Arnold Fox and Barry Fox, *Wake Up! You're Alive* (Deerfield Beach, FL: Health Communications, 1988), 75.

71. McMillen, *None of These Diseases*, 124.

72. Tom W. Smith, "Altruism and Empathy in America: Trends and Correlates," National Opinion Research Center, University of Chicago, February 2004.

73. Mary Carpenter, "Modern-Day Faith Healing: Why Doctors Are Listening, Not Laughing," *Self* (September 1987): 202–5.

74. Blair Justice, "Think Yourself Healthy," *Prevention* (June 1988): 31–32, 105–8.

75. Ibid.

76. Ibid.

77. Blair Justice, *Who Gets Sick: Thinking and Health* (Houston, TX: Peak Press, 1987), 257.

78. Justice, "Think Yourself Healthy."

79. Fox and Fox, *Wake Up!* 85.

80. Justice, *Who Gets Sick?* 258.

81. Emmy Werner and Ruth S. Smith, *Vulnerable But Invincible*, (New York: Adams Bannister Cox, 1989), 18–189.

CHAPTER 16

The Healing Power of Optimism

Every good thought you think is contributing its share to the ultimate result of your life.

—Grenville Kleiser

- Define *optimism*.
- Discuss the characteristics of optimists.
- Understand how optimism influences health.
- Discuss the impact of optimism on immune function and healing.
- Understand the influence of optimism on mental health and performance.

According to *Webster's Dictionary,* optimism is "an inclination to anticipate the best possible outcome." It is *not* the same as "positive thinking." It is a positive outlook, regardless of the situation or circumstances—not what happens, but our hopeful interpretation of what has happened. To redefine it psychologically, optimism is "the tendency to seek out, remember, and expect pleasurable experiences. It is an active priority of the person, not merely a reflex that prompts us to 'look on the sunny side.'"[1] From a physiological point of view, new research is exploring the concept that optimism has a biological basis, which scientists are beginning to identify in the brain.[2]

More than 30 years of research and more than 500 scientific studies have shown that a person's outlook, particularly when under stress or experiencing adversity, influences mood, performance, and even health.[3] Those studies indicate that optimists live longer, and they probably enjoy better health along the way as well. They even do better when they *do* get sick: studies show that people who are optimistic are also much less bothered by symptoms of illness.[4] Scientific evidence suggests that optimism has a specific effect on the physiological functioning of the body. In a real, physical sense, optimists are healthier. Their immune systems are stronger. And, as a group, they do live longer.

Who Are Optimists?

Optimists are people who generally believe that good, rather than bad, things will happen to them. They experience daily events in a more positive way, and they expect positive outcomes in a broad variety of situations.[5] They believe that the future will work out well; they approach the world in an active, productive way. They take reality into account, but they do everything possible with the reality they find. Optimism has a lot to do with other positive qualities as well, such as happiness, self-efficacy, and hardiness.

Research shows that an optimistic bias is far more common than was once considered. Depending on how optimism is measured, studies show that an estimated 80 percent of people have the characteristics of optimism.[6] The community of psychotherapy is realizing that normal, healthy individuals do downplay their faults and the negative things that happen to them—and that the people who lean toward optimism are the most healthy, both physically and mentally.

According to psychologists Shelley Taylor of UCLA and Jonathon Brown of Southern Methodist University in Dallas, research shows that most people view themselves in an optimistic light. "They judge themselves to be nicer, smarter, more charming, and prettier than even their closest admirers judge them to be," the psychologists assert. "Normal, healthy people see themselves more kindly than does the cold eye of the camera or even the caring eyes of family and friends. They think they're more talented and able than they are."[7]

Even aside from improving health, optimism is a positive force. "Optimism galvanizes people," says University of Michigan psychologist Christopher Peterson. "It sets you in motion. To be optimistic in the true sense is not to wear a smile button, but to be a problem-solver."[8]

Researchers think that "dispositional optimism," the belief that one's outcomes will be positive instead of negative, may be "hardwired" into the brains of some people. Suzanne C. Segerstrom—associate professor at the University of Kentucky and a researcher on optimism and immunity—says that 25 percent of dispositional optimism comes from genetic influences, and at least 50 percent results from life experience. (The other 25 percent can't be measured, she says.)[9]

The theory about optimism being hardwired into the brain has received increasing support. In a study conducted at New York University, researchers had people think about both positive and negative past and future events while their brain activity was recorded using magnetic resonance imaging (MRI). One brain area—the rostral anterior cingulated—was so consistently linked to optimism that it surprised the study director. "You can see it in all the subjects, indicating that it's probably very fundamental to human nature," said Tali Sharot, a postdoctorate fellow at University College London, who conducted the research.[10]

The "experts" used to believe that it was important to have a cold, hard perception of reality. Psychologist Sidney Jourard once wrote, "The ability to perceive reality as it 'really is' is fundamental to effective functioning. It is considered one of the two preconditions to the development of health." Psychologist Robert Ornstein and physician David Sobel say that modern psychology and clinical research contradicts this—and that healthy people are not accurate perceivers of reality. "Expecting to be pleased, healthy people cultivate a set of illusions. They inflate their own importance and have an exaggerated belief in their ability to control their destiny."[11]

While a significant amount of research has been done on optimism, there are still four unresolved issues in regard to the influence of optimism on health:[12]

1. Should optimism and pessimism be considered as polar ends of a single dimension— attitude—or should they be considered as two separate dimensions?

2. How important is optimism in promoting health? What unique effects does it have, as considered separately from all other influences?

3. How are the effects of optimism related to health?

4. Can specific health behaviors change or mediate the relationship between optimism and health?

Characteristics of Optimists

Seven-year-old Kealan Jewell is positive about everything. She unabashedly declares she's one of the most popular girls in her class. When asked what she wants to be when she grows up, she doesn't think twice. "I'm going to be an artist," she says. "I'd like to write a book, but I can't find the time."[13]

Kealan is an optimist, as are most other children her age. So was American philosopher Henry Thoreau, who used to lie in bed for a few minutes every morning to think positive thoughts. He would remind himself that he was healthy, that his mind was alert, that his work was interesting, that the future looked bright, and that many people trusted him. When he got out of bed, he entered a world filled with the kind of positive, good people and opportunities that he expected—a kind of "self-fulfilling prophecy."

It usually is easy to tell the difference between an optimist and a pessimist. Optimists experience the same kinds of hard knocks in life as do pessimists, but the optimists look on those hard knocks as being very temporary. Optimists see challenges, not obstacles. When the going gets tough, the optimist generally gets tougher, persevering through the difficulty.

The optimist has an entirely different explanation for things. The optimistic driver acknowledges (or "blames") the reduced visibility, the slick and snow-packed streets, and other adverse conditions for his accident. Then he realizes he hasn't had much experience on snowy roads and tells himself that he'll have to be more careful until he gets more experience. The pessimistic driver, on the other hand, blames himself. His internal reasoning goes something like this: "I'm such a poor driver. I'll never learn to drive safely. Every time I try something new, I screw it up."[14]

Optimists have a number of qualities in common. Probably the most common is that they see the good in situations and truly expect things to go their way. According to Michael Scheier, professor of psychology at Pittsburgh's Carnegie Mellon University, researchers are finding that "anticipating a favorable outcome leads an optimist to do things that actually determine the final outcome. Optimists expect things to turn out well, but they also do things that can change the course of events."[15]

In addition, optimists see events in their lives as controllable—an apt attitude because, says Scheier, optimism comes from the Latin word *ops*, meaning "power." When something bad does happen, optimists are not defeated. Instead, they make a plan of action, follow it, and work quickly before the situation gets out of hand. They expect that they will be able to handle anything that comes along (and they are usually right).

When something bad happens, optimists view it as an isolated occurrence rather than as part of a general trend or life pattern. In day-to-day events, in fact, optimists dismiss the bad and instead internalize the good. They interpret events and circumstances in their favor, a trait that helps them stay positive even when confronted by situations they truly cannot control (such as the death of a loved one).

All this cheerfulness is not to say that optimists can't face reality or see when they're "in over their heads"; optimists express acceptance or resignation when needed. University of Miami psychologist Charles Carver says that researchers "don't want to imply that people should put on a happy face and go around being mindlessly cheerful all the time. Even optimists have occasional doubts or fail sometimes. By resignation, we mean the ability to say, 'I'm not going to pretend this isn't happening, but if I have to put up with it, I will.'"[16] Scheier maintains that they have the instinct to know when to charge forward or when to back off—and their optimistic attitude helps them cope far more effectively when situations come up.

How Optimism Influences Health

A growing body of evidence gives increasing credibility to the idea that optimism and positive emotions promote health. Even positive denial can be health promoting. Psychologist Richard Lazarus believes that a sense of "positive denial"—a refusal to believe in something negative, as long as it is not carried to the extreme—helps keep hopes up, sustains morale, improves health, and reduces anxiety.[17] But researchers who have conducted studies on attitude and beliefs agree with one basic principle: a positive attitude and belief in the body's own healing abilities can certainly supplement medical treatment but should never replace it. Leading researchers emphasize that the best possible outcome results when optimism and positive thinking work hand-in-hand with the medical treatment offered by competent physicians.

Exactly what role can optimism play? For one thing, it appears that an optimistic attitude can actually protect a person from getting sick in the first place. In a study of armed services veterans who had graduated from Harvard University, researchers found that the men who were the most optimistic in their original writings had the best health 40 years later. Their own perception of their experiences was significantly associated with later physical and mental illness; those with an optimistic outlook were healthy, and those with a gloomy outlook were ill (or dead).[18]

In writing down their experiences during World War II, the pessimists, who were in worse health at the end of the study, penned remarks like, "Giving orders was sometimes very hard, if not impossible, because I always had this problem of dealing with men under me, even later in the war when I had the appropriate rank."

The healthy optimists, on the other hand, recorded sentiments such as, "During the war I was occasionally bored, because anyone who's ever been on a ship is bored to tears." The optimist, even though he had a bad experience, didn't blame it on his own shortcomings. He was bored, but isn't everyone bored on a ship?

In summing up the study, researchers wrote, "If you always go around thinking, 'It's my fault, it's going to last forever, and it's going to undermine everything I do,' then when you do run into further bad events, you become at risk for poor health."[19]

Optimism has been shown to have an impact on all kinds of disease conditions, including those as serious as cardiovascular disease. One study involving older men who had no overt cardiovascular disease when the study began showed that those who were optimistic had a lower incidence of coronary heart disease.[20] Other studies showed that those with low levels of pessimism had a reduced risk of heart disease.[21] A large-scale study in Finland showed that optimism was related to better general health behavior and to the reduced risk of cardiovascular disease.[22]

Research results released from Harvard University showed that optimistic coronary bypass patients were only half as likely to be admitted back into the hospital; optimists had lower blood pressure; the most pessimistic men were twice as likely to develop heart disease; and highly pessimistic men were three times more likely to develop hypertension.[23]

Dispositional optimism, defined earlier, plays a huge role in changing cardiovascular health behaviors.[24] Optimists, say the researchers, are more likely than pessimists to believe that good outcomes are attainable and bad outcomes are avoidable, so the optimists put forth greater effort to attain the desired outcome.[25]

Various studies have provided "compelling evidence"[26] that dispositional optimism contributes to greater success among cardiac patients. The May 2008 *Harvard Health Letter* calls the positive feelings that protect heart health "emotional vitality." In a study conducted at the University of Massachusetts Medical Center, patients in a cardiac rehabilitation program were studied to determine which ones were most successful in making the behavioral changes needed to protect their cardiac health. Those who were most optimistic at the beginning of the program had the greatest success in reducing levels of saturated fat, increasing aerobic exercise capacity, reducing body fat, and generally lowering their cardiac risk.[27] Optimism has also been shown to reduce blood pressure and to improve pulmonary function.[28]

The key to better health in the optimistic cardiac patients may come from the influence of optimism on the manufacture and release of certain hormones in the body. Optimism reduces the quantity of stress hormones, for example—and fewer stress hormones reduces the risk of heart disease.[29]

While study findings are mixed and research scientists are divided, it does appear that optimism can even make a difference in illnesses as grave as cancer. A University of California–Los Angeles research team launched a national survey of cancer specialists in an attempt to find out which psychosocial factors were most important in helping patients overcome the disease. A total of 649 oncologists responded to the survey and reported on their experiences in treating more than 100,000 cancer patients. More than 90 percent of the physicians who responded to the survey said that the most significant factor in effective treatment was the attitude of hope and optimism.[30]

A number of studies confirm that point of view. Women undergoing chemotherapy for ovarian cancer were monitored both for emotional status and physical response to the chemotherapy. Those who were optimistic experienced less anxiety, depression, distress, and perceived stress. Those with the highest degree of dispositional optimism at the start of the chemotherapy experienced the greatest drops in the protein marker for ovarian cancer (CA-125)—though none of the patients' CA-125 levels returned to normal during the study.[31]

Scientists studied women who had undergone mastectomies for breast cancer; they recorded psychological responses three months after the surgery and then assessed the women's health 5, 10, and 15 years later. They found that the woman's attitude was a better predictor of survival than were more traditional factors, such as the size of the tumor, the severity of the tumor, or the woman's age. A second study showed that the women who felt most helpless after breast cancer were the ones most likely to relapse or die within five years of diagnosis.[32]

Dr. G. Frank Lawlis and Jeanne Achterberg, a husband-wife team at the University of Texas Health Science Center in Dallas, conducted a series of studies showing that optimism and positive attitude have an impact on cancer.[33] In their studies, Lawlis and Achterberg studied the personalities of 200 terminal cancer patients. They found that certain personality traits were common to those who lived much longer than they had been expected to live: The survivors utterly refused to give up. They were open to new ideas. They rejected their role as invalids. They refused to accept the limits of their illness. And, most important, they were optimistic. They believed in themselves, in their ability to beat the cancer.

Other studies indicate that optimism may not impact the course of cancer. Research done at the Peter MacCallum Cancer Centre in Melbourne, Australia, and published in the scientific journal *Cancer* found that those who remained optimistic during their treatment for lung cancer did not have any advantage when it came to survival. A determined fighting spirit was no guarantee that the patients would not die as a result of the cancer.[34]

While the study did not bring good news for the optimists, some researchers maintained it brought relief for many patients who could not "put on a brave face" while fighting the disease. "This study tells people it's okay to grieve after a diagnosis of cancer. The patients I worry about are those who have no reaction and go straight into fighting spirit mode, because that's not realistic," said Dr. Amanda Ramirez of Cancer Research UK. "Having hope and being optimistic is very important from a quality of life point of view, rather than a quantity of life point of view."[35]

A study of people with head and neck cancers done at the University of Pennsylvania in 2007—a study claiming to be larger and more comprehensive than others done to date—showed no relationship between optimism and surviving the cancer longer. Psychology professor James C. Coyne, who headed up the study, reacted in much the same way as Ramirez did to the Melbourne study. Patients, he says, "have the potential of being blamed" for not being optimistic enough. "Some people just go out cranky and they do it with a roar. More power to them." He notes that there are individual differences to how people react to a disease over which they have little control, "and that's okay."[36]

Optimism even seems to play a role in illnesses like the flu and the common cold. Psychologist Christopher Peterson studied students at Virginia Tech in Blacksburg, Virginia. He reported that pessimistic students were ill twice as many days and had four times as many doctor visits over the course of a year compared with optimistic students.[37] Peterson expressed particular interest in the fact that 95 percent of all the ill students had infectious diseases—the common cold, sore throats, flu, pneumonia, ear infections, venereal diseases, and mononucleosis. Apparently the pessimistic students were less able to fight infection. "This suggests that how we view things may directly affect our immune system," he says.[38] The pessimists, he points out, may have been more likely to get colds and other illnesses in part because they were less apt to seek medical advice or take simple medical precautions.

Peterson was able to confirm his theories with results from several other studies. In one study,[39] he and his colleagues studied summer school students at the University of Michigan. Again, he assessed general style to determine whether each student was pessimistic or optimistic. Then researchers carefully followed the health of each student, asking for an assessment on a daily basis. Again, the pessimists were the most ill—and 95 percent of the reported symptoms were from colds or the flu, suggesting a breakdown in the ability to resist infectious diseases.

In a similar study, in which Carnegie Mellon researchers found that optimistic students reported fewer ills, researchers wrote, "Pessimists, as a rule, care less about their health. In addition, pessimists blame themselves for their failures but then do little to further improve their lot. Optimists, on the other hand, view failures as problems that can be fixed. They meet their problems head on, form a plan of action, and achieve results."[40]

The impact of optimism on health may be due to the tendency of optimists to take control, proactively engage in improving their conditions, attend to health threats, and engage in health-promoting behaviors. Researchers point out that optimism influences health-promoting behavior because optimists focus on problems and work to solve them rather than avoiding those problems. When they think something is attainable, optimists will continue to strive toward their goal, even when progress is difficult or slow.[41] Still other researchers believe that the healthier behaviors among optimists is due to the agreeable nature and conscientiousness that is generally part of optimism.[42]

Studies have shown that those who are most optimistic in their outlook also pay the greatest attention to health risks and threats. Research at the University of Maryland showed that people who are optimistic about their health and their future in general are much more likely to pay attention to information about health risks or threats to health and to act positively on that information.[43] Lisa Aspinwall, who conducted the study, said that the optimists "are people who aren't sitting around wishing things were different. They believe in a better outcome, and that whatever measures they take will help them to heal."[44]

The health benefits of optimism may also be due to the fact that optimistic people tend to attract a larger and stronger social network, which in turn provides the health benefits of social support, and to have better coping strategies in difficult situations.[45] Some researchers think that it may not be the optimism at all, but other factors—such as socioeconomic status, social support, and access to services, which can all contribute to optimism—that actually cause the health benefits sometimes attributed to optimism.[46]

Some believe that optimists are unrealistic in their outlook, ignoring or avoiding the very real negative factors that surround them. The results of several fascinating studies show, however, that optimists are generally very realistic about their situations; but, instead of reacting with a negative outlook, they proactively work to cope with difficult situations and bring about positive change. In one study, researchers collected information from 3,000 people living in high-rise public housing in more than two dozen neighborhoods. According to Michael Greenberg, professor and co-director of the New Jersey Graduate Program in Public Health at Rutgers University:

> Network television, newspapers, public policy documents, and scholarly studies tell Americans that high-rise, public housing projects in Chicago, Detroit, New York City, and other cities are places where nightmares are born and lived. Residents are characterized as terrorized by gangs, unable to move around within their buildings because of unlit hallways and malfunctioning elevators, afraid that their children will become victims of illegal drugs and stray bullets, unfairly treated by police and the judicial system, and subjected to numerous other indignities and risks that cumulatively cause hopelessness.[47]

These conditions challenge dispositional optimism—the "expectation that people will work for a positive outcome even under difficult conditions."[48] Greenberg's study, which canvassed more than two dozen neighborhoods, was part of an ongoing project aimed at understanding how residents of decaying, crime-ridden neighborhoods characterize their environment. Specifically, Greenberg and his colleagues designed their study to do the following:

- Determine the degree to which optimism (and the health-related behaviors associated with it) existed in high-rise public housing.

- Determine whether optimists realized the severity of the problems that existed in their housing.

- Determine whether optimists were more likely to engage in behavior that would protect their own health and the health of others in the housing.

Before he began his formal study, Greenberg spanned a period of three years during which he had informal conversations with more than four dozen people who

> . . . lived adjacent to a massive rat-infested trash pile or an unremediated hazardous waste site, or across the street from houses that were stripped of their aluminum siding and copper pipes and then burned by drug-addicted arsonists. Rather than cringing in fear at their difficult neighborhood conditions, some residents felt they could control their local environment. They welcomed the challenge of improving the neighborhood, spoke about activities . . . to improve the neighborhood, and expected, or at least hoped, for a positive outcome. . . . These kinds of responses are associated with dispositional optimism.[49]

These informal conversations—using people "who were interviewed because they were standing outside when the author was in the neighborhood rather than being scientifically selected"—led Greenberg to wonder how dispositional optimism impacted the residents of these projects. For his formal study, Greenberg chose a controversial high-rise public housing project in central New Jersey. At the time of the study, the project had been threatened with demolition for about a decade; more than 200 of the units were occupied, and the project was surrounded by a bridge, a heavily used highway, and a group of low-rise housing units occupied primarily by lower-middle-income blacks and

Hispanics. As a foundation for his survey, Greenberg relied on questions in the U. S. Department of Commerce's biannual American Housing Survey for the United States. Survey respondents were asked first to indicate whether certain potentially harmful situations existed in the project (such as crime or decaying conditions). Then they were asked whether they were willing or able to take action on their own behalf or on behalf of the neighborhood. A standard test was used to determine whether each survey respondent was an optimist or a pessimist.

Here's what Greenberg found: Optimists and pessimists identified about the same number and types of problems and amenities in the neighborhood. Their rating of neighborhood quality was almost identical, too. In other words, the optimists didn't minimize the serious problems that existed in their housing project. However, the optimists were much more likely to attend a public meeting, participate in a church or civic function, and in other ways engage in neighborhood activities that helped them cope with extremely difficult conditions. They were also more likely to proactively engage in trying to solve the problems than to withdraw, which was the course of action typically chosen by the pessimists.[50]

Optimism and Healing

Not only can optimism help keep a person healthy, but it can also boost the body's own mechanisms to speed the healing process. It can even result in people *feeling* better, even when they are ill.[51] Anxious to see exactly how much power the mind has over the body, researchers decided to look at the example of warts. Viral warts are controlled by the immune system. When the immune system does not work to control the virus, warts appear. Researchers at Boston's Massachusetts General Hospital hypnotized patients with intractable warts and told them, under hypnosis, that the body would heal itself. In almost all the cases, the body did just that; the warts disappeared.

Psychologist and avid skier Lonnie Barbach pulled the ligaments in her left knee and spent a painful six weeks on crutches. Two years later, she injured her right knee in the same way—skiing—and to the same extent. This time she pulled all her optimism to the fore and used mental training to imagine that her ligaments were tightening and that the pain, soreness, and swelling were diminishing. Without using crutches, she was completely healed in less than three weeks.[52]

Optimism can make a big difference in surgical outcomes, too. In a study conducted by Dr. Charles S. Carver of the University of Miami and Dr. Michael F. Scheier of Carnegie Mellon University, coronary bypass surgery patients were questioned the day before surgery and again one week after surgery. Based on the results of the first interview, researchers categorized each patient as being an optimist or a pessimist. While their mental attitudes were different, their physical conditions were similar, and the outlook for their recovery was the same.[53]

Not everyone had the same results after surgery, however. The optimists were busy making plans for the time when they would be released from the hospital; after surgery, they sought information about what they could do to improve their recovery. The pessimists, on the other hand, took an "observer" stance and were much less involved in helping themselves. Although the outlook was the same for all patients, the optimists had a much speedier recovery, marred by fewer complications. In summing up the study, Carver concluded that "optimists may experience more success because they deal with their problems earlier than pessimists do, and in a more direct, goal-oriented way. . . . They use a strategy for coping that is most adaptive and least dysfunctional."[54]

Optimism may make such a difference to recovery that some hospitals have begun using aids to boost it—such as an "artificial window" that provides a peaceful scene as well as simulating the change between day and night. Stanford was the first medical facility in the country to use the window, a four-by-five-foot computer-controlled light box behind a blowup of a slide shot by California nature photographer Joey Fischer. Fischer saw the need for the "window" when his own father had a heart attack and spent many hours counting holes in the hospital ceiling tiles because there was nothing else to look at. In the window is a peaceful pasture topped by billowing clouds; an electronic digital timer produces 650 separate light changes every twenty-four hours, mimicking dawn to twilight.[55]

Imaging

A positive personality and mindset can do even more. Researchers now believe that a positive practice called imaging may mobilize the body's physical resources. Positive imaging—the ability to concentrate on images that represent the body's fight against disease—is a newly recognized and little-understood phenomenon that has begun to attract considerable attention in the medical profession. It was first used as a therapy to treat illness by Dr. O. Carl Simonton, with the Cancer Counseling and Research Center in Fort Worth, Texas. Although scientists and researchers don't understand its effects on the immune system, one thing is obvious: it can sometimes help, even when the odds for recovery seem bleak. As we understand it, positive imaging seems to be an example of the power of the mind over the body.

Impressed by Simonton's results and curious about the effect of imaging on the immune systems of cancer victims, George Washington University biochemist Nicholas Hall began teaching the system of positive imaging to his patients. One of Hall's patients was a man with prostate cancer that had metastasized to the bone marrow. Hall taught his patient imaging, and the patient was tested one to two times a week while he was practicing it. While the patient was practicing imaging, his white blood cell count was up and his body produced greater amounts of thymosin, a thymic hormone that might help regulate the immune response. When instructed to stop imaging, the patient's white blood cell count dropped severely, and thymosin was almost undetectable in his body. Research has found that imagery can help reduce pain and stress, alter the course of disease, and improve patients' outlook on their illness.[56]

Psychologist Patricia Norris, clinical director of the Biofeedback and Psychophysiology Center at the Menninger Foundation, relates a remarkable story about positive imaging.[57] Anna, who had a malignant tumor growing rapidly at the back of her neck, had been given only three months to live. The cancer had virtually crippled her: she was hunched over, her head was forced painfully to one side, and her right arm was paralyzed and contracted. Her doctor had instructed her to do the sensible thing: go home and make the necessary arrangements for the futures of her young children.

Norris instructed Anna in positive imaging. Anna began to visualize her tumor as a dragon on her back; she imagined her white blood cells to be knights that were attacking the tumor with swords.

A year later, Norris saw Anna again. A remarkable change had taken place: her arm was fully mobile, and the tumor had shrunk. The next time the two met, Anna was in total remission. (Note: Although imaging may be helpful in some circumstances, it should never replace appropriate and proven medical treatment.)

Optimism: A Boost to Immunity

As discussed in the early chapters of this book, emotions can impact the immune system—and optimism is one of the emotions that seems to have the strongest ties. In his work over several decades, psychologist Martin Seligman found real physiological differences between pessimists and optimists. In one study, he and his colleagues measured the disease-fighting cells in the blood of 300 people whose average age was 71. The optimists had the healthier immune systems.[58]

People who have a more optimistic outlook do seem to have a healthier immune system and are especially better at adapting to the environment, according to Rosalind Wright, an assistant professor at Harvard Medical School who has studied the impact of optimism on pulmonary health. Wright believes the impact of optimism on immunity has to do with the fact that optimistic people produce fewer stress hormones—and stress hormones are known to weaken the immune system.[59] The results of several studies show that optimistic people experience less stress following major life events, such as a death or major illness in the family.[60]

One study conducted at Harvard University[61] tested healthy first-year law students. Those who were judged to be optimistic were the ones who felt confident when they thought about law school, who expected to succeed, and who had positive evaluations about their abilities. Those who were optimistic at the beginning of the school year had stronger immunity midsemester—including more helper T cells and greater natural killer cell response.

Other studies have yielded similar results. At the Medical Illness Counseling Center in suburban Maryland, 10 cancer patients added guided imagery to their conventional chemotherapy treatment in an attempt to mobilize their own defenses against their cancers. After a year, all 10 were still alive, and blood tests showed that their white blood cells had multiplied to fight the cancer cells.[62]

In a study at Michigan State University, patients used a combination of imagery and relaxation coupled with the optimistic belief that their treatment would work. Among those in the study, patients were able to cause an average of 60 percent of their white blood cells to leave the bloodstream and enter the surrounding tissue.[63]

In another study at Harvard, a group of people imagined that their T cells were attacking cold and flu viruses. That imagery—boosted by optimism—caused both T cell counts and immunoglobulin A counts to increase, multiplying the strength of the immune system.[64]

The ability of optimism to boost the immune system may hold benefits for victims of acquired immune deficiency syndrome (AIDS), which ordinarily knocks out the body's immune system. New York psychologist Lewis Katoff maintains that positive thinking plays "an important role" in helping AIDS victims survive longer. Katoff, reporting on the first-ever study of the attitudes of AIDS victims who have survived three years or longer, said of the victims that they "are not depressed. They refuse to give up."[65]

Optimism's Effect on Mental Health and Performance

In addition to better physical health, optimists score better on performance and mental health, especially in resisting the effects of stress. Writing about some of the greatest entrepreneurs of our day, *Success* editor Scott DeGarmo penned the sentiment that "learning how to rebound with optimism is part of adapting to a world of constant change." Optimism, he says, is one of the key characteristics of the men and women who change the shape of the nation through their entrepreneurial ventures. He quotes Ralph Waldo Emerson in saying that these optimists display "a wild courage, a stoicism not of the schools but of the blood."[66]

Martin Seligman, who has studied optimism extensively, says that the "link between optimism and performance is basically persistence. Optimists keep at it; pessimists give up and fail, even if they have equal talent. And because optimists are always hopeful about the outcome, they tend to take more risks and try more new things."[67]

Seligman has shown that optimists are more successful and perform better than pessimists in almost all fields, including education, business, sports, and politics. He successfully predicted that Bush would face Dukakis in the 1988 presidential campaign long before the crowded field of contenders was narrowed, and he made his prediction based solely on optimistic characteristics. "Forget about the deficit and prayer in schools," one researcher summed. "A leading determinant for political wins is the level of optimism candidates convey. Dukakis and Bush came out on top, based on careful analysis of their stump speeches. Alexander Haig, on the other hand, was at the bottom of Seligman's list of optimistic traits (as was Gary Hart), and the first to withdraw."[68]

Seligman has long been convinced that optimists perform so much better than pessimists in almost every way that optimism should be taken into account when hiring personnel. He was able to convince insurance giant Metropolitan Life that his theory was right—and he developed a twenty-minute written examination to screen applicants for the trait of optimism. Metropolitan Life then administered the test to 15,000 recruits, many of whom had failed the industry examination the first time. The examination separated the optimists from the rest of the pack, and Metropolitan Life hired a new sales force based on optimism.

The new hiring strategy was an unfailing success. By the end of the first year, the optimists were outselling the others by 20 percent. By the end of the following year, they were outselling the others by 50 percent.[69]

Optimism is also one of the best-known buffers against the deleterious effects of stress. Studies have shown that people who meet stress head-on with a sense of optimism and control don't get ill as often as those who meet stress with pessimism. Or, as one writer so aptly put it, "Winners are healthier than whiners."[70]

Researchers at Ohio State University studied more than 200 adults who had been categorized as optimists or pessimists based on scientifically accepted questionnaires. They found that those who were optimists had far less stress, less anxiety, and fewer health problems a year after they were initially categorized. Even more important than being optimistic, says study lead author Susan Robinson-Whelan, it may be crucial to not be pessimistic.[71]

Optimists do better under stress because they're less likely to believe that the source of stress is all-encompassing or overwhelming. They're less likely to turn to drugs or alcohol in an attempt to escape from stress. They're more likely to make recommended changes when ill and more likely to follow prescriptions by a physician. They're more likely to take better care of themselves in general—a boon no matter what the source of stress.

Another reason why optimists fare better under stress than pessimists is the trait called dispositional optimism, which we discussed earlier. According to researchers from Carnegie Mellon University, optimists view the world more positively

> . . . for the simple reason that they take more positive actions to improve it. They were found to deal with stressful situations by focusing directly on the problem at hand. They tended to "positively reinterpret" a difficult situation, focusing on what they could learn from it or the discovery of some new truth about life. Pessimists, by contrast, tended to deal with stress by attempting either to disengage from it, to deny it, or simply to complain about it—techniques poorly suited for achieving positive results.[72]

Optimists and Longevity

There's a real physiological reason why optimists live longer, and researchers believe that it lies in a complex set of "messages" that the mind sends to the body. As a result of his work with thousands of critically ill patients, Yale surgeon Bernie Siegel believes the following:

> The body responds to the mind's messages, whether conscious or unconscious. In general, these may be either "live" or "die" messages. I am convinced we not only have survival mechanisms, such as the fight-or-flight response, but also a "die" mechanism that actively stops our defenses, slowing our body's functions and bringing us toward death when we feel our life is not worth living.[73]

Optimists, it seems, give consistent "live" messages to the body—and, as a result, live longer. Results of a number of studies have confirmed the theory that people with a cheerful outlook on life generally get to enjoy life longer.

In one study, researchers pored through the pages of *The New York Times* and the *Philadelphia Inquirer* analyzing the quotes of all the Baseball Hall of Fame players who played major league baseball between the years 1900 and 1950. Based on the players' comments about the game, researchers were able to tag which were optimists and which were pessimists. The pessimists—those who ascribed their success as being short-lived or due to luck—lived significantly shorter lives than the optimists.[74]

How you perceive your health to be (whether your perception is or is not accurate) also seems to have a significant bearing on how long you will live. People who believe that they are in bad health—even if they are, in reality, in good or excellent health—have an increased mortality risk. Those who believe that their health is good are literally at a reduced risk of dying, even if "objective" measures (such as medical examinations and laboratory tests) show that they are actually in poor health.

Researchers in one study tracked 6,298 adults in Alameda County, California, for nine years. Men who were "health pessimists" (believed they were in poor health) had two times the mortality risk of men who were "health optimists." The mortality risk among women was a striking five times higher for those pessimistic about their health.[75]

Conclusion

With all the evidence that optimism is an important health factor, it's essential to remember that the link between emotion and immunity "is robust. But it is also intricate and filled with surprises that open a dramatic new window on the nature of emotional health."[76] Some of those surprises? Short-term stress may actually prime the immune system, making us stronger. And too much optimism can actually weaken immunity. The best combination, say the researchers, is "optimism seasoned by reality"—not the blind kind of optimism that suggests we will thrive no matter what, and not the renegade type of optimism that causes us to push so hard that we end up getting sick or that we refuse to disengage from stressful situations.[77]

Simply stated, says University of Kentucky's Suzanne Segerstrom, behaving like an optimist can be good for your body in the long run but may cost a lot in the short run. "No personality type is a magic bullet for health, and optimism has its Achilles' heel," she says. "Most of the time, optimism and its typical coping style are associated with better immune function, but it's also important to recognize that that isn't always true."[78]

Seasoned with reality and in the right dose, we know that optimism can be a powerful factor in life. It can be a potent determinant in how healthy we are and how long we live. An increasing number of physicians who are "in the trenches" with patients every day continue to express the firm belief that optimism, more than almost any other attitude, can open the way to health and healing. And even if an optimist can't overcome disease, an optimistic outlook ensures a greater quality of life in the meantime.

Interested in becoming more optimistic? Researchers suggest the following ways to boost your optimism:

- Realize you may need to make a lifestyle change.
- Start small by choosing one area of your life in which to become more optimistic, and then become aware of the way you think in relation to that area.
- Take a good, hard, critical look at your beliefs about yourself and about that area of your life: How realistic are these beliefs?
- Set goals that are small enough to achieve quickly, and then reward yourself when you meet those goals.
- It's important to reward yourself when you reach even the most modest goal.
- Seek out optimistic people; seek a good friend.
- "Play" at being optimistic; stay flexible.[79]

In the book *Mind/Body Medicine: How to Use Your Mind for Better Health*, editors Daniel Goleman and Joel Gurin suggest the following ways to raise an optimistic child:

- Be consistent, positive, and responsive.
- To the extent that you can, "program" the child's world to be consistent, positive, and responsive.
- Give the child responsibility; encourage independence, and involve the child in a variety of age-appropriate activities.
- Set realistic goals and encourage problem solving.
- Teach the child not to generalize from specific failures; instead, help the child see failure as a challenge to do better next time.
- Encourage humor as a way of coping.
- If the child expresses pessimistic views, challenge them.
- As best you can, screen the child's peers and teachers for pessimistic tendencies.
- And, finally, be a role model yourself of realistic optimism.[80]

Norman Cousins, the former *Saturday Review* editor whose own experiences with healing formed the foundation for his remarkable work with others, says:

> Yes, I know that my optimism can be carried too far—but I also know that no one is smart enough to fix its limits; and that it is far better to pursue a remote and even unlikely goal than to deprive oneself of the forward motion that goals provide. My life has been an education in these essentials, and I could no more turn away from them than I could deny my own existence. . . . Some people may interpret the effort as overwrought do-goodism; but the risk is worth taking nonetheless, for every once in a while it happens that hope can rekindle one's spirits, create remarkable new energies, and set a stage for genuine growth. At least nothing I have learned is less theoretical than the way the entire world seems to open up when courage and determination are connected to truly important aims.[81]

WHAT DID YOU LEARN?

1. How does optimism influence health and healing?
2. How would you describe an optimist?
3. What is optimism's effect on immune system strength, mental health, and longevity?

ENDNOTES

1. Robert Ornstein and David Sobel, *Healthy Pleasures* (Reading, MA: Addison-Wesley Publishing Company, 1989), 149.
2. Emily Anthes, "How Do You See This Glass?" *The Boston Globe* (June 2, 2008): 1–2.
3. "Optimism," *Spirituality and Health*, http://www.spiritualityhealth.com/newsh/items/selftest/item_236.html, accessed June 2, 2008.

4. M. F. Scheier and C. S. Carver, "Optimism, Coping, and Health: Assessment and Implications of Generalized Outcome Expectancies," *Health Psychology* 4, no. 3 (1985): 219–47.

5. Mika Kivumaki et al., "Optimism and Pessimism as Predictors of Change in Health After Death or Onset of Severe Illness in Family," *Health Psychology* 24, no. 4 (2005): 413–21.

6. Anthes, "How Do You See This Glass?"

7. Ann Ranard, "The World Through Rose-Colored Glasses," *Health* (August 1989): 58.

8. Carolyn Jabs, "New Reasons to Be an Optimist," *Self* (September 1987): 170–3.

9. S. C. Segerstrom, "Optimism and Immunity: Do Positive Thoughts Always Lead to Positive Effects?" *Brain, Behavior, and Immunity* 19, no. 3 (2005): 195–200.

10. Sarah Kliff, "This Is Your Brain on Optimism," *Newsweek* (October 24, 2007): 1–2.

11. Ornstein and Sobel, *Healthy Pleasures*, 169.

12. Joel E. Milam et al., "The Roles of Dispositional Optimism and Pessimism in HIV Disease Progression," *Psychology and Health* 19, no. 2 (April 2004): 167–81.

13. Example is from Ranard, "The World Through Rose-Colored Glasses," 58.

14. Joan Borysenko, *Minding the Body, Mending the Mind* (Reading, MA: Addison-Wesley Publishing Company, 1987), 120.

15. Sharon Faelten, David Diamond, and the editors of *Prevention* magazine, *Take Control of Your Life: A Complete Guide to Stress Relief* (Emmaus, PA: Rodale Press, 1988), 306.

16. Ibid.

17. T. P. Hackett and N. H. Cassem, "Development of a Quantitative Rating Scale to Assess Denial," *Journal of Psychosomatic Research* 18 (1974): 93–100.

18. Bruce Bower, "Pessimism Linked to Poor Health," *Science News* (July 23, 1988).

19. From Ornstein and Sobel, 167.

20. L. D. Kubzansky, D. Sparrow, P. Volkonas, and I. Kawachi, "Is the Glass Half Empty or Half Full? A Prospective Study of Optimism and Coronary Heart Disease in the Normative Aging Study," *Psychosomatic Medicine* 63 (2001): 910–6.

21. J. Dykema, K. Bergbower, and C. Peterson, "Pessimistic Explanatory Style, Stress, and Illness," *Journal of Social and Clinical Psychology* 14 (1995): 357–71, cited in Kivumaki et al., 2005.

22. P. V. Ylostalo, E. Ek, J. Laitinen, and M. L. Knuuttila, "Optimism and Life Satisfaction as Determinants for Dental and General Health Behavior—Oral Health Habits Linked to Cardiovascular Risk Factors," *Journal of Dental Research* 82, no. 3 (2003): 194–9.

23. "Why Optimists Enjoy Better Health," *Harvard Men's Health Watch*, April 30, 2008.

24. James A. Shepperd, JoAnn J. Maroto, and Lori A. Pbert, "Dispositional Optimism as a Predictor of Health Changes Among Cardiac Patients," *Journal of Research in Personality* 30 (1996): 517–34.

25. M. F. Scheier and C. S. Carver, "A Model of Behavioral Self-Regulation: Translating Intention into Action," pp. 303–46 in Louise Berkowitz, ed., *Advances in Experimental Social Psychology,* vol. 21 (New York: Academic Press, 1988).

26. Shepperd, Maroto, and Pbert, "Dispositional Optimism," 1996.

27. Ibid.

28. Kivumaki et al., "Optimism and Pessimism as Predictors of Change," 413.

29. Pat Hagan, "Is Optimism the Key to Good Health?" *BBC News* (January 2, 2005).

30. Norman Cousins, *Head First: The Biology of Hope* (New York: E. P. Dutton, 1989), 217.

31. Janet S. de Moor et al., "Optimism, Distress, Health-Related Quality of Life, and Change in Cancer Antigen 125 Among Patients with Ovarian Cancer Undergoing Chemotherapy," *Psychosomatic Medicine* 68 (2006): 555–62.

32. Hagan, "Is Optimism the Key to Good Health?"

33. E. Frank Lawlis and Jeanne Achterberg, *Imagery and Disease* (Champaign, IL: Institute for Personality and Ability Testing, 1984).
34. Hagan, "Is Optimism the Key to Good Health?"
35. Ibid.
36. "Optimism Helps Quality, Not Length, of Life for Cancer Patients," *The Wall Street Journal* (October 22, 2007).
37. Adam Khan, "Optimism Is Healthy," http://www.youmeworks.com/optimismishealthy.html, accessed June 2, 2008.
38. Jabs, "New Reasons to Be an Optimist," 171.
39. Benita Jackson, Robert M. Sellers, and Christopher Peterson, "Pessimistic Explanatory Style Moderates the Effect of Stress on Physical Illness," *Personality and Individual Differences,* 32, no. 3 (February 2002): 567–73.
40. Devera Pine, "Cruising Attitude," *Health* (August 1987): 20.
41. Karina Davidson and Kenneth Prkachin, "Optimism and Unrealistic Optimism Have an Interacting Impact on Health-Promoting Behavior and Knowledge Changes," *Personality and Social Psychology Bulletin* 23, no. 6 (June 1997): 617–25.
42. David K. Ingledew and Stuart Brunning, "Personality, Preventive Health Behaviour and Comparative Optimism about Health Problems," *Journal of Health Psychology* 4, no. 2 (1999): 193–208.
43. Lisa G. Aspinwall and Susanne M. Brunhart, "Distinguishing Optimism from Denial: Optimistic Beliefs Predict Attention to Health Threats," *Personality and Social Psychology Bulletin* 22, no. 10 (October 1996): 993–1003.
44. Adam Khan and Klassy Evans, *Self-Help Stuff That Works*, 3rd Edition (YouMe Works, January 1999), 12–4.
45. Kivumaki et al., "Optimism and Pessimism as Predictors of Change," 413.
46. Nadine Smity, Anne Young, and Christina Lee, "Optimism, Health-Related Hardiness and Well-Being Among Older Australian Women," *Journal of Health Psychology* 9, no. 6 (2004): 741–52.
47. Michael Greenberg, "High-Rise Public Housing, Optimism, and Personal and Environmental Health Behaviors," *American Journal of Health Behavior* 21, no. 5 (September/October 1997): 388–98.
48. Ibid.
49. Ibid.
50. Ibid.
51. Kymberley K. Bennett and Marta Elliot, "Pessimistic Explanatory Style and Cardiac Health: What Is the Relation and the Mechanism that Links Them?" *Basic and Applied Social Psychology* 27, no. 3 (September 2005): 239–48.
52. Bernie Zilbergeld and Arnold A. Lazarus, "Use Your Head," *Shape* (June 1988): 115, 146–52.
53. Clive Wood, "Optimism and Health: Expecting the Best," *Mind/Body/Health Digest* 1, no. 3 (1990): 3.
54. Ibid.
55. Jean Seligman and Linda Buckley, "A Sickroom with a View," *Newsweek* (March 26, 1990): 61.
56. Rebecca Stephens, "Imagery: A Strategic Intervention to Empower Clients," *Clinical Nurse Specialist* 7, no. 4 (1993): 170–1.
57. *Applied Psycho-physiology and Biofeedback.* 11, no. 1 (March 1986).
58. Ranard, "The World Through Rose-Colored Glasses," 59.
59. Anthes, "How Do You See This Glass?"

60. Kivumaki et al., "Optimism and Pessimism as Predictors of Change."
61. Suzanne C. Segerstrom, Shelley E. Taylor, Margaret E. Kemeny, and John L. Fahey, "Optimism Is Associated with Mood, Coping, and Immune Change in Response to Stress," *Journal of Personality and Social Psychology* 74, no. 6 (June 26, 1998): 1252–65.
62. Will Stapp, "Imagine Yourself Well," *Medical Self-Care* (January/February 1988): 27–30.
63. Ibid.
64. Ibid.
65. "Expert Hopeful About AIDS Therapy," *Deseret News* (June 20, 1991): A8.
66. Scott DeGarmo, "Optimism: The Secret Weapon," *Success* (July/August 1987): 4.
67. Eric Olsen, "Why Optimists Win," *Success* (December 1988) 32.
68. Ibid.
69. Jill Neimark, "The Power of Positive Thinking," *Success* (September 1987) 38–47.
70. Faelten et al., *Take Control of Your Life*, 309.
71. Julia Van Tine, "Become an Optimist," *Prevention* 50, no. 6 (June 1998): 32.
72. "Squelching Stress with Optimism," *Men's Health* (September 1987): 3, summarizing information from the *Journal of Personality and Psychology* 51, no. 6 (1987).
73. Editors of *Prevention* Magazine Health Books, *The Complete Book of Cancer Prevention* (Emmaus, PA: Rodale Press), 495.
74. Ornstein and Sobel, *Healthy Pleasures*, 168.
75. Blair Justice, "Think Yourself Healthy," *Prevention* (June 1988): 31–2, 105–8.
76. Paul Raeburn, "A Case for Double-Edged Optimism," *Psychology Today* (January 2007).
77. Ibid.
78. Suzanne C. Segerstrom, "Optimism and Resources," *Personality* 41, issue 4 (August 2007): 772–86.
79. David Burns, *Feeling Good* (New York: Avon Books–HarperCollins, 1999).
80. Daniel Goleman and Joel Gurin, eds., *Mind/Body Medicine: How to Use Your Mind for Better Health* (New York: Consumer Reports Books, 1993), 364.
81. Cousins, *Head First*, 68–9.

Explanatory Style and Health

An optimist may see a light where there is none, but why must the pessimist always run to blow it out?

—Michel de Saint-Pierre

- Define *explanatory style*.
- Describe the effects of explanatory style.
- Understand the effects of explanatory style on physical and mental health.
- Discuss the effects of explanatory style on immune function.

It's the first baseball game of the summer, but the sultry afternoon is unusually hot for June. The sun hangs lazily above the western horizon and you absentmindedly wipe the moisture from your forehead with the back of your hand. In an effort to get some relief from the heat, you lift your frosty soft drink to your lips. Take a look at it. Is it half empty? Or is it half full? Your answer reveals what researchers call your explanatory style—and it can help determine your physical and mental health.

What Is Explanatory Style?

Explanatory style is the way in which people perceive or explain the events in their lives. It's the habitual way in which people explain the bad things that happen to them. In reality, it's a habit—a way of thinking that people use when all other factors are equal and when there are no clear-cut right and wrong answers.

The concept of explanatory style was proposed in 1978 as an extension of the classical theory of learned helplessness or hopelessness.[1] According to Martin E. P. Seligman, "Explanatory style is much more specific and scientifically testable than mood. It focuses on three dimensions of our accounting for the good and bad events in our lives. Pessimists attribute bad events, such as the loss of a job, the breakup of a marriage, or a falling-out with a friend, to causes that are long-lasting or permanent, that are pervasive and affect everything they do, and that are their own fault. Optimists see the causes of such events as temporary, limited to the present case and the result of circumstances, bad luck, or other people's actions. A pessimist sees success at work, in love, or in friendship as due to luck; an optimist, as due to his or her own efforts and skill."[2]

Imagine that a driver skids into a school bus on a snowy day. The person with the pessimistic explanatory style moans, "I am the world's worst driver! It is beyond my ability to drive safely. I always foul things up!" The person with the optimistic explanatory style thinks, "I'm just a beginner, and beginners have to expect a banged fender once in a while. I'll have to be extra careful until I'm a little more practiced. Besides, these roads sure are slick! And the snow made it so it was difficult to see exactly where I was and how far I had to stop."[3]

The person with the pessimistic explanatory style interprets one negative event as an "omen," a sign as to how the rest of his or her life will turn out. The person with the optimistic explanatory style sees an isolated bad event as just that: isolated.

People with a pessimistic explanatory style can be identified by three thought patterns that give clues about what they're thinking in their conversation:

1. Pessimists assume the problem is stable, as unchangeable or never-ending. They are sure "it will never go away" instead of "it's a one-time thing." The pessimistic snowy-day driver, for example, believes that "I'll never learn to drive safely" in the snow.

2. Pessimists believe the problem is global, that it affects a broad spectrum of activities instead of an isolated incident.[4] The snowy-day driver opines, "Every time I try something new, I screw it up." A pessimist believes that a bad event "is going to ruin my whole life" instead of seeing a bad event as something with a specific cause that "has no bearing on the rest of my life."

3. Pessimists internalize everything. They believe everything is "my fault." The snowy-day driver is convinced that the accident happened because "I'm a bad driver." In contrast, the person with an optimistic explanatory style ascribes the accident to slick roads, poor visibility, some other adverse weather conditions, or merely a spot of bad luck—being in the wrong place at the wrong time.

To sum it up, pessimists tend to attribute their problems to permanent personal inadequacies that undermine everything they do; those with a pessimistic explanatory style are much more prone to depression. Optimists usually view a setback as a one-time thing attributable to bad luck, some external factor, or at least to a specific cause that can be remedied.[5] Optimists take broad credit for good outcomes and narrow responsibility for bad outcomes; pessimists, on the other hand, blame themselves broadly for bad outcomes and attribute good outcomes to external factors.[6]

University of Pennsylvania psychologist Martin Seligman describes it neatly: "Explanatory style is a theory about your past, your future, and your place in the world."[7] Once you've formulated your theory, he adds, you tend to find evidence for it in any situation that comes along.

While optimism and pessimism generally fall somewhere along a continuum, there are fairly specific differences between those with an optimistic explanatory style and those with a pessimistic explanatory style.[8] Those with an optimistic style:

- Adopt an internal locus of control when things go well and an external locus of control when things go badly
- Are hopeful
- Work hard and persist in order to overcome obstacles
- Seek advancement
- Inspire others
- Are bold and adventurous
- Explore, seize possibilities, and discount or dismiss risks
- Recover quickly from setbacks
- Are unlikely to suffer from depression

Though all that seems rosy, there can actually be a negative side to unbridled optimism. Unwarranted optimism can result in an unearned or undeserved sense of pride. Too much optimism can cause people to avoid responsibility, take unwise risks, become reckless, or make unrealistic plans. It can also result in aggrandizement and egotism.

Those with a pessimistic style:

- Adopt an external locus of control when things go well and an internal locus of control when things go badly
- Have a keen sense of reality
- Are skeptical and defensive
- Are cautious and timid
- Highlight and emphasize risks, seeking to protect themselves and others
- Are conservative
- Recover slowly—if at all—from setbacks, and tend to wallow in defeat

Excessive pessimism can result in unwarranted fear, anxiety, guilt, or shame. It can also cause inaction, passive behavior, and depression.

Paul Rosch, president of the American Institute of Stress, used the example of a roller-coaster ride to illustrate the difference between someone with an optimistic and a pessimistic explanatory style: "Look at how two people might experience a roller-coaster ride. One has his back stiffened, his knuckles are white, his eyes shut, jaws clenched, just waiting for it to be over. The wide-eyed thrill seeker relishes every plunge, can't wait to do it again."[9]

How Permanent Is Explanatory Style?

Once you've developed an explanatory style, are you stuck with it forever? This question evokes considerable controversy among the nation's leading researchers. Many believe that we stick to one explanatory style throughout our lives. Some evidence does exist to support that notion.

Other research indicates that explanatory style is learned, not inherited—and, as a learned behavior, there is the potential for change. According to research, there are three main sources from which we learn explanatory behavior:[10]

1. The mother (or other primary caregiver). If a mother consistently blames herself or her child when bad things happen, the child will pick up on those cues and develop a pessimistic explanatory style.

2. Other adults who care for, discipline, teach, and criticize a child (including parents, teachers, and other influential adults). If these consistently blame the child, his personality, or his character when bad things happen, the child quickly learns to use personal and permanent explanations when things go wrong.

3. Tragic life crises. A child who experiences a crisis—loss of a parent, the divorce of parents, extreme poverty, abuse, or loss of the home—will notice whether the crisis gets resolved after an appropriate period of time or whether the effects appear likely to last forever. A child who sees that adversity is temporary and can be overcome tends to develop an optimistic explanatory style.

The University of Pennsylvania, psychologist Martin Seligman, doesn't think that explanatory style—of even bad events—has to stay the same. Seligman, a pioneer in psychoneuroimmunology research, is convinced that explanatory style, which is basically a belief system, can be changed. Results of his work demonstrate that people can be trained to change their outlook.[11]

What Are the Effects of Explanatory Style?

Regardless of whether researchers believe that a basic explanatory style can be changed, they do agree on one thing: explanatory style has an extremely powerful influence on health and wellness. According to research found in *Health and Optimism*, certain kinds of thoughts are more powerful in predicting health and wellness:

- Manifest thoughts and beliefs
- Explanations for setbacks and disappointments
- What someone thinks about the real world—its events, their causes, and their aftermath
- Thoughts that are responsive to other people
- Beliefs that lead to action[12]

Explanatory style, says Seligman, works like a self-fulfilling prophecy. The way a person "explains events in his life can predict and determine his future," Seligman explains. "Those who believe they are the masters of their fate are more likely to succeed than those who attribute events to forces beyond their control."[13]

In referring to explanatory style, William Wilbanks, professor of criminal justice at Florida International University, refers to "the New Obscenity. It's not a four-letter word, but an oft-repeated statement that strikes at the very core of our humanity. The four words are: 'I can't help myself.'"[14] This kind of explanatory style, says Wilbanks, "sees man as an organism being acted upon by biological and social forces, rather than as an agent with a free will. It views offenders not as sinful or criminal but as 'sick.' By ignoring the idea that people face temptations that can—and should—be resisted, it denies the very quality that separates us from the animals."

The Influence of Explanatory Style on Health

Yale surgeon Dr. Bernie Siegel maintains that a negative explanatory style is harmful to the body. On the other hand, he says, an optimistic explanatory style and the positive emotions it embraces—such as love, acceptance, and forgiveness—stimulate the immune system and kick the body's own healing systems into gear. An optimistic explanatory style sends "live" messages to your body and helps promote the healing process.[15]

Interestingly, people with an optimistic explanatory style often believe that they are less at risk for serious health problems. Research that measured explanatory style among adults also shows that those with an optimistic explanatory style also believe that they are better able to prevent health problems.[16] Research shows that our own opinion about the state of our health is an even better predictor of health than objective factors, such as what a physician can determine through laboratory tests. It's even a better predictor than behaviors, such as cigarette smoking. For example, people in one study who smoked cigarettes were twice as likely to die during the next twelve years as people who did not smoke. But people who thought they were in "poor" health were seven times as likely to die as those who thought they were in "excellent" health.[17]

Although it's essential to have an optimistic explanatory style, says Siegel, it's also crucial to use that explanatory style to deal with the realities in life:

> Learning to let go of negative emotions is the key. The person who smiles on the outside and is hurting on the inside is not dealing with himself or his life. All his "live" mechanisms are told to stop working. Doctors see examples of this every day. You are making rounds at the hospital and you ask a patient how she's doing and she says "Fine." But you know she's not doing fine. Her husband ran off with another woman. Her son is on drugs. And she has cancer. But still she says, "Fine." When I find a person who answers, "Lousy," I say, "That's wonderful! You want to get better so you're dealing with the truth. If your mind and body are feeling lousy and you're relating to that, you'll ask for help."[18]

Impact on Mental Health

According to the most recent research, explanatory style can have a tremendous impact on mental health—and the explanatory style that is considered "normal" is probably much more optimistic than what researchers once believed it was. According to researchers writing in the *Psychological Bulletin*, it was once considered "normal" for people to have accurate perceptions of themselves, the world, and their future; this was a quality considered essential for good mental health. Recent research, however, indicates that "overly positive" evaluations of self, "exaggerated" perceptions of control, and "unrealistic optimism" are characteristic of normal human thought.[19] (See Chapter 16 for a further discussion of this.)

The kind of optimistic explanatory style that researchers describe helps promote other aspects of mental health—the ability to care about others, the ability to be happy or contented, and the ability to engage in productive or creative work—because it "distorts" incoming information in a positive direction and dilutes negative input until it is no longer threatening. All in all, say researchers, an optimistic explanatory style helps people adapt in a healthy way when something negative or stressful happens.

A pessimistic explanatory style, on the other hand, can lead to depression. Princeton University psychologists Susan Nolen-Hoeksema and Joan Girgus demonstrated that explanatory style was a much more important factor in depression than was mood—and that explanatory style is much more permanent than mood. In their study, Nolen-Hoeksema and Girgus repeatedly tested third, fourth, and fifth graders on both mood and explanatory style. The kids who started out in a momentarily happy mood but who had a pessimistic explanatory style were depressed within three months of the time the study began. The ones who had an optimistic explanatory style but who were depressed for some reason in the month the study began tended to bounce back and feel upbeat and happy three months later.[20]

A pessimistic explanatory style can also lead to other negative mental states, including anger. Research that looked at students in their first year of high school found that pessimistic explanatory style was directly related to higher and more intense levels of anger among both young men and young women. Among the young men, it was also related to more frequent episodes of destructive school behavior, though that correlation was not seen among the young women.[21]

According to researchers, a pessimistic explanatory style can lead to anxiety, eating disorders, and a number of emotional problems. It also leads to what researchers call dysphoria—a variety of negative emotional states that cause you to "just feel bad." That dysphoria can take the form of depression, anxiety, guilt, anger, or hostility.[22]

Impact on Physical Health

A growing body of evidence suggests that explanatory style can be a potent predictor of physical health. In one study involving 234 college students at a midsized western university, researchers found that a pessimistic explanatory style was strongly related to experiences of illness—those with a pessimistic explanatory style had much higher rates of illness.[23] A pessimistic explanatory style can also cause other factors to have a more pronounced impact on health. One study involving college students showed that stress had an even more negative impact on health—leading to even greater risk of physical illness—when coupled with negative explanatory style.[24]

Explanatory style also affects the way the body reacts to surgery. After years of medical practice, one surgeon vowed that he would never operate on a patient who believed he (or she) would die because that's what always happened. In one study designed to measure the impact of explanatory style on surgical outcomes, researchers asked patients six to twelve months before their surgery was to take place to rate their expectations of surgery and the problems associated with surgery.[25] The patients' attitudes and expectations about the surgery (their explanatory style) turned out to be powerful predictors. The patients who expected fewer problems had better outcomes. The ones who expected more problems got exactly that. Two years later they had physical problems, dissatisfaction with the surgery, and mood disturbances.

People with pessimistic explanatory styles have a tendency to blame themselves for anything bad that happens to them. That tendency can interfere with health, recovery, and healing. In one study, researchers analyzed the hospital reports of people who were hospitalized for the treatment of acute burns. People with pessimistic explanatory styles tended to blame themselves for the burn—and also had more pain, greater depression, and less compliance with the instructions of nurses and physical therapists.[26]

University of Georgia Researcher James Dabbs studied a group of male college students to determine the effects of explanatory style on health. He found that the optimists in the group had a higher level of the male hormone testosterone, which, he says, provides evidence that optimism and explanatory style influence our secretion of hormones.[27]

Attitude and explanatory style can even impact the circulatory system and the outlook for people with coronary heart disease. Sophisticated instruments and testing procedures have enabled researchers to watch the brain in action. Blood flow in the brain literally changes as thoughts, feelings, and attitudes change. The results of a variety of studies show that people with pessimistic explanatory styles are at increased risk of atherosclerosis, blockage of coronary arteries, and heart attack.

Study results reported to the Society of Behavioral Medicine by Dr. Daniel Mark, a Duke University heart specialist, followed up on 1,719 men and women who had undergone heart catheterization, a common procedure to check for clogging of the arteries. All of the people in the study had heart disease. Those with pessimistic explanatory style (the ones who doubted they would recover) fared much more poorly than those with an optimistic style. Of the pessimists, 12 percent were dead within a year—more than twice as many as the 5 percent of the optimists. In summing up the study, Mark emphasized that "the mind is a tremendous tool or weapon, depending on your point of view."

In another study, researchers found that those with an optimistic explanatory style also had much better results following coronary bypass surgery. One of the most dangerous complications following coronary bypass surgery is high blood pressure. In this study, people with optimistic explanatory styles had better attitudes about the surgery, had more favorable pulse rates after surgery, and had less hypertension after surgery. High blood pressure following surgery was reduced from 75 percent to less than 45 percent among those with healthy attitudes. An optimistic explanatory style also strongly affects the pace of recuperation, the incidence of complications, and the overall outcome of the surgery.[28]

Explanatory style may even enable researchers to predict which people will get sick. In one study, Martin Seligman and his colleagues at the University of Pennsylvania rated 172 undergraduate students on what kind of explanatory style they had. The researchers then predicted which ones would get sick. After a month, they found their predictions were right on. A year later, their predictions still held true.[29]

People with an optimistic explanatory style have better health for a number of factors. Some of those factors include stronger immunity, good social support, and a willingness to continue better health habits.[30] Another reason, say researchers, is that people with a pessimistic explanatory style generally react to illness with helplessness and a lack of fighting spirit—factors that have in themselves been linked to poor health.[31]

A Healthy Style, a Healthy Immune System

As alluded to earlier, one of the reasons an optimistic explanatory style leads to better health may be that an optimistic style tends to increase the strength of the immune system. Robert Good, former president and director of the Memorial Sloan-Kettering Cancer Hospital in New York, maintains that an optimistic explanatory style and the positive attitude it fosters can actually alter our ability to resist "infections, allergies, autoimmunities, or even cancer."[32]

According to researchers, the hypothalamic control center of the brain—the part that is involved in attitudes and outlook—is directly "wired" to the immune system. If a portion of the hypothalamus is electrically stimulated, antibodies increase; if it is cut, immune activity is depressed. The same thing happens in response to thoughts, beliefs, and imaginations, things that are "not ephemeral abstractions but electrochemical events with physiological consequences."[33] Siegel mirrors that belief and points out that positive emotions and attitudes actually stimulate the immune system.

Michael A. Lerner, the founder of Commonweal, a cancer hospice in southern California, and a MacArthur Foundation Genius Award winner, says the attitudes linked to an optimistic explanatory style can even boost the immune system enough to defeat cancer: "Attitudes themselves have a very potent effect on the immune system. You become different than the person who developed the cancer. Becoming a different personality may change the environment the cancer grew in; it may become so inhospitable that the cancer shrinks."[34]

Explanatory style may have enough influence over the immune system to affect even infectious disease resistance. Apparently, optimistic explanatory style may not have as much preventive effect as pessimistic explanatory style has a deleterious effect on the immune system. Using a questionnaire considered to be the predominant measure of explanatory style, Brennan and Charnestski first determined what kind of explanatory style each person in the study had. They then took samples of saliva from each study participant and measured the amount of immunoglobulin A (Ig-A), a primary determinant of immunity to infectious disease. Those with optimistic explanatory style didn't necessarily have higher levels of Ig-A, but those with pessimistic explanatory style had much lower levels of Ig-A in their saliva, leading researchers to conclude that pessimistic explanatory style is related to both immune system deficits and poor health.[35]

In one study, psychologist Stanislav Kasl and his colleagues at Yale University followed the development of infectious mononucleosis among a group of West Point cadets.[36] During a four-year period, all cadets entering West Point were given blood tests that screened for the presence of antibodies to the Epstein-Barr virus, the agent that causes mononucleosis. The cadets were also given interviews that included questions about their outlook, their expectations, and their family backgrounds.

About one in five of the susceptible cadets were infected—but only about one-fourth of those actually got sick. The ones who did get sick had a number of threads in common, including a pessimistic explanatory style, high expectations (usually centered in pressure from parents), and poor academic performance.

In a separate set of studies, researchers conducting studies at Yale University and the University of Pennsylvania compared immune function and explanatory style among a group of elderly people. According to the researchers, people with a pessimistic explanatory style had suppressed immune function.[37] Specifically, said the researchers, the ratio of helper T cells and suppressor T cells was low, as was the number of lymphocytes, which arm the body for waging war against infection or disease.

According to research, a pessimistic explanatory style can depress immunity. Scientists from the University of Pennsylvania, Yale University, and Sydney's Prince of Wales Hospital involved elderly men and women in a study designed to determine the effect of explanatory style on immunity. According to researchers, those with a pessimistic explanatory style had a lower ratio of helper T cells to suppressor T cells and had a poorer T cell response when their immune system was challenged.[38]

One technique that uses an ABCDE mnemonic was developed by Dr. Albert Ellis to help people overcome a tendency to pessimism:[39]

- **Adversity:** when adversity happens—as it always will—think about what caused it.
- **Belief:** determine how you explain the failure to yourself.
- **Consequences:** If you have a negative belief (pessimistic explanatory style) about what caused the event, realize those negative beliefs will have consequences—you might feel shame, get depressed, or feel overwhelmed.
- **Dispute** your negative beliefs. Create more accurate, objective beliefs to explain the adversity.
- **Energize** yourself through your new optimistic outlook.

To sum up the research, scientists have found direct evidence that a pessimistic style and a sense of helplessness may depress the immune system and decrease resistance. An optimistic style that allows for a sense of control boosts immunity. The end result does indeed depend on whether you see the glass as half full or half empty.

WHAT DID YOU LEARN?

1. What is *explanatory style*?
2. What are the health effects of explanatory style?
3. How does explanatory style affect the immune system?

ENDNOTES

1. Francis X. Brennan and Carl J. Charnetski, "Explanatory Style and Immunoglobulin A (IgA)," *Integrative Physiological and Behavioral Science*, (October 2000).
2. Morton Hunt, "Don't Worry, Be Happy," *Longevity* (December 1991): 80.
3. Example is from Joan Borysenko, *Minding the Body, Mending the Mind* (Reading, MA: Addison-Wesley Publishing Company, 1987), 120.
4. Christopher Peterson, George E. Vaillant, and Martin E. P. Seligman, "Pessimistic Explanatory Style Is a Risk Factor for Physical Illness: A Thirty-Five-Year Longitudinal Study," *Journal of Personality and Social Psychology* 55, no. 1 (1988): 23.
5. Carolyn Jabs, "New Reasons to Be an Optimist," *Self* (September 1987): 170–3.

6. "Learned Helplessness," *Emotional Competency,* http://www.emotionalcompetency.com/helpless. htm, accessed July 2, 2008.

7. Jabs, "New Reasons to Be an Optimist."

8. Characteristics in the two following bulleted lists from "Learned Helplessness," *Emotional Competency.*

9. "Good Stress: Why You Need It to Stay Young," *Prevention* (April 1986): 28–32.

10. "Learned Helplessness," *Emotional Competency.*

11. Martin E. P. Seligman, *Learned Optimism* (New York: Alfred A. Knopf, 1991), 178.

12. Christopher Peterson and Lisa M. Bossio, *Health and Optimism* (New York: Free Press, 1991), 60.

13. Seligman, *Learned Optimism.*

14. William Lee Wilbanks, "The New Obscenity," *Reader's Digest,* December 1988, 23.

15. "Mind over Cancer: An Exclusive Interview with Yale Surgeon Dr. Bernie Siegel," *Prevention* (March 1988): 59–64.

16. Christopher Peterson and Mechele E. De Avila, "Optimistic Explanatory Style and the Perception of Health Problems," *Journal of Clinical Psychology* 51 (1):128–32, 2006.

17. Larry Dossey, *Meaning and Medicine: A Doctor's Tales of Breakthrough and Healing* (New York: Bantam Books, 1991), 16.

18. "Mind over Cancer."

19. S. E. Taylor and J. D. Brown, "Illusion and Well-Being: A Social Psychological Perspective on Mental Health," *Psychological Bulletin* 103(2): 1988, 193–210.

20. Nan Silver, "Do Optimists Live Longer?" *American Health,* November 1986, 50–53.

21. Peter Boman, Douglas C. Smith, and David Curtis, "Effects of Pessimism and Explanatory Style on Development of Anger in Children," *School Psychology International* 24 (1): 80–94, 2003.

22. Peterson and Bossio, *Health and Optimism,* 106.

23. Kymberley K. Bennett and Marta Elliott, "Explanatory Style and Health: Mechanisms Linking Pessimism to Illness," *Journal of Applied Social Psychology,* no. 32 (7): 1508–26, 2006.

24. Benita Jackson, Robert M. Sellers, and Christopher Peterson, "Pessimistic Explanatory Style Moderates the Effect of Stress on Physical Illness," *Personality and Individual Differences* 32 (3): 567–73, February 2002.

25. H. Asuman Kiyak, Peter P. Vitaliano, and Jeffrey Crinean, "Patients' Expectations as Predictors of Orthognathic Surgery Outcomes," *Health Psychology* 7 (3): 1988, 251–68.

26. Janice K. Kiecolt-Glaser and D. A. Williams, "Self-Blame, Compliance, and Distress Among Burn Patients," *Journal of Personality and Social Psychology* 53 (1): 1987, 187–93.

27. Peterson and Bossio, *Health and Optimism,* 99.

28. Joseph Lederer, "Surgery: A Mind-Body Event," *Mind/Body/Health Digest* 1 (4): 1–4.

29. Dossey, *Meaning and Medicine.*

30. Seligman, *Learned Optimism,* 173–74.

31. Emily H. Lin and Christopher Peterson, "Pessimistic Explanatory Style and Response to Illness," *Behavioral Research Therapy* 28 (3): 1990, 243–48.

32. Blair Justice, "Think Yourself Healthy," *Prevention,* May 1988, 27–32, 102, 107.

33. Ibid.

34. Daniel Goleman, "The Mind over the Body," *New Realities,* March/April 1988, 14–19.

35. Francis X. Brennan and Carl J. Charnetski, "Explanatory Style and Immunoglobulin A (IgA)," *Integrative Physiological and Behavioral Science,* October 2000.

36. Robert Ornstein and David Sobel, "The Healing Brain," *Psychology Today,* March 1987, 48–52.

37. Leslie Kamen-Siegel, Judith Rodin, Martin E. P. Seligman, and John Dwyer, "Explanatory Style and Cell-Mediated Immunity in Elderly Men and Women," *Health Psychology* 10 (4): 1991, 229–35.

38. Ibid.

39. "Learned Helplessness," accessed July 2, 2008.

CHAPTER 18

Locus of Control, Self-Esteem, and Health

How shall I be able to rule over others when I have not full power and command over myself?

—François Rabelais

We can secure other people's approval, if we do right and try hard; but our own is worth a hundred of it.

—Mark Twain

LEARNING OBJECTIVES

- Relate how locus of control has been recognized throughout history.
- Discuss the factors that impact locus of control.
- Describe how locus of control and hardiness are related.
- Understand the influence of locus of control on health.
- Describe how control mitigates the effects of stress.
- Understand the effects of control on immunity and healing.
- Define *self-esteem*.
- Understand what factors impact self-esteem.
- Describe the impact of self-esteem on the body.
- Define *self-efficacy*, and understand how it differs from self-esteem.

Locus of Control

Noted psychologist Martin Seligman paints for us what he calls the infant's "dance of development." In it, the good mother mirrors and responds to the actions of her infant son or daughter. The baby smiles, and the mother smiles. The baby coos or gurgles with delight, and the mother does the same. The baby cries with hunger, and the mother responds with the warm sweetness of milk. Through this "dance of development," Seligman says, infants learn that they have control. And, through the sense of control that results, infants learn that they can ensure their own survival.[1]

What Does *Locus of Control* Mean?

What, exactly, is a sense of control, and why is it so important to health? The concept of a locus of control originated in the 1950s with the work of Julian Rotter; it involves the belief that our own actions will be effective enough to control or master the environment.[2] Control does not mean that we need to control everything around us—such as other people, the environment, or our circumstances, whether good or bad. Control does entail a deep-seated belief that we can impact a situation by how we look at the problem.[3] We can choose how we react and how we respond. If we regard a loss with gloom and doom, we allow it to hurt us; if we view it as a chance for growth and opportunity, we minimize its ability to hurt us.

Suzanne O. Kobasa and Salvatore Maddi, renowned for their research into what makes us "hardy" and able to resist disease, theorize that a sense of control is crucial to health. They say that those "high in control believe and act as if they can influence the events of their experience, rather than being powerless in the face of outside forces." That kind of attitude allows people to take responsibility and act effectively on their own.[4]

Regarding a sense of control, it's not an "either/or" proposition but rather a continuum. At one end of the continuum is the "external locus of control"; at the opposite end is the "internal locus of control." Where a person is along the continuum influences his or her health.

People with an external locus of control believe that the things that happen to them are unrelated to their own behavior—and, subsequently, beyond their control.[5] At the opposite end of the spectrum are the people with an "internal locus of control." These people believe that negative events are a consequence of personal actions, and can thus be potentially controlled.[6] As S. I. McMillen defines them, "Internals believe that their own actions have a large influence on what happens to them. If they get fired from a job, internals believe that when they go out to look for a job they will be able to find one. They do not give up; rather, they hope for a brighter future."[7]

An excellent example is a college student. The one with an internal sense of control believes that she got good grades because she worked hard, studied when her friends were out partying, applied herself, and refused to give up. She's apt to study hard and apply herself again. The one with an external sense of control believes his bad grade in physics was the fault of a teaching assistant who designed poor tests, a professor who graded capriciously, and a string of bad luck. He's not likely to study hard and apply himself; after all, according to his belief system, his level of hard work really has no impact on his grades. As researcher Phillip Rice so aptly put it, "If the theme song of the external is 'Cast Your Fate to the Winds,' the theme song of the internal is 'I Did It My Way.'"[8]

Bringing those definitions together, then, a *health locus of control* is the degree to which we believe our health is controlled by internal or external factors. The most healthful attitude, of course, is one in which we believe that our health is directly the result of our behavior—because then we are free to change factors within our control to influence the outcome of our health.

Research findings have summarized the differences between those with an internal and an external locus of control. Those with an internal locus of control:

- Are more likely to work for achievements
- Will more willingly tolerate a delay in reward
- Generally plan for long-term goals
- Lower expectations of success and re-evaluate future performances after failing at a task
- Are better able to resist coercion
- Can more easily tolerate ambiguity
- Are less prone to depression, helplessness, and anxiety
- Realize greater benefits from social supports
- Prefer games based on skill
- Are more prone to guilt
- Are more willing to take risks
- Are more likely to embark on self-improvement programs
- Recover more rapidly in terms of mental health when adjusting to a physical disability

Those with an external locus of control:

- Are more likely to lower their goals if an achievement appears too daunting
- Raise their expectations after failing at a task
- Are less likely to tolerate delayed gratification
- Are more prone to plan for short-term goals but avoid planning for long-term goals
- Are more prone to learned helplessness and depression
- Are less willing to take risks
- Are less likely to work on self-improvement programs or tasks
- Prefer games based on chance or luck

A Brief History of Control

Philosopher and researcher Leonard Sagan—an epidemiologist at Stanford University—believes that an external locus of control dominated many cultures throughout a significant period of the world's history. As he states,

> Almost universally, the social adjustment to poverty and helplessness has been the adoption of a fatalistic, authoritarian world view: "These events are out of our hands, they are in the hands of God." Children are taught that bad outcomes are the result of forces beyond their control, that life must be lived in the present, since, in an incalculable world, individual effort counts for naught.

[This] pervading sense of helplessness dominated the human condition throughout history—until the Enlightenment. The Enlightenment encouraged the attitude that all natural phenomena operate in conformance with universal physical-chemical properties and are predictable, not the result of whimsical divine forces. If men could understand those principles, they could control their environment and their destiny. These were heady and revolutionary thoughts, unique in human history.[9]

As mentioned earlier, the locus of control concept evolved in the 1950s from the work of Ohio State University researcher Julian B. Rotter, who developed a framework known as the *social learning theory* of personality.[10] Basically, that theory said that in order for behavior to occur in any given situation, the person needs to believe that the behavior will be reinforced—and that the reinforcement will be of value. The reinforcement is a consequence that immediately follows the behavior; it can either add to the positive or take away some of the negative.

Students studying under Rotter developed a theory of what they called *expectancy shifts*. Those with a "typical expectancy shift" believed that a success would be followed by another success, and a failure would be followed by another failure—and they attributed the outcome of success or failure to their own abilities (what we now know as an internal locus of control). Those with an "atypical expectancy shift" believed that success would be followed by failure, and failure would be followed by success—and they attributed these outcomes to luck or chance (what we now know as an external locus of control).

In 1966, Rotter summarized a decade of previously unpublished work of his and his students in a paper published in a professional journal.[11] During the next two decades, other researchers added to Rotter's model; for example, one pointed out that there are both stable and unstable factors in each type of belief. (For an internal locus of control, for example, ability would be a stable cause, while effort would be an unstable cause; for an external locus of control, difficulty of the task would be a stable cause, while luck would be an unstable cause.) In later articles, Rotter discussed misconceptions about his work and criticized some of what he saw as misguided attempts of others in trying to use the internal/external locus of control construct.[12]

Taking it a step further, another group of researchers proposed what they called *attributional style*. Basically, it said that people explained successes and failures in their lives based on three things: whether the factors were within or outside their control; whether the factors were short term or long term; and whether these factors affected all situations in their lives.

The concept of control is important to health, and its best-known application has been in the area of health psychology. Sagan maintains that life expectancy increased by more than 30 years during the last century because we have more control over our lives—due to factors like police and fire departments, insurance against loss, and a steady and reliable food supply. Because "we can foresee, avoid, and mitigate problems," he points out, "we have more resources to adapt and cope with them."[13] We have a greater sense of control over our environments.

What Is the Source of Control?

Research shows that an internal locus of control is strongly influenced by nurturing and accepting parents who provide consistent discipline; it is also related to higher socioeconomic status, with its variety of available resources.[14] Parental behavior patterns—such as being demanding of conformity or being overly critical and strict—are more common in lower socioeconomic families and may reflect a feeling of low control and insecurity among the parents, which can shape the personality development in the child and lead to an external locus of control.[15]

In addition to the influence of parents, a sense of increased control can come from a variety of sources:

1. Gaining information: people who are informed about a situation feel an increased sense of control because the situation becomes predictable and manageable

2. Adopting a less pessimistic outlook

3. Placing faith in someone or something we deeply trust

4. Learning new coping skills

5. Building a stronger support system

6. Being prepared: when people feel prepared for something, they perceive a much greater ability to control even a difficult situation[16]

The impact of preparation is illustrated beautifully by a study conducted on a Special Forces unit in Vietnam that was expecting an enemy attack.[17] An Army psychiatrist, researcher Peter Bourne, lived in the camp with the men and took blood samples daily. He measured the amount of an adrenal hormone that is normally present when a person is under extreme stress. It's difficult to imagine any situation much more stressful than anticipating an enemy attack in a war zone—but, to Bourne's surprise, the hormone levels of the men indicated that they were not experiencing any elevated stress. Other tests showed that the men had lower levels of anxiety and depression than even the basic recruits who were entering training.

What enabled these soldiers to rally so valiantly in such difficult circumstances? Bourne believes it was their sense of control. They gained that sense of control, he believes, by being prepared. The soldiers coped with the threat of impending battle by engaging in "a furor of activity," maintaining their equipment and building their defenses.

Only three men in the unit showed elevated stress hormones. They were the two officers and the radio operator who had to receive—and respond to—orders from a distant command post over which they had no control.

Hardiness and Control

Psychologists Suzanne Kobasa and Salvatore Maddi first developed the now-well-accepted theory that people who are able to stay healthy even while under stress have behaviors and personalities marked by "hardiness." One of the key components of hardiness, say the pair, is a sense of control. Dr. Arthur Schmale, a University of Rochester researcher, was one of the first to identify the importance of control; his research, paired with the work of Kobasa and Maddi, demonstrates the importance of control as a factor in health and well-being (see Chapter 8).

As a classic example, Schmale cites the case of a woman who was diagnosed with leukemia.[18] Her diagnosis came shortly before her husband's death from tuberculosis. She told her physician that she hoped to live until her son—then aged ten—was grown up and settled.

The course of leukemia can be charted by measuring red blood cell count; as her physician measured her red blood count over the years, he was interested to note a trend. At times when she felt in control, her disease lapsed into remission. At other times, when she felt that she was losing control, her disease intensified.

The leukemia soared, for example, as she entered menopause. It intensified, too, when she finally admitted that her second marriage was failing. It even came and went during various times of the year. For example, her disease became much worse every year about the time her physician was scheduled to take his annual summer vacation. Possibly she felt a dangerous loss of control in contemplating his absence.

The worst period of her disease occurred when her son left home to join the Army. Her condition became so critical that, for the first time since becoming ill, she required blood transfusions to stay alive. The four years while her son was in the military were extremely difficult for her. According to her physician, she required almost constant medical treatment and various hospitalizations just to keep the disease under control. When her son was released from the military, he announced that he was engaged to be married. Shortly afterward, she died. As her physician related, she would now have almost no control in her relationship to him.

According to Kobasa and Maddi and the other researchers who have since studied hardiness, it is earmarked by a sense of control. The control that characterizes hardiness is a belief that we can influence events coupled with a willingness to act on that belief rather than just be a victim of circumstances. It is not a desire or a need to be in control of situations or to control other people.

The Influence of Control on Health

The results of a host of studies show the importance of control. First, of course, is the concept itself. Those with an external locus of control believe that their health is either controlled by powerful others (such as medical professionals) or is determined by fate, luck, or chance. Health history can actually play a role, too: women with a history of frequent childhood illness or accidents are more likely to have an external sense of control regarding their health; they have little belief that they can control their health. Those who have experienced serious illness of a family member generally feel the same way.

While there is some disagreement among experts, researchers have fairly conclusively shown that those with an internal locus of control, on the other hand, believe that their health is the direct result of their own behaviors—and are more likely to adopt positive health behaviors as a result.[19] A study in Wales involving almost 12,000 people showed that those with an internal locus of control were much more likely to practice positive health behaviors, as measured by smoking, alcohol consumption, exercise, and diet.[20] In another study involving 7,000 university students from throughout Europe, researchers found that those with an internal locus of control were more likely—and those with an external locus of control were less likely—to engage in a number of positive health behaviors, including exercise, eating breakfast, brushing their teeth, wearing seatbelts, and eating a healthy diet that included fruits and fiber and limited salt and fats.[21] The "internals" were also less likely to smoke and had much lower alcohol consumption. It is widely accepted that an internal locus of control is significantly associated with knowledge about disease, the ability to stop smoking, the ability to lose weight, adherence to a medical regimen, effective use of birth control, getting preventive immunizations and vaccinations, getting regular dental check-ups, and wearing seat belts.[22]

As a whole, people with a greater sense of control are at less risk of illness. Research demonstrates that people who believe they have poor control over what happens in their lives are more likely to suffer from chronic illness.[23] One study showed that rheumatoid arthritis patients who had an internal locus of control had less pain and greater function than those with an external locus of control.[24] As new research is completed, scientists are realizing that an internal locus of control has an even more profound role in protecting health than we once thought.

Former *Saturday Review* editor Norman Cousins, renowned for his work linking attitudes and health, maintains that, in general:

> Anything that restores a sense of control to a patient can be a profound aid to a physician in treating serious illness. That sense of control is more than a mere mood or attitude, and may well be a vital pathway between the brain, the endocrine system, and the immune system. The assumed possibility is that it may serve as the basis for what may well be a profound advancement in the knowledge of how to confront the challenge of serious illness.[25]

A sense of control can affect health and well-being in a number of ways. Studies show that people with little sense of control—those who see their lives and futures controlled by luck or fate—suffer much greater psychological distress. These people, who believe that nothing they do will significantly change their circumstances or their reliance on "luck," have higher levels of depression and anxiety and are much less effective in dealing with chronic pain.[26]

A pilot study of long-term AIDS survivors conducted by Dr. George Solomon found that the survivors had a number of psychosocial characteristics in common—many of which pointed to an increased sense of control over their situation. The survivors were assertive, able to nurture themselves, actively involved with others who had the disease, and able to communicate openly about their needs, according to Caryle Hirshberg. In addition, says Hirshberg, the long-term AIDS survivors in the study took personal responsibility for the disease but did not perceive it as a death sentence; felt they could influence the outcome of the disease; had a sense of purpose; and took control by altering their lifestyles. Finally, many of the long-term AIDS survivors had successfully overcome a previous life-threatening illness—something that would certainly impart a sense of control.[27]

Control and Cardiovascular Health

Authorities on heart disease gathered in a forum on coronary-prone behavior concluded that slowing of the heart—which is seen in many situations in which people feel they have lost control—causes death, even though there are no apparently fatal physiological changes in the heart itself.[28]

Taking control, on the other hand, can have the opposite effect on health. According to a study reported in *Clinical Psychiatry News,*[29] researchers at the University of Connecticut School of Medicine observed a group of more than 200 heart attack survivors for eight years. The researchers noted that the patients who accepted the responsibility for their heart attacks had fewer second attacks than patients who blamed their genes, their spouse, or other factors. According to study leader Glenn Affleck, "The value in accepting responsibility for a heart attack could stem from its being a sign of taking control. Passing the buck, on the other hand, could be indicative of the very sort of thinking that may contribute to heart attacks in the first place—namely, feeling a lack of control. This, in turn, could lead to a feeling of helplessness in making adaptive lifestyle changes."

An internal locus of control has been shown to help people increase their physical activity, bring their weight closer to normal levels, and stop smoking—all of which have been shown to improve cardiovascular health.[30] Studies among heart attack patients showed that those with an internal locus of control were less depressed and more cooperative throughout the time they were being treated in the intensive care unit. On three of the most important measurements following heart attack, those with an internal locus of control did consistently better; in addition, their peak body temperature was lower, and they spent less time in the intensive care unit and in the hospital than did those with an external locus of control.[31]

Biochemical Imbalances

One reason why control has such a profound influence over health is that a lack of control disturbs the biochemical balance in the brain and body. An internal locus of control has a significant influence over the body's release of hormones, which has been found to be a powerful determinant of health. Three of the hormones influenced by a lack of control are:

- Serotonin, which regulates moods, relieves pain, and helps control release of the powerful pain-killing brain chemicals, the endorphins
- Dopamine, which is largely responsible for a sense of reward or pleasure
- Norepinephrine, which causes depression when depleted

Both norepinephrine and dopamine are critical to relaying nerve impulses from one neuron to another; they are essential to the nervous system's ability to "communicate" among its many cells. All three of these hormones are essential to activity, appetite, moods, sleep, sex, reinforcement, reward, and pleasure, and they play an important role in healthy mental functioning.[32]

When we feel little sense of control, the levels of norepinephrine, dopamine, and serotonin drop.[33] As a result, a disturbance in our sense of control can also seriously disturb our mental functioning, appetite, mood, sleep, sex drive, and senses of reinforcement, reward, and pleasure.

Furthermore, when we have little internal locus of control, the level of corticosteroids in our bloodstream soars. The corticosteroids, released by the body during stress, cause a variety of physical damage. They lower our resistance to disease and suppress the body's manufacture of norepinephrine, dopamine, and serotonin—making lack of control a double-edged sword.

Lack of Control Versus Stress

A lack of control may have an even stronger influence over health than do high levels of stress. Turning to a situation in which people often have little control, the workplace, researchers have found that those with little control suffer more severe health problems than do those with high levels of stress.

Researcher Rena Pasick, with the University of California School of Public Health, studied almost 800 working adults in Alameda County, California. She found a "significant association" between the amount of control on the job and health status.[34]

For example, upper-level management and other white-collar employees have been considered at highest risk because of the amount of stress and responsibility they have. However, Pasick's study showed that they actually enjoy better health than those they supervise or than blue-collar workers in general. This is because they have more control.[35]

Various studies among work populations have shown that lack of control can be deleterious to health. People with little control but high demands have more than three times the risk of heart disease and chronically escalated blood pressure than do people with few demands but a high level of control. Robert Karasek, an industrial engineering professor at Columbia University, has found that people who have little control over their jobs have higher rates of heart disease than do people who can dictate the style and pace of their work. Worst off are those whose work makes substantial psychological demands but offers little opportunity for independent decision making—occupations such as telephone operators, waiters, cashiers, cooks, garment stitchers, and assembly-line workers. According to Karasek, the combination of high demands and low control appears to raise the risk of heart disease as much as "smoking or having a high cholesterol level."[36]

According to researchers with the Framingham Heart Study, women clerical workers and others with little control have twice as much heart disease as women in occupations with higher levels of control.[37] The Framingham researchers suggest that the clerical workers and others with a low sense of control "experience severe occupational stress, including a lack of autonomy and control over the work environment, underutilization of skills, and lack of recognition of accomplishments."[38]

In another study of the link between control and heart disease, researchers found that heart disease is greater among waiters and assembly-line workers than among managers who are faced with equally high stress and demands but who have more control and decision-making ability.[39]

The Stress-Buffering Power of Control

A person in a stressful situation who believes that he or she has some control over the situation suffers far less physiological damage normally associated with stress. Control also acts as a buffer against stress when we believe we have control, even if we really don't.

In one study,[40] individuals were placed in booths and asked to perform arithmetic problems in their head. To make the situation even more stressful, researchers piped noise into the booths. Half of the people in the study were able to control the noise level by turning a knob in the booth; the other half were dependent on the first half for volume control. Both groups were exposed to an identical level of noise; the only difference between the two was the ability to control the volume of noise. At the end of the experiment, researchers took blood samples and studied the level of stress hormones in the blood. The people who did not have a knob to turn had much higher levels of cortisol, a major stress hormone. According to the research authors, "The ability to control external stress has a large influence on how much internal stress we experience."

The stress-buffering effects of control have been observed in a wide variety of situations, and the ability of control to buffer stress has even been seen in the most stressful conditions, such as those endured by hostages and prisoners of war. Those who have been able to maintain hardiness and survive their ordeals, according to researchers, are those who have somehow been able to achieve some sense of control, even in prison. National Institute of Mental Health psychologist Julius Segal found that one of the hostages in Iran "achieved this by saving a bit of food from his meals and then offering it to anyone who came into his cell. That simple coping strategy had the effect of turning the cell into a living room, the hostage into a host welcoming visitors."[41]

The Influence of Control on Immunity and Healing

One reason why a lack of control may lead to poor health is its impact on the immune system. According to research, control may have a significant effect on the function of the body's immune defenses. People who feel powerless, helpless, and out of control generally have compromised immunity, whereas those who feel a sense of control have healthier immune systems.

Physicians tested women with early-stage breast cancer. Those who felt some control over their lives and their disease were compared with women who felt a distressing lack of control. The women with control had a far greater level of natural killer cell activity—a much stronger immune system.[42]

A sense of control also appears to trigger the body's internal healing mechanisms. Several different studies with patients about to undergo surgery demonstrate that a sense of control can have a significant effect on the healing process. In one, 100 lung transplant patients were measured for their locus of control. Those with a high internal locus of control healed better and lived longer after their lung transplant than did the patients with a low internal locus of control. [43]

A similar experiment conducted by psychologists at the University of Iowa School of Medicine involved patients about to undergo coronary bypass surgery. The patients in the group that had received enough information to give a sense of control "fared significantly better on all counts. There was less hypertension, anxiety, and pain." A greater sense of control "proved to be the most powerful predictor of recovery without complication."[44]

Studies at other hospitals have had the same result: patients with a sense of control heal more quickly and with fewer complications. All of the studies combine to show us the power of an internal locus of control. With it, we may have improved immune function, have the ability to fight disease, and recover more quickly when illness does strike. Control may possibly be the weapon researchers were referring to when they told us, "You carry with you the most powerful medicine that exists. Each of us has it if we choose to use it, if we learn to use it."[45]

Self-Esteem

American humorist and author Samuel Clemens—the legendary Mark Twain—believed that it's a hundred times more valuable to approve of ourselves than to have the approval of others. A century after he penned that advice, it is proving to be true.

In his book *Honoring the Self,* psychologist Nathaniel Branden calls self-esteem the reputation we have with ourselves; when we believe that we are bad or unworthy, the reputation is poor, and low self-esteem is the result.[46]

We stand in the midst of an almost infinite network of relationships: to other people, to things, to the universe. And yet, at three o'clock in the morning, when we are alone with ourselves, we are aware that the most intimate and powerful of all relationships and the one we can never escape is the relationship to ourselves. No significant aspect of our thinking, motivation, feelings, or behavior is unaffected by our self-evaluation.[47]

According to a growing body of evidence, a healthy self-esteem is one of the best things we can do for overall health, both mental and physical. A good, strong sense of self can apparently help boost the immune system, improve heart function, protect against disease, and aid in healing.

What Is Self-Esteem?

Self-esteem is the core belief we have about ourselves—a sense of positive self-regard, or the degree to which we like or dislike ourselves.[48] It's a way of viewing ourselves as good people who are well in all aspects. It's a sense of feeling good about our capabilities, physical limitations, goals, place in the world, and relationship to others. Self-esteem is a powerful element: our perceptions about ourselves are what set the boundaries for what we can and cannot do. Self-esteem can be called the blueprint for behavior.

Self-esteem should not be confused with self-concept. Self-concept is a broad term used to encompass all the ways we evaluate ourselves in comparison to those around us. It refers to the way we compare ourselves physically, mentally, and socially. Self-esteem contributes to, but is not the same as, self-concept.[49] Instead, self-esteem is characterized by a powerful source of inner strength—the willingness to cope with the basic challenges of life, knowing we are more than our problems, learning to discriminate, and having self-acceptance and self-responsibility.[50]

A sense of high self-esteem means we appreciate ourselves and our personal worth. We have a positive attitude, see ourselves as competent, and feel in control of our lives. The value we assign to ourselves, self-esteem, begins in childhood and is generally based on five factors—two physical and three psychological. The physical factors that determine our self-esteem are (1) our appearance (the way we look) and (2) our physical abilities. The psychological determinants of self-esteem are (1) how well we do in school (our perceived intelligence), (2) how confident we are in social situations, and (3) how we regard ourselves.[51] Research by Finnish scientist Mirja Kalliopuska suggests that empathy—the ability to put oneself in the place of other people and appreciate their feelings—may also be linked to self-esteem.[52]

Researchers have been able to identify what constitutes a healthy self-esteem. One of the most focused definitions was presented by Leonard Sagan in his examination of the factors that influence health and wellness in the world's various nations. In his comprehensive work, *The Health of Nations,* Sagan writes that those with a high level of self-esteem also have an inner locus of control:

> They are confident of their ability to make competent decisions. They do not rely solely on traditional authority for guidance, but are able to acquire and evaluate information and make decisions independently. In contrast with traditional people who believe that outcomes are determined by gods, chance, or persons of influence, healthy people believe that their decisions can be efficacious in determining outcomes—that is, they believe that what they think and do will matter.[53]

In his definition of healthy people, Sagan pointed out a vital characteristic among those with high self-esteem. Although healthy people have high regard for themselves, he said,

> They are not self-indulgent or preoccupied with their personal identity or welfare. Rather they are committed to goals other than their own personal welfare. Goals may be global in scope or quite modest; most important, however, they are not egotistical in nature but will benefit others. Healthy people are compassionate, they have a strong sense of community. I believe that these qualities are in a state of decline in the United States, and it may not be a coincidence that evidence of worsening health is appearing at the same time that Americans are preoccupied with "self-realization."[54]

In summary, he says, those with a healthy self-esteem have confidence in themselves and their ability to control their own lives; those who have low self-esteem tend to view themselves as passive victims—and are much more prone to illness and the stress of difficult life situations.

There is evidence that the way we think about ourselves may cause us to take better care of ourselves. However, there are mixed findings regarding self-esteem and positive health behaviors, and some controversy exists among researchers. Some have found that those with strong self-esteem are less likely to engage in destructive behavior such as violence, child abuse, crime, and alcohol and drug abuse; they have found that young girls who have high self-esteem are less likely to get pregnant as teenagers.[55] Some researchers have also found that low self-esteem among adolescents leads them to engage in self-destructive or health-harming behaviors, such as substance abuse, early sexual activity, eating disorders, and suicidal thoughts.[56] In contrast, others who have reviewed the studies that have been done maintain that self-esteem has little association with health behavior[57]—and that it does *not* seem to prevent adolescents from engaging in substance abuse, drinking, smoking, or early sexual activity. In fact, they maintain that high self-esteem in adolescents may encourage experimentation with some of these behaviors; but, in the end, they say, the effect of self-esteem is probably negligible. The one exception they have found is with eating disorders: in studies across the board, girls and women with high self-esteem are less likely to become bulimic.

Health behaviors aside, when you have a strong sense of self-esteem, the exhilarating feeling that you are worthwhile can have a positive influence on your health. A variety of studies have shown a strong correlation between self-esteem and health. When the California Department of Mental Health surveyed 1,000 Californians, they found that the healthiest ones cared most for others—and for themselves. Researcher James Lynch suggests that people with high self-esteem do take better care of their bodies.

People with positive self-esteem view themselves as good people who are well in all aspects of life. They have a physical, mental, social, emotional, and spiritual balance that enables them to achieve an equilibrium that acts as a buffer against stress and difficult life situations.

Where Does Self-Esteem Come From?

The formation of self-esteem begins early in life. Some of the first ingredients that make up self-esteem are the messages we receive during childhood from our parents, our other relatives, our teachers, and our friends. The family is particularly important in the development of self-esteem; parents are the most significant influence on a child's self-esteem,[58] and parents who have strong self-esteem generally nurture high self-esteem in their children.[59]

Self-esteem depends partly on physical limitations—whether we are overweight, hard of hearing, or incapable of speaking without stuttering. It is influenced by social class, socioeconomic status, and cultural restrictions. And it depends to a great extent on how much love we feel from those around us—how much acceptance, how much compassion, how much we are able to identify and feel identified with. Those in unhappy marriages, for example, suffer not only from lower happiness and life satisfaction but also tend to have lower self-esteem.[60]

So far, the factors that influence self-esteem seem to be largely beyond our control. We can't determine how our third-grade teacher deals with us, for example, nor can we change the fact that a mother's problem pregnancy left us severely visually impaired. However, each of us can control one large factor in self-esteem: it's the way we communicate with our self-esteem, the words we say about ourselves, that may have a powerful effect not only on our minds but also on our bodies.

Psychologist Susan Jeffers likes to use a demonstration to impress people with the importance of what they're communicating to their self-esteem.[61] Whenever she gives a talk, she invites a volunteer from the audience to come up to the front. She has the volunteer make a fist and extend his or her right arm in front of the body, angled down to the left for strength. She then asks the volunteer to resist as powerfully as possible while she tries to push down on the arm. She relates that she's never "won" this initial trial.

She then asks the volunteer to stand at ease, close his or her eyes, and repeat ten times aloud, "I am a weak and unworthy person." She encourages the volunteer to really feel the words while speaking them. She then asks the volunteer to open his or her eyes, assume the original posture, and resist her efforts to push the same arm down.

"I wish I had a camera to record the expression on my volunteer's face as I press his arm and it gives way," Jeffers exclaims. "A few object, 'I wasn't ready!' So I do it again."

Once again, Jeffers has the volunteer close the eyes, stand at ease, and repeat aloud a different set of words: "I am a strong and worthy person." Jeffers says that, to everyone's surprise, she once again cannot budge the arm.

She concludes that she can run this experiment backward and forward almost any number of times, and "it makes no difference if I leave the room while he speaks and I don't know what he has said: Weak words mean a weak arm; strong words mean a strong arm."

Jeffers explains this phenomenon by stating,

> It is as though the inner self doesn't know what is true and false, and believes the words it is told without judging them. . . . We can control our self-esteem by speaking to it. I think the conclusion is obvious: Stop feeding yourself negative words, and start building yourself up with positive ones.[62]

The Impact of Self-Esteem on the Body

A fascinating finding has emerged from the research on self-esteem and the body: self-esteem and health appear to be connected in a continual cycle. Researchers studied almost 800 older adults in the Durham–Raleigh–Chapel Hill area of North Carolina who were transitioning into retirement as part of the Carolina Health and Transition Study. The adults were rated on level of self-esteem and on functional health, which was measured by their difficulty in performing seven activities. During the two years of the study, they found that good health enhances self-esteem: the better the health, the higher the self-esteem. They also found out that strong self-esteem impacts health: the stronger and higher the self-esteem, the better the health.[63]

How can self-esteem impact physical health? Whether people do or do not get sick—and how long they stay that way—may depend in part on how strong their self-esteem is. Researchers have gone so far as to brand self-esteem as "a social vaccine"—a dimension of personality that "empowers people and inoculates them" against a wide spectrum of self-defeating behaviors.[64] A growing body of evidence indicates that low self-esteem is often a factor in chronic pain, for example. Several studies show that recovery from infectious mononucleosis is related to "ego strength"; the higher the self-esteem, the more rapid the recovery.[65]

The level of self-esteem we have appears to be a crucial factor in how we respond to stress, regardless of personality type. Self-esteem is so powerful an influence on health that it even impacts the way we react to life events—situations in life that researchers have determined cause stress. Many are negatives, such as the death of a loved one, divorce, a jail term, or assuming a new debt. However, researchers have found that positive life events—such as getting married, getting a new job, or giving birth—are also sources of stress. Whether these stressors cause a person to become ill depends on many factors, including one's ability to cope with the stress.

In their research in life events, scientists have found that self-esteem has significant influence on how positive life events impact our health. If we've got strong self-esteem, the outlook is good: the more positive life events, the better our health. But if our self-esteem is poor, our health can decline in direct proportion as our life becomes peppered with more positive life events.[66] This may be because we believe we are not worthy of positive life events.

Results of various studies show that positive self-esteem helps protect health. An interesting study took place among Arizona's Pima Indians, who have long been known to have high rates of obesity and diabetes. Researchers divided them into two groups: an "action group," which had a familiar mix of treatments aimed at nutrition and exercise, and a "pride group," which received printed information about nutrition and exercise but which had regular discussions with local leaders about Pima history and culture. At the end of a year, there were many problems in the "action group," but the "pride group" had either less deterioration or had actual improvement as far as weight, waist circumference, blood glucose levels, and insulin levels. Researchers tentatively concluded that increasing pride in their identity had a greater favorable impact on health behaviors and risk than did focusing on how to change diet and exercise.[67]

One reason behind its protective nature may be its effect on the immune system. One study that gives a glimpse of the self-esteem/immunity link was conducted by psychiatrist J. Stephen Heisel and his colleagues at McLean Hospital. They studied 111 college students who had completed the Minnesota Multiphasic Personality Inventory (MMPI), a 566-item questionnaire that describes personality and other measures of mental health, such as level of depression. In analyzing the students' scores, he found that those with the highest self-esteem were also the ones with the strongest natural killer-cell activity. High self-esteem seemed to provide a boost to the immune system and give students stronger immunity against disease.[68]

Researchers have also found a possible connection between poor self-esteem and premature death from coronary heart disease. Researchers from McGill University in Montreal gave thorough psychological questionnaires to 200 men recovering from heart attack. Over the next five years, the men who reported feeling "useless" or unable to "do things well" were nearly four times as likely to die from coronary disease as men with higher self-esteem. That association remained strong even after researchers adjusted for other factors.[69]

Self-Efficacy: Believing in Yourself

An important part of self-esteem is what psychologists call self-efficacy, one of the components of self-esteem that apparently leads to both psychological and physical well-being. Self-efficacy is your perception of your own ability to do a specific task and to overcome the difficulties inherent in that specific task.[70] Dr. Albert Bandura of Stanford University says that self-efficacy is not related to your skills but to what you think you can do with the skills you have.[71] It's your belief in yourself, your conviction that you can manage the adverse events that come along in your life.

People tend to pursue tasks they know they can accomplish and avoid those they believe exceed their capabilities.[72] In other words, your sense of self-efficacy generally influences what you will and will not try to do. For example, if you believe that you can learn a new software program recommended by an associate, you'll plunge in with gusto. If you believe that you have real problems learning software, you'll be unlikely to try—unless you're required to for a class or for your job. Self-efficacy also influences how much effort you'll make while trying something new and your persistence in overcoming any obstacles.[73]

Self-efficacy is measured by:

- **Magnitude**—the judgment a person has about the ability to accomplish a number of things; a person with high magnitude believes she can accomplish everything on a list, for example, and will feel capable of doing even the most difficult things on the list.

- **Strength**—confidence about the ability to perform any single thing.

- **Generality**—how many areas the person feels confident in. The extent to which a person feels confident in the ability to do one thing will affect whether he feels confident in being able to do other related things.[74]

Just as with self-esteem, various factors combine to determine how strong your self-efficacy is:

1. **Past performance.** If you've handled things well in the past, your faith in yourself is bolstered, and you are more likely to feel confident about facing any new situations.

2. **Vicarious experience.** This means keeping your eyes open and watching what goes on around you. You see how a friend deals with the death of her spouse. You watch what happens to a coworker when he loses several big accounts and then gets fired. You watch a television documentary about a midwestern farm family that faces seemingly insurmountable odds but emerges with spirit and courage after losing farm, home, and source of income. You read a magazine article about a young mother who faces with great courage the task of caring for her severely handicapped baby. You take all of that in, and the message comes through: If they can do it, so can I. You gain strength from their strength, courage from their courage. You make the unspoken commitment that when your time comes, you'll rally, too.

3. **The encouragement of others.** It's much easier to believe in yourself when the people around you are cheering you on.

Self-efficacy is an important component of self-esteem because it can, in a very real way, predict your behavior. It determines your level of effort: If you really believe you can succeed, you're apt to keep on trying. It endows you with perseverance in the face of failure: If you really believe in yourself, you're less likely to give up. Your level of self-efficacy determines whether you will help yourself or hinder yourself. It determines, too, how well you will react to stress: if you are low in self-efficacy, you may become overwhelmed by stress because you become convinced that your life, or a particular situation, is unmanageable.

To sum it up, people with solid self-efficacy believe they'll come out on top—so they usually do. Bandura has identified three landmark characteristics of people with high self-efficacy:

1. They believe the intended outcome of a given behavior is of value to themselves.

2. They believe that performing the behavior will lead to that outcome.

3. They believe that they can successfully perform the behavior.[75]

As Bandura says, "When beset with difficulties, people who entertain serious doubts about their capabilities slacken their efforts or give up altogether, whereas those who have a strong sense of efficacy exert great effort to master the challenges."[76]

Psychologist Blair Justice gives an example of the difference that self-efficacy can make in one of the most stressful situations: the relocation of an elderly person from one place to another or from one institution to another. A marked increase in death rate often occurs, he says, usually within the first three months after relocation. When a home for the elderly in Chicago was closed, Justice writes, "The mortality rate was substantially lower for those who accepted the news of relocation philosophically but not with a sense of defeat or helplessness."[77] Those who became angry about the move fared almost as well—possibly because their anger mobilized them "to take care of themselves by eating, keeping as active as possible, and not giving up."

Self-efficacy is also a predictor of health behaviors. For example, people who believe they can quit smoking are much more likely to actually quit. In one study of more than 800 smokers, those with the greatest self-efficacy moved most quickly—and most surely—from a stage of just thinking about quitting to actually quitting during the six-month period of the study.[78] Research also shows that self-esteem and self-efficacy are related to more positive health behaviors in young adults[79] and that healthy self-esteem acquired early in life can significantly impact key long-term preventive health behaviors.[80] Self-efficacy has also been positively related to many other health behaviors, including:

1. **Exercise.**[81] In one study involving more than fifty men who had suffered heart attacks, those with the highest self-efficacy did best on treadmill tests and were the ones who followed up most consistently at home.[82] In another study involving men and women with chronic obstructive pulmonary disease, those with the highest self-efficacy did best in following a program of walking, which helped control their disease symptoms.[83]

2. **Weight loss and nutrition.**[84] In one study of 179 men and women aged 20 to 60, those with the highest self-efficacy followed through with a program of exercise and nutrition that led to weight loss.[85] In another study involving almost 200 men and women from three different ethnic groups (white, Hispanic, and black), self-efficacy was the highest predictor of who would follow exercise and nutrition guidelines and actually lose weight.[86]

3. **Persistence in following physician orders following heart attack and other cardiac disease.**[87] Interestingly, one study of 411 men and women from different ethnic groups found that those with the highest self-efficacy also had the lowest risk for cardiac disease, probably because of positive health behavior.[88]

4. **Consistency in using contraceptives.**[89]

Self-efficacy can actually cause physiological changes in the body. When under stress of any kind, the brain releases chemicals called catecholamines, which trigger a complex set of physiological reactions enabling a person to meet the challenge of the stress (the classic fight-or-flight syndrome). By measuring the levels of catecholamines in the blood, researchers can determine the degree of stress.

Bandura and his colleagues selected twelve women who had arachnophobia and measured the level of catecholamine secretion when the women were faced with situations that frightened them—looking at a spider, putting a hand in a bowl with a spider, or allowing a spider to crawl on a hand. When women felt that they could handle a situation, catecholamine levels were low; when they felt that a situation was more than they could handle (in other words, when their self-efficacy was low), catecholamine levels shot up.

Bandura and his colleagues at Stanford worked with the women to bolster their level of self-efficacy regarding spiders. The women gained confidence, and some began to believe that they could manage an encounter with a spider. When that happened, says Bandura, catecholamine levels stayed low. Stress was eased, and the women did not suffer the physiological reactions as before.[90]

The real power of self-efficacy on health is demonstrated quite simply. If you want to get a fairly accurate prediction of how healthy someone is or will be, ask people how healthy they think they are. Researchers have found that "self-rated" health—much the same as self-efficacy—determines to a large extent how healthy a person will actually be. Some studies have even shown that asking that simple question will tell you more about a person's health than an entire battery of sophisticated laboratory tests.

Ornstein and Sobel report on a seven-year study carried out in Manitoba, Canada. More than 3,500 elderly people were asked, "For your age would you say, in general, your health is excellent, good, fair, poor, or bad?" Researchers conducting the study also sought health reports from physicians that gave detailed records on illnesses, surgeries, hospitalizations, and other medical problems. When researchers correlated actual health at the end of the study with self-ratings and medical observations seven years earlier, they found the self-ratings to be more accurate and predictive than the health measures from the physicians. Even more surprisingly, "Those who were in objectively poor health by physician report survived at a higher rate as long as they believed their own health to be good."[91] The only thing more powerful than self-rated health, in fact, was increasing age.

Belief in oneself is one of the most powerful weapons we have in protecting our health and living longer. It has a startling impact on wellness. And we are able to harness it to our advantage. As Madeline Gershwin said, "What wise people and grandmothers have always known is that the way you feel about yourself, your attitudes, beliefs, values, have a great deal to do with your health and well-being."[92]

WHAT DID YOU LEARN?

1. What is the meaning of *locus of control?*
2. What is the major source of control?
3. What is the relationship between hardiness and locus of control?
4. How does locus of control affect stress, immunity, and healing?
5. What are the characteristics of self-esteem?
6. How does self-esteem develop?
7. What is *self-efficacy,* and how does it impact health?

ENDNOTES

1. Joan Borysenko, *Minding the Body, Mending the Mind* (Reading, MA: Addison-Wesley Publishing Company, 1987), 22.
2. Phillip L. Rice, *Stress and Health: Principles and Practice for Coping and Wellness* (Monterey, CA: Brooks/Cole Publishing Company, 1987), 109.
3. Blair Justice, *Who Gets Sick: Thinking and Health* (Houston, TX: Peak Press, 1987), 61–2.
4. Aaron Antonovsky, *Unraveling the Mystery of Health: How People Manage Stress and Stay Well* (San Francisco: Jossey-Bass, 1987), 36–7.
5. H. M. Lefcourt, *Locus of Control: Current Trends in Theory and Research* (Hillsdale, NJ: Erlbaum, 1976), 29.
6. Ibid.

7. S. I. McMillen, *None of These Diseases,* rev. ed. (Old Tappan, NJ: Fleming H. Revell Company, 1984), 177–8.
8. Rice, *Stress and Health,* 109.
9. Leonard A. Sagan, *The Health of Nations* (New York: Basic Books, 1987).
10. H. M. Lefcourt, *Locus of Control: Current Trends in Theory and Research* (New Jersey: Lawrence Erlbaum Associates, 1976).
11. Julian B. Rotter, "Generalized Expectancies of Internal versus External Control of Reinforcements," *Psychological Monographs* 80, 1966.
12. Julian B. Rotter, "Some Problems and Misconceptions Related to the Construct of Internal versus External Control of Reinforcement," *Journal of Consulting and Clinical Psychology* 43 (1975): 56–67; and Julian B. Rotter, "Internal versus External Control of Reinforcement: A Case History of a Variable," *American Psychologist* 45 (1990): 489–93.
13. Tony Eprile, "Longevity Tied to Self-Mastery," *Omni Longevity* 2, no. 10 (1988): 109–11.
14. Amy Mackey, "Power, Pessimism, and Prevention," http://www.units.muohio.edu/psybersite/control/health.shtml, accessed June 4, 2008.
15. "Locus of Control and Cardiovascular Health," *Job Stress Network,* http://www.workhealth.org/risk/rfblocus.html, accessed June 4, 2008.
16. Justice, *Who Gets Sick,* 145.
17. P. G. Bourne, R. M. Rose, and J. W. Mason, "17–OHCS Levels in Combat: Special Forces 'A' Team Under Threat of Attack," *Archives of General Psychiatry* 19 (1968): 135–40.
18. Case cited in Steven Locke and Douglas Colligan, *The Healer Within* (New York: E. P. Dutton, 1986), 96.
19. Pamela Williams-Piehota et al., "Matching Health Messages to Health Locus of Control Beliefs for Promoting Mammography Utilization," *Psychology and Health* 19, no. 4 (August 2004): 407–23.
20. Paul Norman, Paul Bennett, Christopher Smith, and Simon Murphy, "Health Locus of Control and Health Behaviour," *Journal of Health Psychology* 3, no. 2 (1998): 171–80.
21. A. Steptoe and J. Wardle, "Locus of Control and Health Behaviour Revisited: A Multivariate Analysis of Young Adults from 18 Countries," *British Journal of Psychology* 92, no. 4 (November 2001): 659–772.
22. Mackey, "Power, Pessimism, and Prevention."
23. W. Stelmach, K. Kaczmarczyk-Chalas, W. Bielecki, and W. Drygas, "The Association Between Income, Education, Control over Life and Health in a Large Urban Population of Poland," *International Journal of Occupational Medicine & Environmental Health* 17, no. 2 (2004): 299–310.
24. M. J. Cross et al., "Patient Self-Efficacy and Health Locus of Control: Relationships with Health Status and Arthritis-Related Expenditure," *Rheumatology* 45, no. 1 (2006): 92–6.
25. Norman Cousins, *Head First: The Biology of Hope* (New York: E. P. Dutton, 1989), 120.
26. J. E. Crisson and F. J. Keefe, "The Relationship of Locus of Control to Pain Coping Strategies and Psychological Distress in Chronic Pain Patients," *Behavioral Medicine* 35, no. 2 (1988): 147–54.
27. Caryle Hirshberg, "Spontaneous Remission: The Spectrum of Self-Repair," *The Psychology of Health, Immunity, and Disease,* vol. B, 186, in *Proceedings of the Sixth International Conference of the National Institute for the Clinical Application of Behavioral Medicine* (Mansfield Center, CT: NICABM).
28. National Institutes of Health, *Proceedings of the Forum on Coronary Prone Behavior* (Bethesda, MD: National Institutes of Health, Department of Health, Education, and Welfare Publication #78–1451), June 1987, 162.
29. As reported in "Health Briefs," *Executive Fitness* (November 1987): 8.

30. "Locus of Control and Cardiovascular Health," *Job Stress Network*.

31. Ibid.

32. H. S. Akiskal and W. T. McKinney, "Overview of Recent Research in Depression," *Archives of General Psychiatry* 32 (1975): 285–305.

33. P. Ahluwalia, R. M. Zacharko, and H. Anisman, "Dopamine Variations Associated with Acute and Chronic Stressors" (presentation at the Annual Meeting of the Society of Neuroscience, Dallas, TX, October 20–25, 1985).

34. W. Vale, J. Spiess, C. Rivier, and J. Rivier, "Characterization of a 41-Residue Ovine Hypothalamic Peptide that Stimulates Secretion of Corticotropin and Beta-Endorphin," *Science* 213 (1981): 1394–7.

35. Ibid.

36. Claudia Wallis, "Stress: Can We Cope?" *Time* (June 6, 1983): 48–54.

37. S. G. Haynes, "Type A Behavior, Employment Status, and Coronary Heart Disease in Women," *Behavioral Medicine Update* 6, no. 4 (1984): 11–5.

38. Ibid., 13.

39. R. A. Karasek et al., "Job, Psychological Factors, and Coronary Heart Disease," *Advances in Cardiology* 29 (1982) 62–7.

40. U. Lundberg and M. Frankenhaeser, "Psychophysiological Reactions to Noise as Modified by Personal Control over Stimulus Intensity," *Biological Psychology* 6 (1978): 51–8.

41. Wallis, "Stress: Can We Cope?"

42. Sandra M. Levy, *Emotional Expression and Survival in Breast Cancer Patients: Immunological Correlates* (paper presented at the Meetings of the American Psychological Association, Anaheim, CA, August 1983).

43. Eileen J. Burker, Donna M. Evon, Joseph Galanko, and Thomas Egan, "Health Locus of Control Predicts Survival After Lung Cancer," *Journal of Health Psychology* 10, no. 5 (2005): 695–704.

44. Justice, *Who Gets Sick*, 310–1.

45. R. S. Eliot, "Cognitive and Behavioral Stress Management Considerations" (presentation at a Conference on Stress and the Heart of the American College of Cardiology, Jackson Hole, WY, July 1986).

46. Nathaniel Brandon, *Honoring the Self: Self-Esteem and Personal Tranformation* (Bantam, 1985).

47. Joan Borysenko, *Guilt Is the Teacher, Love Is the Lesson* (New York: Warner Books, 1990), 45.

48. M. Rosenberg and H. B. Kaplan, *Social Psychology of the Self-Concept* (Arlington Heights, IL: Harlan Davidson, 1982).

49. Rice, *Stress and Health*, 111.

50. Nathaniel Branden, "Living with Self-Esteem," *Lotus* (Fall 1992).

51. Rice, Stress and Health.

52. *Psychological Reports* 70: 1119–22.

53. Sagan, *The Health of Nations*, 187.

54. Ibid.

55. Tracy Turner, "Self-Esteem," *BBC Health* (September 2006), http://www.bbc.co.uk/health/conditions/mental_health/emotion_esteem.shtml, accessed June 4, 2008.

56. Rob McGee and Sheila Williams, "Does Low Self-Esteem Predict Health Compromising Behaviours Among Adolescents?" *Journal of Adolescence* 23, no. 5 (October 2000): 569–82.

57. R. F. Baumeister, J. D. Campbell, J. I. Kreuger, and K. D. Vons, "Does High Self-Esteem Cause Better Performance, Interpersonal Success, Happiness or Healthier Lifestyles?" *Psychological Science in the Public Interest* 4, no. 1 (2003): 1–44.

58. Sabra L. Katz Wise and Ralph Poore, "Self-Esteem," *Healthwise* (January 3, 2007): 10.

59. Turner, "Self-Esteem."

60. Vicki Fong, "Unhappy Marriages Detrimental to Self-Esteem and Health," *Medical News Today* (January 27, 2006).
61. Described in Susan Jeffers, "Building Your Self-Esteem: Your Positive Words Will Make You Strong," *Success* (October 1987): 72.
62. Ibid.
63. Donald C. Reitzes and Elizabeth J. Mutran, "Self and Health: Factors That Encourage Self-Esteem and Functional Health," *The Journal of Gerontology* 61 (2006): S44–51.
64. Turner, "Self-Esteem."
65. S. Michael Plaut and Stanford B. Friedman, "Biological Mechanisms in the Relationship of Stress to Illness," *Pediatric Annals* 14, no. 8 (1985): 563–7.
66. Barbara R. Sarason, Irwin G. Sarason, and Gregory R. Pierce, *Social Support: An Interactional View* (New York: John Wiley & Sons, 1990), 164.
67. Michael Marmot, "Self Esteem and Health," *British Medical Journal* 327, no. 7415 (September 13, 2003): 574–5,.
68. "Research Strengthens Link Between Poor Mental and Physical Health," *Sexuality Today Newsletter* (November 24, 1986): 4.
69. "Danger from Depression," *Consumer Reports on Health* (August 1992): 63.
70. Rayane AbuShaba and Cheryl Achterberg, "Review of Self-Efficacy and Locus of Control for Nutrition- and Health-Related Behavior," *Journal of the American Dietetic Association* 97, no. 1 (October 1997): 1122–32.
71. Albert Bandura, *Social Foundations of Thought and Action* (Englewood Cliffs, NJ: Prentice Hall, 1986).
72. AbuShaba and Achterberg, "Review of Self-Efficacy."
73. Ibid.
74. Ibid.
75. Aaron Antonovsky, *Unraveling the Mystery of Health: How People Manage Stress and Stay Well* (San Francisco: Jossey-Bass Publishers, 1988), 59.
76. "Self-Efficacy," *University of California Berkeley Wellness Letter* 3, no. 8 (1987): 1–2.
77. Justice, *Who Gets Sick*. 144–5.
78. J. O. Prochaska and C. C. DiClemente, "Self-Change Processes, Self-Efficacy and Decisional Balance Across Five Stages of Smoking Cessation," in A. R. Liss, ed., *Advances in Cancer Control: Epidemiology and Research* (New York: Alan R. Liss, 1984): 131–40.
79. Sarah E. Lowery et al., "Body Image, Self-Esteem, and Health-Related Behaviors Among Male and Female First Year College Students," *Journal of College Student Development* (November/December 2005): 612–23.
80. Erik T. Huntsinger and Linda J. Luecken, "Attachment Relationships and Health Behavior: The Mediational Role of Self-Esteem," *Psychology and Health* 19, no. 4 (August 2004): 515–26.
81. R. Desharnais, J. Bouillon, and G. Gordin, "Self-Efficacy and Outcome Expectation as Determinants of Exercise Adherence," *Psychological Reports* 59 (1986): 1155–9.
82. AbuShaba and Achterberg, "Review of Self-Efficacy."
83. R. M. Kaplan, C. J. Atkins, and S. Reinsch, "Specific Efficacy Expectations Mediate Exercise Compliance in Patients with COPD," *Health Psychology* 3 (1984): 223–48.
84. AbuShaba and Achterberg, "Review of Self-Efficacy"; N. Bernier and J. Avard, "Self-Efficacy Outcome and Attrition in a Weight Reduction Program," *Cognitive Therapy Research* 10 (1986): 319–38, 1986; and R. S. Weinberg et al., "Effects of Pre-Existing and Manipulated Levels of Self-Efficacy on Weight Loss in a Self-Control Program," *Journal of Research Perspectives* 18 (1984): 352–8.
85. M. H. Weitzel, "A Test of the Health Promotion Model with Blue-Collar Workers," *Nursing Research* 38 (1989): 99–104.

86. M. H. Weitzel and P. R. Waller, "Predictive Factors for Health-Promotive Behaviors in White, Hispanic, and Black Blue-Collar Workers," *Family and Community Health* 13, no. 1 (1990): 23–34.

87. AbuShaba and Achterberg, "Review of Self-Efficacy"; C. K. Ewart, C. B. Taylor, L. B. Reese, and R. F. Debusk, "Effects of Early Postmyocardial Infarction Exercise Testing and Self-Perception and Subsequent Physical Activity," *American Journal of Cardiology* 51 (1985): 1076–80; and C. B. Taylor et al., "Raising Spouse's and Patient's Beliefs Perception of His Cardiac Capabilities Following a Myocardial Infarction," *American Journal of Cardiology* 55 (1985): 635–8.

88. M. A. Winkleby, J. A. Flora, and H. C. Kraemer, "A Community-Based Heart Disease Intervention: Predictors of Change," *American Journal of Public Health* 84, no. 5 (1994): 767–72.

89. Albert Bandura, "Social Cognitive Theory and Exercise of Control of HIV Infection," in J. Peterson and R. DiClemente, eds., *Preventing AIDS: Theory and Practice of Behavioral Interventions* (New York: Plenum Press, 1993), 25–51.

90. Robert Ornstein and David Sobel, *The Healing Brain* (New York: Simon & Schuster, 1987), 249.

91. Cited in Ornstein and Sobel, *The Healing Brain*, 246–8.

92. Ibid., 249–50.

CHAPTER 19

The Healing Power of Humor and Laughter

With the fearful strain that is on me night and day,
if I did not laugh I should die.

—Abraham Lincoln

The art of medicine consists of keeping the patient amused
while nature heals the disease.

—Voltaire

LEARNING OBJECTIVES

- Discuss professional trends toward using humor in healing.
- Understand the physical and psychological benefits of humor.
- Discuss the physiology of laughter.
- List the ways in which laughter is a form of exercise.
- Discuss the physical and psychological benefits of laughter.
- Understand how laughter contributes to pain relief.

Mark Twain once penned the sentiment that "against the assault of laughter nothing can stand." What the great American humorist and author believed more than a hundred years ago is being shown true today by some of our most gifted scientists: a sense of humor, and the laughter that accompanies it, can actually banish pain and keep us well.

They may not have had the scientific proof to back up their suppositions, but even early physicians recognized the healing power of humor. The famous seventeenth-century physician Thomas Sydenham said that "the arrival of a good clown exercises more beneficial influence upon the health of a town than twenty asses laden with drugs."[1]

Webster's Dictionary defines humor as the quality that appeals to a sense of the comical or absurdly incongruous. Humor involves cognitive, emotional, behavioral, psychophysiological, and social aspects. The term *humor* can refer to a stimulus that is meant to produce a humorous response (such as a joke or a funny movie), a mental process (the perception of something amusing), or a response (laughter).[2] What we generally refer to as a "sense of humor" is a psychological trait that brings with it the ability to bring happiness both to your own life as well as to the life of others. (It's important to understand that there is also bad—or unhealthy—humor as well: any time humor is used to hurt someone, lower another person's self-esteem, or bring tears of sadness, it is not a healthy kind of humor.)[3] According to Loretta LaRoche of Boston's Deaconess Hospital, good humor is "the ability to feel inner joy, peace, and harmony within yourself and your surroundings—to discover that we are all part of a divine comedy."[4] Humor is a way of looking at things that helps to dissipate stress and accentuate the positive. "When we become too serious," says LaRoche, "we help create the components for stress, rigid thinking, helplessness, cynicism, and hardening of the attitude."[5]

Humor has been used across the span of cultures to make people feel better. A number of American Indian tribes—the Zunis, Crees, Pueblos, and Hopis among them—had ceremonial clowns whose sole purpose was to provide humor for their tribesmen. According to accounts, they were called in "to entertain and heal the sick with their hilarity, frightening away the demons of ill health."[6]

Humor has been widely used in traditional medicine in a number of cultures. Dr. Rosita Arvigo, who practiced in Belize under the tutelage of the great Mayan healer Don Elijio Panti, remembers that he was the "funniest man I ever knew," a man who referred to himself as "the doctor clown." Given the choice between being a doctor and a clown, he said, he would choose a clown. He believed laughter was extremely important in medicine—and greeted his patients by teasing them, doing hilarious dances, and performing crazy gestures until they were wild with laughter. She remembers that one of his lessons for contemporary physicians would be

> . . . that a person's spirit needs to be uplifted as much as the body needs to be healed. And without an uplifted spirit I don't think there is enough energy within the body, enough vital force or what the Maya call ch'ulel [known as prana or chi in other cultures] for a person to properly and completely experience healing.[7]

One of the most renowned uses of laughter in our day occurred when former *Saturday Review* editor Norman Cousins incorporated it into a program to treat ankylosing spondylitis, a debilitating connective tissue disease. Cousins employed funny movies and books to relieve the pain of the disease.

"Ten minutes of genuine belly laughter had an anesthetic effect and would give me at least two hours of pain-free sleep," Cousins relates. "When the pain-killing effect of the laughter wore off, we would switch on the motion picture projector again and, not infrequently, it would lead to another pain-free sleep interval."[8] Indeed, claims Cousins, of "all the gifts bestowed by nature on human beings, hearty laughter must be close to the top. The response to incongruities is one of the highest manifestations of the cerebral process."

Professional Trends Toward Humor

While humor is a very complex concept, researchers are providing scientific proof that laughter (along with a sense of humor) can literally make a person feel better. Based on the scientific evidence proving laughter's health benefits, hospitals and medical clinics are utilizing laughter in unique ways to promote the health of patients.[9] The result is "therapeutic humor," defined as "any intervention that promotes health and wellness by stimulating a playful discovery, expression or appreciation of the absurdity or incongruity of life's situations."[10]

In studies involving cancer patients who are using at least one additional therapy to deal with their cancer, humor rates high on the list—50 percent of the patients in one rural midwestern treatment center were using humor, as were more than a fifth of the breast cancer patients in a Tampa Bay area study group. In a third study, in which humor is one of the most popular therapies, the cancer patients said that humor plays a role in their spirituality and their perception of the meaning of life, and for them it is an important coping strategy.[11]

One of the prototypes for "humor centers" in the nation's hospitals is the Living Room of the William Stehlin Foundation for Cancer Research at Houston's St. Joseph's Hospital. The room is filled with greenery and furnished with comfortable, overstuffed pieces. Patients are free to go to the room as often as needed for "comic relief" from the severity of their illness.

The "humor room" at Schenectady's Sunnyview Hospital and Rehabilitation Center boasts a poster reminding patients to take a "humor break" from illness. In the room, patients can check out funny movies, humorous tapes, and funny books. They are also given access to proven "mirth makers," such as balloons, clown noses, and bottles of bubble soap. At DeKalb General Hospital in Decatur, Georgia, patients can spend part of their recovery time in a brightly painted "Lively Room" stocked with funny games, tapes, and movies. Laurel and Hardy movies are shown in the Living Room of Orlando's Humana Hospital Lucerne.

Leslie Gibson, creator of the Comedy Cart Connection at Morton Plant Hospital in Clearwater, Florida, points out that being hospitalized puts people at the highest level of stress—and that humor is a natural remedy. "The loss of control often places patients in fearful, compromising situations. Besides promoting healing, humor is an excellent diversionary tool for keeping their minds off their pain."[12]

At the Detroit Medical Center's Children's Hospital of Michigan, clowns from the hospital's Clowns-on-Call program wander the halls, lobbies, and waiting rooms several days a week. These volunteers—mostly people from the community who volunteer on a regular basis—transform themselves into Dr. Ha Choo, Nurse Stefy Scope, and Dr. ICU Giggle. They make their rounds, visiting those patients who need a "clown consult" or a prescription for laughter. Founders of the program say that children with chronic diseases need to know it's okay to laugh—and so do their parents. "We try to make children forget about the hospital and focus on the fun," says Dr. Barry Duel, a pediatric urology fellow also known as Dr. Bee Dee who started the program. "If they're laughing, they're having fun and they can't focus on the pain."[13]

Another innovative program is the Clown Care Unit at Babies and Children's Hospital at Columbia-Presbyterian Medical Center in New York. Researchers there were awarded three pilot research grants to study the value of clown therapy for pediatric heart and cancer patients. Finding that the clowns helped decrease both the physical and psychological distress of patients who were undergoing medical procedures for heart disease and cancer, the program brought in specially trained clowns to work with the children. Researchers found that "the joyful distraction provided by the clowns would increase patient cooperation, decrease parental anxiety, and decrease the need for sedation during anxious moments in the hospital."[14]

The trend toward humor as a way of boosting both physical and mental health has spread to private practice. Increasing numbers of physicians throughout the nation have begun using humor and laughter as a way of easing tension, promoting healing, and even boosting immunity among their patients. Nurses, too, have caught the vision: More than 1,000 nurses joined forces several years ago to organize Nurses for Laughter (NFL). The members, who try to make humor a part of their bedside manner, boast the motto "Caution: Humor may be hazardous to your illness." The nurses work to help patients see some humor in their situations and to bring some life and laughter to the hospital setting, which can too often be sterile and solemn.

Humor is also being used successfully in long-term care facilities. At Regency Healthcare and Rehabilitation Center, a 300-bed nursing facility in Niles, Illinois, staff members act out whodunit mysteries, residents do imitations of John Wayne, and everyone at the facility comes together to put on their own Academy Awards show—with Clark Gable continuing to be a big winner. "Residents face so many challenges and losses—and when things get rough, humor is a coping mechanism," says Kevin M. Kavanaugh, director of community relations for Regency.[15]

Humor is even being used in a setting not normally considered at all funny: hospice care, where people are assisted in the death process. At the VNA Community Hospice in Arlington, Virginia, workers help the patients focus on life—on living each day until they die. At weekly Tuesday night meetings, people gather, have a cup of coffee, and share their experiences, and the room very often fills with laughter as people acknowledge the elements of humor in their stories, struggles, and memories. It's not unusual, say the organizers, to hear people describe uncontrollable laughter at times not usually thought of as funny because humor is often a mechanism that frees them from emotional bondage.

Humor has also been shown to be extremely beneficial to medical professionals who work with terminally ill patients, an extremely difficult job. In a large-scale study, they were asked how they are able to come back to work every day despite the challenges involved in the job. Their answer: humor.[16]

The benefits of laughter on physical and mental health are being noted even in the corporate world. According to a report published in *Newsweek*,[17] some of the nation's largest corporations have instituted humor programs to help develop a sense of humor in employees; the results include an increased employee capacity to deal with stress and an overall improvement in job performance. Management for Safeway Stores, in fact, reports a sharp decrease in the number of debilitating accidents since the stores began holding humor clinics in 1984. Southwest Airlines[18] has incorporated a strategic effort to integrate humor into the workplace in order to create a positive environment for both employees and customers. Other major entities that hold humor clinics or programs for employees include Manville Corporation, Southwestern Bell, IBM, Hewlett-Packard, the U. S. Air Force, Monsanto, the Internal Revenue Service, General Foods, and the Hartford Insurance Group.

Humor in the workplace has a number of important benefits, says Melissa B. Wanzer, professor of communication studies at Canisius College in Buffalo, New York. Employees who see their managers as humor oriented also view them as being more effective, she says. And employees "also reported higher job satisfaction when they worked for someone who was more humor oriented and used humor appropriately and effectively."[19]

The Impact of Humor on Health

The physiological changes that occur from laughter are so effective that laughter may be classed as aerobic activity. And the outlook characterized by a good sense of humor is beneficial to both physical and mental wellness, according to the most recent evidence.

Educator and author John-Roger was traveling with some friends on the lecture circuit. When they arrived at one destination, the plane was late. To make matters worse, everyone else's luggage arrived first. When their luggage finally appeared, one piece of luggage was obviously damaged. Another suitcase had sprung open, and clothing and personal items were spread all over the conveyor belt. The people traveling with John-Roger were becoming increasingly upset.

Finally he turned to the group and said, "Relax, this is funny. In a few weeks we'll be telling stories about tonight and laughing about it. If it'll be funny then, it's funny now."

According to John-Roger, the focus changed. They started looking at the situation "as if it were a Woody Allen movie. When some of the luggage didn't arrive, we smiled. When the car rental agency didn't have our reservation (or cars), we laughed. When we heard there was a taxi strike, we howled."[20]

Antioch University Professor Harvey Mindess, an expert in humor, points out, "Humor at its best encourages a broad perspective on life. It provides a view of the ironies that abound, of the fact that nobody and nothing is as it seems. And recognizing life's zaniness encourages flexibility and adaptability, rather than rigidity and brittleness."[21]

The Physical Benefits of Humor

It is well-accepted in the scientific community that humor is strongly related to good physical health and a sense of well-being, but researchers are reluctant to link any specific disease process to humor. One reason for that reluctance is the possibility that being in good health may naturally cause someone to be in better humor than if he or she were in poor health.[22] So while some researchers hold back in releasing a blanket statement about humor and specific disease processes, research *has* shown that humor has significant impact in various disease conditions. For example, humor has been shown to have a positive effect on people with heart disease. In one study, two groups of people who had experienced heart attacks were followed throughout their cardiac rehabilitation; one group was allowed to view humorous videos or television programs for half an hour a day as part of their standard therapy. That group, the research revealed, suffered fewer arrhythmias, had lower levels of harmful catecholamines in their blood and urine, required less medication, and had fewer heart attack recurrences.[23]

Because the type A personality has been implicated in heart disease, one study looked at the relationship between humor and the type A personality. Researchers found that 40 percent of people with coronary heart disease laughed less frequently and used humor less often during adversity. Basically, said the researchers, the people who laughed more were healthier.[24]

The results of recent research also show that a sense of humor— an attitude of merriment and a point of view that sees the comical in things—can actually promote good health by strengthening the immune system. Something about humor and laughter metabolically "turns on" the immune system and increases its effectiveness in promoting health and resisting infection. Studies have shown that people with a humorous outlook get sick less often and especially suffer from fewer colds and flu infections.[25]

Researchers have long known that stress, including everyday hassles, weakens the immune system. Some of these researchers have compared people with a well-developed sense of humor (those who see humor in their everyday lives) to those who have a poorly developed sense of humor. They found that among those with a well-developed sense of humor, the immune system was not weakened by everyday hassles and problems. Essentially, their immune systems were stronger and better able to handle various threats to health.

In one study, researchers had a group of men watch a 60-minute humor video; they then measured various immune indicators. After watching the video, the men had greater activity among their natural killer cells—the cells that assist in immune surveillance—that lasted for at least 12 hours after watching the video. Researchers determined that, because the effect lasted for 12 hours, daily exposure to humor could prolong the elevation of natural killer cells, adding powerful immune protection.[26]

In a separate study in which people watched an hour-long humor video, there was a significant increase in the number of B cells—cells produced in the bone marrow that are responsible for making immunoglobulins. It also increased the number and activity of natural killer cells, the number and activity level of helper T cells, and the ratio of helper to suppressor T cells.[27]

Humor has also been shown to increase the levels of gamma interferon, a complex immune substance that activates natural killer cells, plays an important role in the maturation of B cells, and has significant impact on the growth of cytotoxic T cells. Essentially, gamma interferon tells different components of the immune system when to become more active and regulates and promotes levels of coordination between various cells of the immune system.[28]

In another study, people were randomly assigned to watch either a humorous or a distracting video. Those who watched the humorous video had greater stress reduction and elevated natural killer cell activity. The investigators who conducted the study observed that "the amount of mirthful laughter was the major contributing factor for the increased immune function seen in these subjects, rather than the reduced stress levels."[29]

One interesting study showed that mothers with newborn infants who used humor to cope with the stresses of caring for a new baby had significantly fewer upper respiratory infections. Their babies also had significantly fewer upper respiratory infections because the mothers who used humor had higher levels of immunoglobulin A in their breast milk, which protected their infants.[30]

Finally, research has shown that healthy people who watch a sixty-minute humorous video have elevations in growth hormones and important decreases in stress hormones—including cortisol, dopamine, and adrenaline. The implication of these findings is that humor could reverse some of the classical physiological changes that occur during stress.[31]

The Psychological Benefits of Humor

A sense of humor has tremendous psychological benefits as well and correlates positively to quality of life. Humor helps replace distressing emotions with pleasant ones, enhances the ability to connect with other people, increases energy, and makes people feel good. It also helps increase hope, as shown by researchers at Texas A&M University, which can lead to increased feelings of well-being.[32] In one study, humor was shown to boost a number of factors that are related to psychological health, such as optimism and self-esteem. The same study found that those who did not score well on a scientific scale that measures humor were much more likely to show signs of psychological distress, such as depression.[33]

In essence, a good sense of humor is correlated with increased self-esteem and decreased depressive personality attributes. Most of the research that has been done so far indicates that humor does reduce depression—either by directly moderating the depression itself, moderating depressive personality factors, or buffering the ability of life events to cause depression. The link between humor and clinical depression is less clear and will require more research to determine whether the depression itself reduces a sense of humor.[34]

Researchers conducting a wide array of studies have found that, in addition to enhancing self-esteem, a humorous outlook on life can have far-reaching benefits, including promoting creativity, improving negotiating and decision-making skills, maintaining a sense of balance, improving performance, bestowing a sense of power, relieving stress, and improving coping abilities.

Promoting Creativity   People with a good sense of humor are generally more creative—and tend to have much more creativity in the way they approach life's problems. Edward de Bono, the world's leading authority on creativity, says that humor and the creative process are actually one and the same thing. With both, he says, the brain recognizes the value of the absurd or the creative idea only in hindsight because, before that, both seem "crazy." The hallmarks of creative thinkers, then, are the willingness to play with ideas and to risk foolishness without fear.[35]

Improving Negotiating and Decision-Making Skills   A good sense of humor apparently improves the ability to negotiate and to make decisions. Researchers who wanted to measure the impact of humor on negotiating situations set up a role-playing situation in which paired volunteers played the roles of buyers and sellers of appliances.[36] The volunteers were given a range of alternatives and were told to achieve the highest profit (the sellers) or the best deal (the buyers). The pairs who read funny cartoons prior to negotiations—of the

B.C. and *New Yorker* variety—did best. During the face-to-face negotiation involved in the role playing, they were less anxious, had fewer contentions, and were better able to reach a solution that pleased both the "buyer" and the "seller."

Maintaining a Sense of Balance   Renowned American clergyman Henry Ward Beecher wrote that a person without a sense of humor "is like a wagon without springs—jolted by every pebble in the road." Indeed, a sense of humor helps us achieve and maintain that delicate balance that puts life in perspective. We all suffer stress; we all endure heartache; we all struggle with situations that are less than perfect. Viewed through a sense of humor, it all seems okay. We don't take things too seriously, and we are able to coast through situations that would otherwise tip us precariously off balance.[37]

Improving Performance   Humor helps to improve both group and individual performance. The greatest benefits occur, says University of Tennessee psychologist Howard Pollio, when the humor is directly related to the task at hand.[38]

Bestowing a Sense of Power   A sense of humor can give us a sense of power. According to "jollyologist" Allen Klein, laughter helps us to transcend our predicaments.[39] He gives the example of Anatoly Sharansky, the Russian human rights advocate who was confined for nine years in Soviet prisons. His prison sentence included 16 months of solitary confinement and the constant threat of the death penalty.

Klein relates that Soviet police constantly threatened Sharansky with the rastrel (the "firing squad"), knowing that Sharansky's greatest battle was against fear. Sharansky managed to win the war against fear through humor. He started actually joking about the firing squad and talking about it on a daily basis.

"You make jokes fifteen to twenty times," Sharansky remembers, "and the word becomes like any other word. The ear gets accustomed to it, and it no longer prompts fear."

Klein relates a second example involving eighteenth-century philosopher Moses Mendelssohn. While walking down the streets of Berlin one day, he accidentally collided with a plump Prussian officer. "Swine!" the officer bellowed. Mendelssohn, knowing that a reprisal would invite punishment from the officer, decided on a different approach—one laced with humor. He smiled, tipped his hat, and replied, "Mendelssohn." As Klein points out, humor can turn any situation around—and can give us a feeling of power over our circumstances.

Relieving Stress   Numerous studies have shown that people who withstand even tremendous stress without becoming brittle, bitter, and broken have several traits in common: they are altruistic (they actively care about the welfare of others), they get plenty of support from friends and the community, and they gain control over difficult situations with humor.[40]

Humor has been demonstrated in a wide variety of studies to help alleviate the effects of stress. In one, researchers showed that people with a good sense of humor don't get as stressed to begin with. They placed an old tennis shoe, a drinking glass, and an aspirin bottle on a table and asked volunteers to make up a three-minute comedy routine using the objects on the table. Results of the study showed that the volunteers who wrote the funniest routines were those who were least likely to become tense, depressed, angry, fatigued, or confused when stress occurred in their lives.[41]

In one study, volunteers were shown a film about an industrial accident—a decidedly unfunny topic. Half the volunteers were asked to come up with a comical dialogue during the film; the other half were asked to give a straightforward report about the film afterward. Researchers were able to measure far less of the stress response in the bodies of those who came up with the comical dialogue—even among those who researchers characteristically would have categorized as "not funny."[42]

Results of that survey show not only that humor helps relieve stress but also that it can be learned, even by those who may not consider themselves to have a great sense of humor. Study author Michelle Newman says that the study "suggests that the way we perceive ourselves may not necessarily reflect how capable we are of using humor to cope. It challenges the notion that using coping humor is an unchangeable trait rather than an acquired skill." According to Newman, the study results show that you can "rethink the situation to decide if it's really a big deal or if you can handle it. And it may help you distance yourself enough from a situation to calm down."[43]

Humor has been shown repeatedly to be a tool that helps relieve the stress of illness, terminal disease, and hospitalization. Lenore Reinhard, coordinator of the humor program at Schenectady's Sunnyview Rehabilitation Hospital, says she has seen repeated evidence that humorous books and tapes really help relieve the stress of being confined to a hospital. She remembers one patient in his forties who was under significant stress and who was not helped by relaxation tapes.

"I suggested that he check out some of our humor tapes—we have Woody Allen, Bill Cosby, 'Father' Guido Sarducci, George Burns, Rodney Dangerfield, Mel Brooks, and others," she relates. "Several weeks later, after he left, I checked the sign-out book—he'd borrowed nine tapes. They really helped him relax and get his mind off the very difficult situation he was in."[44]

Norman Cousins points out that humor neutralizes emotionally charged stress and is especially helpful for people who are facing serious or terminal illness. He says that humor "accomplishes one very essential purpose. It tends to block deep feelings of apprehension and even panic that all too frequently accompany serious illness." In addition, he says, it frees concentration on the body and enables healing to begin.[45]

Improving Coping Abilities   Lawrence Mintz, a professor of American studies at the University of Maryland, believes that "humor is the way we cope with living in an imperfect world with imperfect selves. When we can't win, the best thing to do is to laugh about it."[46]

Antioch University professor Harvey Mindess agrees that humor is "a great coping mechanism. When a client of mine is very anxious about something, I try to get him to break out of his anger or fear by laughing at himself."[47]

As early as the turn of the twentieth century, eminent psychoanalyst Sigmund Freud touted humor as one of the only socially acceptable ways to release pent-up frustration and anger, and he hailed it as a way to preserve the emotional energy that would normally be required to cope with a stressful situation. "The essence of humor is that one spares oneself the effects to which the situation would naturally give rise," he explained, "and overrides with a jest the possibility of such an emotional display."[48]

Allen Klein cites the examples given by psychologist Samuel Janus and scientists Seymour and Rhoda Fisher of famous "funny people" who used humor to cope with deep psychological pain. In Klein's book, *The Healing Power of Humor,* he points out that Totie Field's mother died when she was five, David Steinberg's brother was killed in Vietnam, Jackie Gleason's father deserted him, W. C. Fields ran away from home because his father was going to kill him, Dudley Moore was born with a clubfoot, Art Buchwald's mother died when he was very young, and Carol Burnett's parents were both alcoholics who fought constantly.

"Charlie Chaplin, too, found solace in humor," Klein writes. "Raised in one of the poorest sections of London, he was five years old when his father died of alcoholism; after that his mother went mad. Chaplin used these gloomy memories in his films and turned them into comedic gems. Who could forget the scene in Gold Rush, for example, where he eats a boiled leather shoe for dinner because no other food is available?"[49]

Laughter: The Best Medicine

Laughter as medicine is probably as old as humankind. One of the earliest written accounts recognizing the healing power of humor is found in the Bible, in which King Solomon remarked that "a merry heart doeth good like a medicine."[50] Members of royal courts around the world and throughout the ages have valued the court jester—the colorful clown who provided the humor that made governing a palatable job.

Henri de Mondeville, a thirteenth-century surgeon, told jokes to his patients as they emerged from operations. Sixteenth-century English educator Richard Mulcater prescribed laughter for those afflicted with head colds and melancholy; a favorite "cure" was being tickled in the armpits. Humor was even used by ancient Americans: Ojibway Indian doctor-clowns, the Windigokan, used laughter to heal the sick.[51]

Psychologist Robert Ornstein and physician David Sobel recite the scientific definition of a laugh as "a psychophysiological reflex, a successive, rhythmic, spasmodic expiration with open glottis and vibration of the vocal cords, often accompanied by a baring of the teeth and facial grimaces."[52] While laughter often goes along with humor or happiness, it is *not* the same as either one—instead, it is the physical and physiological response to humor (something funny), and it often *results in* a feeling of happiness.[53]

Is it possible that happiness and health are linked because people who are healthy are therefore happy about it? Obviously someone would be happy about being healthy. But researchers believe that happy people actually promote their own good health as a result of the physiological benefits of being happy.[54]

Long considered helpful to the healing process, laughter has been shown to exercise the cardiovascular system, improve breathing, increase oxygen flow throughout the body, boost the level of endorphins, improve pain tolerance and reduce pain, strengthen the immune system, tone the internal organs, and improve optimism and a healthy outlook—all without any adverse side effects.[55]

The Physiology of Laughter

Laughter may seem simple, but it's actually a complex physical process. Scientists have found that there are actually two different kinds of laughter: laughter in response to a humorous stimulus (the spontaneous response to a hilarious scene in a movie, for example) and laughter that is "self-generated," or strategic (laughter that makes someone else like you, that smoothes over an awkward spot in a conversation, or that covers up embarrassment).[56] Regardless of its type or source, a good laugh works the same in the body. According to studies reported in the *Journal of the American Medical Association,* laughter does the following:

- **Breathing:** increases the breathing rate, increases the amount of oxygen circulated through the blood, and clears mucus from the lungs

- **Muscles:** provides limited muscle conditioning, provides muscle relaxation, and breaks the pain/spasm cycle common to some muscle disorders

- **Cardiovascular system:** temporarily increases the heart rate and blood pressure, increases circulation, and increases the amount of oxygen delivered to all body cells[57]

Stanford Medical School psychiatrist William Fry, Jr., says that laughter is valuable for strengthening the heart muscle and, he says, just 20 seconds of laughter is the cardiovascular equivalent of three minutes of strenuous rowing.[58] In fact, he said, it took him ten minutes on a rowing machine to get his heart to the rate it was at after just one minute of hearty laughter.[59]

Consider this description, published in a scientific journal around the turn of the twentieth century:

> There occur in laughter and more or less in smiling, clonic spasms of the diaphragm in number ordinarily about eighteen perhaps, and contraction of most of the muscles of the face. The upper side of the mouth and its corners are drawn upward. The upper eyelid is elevated, as are also, to some extent, the brows, the skin over the glabella, and the upper lip, while the skin at the outer canthi of the eye is characteristically puckered. The nostrils are moderately dilated and drawn upward, the tongue slightly extended, and the cheeks distended and drawn somewhat upward; in persons with the pinnal muscles largely developed, the pinnae tend to incline forwards. The lower jaw vibrates or is somewhat withdrawn (doubtless to afford all possible air to the distending lungs), and the head, in extreme laughter, is thrown backward, until (and this usually happens soon) fatigue-pain in the diaphragm and accessory abdominal muscles causes a marked proper flexion of the trunk for its relief. The whole arterial vascular system is dilated, with consequent blushing from the effort on the dermal capillaries of the face and neck, and at times of the scalp and hands. From this same cause in the main the eyes often slightly bulge forwards and the lachrymal gland becomes active, ordinarily to a degree only to cause a "brightening" of the eyes, but often to such an extent that the tears overflow entirely their proper channels.[60]

Laughter as Exercise

Laughter is one of the best exercises around, and one of the nicest things about it is its simplicity. It requires no special training. It requires no special equipment. You don't have to do it at the gym or on the track or on a Nautilus machine. All you need, in fact, is a sense of humor.

Stanford Medical School's William Fry likens laughter to a form of physical exercise—it causes huffing and puffing, speeds up the heart rate, raises blood pressure, accelerates breathing, increases oxygen consumption, gives the muscles of the stomach and face a workout, and relaxes the skeletal muscles that aren't used in laughing (in one study, people using a biofeedback device were able to relax muscles more quickly after watching funny cartoons than after look at beautiful scenery[61]). Twenty seconds of laughing can double the heart rate for three to five minutes, he adds.[62] While laughter should not be used as a substitute for aerobic exercise, it should be valued for its beneficial effects on the entire body.

Laughter provides what some experts have called "a total inner body workout"—and more and more researchers are finding out exactly what it is about a laugh that is so good for us.

In brief, he says that something you see or hear or think of sets off "a massive brain reaction." Nerve fibers in the involuntary nervous system trigger a snowballing cycle of discharges in the brain stem. "Your neural circuits reverberate with the news: something is funny."[63]

Your humor is then converted into electrical and chemical impulses that wash through the frontal lobes of the brain, go over the motor centers of the brain, and land smack in the center of the cerebral cortex. The cortex then hands out an order to the body: Laugh!

"A laugh," Brody writes, "can run anywhere from a half-second giggle or guffaw to a 60-second belly burster, a memorable earthquake down in your abdomen, with many variations in between."[64] Fry, who has studied laughter extensively, estimates that people in good spirits let loose with as many as 100 to 400 laughs a day.

Once you're ready to laugh, the muscles in your face that control expressions start to contort, says Brody. Muscles throughout your body contract like fists. Your vocal cord muscles, designed for intelligible sound, cannot coordinate. Your glottis and larynx open, relaxed and ready to vibrate. Your diaphragm tenses up in anticipation of respiratory spasms. According to Brody, "Air in your body billows until you feel pressure building in your lungs. Trying to hold in a laugh is no less than a violation against nature—rarely successful."

Once the laugh gets into full gear, writes Brody, "your breathing is interrupted for a station break. Your lower jaw vibrates. A blast of air gusts into your trachea, flinging mucus against the walls of your windpipe. Pandemonium! Out comes your laugh, in some cases clocked at 170 miles an hour. You issue a strange machine-gun sound, almost a violent bark."

Once in the throes of a full-bodied laugh, your body bucks. Your torso is flexed. Your arms flail, your hands slap your thighs. "Your lacrimal glands squeeze out tears, giving your eyes a mirthful sheen. You puff and rasp with symphonic regularity. You can hardly stand so much glee coursing through you. You're wobbly in the knees, wheezing like an asthmatic. Pleading for mercy, you collapse on the nearest sofa. Sounds like fun, no?"[65]

The complicated combination of physiological reactions makes laughing what some researchers have called "inner jogging." Your metabolism steps up, and calories are burned off. Your body temperature increases. Your entire system is showered with adrenaline, making you feel good all over. Best of all, the physical effects of laughter endure for up to two hours after you stop laughing.

Laughter is essentially an act of respiration—and the lungs immediately fill with air. Air volume is dramatically increased, and your breathing rate goes up. Because of increased air volume and breathing rate, much more oxygen is delivered to the body than with normal breathing. You also breathe out more carbon monoxide and water vapor, which can encourage bacterial growth if it stays in the lungs. Once you finish laughing, you usually cough—a reaction that finishes clearing out the lungs.

Next, your heart rate increases during laughter, and the increase is in direct proportion to how long and hard you laugh. The entire cardiovascular system is stepped up, and the circulation increases; as a result, the entire cardiovascular system is toned. Fresh nutrients and oxygen go coursing through your arteries. Your blood pressure goes up. When you finish laughing, your heart rate and blood pressure drop to levels below those when you started laughing.

Laughter improves your digestion and may even stimulate enzymes that act as natural laxatives. It stimulates your central nervous system. And it first contracts, and then relaxes, almost all the muscles in your body. When you begin to laugh, at least five major muscle groups begin a rhythmic movement; when you finish laughing, your muscles— especially those of the abdomen, diaphragm, shoulders, neck, and face—are more relaxed than when you started laughing. Laughter not only improves muscle tone but also enables total relaxation of all major muscle groups in your body.

Combining laughter with physical movement—such as waving your arms around while you laugh—doubles the benefit!

The Health Benefits of Laughter

In describing the health benefits of laughter, Norman Cousins—who laughed his way back to health from a painful and debilitating disease—likes to relate the story of an encounter he had in a veterans' hospital. Concerned about the glum spirits of the men on the cancer ward at the hospital in Sepulveda, California, physicians asked Cousins to impress the men with how optimism and good cheer could actually help them feel better and maybe even help them heal. Cousins met with 50 or 60 of the veterans and discussed the role of humor and cheer. Then he told them he hoped they would work together to create an atmosphere conducive to the best medical treatment available.

When Cousins returned to the hospital a few weeks later, he noted that the men had accepted the challenge. He could see the changes immediately. In their meeting that morning, each veteran was asked to tell about something good that had happened to him since the previous meeting. Each one in turn told about something good, with intermittent cheers bursting forth from the others. When each had taken a turn, they all turned to face Cousins. Obviously, they expected him to relate a story as well.

In his book *Head First*, Cousins relates the following experience, which he feels demonstrates the power of laughter:[66]

> "What I have to report is better than good," I said. "It's wonderful. Actually, it's better than wonderful. It's unbelievable. And as long as I live, I don't expect that anything as magnificent as this can possibly happen to me again."

The veterans sat forward in their seats.

"What happened is that when I arrived at the Los Angeles airport last Wednesday my bag was the first off the carousel."

An eruption of applause and acclaim greeted this announcement.

"I had never even met anyone whose bag was first off the carousel," I continued.

Again, loud expressions of delight.

"Flushed with success, I went to the nearest telephone to report my arrival to my office. That was when I lost my coin. I pondered this melancholy event for a moment or two, then decided to report it to the operator.

"Operator," I said, "I put a quarter in and didn't get my number. The machine collected my coin."

"Sir," she said, "if you give me your name and address, we'll mail the coin to you."

"I was appalled."

"Operator," I said, "I think I can understand the reason behind the difficulties of AT&T. You're going to take the time and trouble to write down my name on a card and then you are probably going to give it to the person in charge of such matters. He will go the cash register, punch it open and take out a quarter, at the same time recording the reason for the cash withdrawal. Then he will take a cardboard with a recessed slot to hold the coin so it won't flop around in the envelope. Then he, or someone else, will fit the cardboard with the coin into an envelope, first taking the time to write my address on the envelope. Then the envelope will be sealed. Someone will then affix a twenty-cent stamp on the envelope. All that time and expense just to return a quarter. Now, operator, why don't you just return my coin and let's be friends."

"Sir," she repeated in a flat voice, "if you give me your name and address, we will mail you the refund."

"Then, almost by way of afterthought, she said, 'Sir, did you remember to press the coin return plunger?'"

"Truth to tell, I had overlooked this nicety. I pressed the plunger. To my great surprise, it worked. It was apparent that the machine had been badly constipated and I happened to have the plunger. All at once, the vitals of the machine opened up and proceeded to spew out coins of almost every denomination. The profusion was so great that I had to use my empty hand to contain the overflow.

"While all this was happening, the noise was registering in the telephone and was not lost on the operator.

"Sir," she said, "what is happening?"

I reported that the machine had just given up all its earnings for the past few months, at least. At a rough estimate, I said there must be close to four dollars in quarters, dimes, and nickels that had just erupted from the box.

"Sir," she said, "will you please put the coins back in the box."

"Operator," I said, "if you give me your name and address I will be glad to mail you the coins."

According to Cousins, the veterans "exploded with cheers. David triumphs over Goliath. At the bottom of the ninth inning, with the home team behind by three runs, the weakest hitter in the lineup hits the ball out of the park. A mammoth business corporation is brought to its knees. Every person who has been exasperated by the loss of a coin in a public telephone booth could identify with my experience and share both in the triumph of justice and the humiliation of the mammoth and the impersonal oppressor."

One of the doctors in the room, noticing how relaxed and mobile the men were, asked how many had been experiencing their usual amount of pain when they arrived at the meeting. More than half of the veterans in the room raised their hands. The doctor then asked how many noticed that their pain had receded or completely disappeared. The same hands went up.

The example given by Cousins is just one of the many that doctors and researchers studying laughter are hearing. Because of the physiological changes that take place during laughter, it packs a punch in terms of physical benefits, pain relief, boosts in immunity, and psychological benefits.

Physical Benefits of Laughter

As discussed, Stanford University researcher William Fry concluded that laughter is like a form of physical exercise. According to Fry, laughter also stimulates the sympathetic nervous system, the pituitary gland, and the hormones that relieve pain and inflammation, making it a possible benefit in conditions like arthritis and gout. The results of several studies suggest that laughter reduces allergic reactions, including the symptoms of hay fever.[67]

Laughter has even been shown to reduce food cravings[68] and to help in keeping diabetes under control by regulating spikes in blood sugar levels following a meal and by reducing the risk of diabetic complications. In one study, participants were shown either a funny video or a lecture video during dinner. After the meal, those who had watched the funny video had consistently lower blood sugar levels.[69]

Psychologist Jeffrey Goldstein of Temple University credits laughter with contributing to longevity, and says that results of his research show that laughter works physiologically to reduce stress, hypertension, depression, heart attacks, and stroke. Laughing, says Goldstein, is much like jogging as a physical exercise—and its benefits are just as great. It even burns calories: research at Vanderbilt University shows that 10 to 15 minutes of laughter burns 50 calories.[70]

Cortisol—a stress hormone that increases the risk of both heart disease and diabetes—is reduced by laughter and happiness; in one study, those who were happiest had 32 percent lower cortisol levels when subjected to a stressful mental exercise than did the less happy people.[71] Researchers have even found that the tears you shed during a good laugh have the same chemical composition as the tears you shed during a good cry. Both have been scientifically proven to carry away toxins and the hormones manufactured during stress.

Furthermore, when you laugh, you breathe much more deeply—usually emptying your lungs fully of air, and then drawing in a full, deep breath for the next peal of laughter. That kind of deep breathing rids the lungs of carbon dioxide, better oxygenates the entire body, gets rid of water vapor in the lungs (which, if it remains, can lead to respiratory infection), and helps in relaxation.[72]

Cardiovascular Benefits of Laughter

One clear benefit of laughter is to the cardiovascular system. According to researchers at the University of Maryland School of Medicine, laughter, along with a great sense of humor, protects against heart disease in general and can help prevent heart attack.[73]

Other research released by the American College of Cardiology[74] showed that laughter increases blood flow by more than 20 percent—equivalent to a round of aerobic exercise—and that the effect of laughter on the cardiovascular system lasts as long as 45 minutes. (Contrast that to stress, which *decreases* blood flow by about 35 percent.) In the study, volunteers were shown two 15-minute film clips: one a comedy movie clip, and the other a stressful film sequence. The film clips were viewed 48 hours apart. After watching the comedy clip, 95 percent of the volunteers had better blood flow; but, after watching the stressful film, 70 percent had worse blood flow.

The benefit of laughter seemed to be on the endothelium (the inner lining of the arteries), which regulates the diameter of the blood vessels; damage to the endothelium is one of the factors involved in cardiovascular disease. Researchers found that laughter expanded the endothelium—helping keep the arterial walls fit—while stress narrowed it. While researchers clearly saw the beneficial effect, they're still not sure *why* laughter expands the arteries; hypotheses include the release of endorphins and the preservation of nitric oxide, a natural chemical that helps the arteries expand and that is broken down during stress.

The same research group published a separate study indicating that a good sense of humor may help protect against heart disease.[75] The researchers compared 150 men and women with heart disease to 150 men and women who had no heart problems. All were put in difficult and embarrassing situations. Those with heart disease were much more likely to react to the difficult situations with anger and hostility, while those free of heart disease most often used humor to overcome their embarrassment. Those with heart disease were also less likely to laugh in positive situations and reported a reduced ability to laugh in general. Researchers concluded that laughter is likely to protect the heart—and that the ability to laugh at difficulties can reduce the risk of heart disease.[76]

A six-year study of 2,500 senior citizens found that those who scored the highest on a happiness quiz had far fewer strokes than those who scored the lowest.[77] A study of London civil service employees found that those who reported feeling happy almost every day—including at work and on the weekends—had lower heart rates and were significantly healthier than their less-happy counterparts.[78]

Heart rate variability (HRV) reflects the heart's ability to adapt to changing situations, such as increased mental stress or a session of aggressive physical exercise. A low HRV is a strong predictor of coronary events, including sudden death, while a high HRV is a robust protector of cardiovascular health. Studies have shown that happy people have consistently higher HRVs, which reduces chemicals like cortisol that cause insulin resistance, diabetes, and hypertension—all part of the heart-harming metabolic syndrome, a major risk factor for cardiovascular disease.[79]

Pain Relief Benefits of Laughter

The most well-known example of laughter as an anesthetic is provided by Norman Cousins. When his symptoms of achiness, fatigue, and fever worsened instead of getting better, he sought medical help. The diagnosis was devastating: a potentially life-threatening collagen disease that affected all the connective tissues of the body. Involvement was already so extreme that he was having difficulty merely moving his joints. His physician told him that recovery was not probable.

Instead of merely accepting the prognosis that would have sentenced him to pain and then death, Cousins decided to take things into his own hands. He designed a program of positive thinking, nutritious food—and, as a painkiller, laughter.

Cousins found that laughter was the most effective painkiller he could find. Ten minutes of hearty laughter (usually prompted by old Candid Camera reruns) provided two hours of pain-free sleep. Even more remarkably, he found that inflammation in the tissues was reduced after each laughter session.

A decade later—fully recovered and functioning as a vital, vigorous man—he wrote of his experience. He gave laughter part of the credit for his miraculous recovery. Following his claims, a number of scientists set out to test his theory that laughter could act as an analgesic. Indeed, it was found that laughing does relieve pain; children who watched comedy films were able to relax, which relieved their pain, and to better tolerate what pain they did have.[80] Therapeutic laughter is being used in a number of hospitals, and humorous videos are being incorporated in treatment rooms.

Laughter probably relieves pain for several different reasons. One is distraction; something humorous that makes us laugh draws attention away from the pain, at least temporarily. Another is muscle relaxation. Pain often involves muscle tension—the same kind of muscle gripping and spasm you would experience if you tried to stand on one leg for a long time. When you laugh, the tension dissipates, and the spasms relax.

Laughter also stimulates the brain to release endorphins.[81] These potent natural chemicals have painkilling power estimated to be 200 times that of morphine; they also reduce inflammation and can stimulate the immune system. These are the chemicals responsible for the famed "runner's high"— and researchers believe there may be a very real and similar "laugher's high" that results when these chemicals leave laughers feeling relaxed and good all over.

Laughter and humor can relieve not only physical pain but emotional pain, too. By providing a new perspective and lightening the emotional tension of a situation, laughing can relieve emotional stress and ease psychological pain.

A number of studies on laughter are being conducted throughout the United States and Europe. The results of one study, published in the *Journal of the American Medical Association,* involved only a small group of patients but shows great promise for the role of "humor therapy" in relieving pain.

Dr. Lars Ljungdahl and his colleagues at Sweden's Lyckorna Primary Health-Care Centre chose six women who were incapacitated with an extremely painful muscle-bone disorder. The physicians administered psychological tests to the women before beginning the experiment to determine general psychological well-being.[82]

The women were then given "humor therapy" for 13 weeks. The patients used humorous books, records, and videotapes daily; they also met once a week with nurses who gave lectures on humor and helped the women understand how to better use humor in their everyday lives. The patients were asked to regularly record on separate scales how amused they were and how much pain relief they had.

Ljungdahl said that the women who participated in the study enjoyed "significant relief" from their painful symptoms—and those with the greatest degrees of amusement were also the ones who had the greatest pain relief. Tests administered at the end of the 13-week period also showed that the women had a greater overall sense of well-being.

"Their self-confidence also seemed to increase, they coped more ably with their symptoms, and allowed themselves to be happy and enjoy life regardless of their medical problems," he said. Ljungdahl noted that pain relief was greater during the last seven weeks than during the first six weeks (during the first six weeks, the women learned how to use humor to relieve pain), indicating that laughter had the greatest benefits.[83]

Immunity-Enhancing Benefits of Laughter

All of the research on laughter has revealed what may be one of laughter's most important benefits: It apparently enhances the immune system. Researchers believe that the immune-enhancing powers of laughter are due to two separate aspects of laughter. First, it boosts the production of immune enhancers, including immunoglobulins, natural killer cells, and T cells.[84] Dr. Lee Berk, an immunologist at California's Loma Linda University Medical Center, has conducted studies involving both of these effects of laughter on the immune system. In experiments with students, those who watched humorous videotapes compared with those who didn't had the highest concentrations of lymphocytes, greater natural killer cell activity, and significantly better measures of overall immune system activity. "The changes in the white cell counts and hormones," he says, "have been more surprising than we ever realized."[85]

Second, it suppresses the production of stress hormones that weaken immunity. According to psychologist Robert Ornstein and physician David Sobel, "When confronted with a threatening situation, animals have essentially two choices: to flee or fight. Humans have a third alternative: to laugh."[86]

One series of studies measuring the effects of laughter on stress hormones was carried out by Berk and his Loma Linda University Medical Center colleagues. Berk had five men watch an hour-long comedy video of the comedian Gallagher; he then took blood tests and compared them to test results from five men who did not watch the video.[87]

The five who watched the funny film had lower levels of the stress hormone adrenaline. They also had significantly lower levels of DOPAC (3,4-dihydroxyphenylacetic acid, a metabolite that indicates dopamine activity) and the stress hormone cortisol, which can shut down the body's production of the immune substance interleukin-2. Berk and his colleagues concluded from the studies (and others they conducted on laughter) that laughing definitely has beneficial effects on the immune system—and may even help combat certain diseases.

The message for us is clear. As psychologist Gordon Allport suggested, "I venture to say that no person is in good health unless he can laugh at himself, quietly and privately."[88]

Psychological Benefits of Laughter

Among the psychological benefits of laughter are its ability to diminish fear, calm anger, and relieve depression. Laughter has been shown to improve job performance (especially in jobs that demand creativity), improve marriages and other intimate relationships, synchronize the brains of speaker and audience, and establish or restore a sense of connection between two people.[89] Perhaps the most pronounced psychological benefits of laughter, however, are its ability to relieve stress and its tendency to improve our perspective—on everything from pain to life itself.

Laughter as Stress Relief   Steve Allen, Jr.—the physician son of comedian Steve Allen—believes that "laughter is not only as good a method of stress relief as a massage, a hot bath, or exercise, it's essential to stress relief." Some of the reasons are tied to the physical outcomes: The body doesn't produce stress hormones as efficiently during laughter, and laughter itself physically breaks up tension. Laughter has been shown to reduce at least four hormones associated with the stress response: adrenaline, cortisol, DOPAC, and growth hormone.[90]

Lawrence Peter, author of *The Laughter Prescription*, considers laughter to be an important safety valve. When you laugh, Peters maintains, you get rid of stress-related tension that can otherwise accumulate and damage health.

We've already discussed the fact that laughter helps keep the endothelium (the lining of the arteries) healthy and able to expand, allowing greater blood flow. According to Michael Miller of the University of Maryland, one way in which laughter protects the endothelium is by offsetting the impact of mental stress, which harms the endothelium.[91] Another benefit of reducing mental stress is that laughter reduces the levels of fibrinogen (a measure of inflammation), which also causes the blood to thicken and clot.[92]

The stress-relieving effect of laughter doesn't last just while you're chuckling, either. Experts agree that the ability of laughter to dispel stress lasts long after the laugh—and can even help the person who laughs to build an actual immunity to stress. That's the opinion of *Laughing Matters* magazine editor Joel Goodman, who believes that laughter can "provide immediate relief from life's daily pressures" as well as "build up an immunity to stress for the long haul."[93]

It's important to note that the studies on stress hormones and laughter have produced some conflicting results. While the period following laughter does show a decrease in heart rate, respiratory rate, and blood pressure and a period of general muscle relaxation, more study is needed on the impact of laughter on specific stress hormones, such as adrenaline, noradrenaline, dopamine, and cortisol.[94]

Laughter as New Perspective   According to Yale surgeon Bernie Siegel, renowned for his work in helping patients heal themselves,

> Humor's most important psychological function is to jolt us out of our habitual frame of mind and promote new perspectives. Psychologists have long noted that one of the best measures of mental health is the ability to laugh at oneself in a gently mocking way—like the dear old schoolteacher, a colostomy patient of mine several years ago, who named her stomas Harry and Larry.[95]

Apparently laughter can give us a new perspective on almost anything—even something as real and so distressing as pain. Psychologists Rosemary Cogan and Dennis Cogan of Texas Tech University in Lubbock designed an experiment[96] to see whether laughter would help change the perspective of pain. They randomly assigned students into one of four groups: one listened to a humorous audiotape, one listened to a relaxation tape, one listened to an informative narrative, and the fourth group did not hear a tape.

The Cogans then fastened automatically inflating blood pressure cuffs around the students' arms and subjected the students to the highest level of discomfort that the cuffs could produce.

The students who were able to withstand even the highest pressure without becoming distressed were those who had listened to the humorous tape. Laughter, the Cogans suggest, changes our perspective of discomfort or distress and enables us to withstand many times what we normally could.

As mentioned earlier, it's not too late to "learn" to have humor, even if you feel you don't have that great a sense of humor now. Whenever you can, laugh with friends—you'll find that laughter is contagious, and you're likely to laugh harder and longer than if you're doing the same thing (watching a funny video or listening to a comic) alone. If you want to have more fun in your life, try following these suggestions of Leigh Anne Jasheway, coordinator of health promotion at the University of Texas Health Science Center at Houston:

- Make a pledge to laugh out loud or to make someone else laugh at least ten times every day.
- Once a week, set aside time to call someone who always adds fun to your day.
- Read your favorite comics in the newspaper every day.
- Make regular dates with a friend or your spouse to do any recreation that you both enjoy.
- Do something silly at least once a week.
- Start a humor collection—go for jokes, clippings, cartoons, cards, mugs, books, or videos.
- Share funny items with others, and use stick-on notes that have humorous messages.
- Rent funny movies.
- Try to find the humor in every predicament.
- Keep a "fun first-aid kit"—cram it full of things like modeling clay, bubbles, puzzles, brain teasers, and other things you love to do.
- Finally, recall all the fun you had as a child![97]

Perhaps one of the best suggestions is to create what Loretta LaRoche calls a "humor survival kit"—and one of her best tools, she says, always gets a laugh:

> Buy something silly you can put on (a pair of Groucho Marx glasses are my favorite). Put them on in situations where you tend to awfulize. I wear mine driving through Boston, especially when I have to merge. People always let me in. Food shopping is another favorite. Among others, going to the dentist, the doctor, staff meetings, talking to your mate, the children, a coworker. When things have really reached the limits of your endurance, go into a bathroom, look into the mirror, put on your glasses, and ask yourself this question: "How serious is this?"[98]

WHAT DID YOU LEARN?

1. Is the medical profession finally recognizing humor as a healing modality?
2. What impact does humor have on health?
3. Why is laughter described as the "best medicine"?

ENDNOTES

1. Barbara Powell, *Good Relationships Are Good Medicine* (Emmaus, PA: Rodale Press, 1987).
2. Mary Payne Bennett and Cecile A. Lengacher, "Humor and Laughter May Influence Health. I. History and Background," *Evidence-Based Complementary and Alternative Medicine* 3, no. 1 (January 2006): 61–3.
3. Mary Christelle Macaluso, "Humor, Health, and Healing," *American Nephrology Nurses' Association Journal* 20, no. 1 (February 1993): 14–6.
4. Loretta LaRoche, "Fully Human, Fully Alive with Humor, Compassion, and Love," *The Psychology of Health, Immunity, and Disease,* vol. A, p. 326, in Proceedings of the Sixth International Conference of the National Institute for the Clinical Application of Behavioral Medicine (Hilton Head, SC: 1994).
5. Ibid.
6. Powell, *Good Relationships Are Good Medicine.*
7. Michael J. Balick and Roberta Lee, "The Role of Laughter in Traditional Medicine and Its Relevance to the Clinical Setting: Healing with Ha!" *Alternative Therapies* 9, no. 4, (July/August 2003): 88–91.
8. Norman Cousins, "The Laughter Connection," *East/West* (February 1990): 58.
9. Nick Gallo, "Lighten Up: Laugh Your Way to Good Health," *Better Homes and Gardens* (August 1989): 31.
10. *Association for Applied and Therapeutic Humor,* http://www.aath.org, accessed June 4, 2008.
11. Mary Payne Bennett and Cecile Lengacher, "Humor and Laughter May Influence Health: II. Complementary Therapies and Humor in a Clinical Population," *Complementary Alternative Medicine* 3, no. 2 (June 2006): 187–90.
12. Barbara Graham, "The Healing Power of Humor," *Mind/Body/Health Digest* 4, no. 2 (1990): 2.
13. Laurie Dayton, "Healing with Humor," *Michigan Health and Hospitals* 33, no. 5, (1997): 16.
14. Balick and Lee, "The Role of Laughter," *Alternative Therapies in Health and Medicine* 9, no. 4 (July/August 2003): 88–91.
15. Dorothy Foltz-Gray, "Make 'Em Laugh," *Contemporary Long-Term Care* 2, no. 9, (September 1998): 44–50.
16. "Laughter Is the Best Medicine," *Science Daily* (January 26, 2008).
17. Penelope Wang, Karen Springen, Tom Schmitz, and Mary Bruno, "A Cure for Stress?" *Newsweek* (October 12, 1987): 84–5.
18. "Laughter Is the Best Medicine."
19. Ibid.
20. Peter McWilliams and John-Roger, *You Can't Afford the Luxury of a Negative Thought* (Los Angeles, CA: Prelude Press, 1989), 277.
21. Caryl S. Avery, "Lighten Up," *Self* (September 1988): 150–7.
22. Bennett and Lengacher, "Humor and Laughter. II. Complementary Therapies and Humor."
23. Balick and Lee, "The Role of Laughter."
24. Ibid.
25. Paul E. McGhee, "Humor and Health," *Holisticonline,* http://holisticonline.com/Humor_Therapy/humor_mcghee_article.htm, accessed June 4, 2008.
26. Lee S. Berk et al., "Modulation of Immune Parameters During the Eustress of Humor-Associated Mirthful Laughter," Alternative Therapies in Health and Medicine 7, no. 2 (2001): 62–7.
27. McGhee, "Humor and Health."
28. Ibid.

29. M. Bennet, J. Zeller, and L. Rosenberg, "The Effect of Mirthful Laughter on Stress and Natural Killer Cell Activity," *Alternative Therapies in Health and Medicine* 9, no. 2 (2003): 38–43.

30. McGhee, "Humor and Health."

31. Balick and Lee, "The Role of Laughter."

32. "Humor Can Increase Hope, Research Shows," *Science Daily* (April 13, 2005).

33. James A. Thorson, F. C. Powell, Ivan Sarmany-Schuller, and William P. Hampes, "Psychological Health and Sense of Humor," *Journal of Clinical Psychology* 53, no. 6 (1997): 605–19.

34. Bennett and Lengacher, "Humor and Laughter. II. Complementary Therapies and Humor."

35. C. W. Metcalf and Roma Felible, *Lighten Up* (New York: Perseus Books, 1992), 9–10.

36. Susan Lang, "Laughing Matters—At Work," *American Health* (September 1988): 46.

37. Allen Klein, *The Healing Power of Humor* (Los Angeles, CA: Jeremy P. Tarcher, 1989), 16–7.

38. Lang, "Laughing Matters."

39. Klein, *The Healing Power of Humor,* 4.

40. Metcalf and Felible, *Lighten Up*, 26.

41. Robert Ornstein and David Sobel, *Healthy Pleasures* (Reading, MA: Addison-Wesley Publishing Company, 1989), 218.

42. M. G. Newman, and A. A. Stone, "Does Humor Moderate the Effects of Experimentally Induced Stress?" *Annals of Behavioral Medicine* 18, no. 2 (1996), 101–9.

43. Ibid.

44. Cathy Perlmutter, "Comic Relief," *Prevention* (March 1988): 107.

45. Norman Cousins, *The Healing Heart* (New York: W. W. Norton and Company, 1983), 57–8.

46. Lawrence E. Mintz, ed., *Humor in America: A Research Guide to Genres and Topics* (Wesport, CT: Greenwood, 1988), 19.

47. Harvey Mindess et al., *The Antioch Humor Test: Making Sense of Humor* (New York: Avon, 1985).

48. Ibid.

49. Klein, *The Healing Power of Humor,* 5–6.

50. Proverbs 17:22, King James Version.

51. LaRoche, "Fully Human, Fully Alive."

52. Ornstein and Sobel, *Healthy Pleasures,* 216.

53. Paul J. Rosch, "Do the Health Benefits of Humor and Laughter Have Scientific Support?" *Health and Stress* (November 2005).

54. Ibid.

55. Victoria Anisman-Reiner, "Healing Power of Laughter," *Natural Medicine* (January 31, 2008).

56. "The First Laugh: New Study Posits Evolutionary Origins of Two Distinct Types of Laughter," *Science Daily* (Chicago: University of Chicago Press Journals), November 22, 2005 from http://www.sciencedaily.com/releases/2005/11/051122184228.htm, retrieved October 23, 2008.

57. "Laughter—Can It Help Keep You Healthy?" *Mayo Clinic Health Letter* (March 1993): 6.

58. Metcalf and Felible, *Lighten Up,* 11–12.

59. R. Morgan Griffin, "Is Laughter the Best Medicine?" *WebMD*, http://www.webmd.com, accessed April 7, 2006.

60. George V. N. Dearborn, "The Nature of the Smile and Laugh," *Science*, 2 (1900): 851–6.

61. McGhee, "Humor and Health."

62. Loretta LaRoche, "Laughter and Healing," presented to the Fourth National Conference on the Psychology of Health, Immunity, and Disease and published by the National Institute for the Clinical Application of Behavioral Medicine (Hilton Head, SC: 1992).

63. Metcalf and Felible, *Lighten Up*, p. 59.

64. Robert Brody, "Anatomy of a Laugh," *American Health* (December 1983): 43.
65. Ibid.
66. From Norman Cousins, *Head First* (New York: E. P. Dutton, 1989), 143–5.
67. Judy Tidwell, "The Healing Power of Humor," *Allergies* (November 2004); H. Kimata, "Effect of Humour on Allergen-Induced Wheat Reactions," *Journal of the American Medical Association* 285, no. 6 (2001): 738; and H. Kimata, "Laughter Counteracts Enhancement of Plasma Neurotrophin Levels and Allergic Skin Wheal Responses by Mobile Phone-Medicated Stress," *Behavioral Medicine* 29, no. 4 (2004): 149–52.
68. K. Hayashi et al., "Laughter Lowered the Increase in Postprandial Blood Glucose," *Diabetes Care* 26, no. 5 (2003): 1651–2.
69. Elizabeth Scott, "The Stress Management and Health Benefits of Laughter," *About.com*, http://stress.about.com/od/stresshealth/a/laughter.htm, updated April 22, 2008, accessed June 4, 2008.
70. Griffin, "Is Laughter the Best Medicine?"
71. Rosch, "Do the Health Benefits of Humor and Laughter."
72. McGhee, "Humor and Health."
73. Michelle W. Murray, "Laughter Is the 'Best Medicine' for Your Heart," *University of Maryland Medical Center*, http://www.umm.edu/features/laughter.htm, updated May 11, 2007.
74. "Laughter Helps Blood Vessels Function Better," *Eurekalert*, www.eurekalert.org, March 7, 2005.
75. A. Clark, A. Seidler, and M. Miller, "Inverse Association Between Sense of Humor and Coronary Heart Disease," *International Journal of Cardiology* 80, no. 1 (2001): 87–8.
76. "Hearty Laughter: Health Benefits of Seeing the Funny Side," *NHS Electronic Library for Health*, http://www.pubmedcentral.nih.gov, January 16, 2003.
77. Rosch, "Do the Health Benefits of Humor and Laughter."
78. Ibid.
79. Ibid.
80. M. Weisenberg, I. Tepper, and J. Schwarzwald, "Humor as a Cognitive Technique for Increasing Pain Tolerance," *Pain* 63, no. 2 (1995): 207–212; and "Laughter Tested as Pain Therapy for Children," *RX Laughter* (February 21, 2002).
81. Karen Rutter and Nichol West, "The Healing Power of Humor," Family Services of Western Pennsylvania Employee Assistance Program, November 2004.
82. Lars Ljungdahl, "Laugh If This Is a Joke," *Journal of the American Medical Association* 261 (January 1989): 558.
83. Ibid.
84. L. S. Berk et al, "Modulation of Neuroimmune Parameters During the Eustress of Humor-Associated Mirthful Laughter," *Alternative Therapy Health and Medicine* 7 (2001): 62–72, 74–6; M. P. Bennett et al., "The Effect of Mirthful Laughter on Stress and Natural Killer Cell Activity," *Alternative Therapeutic Health and Medicine* 9, no. 2 (2003): 38–45; and K. Takahashi et al., "The Elevation of Natural Killer Cell Activity Induced by Laughter in a Crossover Designed Study," *International Journal of Molecular Medicine* 8, no. 6 (2001): 645–50.
85. Berk et al., "Modulation of Neuroimmune Parameters During the Eustress of Humor-Associated Mirthful Laughter." *Alternatives to Therapeautic Health Medicine* 7, no. 2 (March 2001): 62–72, 74–6.
86. Ornstein and Sobel, *Healthy Pleasures*, 218.
87. R. Booth, "Laughter and Immunity," *Advances* 6, no. 2 (1996): 5.
88. Gordon W. Allport and Pierre Teilhard de Chardin, "Maturity," *Journal of Religion and Health* 7, no. 2 (April 1968): 141–50.
89. Hara Estroff Marano, "Laughter: The Best Medicine," *Psychology Today*, http://www.psychologytoday.com, accessed online June 6, 2008.

90. McGhee, "Humor and Health."

91. Ibid.

92. Rosch, "Do the Health Benefits of Humor and Laughter."

93. Joel Goodman, ed., *Laughing Matters* (Saratoga Springs, NY: The HUMOR Project, Inc.).

94. Mary Payne Bennett and Cecile Lengacher, "Humor and Laughter May Influence Health: III. Laughter and Health Outcomes," *Evidence-Based Complementary and Alternative Medicine* 5, no. 1 (March 2008): 37–50.

95. Bernie S. Siegel, *Love, Medicine and Miracles* (New York: Harper & Row Publishers, 1986).

96. Rosemary Cagan, Dennis Cagan, "Effects of Laughter and Relaxation on Discomfort Thresholds," *Journal of Behavioral Medicine* 10, no. 2 (April 1987).

97. *Journal of Behavioral Medicine* 10, no. 2 (April, 1987): 139–44.

98. LaRoche, "Laughter and Healing," 331.

CHAPTER 20

The Importance of Nutrition to Mind and Body Health

*All physicians are involved with nutrition,
for it is not the disease that is important,
but the person who has the disease,
and each person is the product of his nutrition.
What is nutrition?
It is the cornerstone of preventive medicine,
the handmaiden of curative medicine
and the responsibility of every physician.*

—Symposium on Nutrition for Physicians[1]

LEARNING OBJECTIVES

- Understand the basic principles of nutrition and how to apply them in making daily food choices.
- Identify the major problems with the typical American diet and lifestyle as they relate to adequate nutrition.
- Understand how nutrition affects the brain and the mind and how the process increases the evidence of a connection between the mind and the body.
- Discuss how nutrition affects physical and mental health.

While it is true that we depend on energy from our thoughts, feelings, and consciousness to fuel the functions of our body, it is also true that we need energy from oxygen and from the nutrients in the food we eat. It is clear that our mental, spiritual, and emotional processes depend on a healthy physical body.

Candice Pert, the Georgetown University researcher who wrote *Molecules of Emotion*,[2] demonstrated that every thought and emotion is also a chemical molecule that has very concrete functions in the network of cellular messengers that course throughout the nervous, endocrine, and immune systems. In other words, you feel emotions like anger and compassion because their molecules have a chemical effect on the 100 trillion cells of your body. That body, in return, must be kept healthy if you hope for optimal expression of your thoughts and emotions—and one of the best ways to keep it healthy is by fueling it with the right nutrition.

Most of your cognitive functions occur in the brain; however, the research of Dr. Pert and others shows that another form of consciousness is made up of the "molecules of emotions" that are found throughout your body. Your entire body, then, helps support the functions of your mind and spirit. Physicians from Mount Sinai School of Medicine believe that consciousness occurs in the cell membrane of each cell in the body, not just in the neurons in the brain.[3] Your brain and each cell of your body depend on the functions of all organs of the body to provide the energy, oxygen, and means to detoxify each cell as the body's metabolism processes molecules. What that means is that the digestive tract, the circulatory system, the liver, the kidneys, and practically every organ system of the body is involved in supporting the higher functions of the brain.

Cell communication is achieved through a network of messengers that act on interrelated receptors on the cell membrane. It's a network that acts as a single functioning unit and is best understood as a whole. In the same way, the mind—what we call the psyche—is tightly interwoven with the nervous, immune, and endocrine systems; it, too, can be regarded as a single functioning network that is best understood as a whole. The hormones produced by these systems not only impact the functioning of the system but also are significantly impacted by what we eat.[4]

The Basic Principles of Nutrition

Before discussing the basic principles of nutrition, it's important to understand why diet and nutrition are so important. Simply, proper and balanced nutrition keeps the body functioning as it should, enabling the various systems of the body to perform as they were designed to. As we also know from important research done during the last several decades, good nutrition supports the mind and the emotions, allowing us to experience total wellness.

One of the basics of physical health is cellular regeneration. Simply put, body cells constantly renew themselves, sloughing off used-up matter and regenerating with fresh matter. The materials the body uses for replacement—which keeps the body healthy and functioning as it should—come from the food we eat and the nutrients we provide the body.[5]

What we eat is also important because it is a major determining factor in how well we are able to resist disease. Some disease conditions have been directly linked to dietary factors; one of the best examples is the link between cardiovascular disease and total serum cholesterol levels, especially low-density lipids in the blood. Obviously there are other factors that contribute to high total serum cholesterol (and high low-density lipoproteins); however, diet is a major one, and it has been strongly implicated in both coronary heart disease and high blood pressure. A diet high in sodium (salt) has also been linked to high blood pressure. Dietary factors have even been implicated in some cancers; some researchers have estimated that the degree to which diet contributes to the incidence of cancer exceeds 40 percent.[6] Cancers that have been especially linked to diet include cancers of the breast, colon, pancreas, and stomach. Diet can be a particular factor in contributing to disease when combined with other risk factors, such as stress.

The Process of Converting Food into Energy

Before food can be used by the body to provide energy for cells and repair tissues, it has to be metabolized—changed into a form that can be absorbed into the blood and used by the body's cells. This portion of metabolism is called digestion.

Digestion begins when food is chewed; various enzymes in the saliva start the actual process of breaking down the food; starches and some fats (such as milk fats) are the first to be broken down. Large, solid pieces of food are shredded and ground into a more manageable form that can be swallowed without causing choking. The process of chewing also breaks open seeds, pods, and kernels (such as kernels of corn) that would otherwise travel undigested throughout the digestive system. Chewing and the saliva that is secreted also make each bite of food slippery enough to be swallowed easily and help soften sharp or rough foods that could otherwise tear the esophagus. As chewed food is swallowed, it passes into the esophagus, where rhythmic, squeezing muscular action called peristalsis moves the food toward the stomach. A powerful circular muscle called a sphincter separates the esophagus from the stomach and prevents food from moving back into the esophagus from the stomach.

The stomach produces a mixture of water, enzymes, and gastric acids that further break down the food; the main nutrient that is broken down in the stomach is protein. A thick coating of mucus protects the stomach and other parts of the digestive system from being corroded by the acids that are produced for digestion. The secretion of these acids and enzymes is controlled by the vagus nerve, which is stimulated by the sight, smell, or even thought of food—so, by the time food reaches the stomach, the stomach already contains the gastric juices needed to help digest the food.

Food is stored in the highly muscular stomach for as long as several hours, while gastric juices and water help change the food into a fine, pastelike substance. At first, food is stored in the broad upper part of the stomach; it is then moved a little at a time into the lowest section of the stomach, where powerful muscular contractions grind and mix the food thoroughly into a substance called chyme. Because the digestive process is well underway, chyme no longer resembles the food that was eaten—fats have been separated, proteins have undergone changes, and starches have started to be split into smaller fragments.

The stomach acts as a type of holding tank; it releases only small amounts of food at a time into the duodenum, the first part of the small intestine. Another powerful muscle, the pyloric valve, controls how much chyme is secreted into the duodenum at any given time. It normally takes several hours for the food from a typical meal to be emptied completely from the stomach.

Enzymes from the pancreas and liver are secreted into the duodenum; pancreatic juices help break down fats, proteins, and starches, and the bile secreted by the liver helps break down fats. The bile produced by the liver is stored in the gallbladder and is secreted from the gallbladder into the duodenum in response to foods that contain fats.

Most of the absorption of food into the bloodstream takes place in the small intestine, where its enzymes finish breaking down the food into its molecular building blocks. Every molecule of nutrient that is absorbed must move through one of the cells of the intestinal lining and into the blood and lymph. The intestinal lining is made up of millions of finger-shaped projections called villi, which are covered with microscopic hairs that trap particles of nutrients; each villi has its own lymph vessel and capillary network, which enable the nutrients to move into either the blood-stream or the lymphatic system. The surface of the small intestine—which is wrinkled into thousands of folds—is actually enormous: spread flat, it would cover almost one-third of a football field, though the total weight of the small intestine is only about five pounds.

The same kind of peristalsis that moves food through the esophagus moves it through the small intestine. Signals from the parasympathetic nervous system speed up the movement of food through the small intestine, while the signals from the sympathetic nervous system slow it down.

Finally, what is left of the food moves into the colon, also known as the large intes-tine. As the matter (made up of fiber and undigested materials) moves through the three sections of colon—ascending, transverse, and descending—minerals and extra water are absorbed into the bloodstream, and only those parts of the food that cannot be digested by the body remain. Fiber is an important element in the diet because it provides the bulk against which the muscles of the colon push to move the waste along. That solid waste (called feces) then moves into the rectum and causes the urge to defecate, which removes the waste from the body.

Achieving Balance in the Diet

Good health, both mental and physical, depends in part on getting the right quantity and balance of nutrients in the diet. Generally, aim for a diet that is low in fat (especially sat-urated fat) and cholesterol and moderate in sugar, sodium, and salt. Your diet should contain plenty of fruits, vegetables, and grains and a variety of sources of proteins. Generally, there are four characteristics that make up a nutritious diet:

- **Quantity**—the body requires different amounts of different nutrients, such as vitamins and minerals; recommended daily allowances are a good guideline that help determine how much of each nutrient (such as calcium, iron, or vitamin C) is needed to maintain optimal health.

- **Balance**—there are approximately 40 nutrients that are needed for good health, and it's necessary to eat the right balance of foods to get all the necessary nutrients.

- **Moderation**—some nutrients (such as sugars, fats, and salts) are required for proper functioning of the body but can be detrimental in large quantities.

- **Calorie control**—the energy (fuel) your food provides should be balanced by the amount of energy you expend in a day; if you eat more energy than you expend, the excess is deposited as fat.

Eating foods in a more natural state—instead of the highly processed and packaged foods that many Americans eat—is also an important part of a balanced diet. Aim for balance by eliminating as many processed foods as possible and replacing those with a variety of fruits, vegetables, grains, beans, nuts, soy products, and water.[7]

Make sure that any nutrition information you get is from a credible source—such as the American Dietetic Association, the U. S. Food and Drug Administration, or the U. S. Department of Agriculture (USDA). Volunteer health agencies—such as the American Cancer Society, the American Heart Association, or the American Diabetes Association—are also considered credible sources of nutrition information. You can generally also rely on your physician or reliable consumer groups, such as the National Council Against Health Fraud or the American Council on Science and Health.

Remember, too, that as people age, their nutritional needs change, partly because the ability to absorb nutrients decreases with age. For example, those over the age of 50 need increased quantities of folic acid, niacin, riboflavin, vitamin B_6, and vitamin B_{12}, among others. Older adults also need increased vitamin E to protect against chronic diseases like heart disease and stroke and more vitamin K to maintain bone health.[8]

A balanced diet is critical to health, and physicians and scientists alike are concerned about today's increased marketing of junk food and fast food—a trend so alarming that some have termed it the next "tobacco." Companies that sell fast food and junk food are spending top dollar to market their wares: Pepsi spends an estimated $2.1 billion a year on marketing, McDonald's spends $1.2 billion, and Coca-Cola puts out $895 million. The dollars are working—Americans spend $110 billion on fast food each year and guzzle 56 *gallons* of soda per person, which amounts to 600 12-ounce cans each. That creates another real concern: young people are getting extremely mixed messages from the media. On the one hand, they are bombarded by advertisements for junk food and fast food—but the same media set up obsessively thin models as the desired body type. The result is an estimated 10 million girls and women, and 1 million boys and men, who are afflicted with eating disorders.[9]

The Typical American Diet

Health objectives for Americans are established every 10 years by the U. S. Department of Health and Human Services; one of the sections of the resulting document, *Healthy People 2010,* specifically addresses nutrition-related health objectives. Some of the objectives set for this decade include, but are not limited to, the following:

- Reducing coronary heart disease deaths

- Reducing cancer deaths

- Decreasing the incidence of type 2 diabetes (adult onset diabetes, which is generally caused by diet and obesity)

- Reducing the incidence of osteoporosis (primarily related to lack of calcium)

- Increasing the prevalence of healthy weight and decreasing the prevalence of obesity

- Reducing growth retardation among low-income children

- Increasing the proportion of people aged two and older who meet the dietary guidelines for fat and saturated fats in the diet

- Increasing the intake of fruit and vegetables to at least five servings a day

- Increasing the intake of grain products to at least six servings a day

- Increasing the proportion of people who meet the recommendation for calcium
- Reducing iron deficiency in children, adolescents, women of childbearing age, and low-income pregnant women
- Increasing the proportion of children and adolescents whose intakes of meals and snacks at school contribute to overall dietary quality
- Increasing the proportion of schools teaching essential nutrition topics

So, how are we measuring up against these goals? According to the USDA, American children eat far too much fat and too few fruits and vegetables,[10] which has led to an epidemic of obesity among the nation's children. Americans in general also eat too much sugar and far too many animal fats.[11] In the past two decades, Americans have increased the amount of sugars, fats, and oils they eat and have sharply increased the soft drinks they consume. Most American adults—especially women and the elderly—get too little calcium, vitamin B_6, vitamin E, magnesium, and zinc.

In the United States today, 65 percent of all Americans are overweight, and more than 31 percent are obese—compared with 23 percent in 1994—a number that will climb to an estimated 366 million in 25 years. An estimated 9 percent are extremely obese. The proportion of American children who are obese has tripled since 1980. The Centers for Disease Control report that American children now have a 33 percent lifetime risk of becoming diabetic—and by 2050, the incidence of diabetes will increase by 165 percent. It is estimated that one-fourth of all American children and one-third of the population at large have a pre-diabetic condition. It has been estimated that the annual cost of overweight and obesity in the U. S. is $122.9 billion—$64.1 billion in direct costs and $58.8 billion in indirect costs related to the obesity epidemic, a sum that is comparable to the economic costs of cigarette smoking. Obesity is considered the second-leading cause of preventable death in the United States.

On the bright side, the same statistics show that during the past two decades, Americans have increased the quantities of fruits, vegetables, grains, and cereals they are eating and have replaced some of the red meat they eat with poultry and fish.

How Nutrition Affects the Brain

The specific nutrients that help the brain to work well are found in high concentration in the Mediterranean diet, which has shaped our genes and determined what fuel we need for optimal function. The new field of nutrigenomics highlights these important concepts,[12] providing exciting opportunities in the field of nutrition.[13]

There is a tendency to think of medical problems, like depression, as being caused by "chemical imbalances" that are due to genetic factors. While it is true that such genes do exist, it is also true that genetic conditions can be moderated by getting proper nutrition, living in clean environments, learning good coping skills, having healthy intimate relationships, and developing a spiritual connection with our fellow people.[14]

As an example, Dr. Linus Pauling showed in the 1960s that nutritional intervention could help most people suffering from depression and schizophrenia,[15] research that has since been corroborated by many other publications. Some speak on the role of nutrition in general, while others address specific micronutrients in the diet. The basic finding is that there is more depression and mental dysfunction when there is poor diet.[16]

For example, vitamin C has been found to help in the treatment of schizophrenia and bipolar disorder.[17] Vitamin E can help in the treatment of stress-related mental dysfunction.[18] Chromium picolinate has been shown to improve depression,[19] as does magnesium, which facilitates more than 400 reactions of enzymes.[20] A "Mediterranean-style" diet—abundant plant foods (with fresh fruit as the typical daily dessert), olive oil as the principal source of fat, moderate amounts of dairy products (principally cheese and yogurt), moderate amounts of fish and poultry, no more than four eggs a week, and low amounts of red meat—has been shown to reduce the risk of Alzheimer's disease.[21]

These findings may create the impression that nutrition and micronutrients can be used to "treat" a medical or behavioral problem. Instead, it's better to conceptualize disease—mental or physical—as being triggered by a lack of these nutrients. Consequently, the beneficial effect of restoring these nutrients is not a "pharmaceutical" one but the result of correcting the deficiency that triggered the problems in the first place.

Essential Fatty Acids

Not surprisingly, essential fatty acids and B-complex vitamins are the nutrients most studied in relation to psychology, the function of the mind, the function of the nervous system, and the moderation of genetic conditions. While genetic predispositions have been implicated in behavioral conditions, it has been shown that nutrients can significantly reduce genetic tendencies, making disorders such as depression less likely.[22]

Essential fatty acids are those fatty acids that the body needs but cannot make in sufficient amounts to meet its physiological needs; two of them—linoleic acid and alpha-linolenic acid—are critical for the body's basic functions but cannot be made in any amount by the body, so they must be supplied completely by the foods we eat. Essential fatty acids are found in plant oils (corn, safflower, cottonseed, sesame, canola, soybean, and sunflower), cold-water fish (salmon, mackerel, tuna, sardines, herring, anchovy, bluefish, lake trout, mullet, sablefish, and menhaden), green leafy vegetables, seeds, nuts (especially walnuts), grains, and breast milk.

Essential fatty acids are critical to cell membrane structure, and phospholipids (fats) in the cell membrane are essential for cell communication. These nutrients keep cell membranes fluid and in good repair; and, because they are necessary to the function of neurotransmitters, they help in treating mental illness.[23] Essential fatty acids are also needed to build the fatty sheath around the axons of neurons, which conducts electrical impulses along the neurons.[24] Keep in mind, too, that 60 percent of the brain is "white matter," or phospholipids. Based upon this research, it is important to include essential fatty acids in the diet.

The following main points about essential fatty acids have been established:[25]

- The ideal ratio of omega-3:omega-6 fatty acids should be 1:1, but the typical American diet is 1:20 because we consume too much corn, sunflower, safflower, and cottonseed oils.
- The less fish in the diet, the greater the incidence of depression.
- There is a lower incidence of seasonal affective disorder (SAD) with a diet higher in fish.

- Depressed people have less omega-3 in their blood and 35 percent less DHA (docosahexaenoic acid; an essential fatty acid) in their adipose (fat) tissue, which is a reflection of long-term intake.

- Depression is an inflammatory disease; both antidepressants and essential fatty acids reduce inflammation.

- A diet deficient in essential fatty acids causes a number of serious problems in cell communication in the tissues of the brain and nervous system.

- Ten grams of omega-3 per day help in the treatment of bipolar disorder; the 2004 Meeting of the American Psychiatry Association determined that only 1 gram of essential fatty acid is the best dose to treat depression.

- Depression in premenstrual syndrome and postpartum depression are helped with 4 grams of the marine oil, Krill.

- Social phobia is helped with 4 grams of eicosapentaenoic acid (EPA), an omega-3 fatty acid.

- Borderline personality disorder improves with 1 gram of EPA.

- Antidepressant drugs work better when mixed with omega-3.

The best study on the antidepressant effects of essential fatty acids consisted of a 12-week randomized, double-blind, placebo-controlled study of 70 patients. There was 50 percent improvement in the depression scores in 53 percent of the patients who took 1 gram of EPA (omega-3). They reported less depression, anxiety, sleep disturbances, lassitude, libido problems, and suicidal ideation.[26]

Recent research on the omega-3 fatty acid DHA shows that it provides brain-boosting benefits in both infants and aging adults and that it improves brain health and function at all ages. It has been shown to help prevent psychiatric and neurological ailments such as depression, post-traumatic stress disorder, and Alzheimer's disease; DHA deficiencies have been linked to anger, hostility, suicidal behavior, and depression. It helps promote nervous system development and critical memory function, increases the production of anti-inflammatory compounds (chronic brain inflammation has been found in both postpartum depression and posttraumatic brain disorder), and reduces aggressive behavior. Docosahexaenoic acid is especially critical for pregnant women: it impacts brain development before birth and results in better brain function, cognitive function, and visual acuity after birth.[27]

B-Complex Vitamins

B-complex vitamins are just as important for function at every level as are essential fatty acids. The B-complex vitamins facilitate the work of every cell in the body, working to help metabolize fats, proteins, and carbohydrates. B-complex vitamins help the enzymes do their job in the body; some also help generate energy, while others help make proteins and build new cells. Because of its effect on proteins in the liver, B-complex vitamins affect not only detoxification in the liver but also our genes and how our neurotransmitters function.[28]

Of the B-complex vitamins, thiamin (vitamin B_1) is found in whole grains, legumes, nuts, pork, and liver. Riboflavin (vitamin B_2) is found in meat, leafy green vegetables, whole-grain enriched breads and cereals, milk, yogurt, cheese, and cottage cheese. Rich sources of niacin (vitamin B_3) include milk, eggs, meat, poultry, fish, whole-grain breads and cereals, and nuts. Vitamin B_6 (pyridoxine) is found in green leafy vegetables, legumes, fruit, whole grains, meat, fish, poultry, and shellfish; vitamin B_{12} (cobalamin) is found in animal products. Rich sources of folate include leafy green vegetables, legumes, seeds, liver, and enriched whole-grain products. Pantothenic acid and biotin are found in most foods.

Under normal conditions, the blood-brain barrier prevents many toxins in the blood from permeating the brain. A lack of thiamine causes the blood-brain barrier to leak, allowing toxins to penetrate the brain more readily. For this reason, some researchers theorize that a lack of vitamin B can cause one's mental health to deteriorate. There is a twofold increase in risk of severe depression with vitamin B_{12} deficiency.[29] Postpartum depression is often due to low levels of vitamin B, and premenstrual syndrome worsens when women are low in B-complex vitamins. The elderly are particularly vulnerable to decreased levels of B-complex: Their diets are notoriously poor, and a decrease in digestive enzymes as they age results in poor absorption of this key nutrient.[30]

Further research into the treatment of depression supports the idea that a B-complex deficiency may be partially responsible for depression. A metabolite of B-complex, S-adenosyl methionine (SAMe)—also called "methyl magic"—became a drug in Europe used to treat depression. A symposium on SAMe held in Santa Barbara, California, made the following points:[31]

- 1,600 mg/day of SAMe is equal to 150 mg of the antidepressant Imipramine, but it causes fewer side effects and starts to work more quickly.

- S-Adenosyl methionine may protect against Alzheimer's disease by making cell membranes more fluid (cell membranes appear to be stiffer in Alzheimer's disease patients).

- In order for SAMe to be used by the body, there needs to be enough vitamin B_{12}, folate, and L-methionine. This explains why people who are deficient in those nutrients develop depression at an earlier age and why the depression is relieved by administering those nutrients. Antidepressant therapy is also potentiated by these nutrients.

Amino Acids

Amino acids, the building blocks of protein, are needed for many functions, including the structuring of the brain and the production of neurotransmitters. The body produces adequate quantities of only about half of the twenty amino acids it needs; the others, called essential amino acids, must be obtained from the foods we eat.

Amino acids are found in beef, pork, poultry, fish, shellfish, eggs, milk, yogurt, cheese, cottage cheese, broccoli, leafy green vegetables, seeds and nuts (walnuts, cashews, sesame seeds, sunflower seeds, and nut butters), and whole grains (oats, rice, cornmeal, barley, and bulgur).

One of the most publicized essential amino acids is L-tryptophan. People who cannot process L-tryptophan well in the brain have lower levels of serotonin; L-tryptophan supplementation has also been shown to be as potent as antidepressant drugs in the treatment of depression.[32] Additionally, L-tryptophan has been found to boost the effectiveness of tricyclic antidepressants.[33]

There were early concerns about L-tryptophan supplementation when it was initially linked to a condition called eusinophilic syndrome. However, scientists have subsequently discovered that the syndrome was caused by the way the amino acid was processed in Japanese laboratories, not by the L-tryptophan itself.[34]

Other amino acids are also helpful in treating and preventing depression. The amino acids glutamine and glycine activate receptors in the brain, in collaboration with specific proteins.[35] In other words, amino acids and proteins are key to the proper functioning of the brain.[36] This, in turn, affects the entire body and its ability to function to its best potential.

Vitamin D and Sunlight

Among the vitamins, vitamin D is unique because it can be produced by the body: When sunlight interacts with one of the cholesterol compounds in the skin, the compound is transformed into a precursor of vitamin D, which is then absorbed directly into the blood. The liver and the kidneys finish converting the substance into vitamin D. As such, vitamin D acts as a hormone—a substance that is produced by one organ (the skin) and that then acts on other organs and tissues. It is a member of a large interacting team of nutrients and hormones that work together in ensuring the function of the bones, intestines, pancreas, kidneys, skin, reproductive organs, and brain. It is also essential in helping the body properly absorb calcium, which is needed for the proper function of all cells and tissues of the body. Vitamin D draws calcium from the blood, digestive tract, and kidneys for the body to use.

Early pioneers in medicine used to treat depression by giving patients cod-liver oil. Those pioneers have been vindicated through our findings about essential fatty acids and additional research[37] showing that light therapy works by restoring serotonin levels in the brain. It turns out that vitamin D is also involved, acting more like a hormone with nearly the same nuclear receptors as thyroid hormone.[38]

Most Americans don't consume foods high in vitamin D (cod-liver oil, salmon, mackerel, sardines, liver, and eggs). They also don't get vitamin D from sunlight: Americans spend 98 percent of their time indoors—and, when they do go out, they tend to use sunblockers, which limit vitamin D synthesis. Furthermore, people who live in higher latitudes don't get enough sunlight, compromising many bodily functions and contributing to diabetes, arthritis, lupus, thyroiditis, psoriasis, and possibly multiple sclerosis.

Alpha-Lipoic Acid

Also known as thioctic acid and lipoic acid, alpha-lipoic acid is a vitamin-like substance and powerful antioxidant that helps produce energy in the body. Part of the first-line defense against free radicals (along with vitamins C and E) and an important factor in aerobic metabolism, it is a coenzyme in the production of cellular energy and has been described at times as the "universal" and "ideal" metabolic antioxidant.

Alpha-lipoic acid neutralizes free radicals in both the fatty and watery regions of cells and plays an important role in the synergism of antioxidants. Because of that, it has tremendous potential in treating a number of conditions in which oxidative damage has occurred. It has been administered intravenously to successfully treat acute and severe liver damage, is being used to treat AIDS, and has been used to treat various cancers for which no effective treatment exists. There is also limited evidence that it can improve glucose utilization and reduce the risk of damage to blood vessels in people with type 2 diabetes.

One side effect of high blood sugar levels in diabetics is damage to the nervous system, a condition called *neuropathy.* Resulting symptoms include burning, sharply cutting pain, prickling sensations, and numbness, most commonly in the legs and feet. A collaborative study between the Mayo Clinic and a medical center in Russia found that ALA significantly and rapidly reduces the frequency and severity of diabetic neuropathy symptoms and to improve circulation to the sciatic nerve, which is critical for nerve function and which is reduced in neuropathy. It has been shown to prevent or slow the development of neuropathy in 70 percent of diabetics and has been used in Germany for more than thirty years to successfully treat neuropathy.[39] Mayo Clinic neurologist Peter Dyck said researchers were "surprised" by the magnitude and rapidity of the response and wrote that "the magnitude of the change is considerable." He also said ALA is "very safe" and causes "no known complications."[40]

ALA has been shown to be effective in a variety of conditions when used in combination with other nutrients. Combined with evening primrose oil, ALA has been shown to lower blood fats. Used in conjunction with carnosine, it has been shown to prevent disorders of cognitive decline, such as Alzheimer's disease. And used with carnosine and acetyl-L-carnitine, it has been shown to reduce atherosclerotic plaque and to play an important role in the prevention of cardiovascular disease.[41]

Studies in the laboratory with mice and rats have shown that ALA may slow the progression of multiple sclerosis (MS), though studies have not been conducted on humans.[42] A study at the University of California–Berkeley showed that ALA enabled older rats to do better on memory tests, improved the function of energy-producing segments of cells, and significantly increased energy.[43]

It is sold as a dietary supplement in the United States. The richest natural source of ALA is red meat; it is especially rich in kidney, heart, and liver. Other good sources of ALA are spinach, broccoli, and potatoes.

The Impact of Wheat Allergies on the Brain

Wheat allergies now afflict 1 in every 100 Americans, due mostly to wheat processing and poor reception by the intestines. The consequences of wheat allergies are far-reaching because of the increased leakiness of the gut, which appears to be correlated with an increased number of autoimmune disorders. In other words, the immune system gets so confused that it starts attacking the body. According to R. McManus and D. Kelleher, a wheat allergy adds to the development of diabetes, anemia, osteoporosis, chronic fatigue, autoimmune disorders, gastrointestinal cancer, dermatitis, miscarriages, irritable bowel syndrome, neurologic symptoms, and behavioral changes.[44]

Wheat allergy causes such a wide variety of symptoms that the *American Journal of Clinical Nutrition* recommends a very high level of suspicion when dealing with gastrointestinal symptoms of any kind.[45] Gluten—a component of wheat, barley, and rye— is hidden in many products, including dairy products; it is in dextrins (sweeteners), natural flavors in potato chips and chewing gum, caramel coloring (in colas and soft drinks,) and the malt flavoring or extract found in corn flakes and rice cereals.

Wheat allergy can even occur without a trace of intestinal inflammation. Most people affected have mild symptoms, but with time, numbness, arthritis, and many other conditions may develop. In fact, gluten allergy has been associated with behavioral problems, changes in personality, and depression.[46] The journal *Lancet* reported that one-third of undiagnosed inflammation of the nerves is caused by wheat allergies.[47] Some of this is due to the antibodies made against the thyroid gland and possibly against insulin (because wheat allergy increases the risk of diabetes).

In addition to triggering behavioral problems, wheat intolerance can trigger migraines, a very common inflammatory condition of the brain.[48] Also, it has been shown that L-tryptophan, the amino acid that enables the body to use serotonin, is decreased in children with wheat allergy.[49]

How Nutrition Affects Physical and Mental Health

Not all diseases are equally influenced by the things we eat: We know that some diseases are not related to nutrition at all, while others are strongly related to nutrition. For example, genetic diseases—such as Down's syndrome or sickle cell anemia—are not caused at all by the foods we eat. On the other hand, a condition like iron-deficiency anemia is directly related to how much iron is in the diet. In between those two extremes, along a sort of continuum, are conditions that are related to some extent or another to nutrition, including diseases like cancer, diabetes, and coronary artery disease.

Along that continuum are conditions that have been established to have some sort of connection to nutrition. We know, for example, that

- Too few essential nutrients (especially proteins) can cause some forms of birth defects, low birth weight, some kinds of physical and mental retardation, growth deficits, poor resistance to disease, susceptibility to some kinds of cancer, and deficiency diseases (such as scurvy and cretinism).

- Too many fats—especially saturated fats—can cause coronary artery disease and certain kinds of cancers.

- Too much sugar can cause dental cavities (caries) and can lead to obesity and its related diseases (such as diabetes, high blood pressure, and certain kinds of cancers).

- Too much sodium (salt) may cause high blood pressure and related diseases of the heart and kidneys.

- Too little calcium can cause loss of bone tissue in adults and may lead to high blood pressure and colon cancer.

- Too little iron causes iron-deficiency anemia.

- Too little fiber in the diet can cause some digestive diseases (including diverticulitis), can cause constipation, and can lead to the development of colon cancer and some other cancers.

- Too much alcohol can cause liver disease and may cause sudden death; because it has no nutrients, it can also cause the diseases associated with inadequate nutrition.

Nutrients have also been shown to affect the functioning of the brain and mental health. Some evidence indicates that mineral-rich foods help protect mental health, while eating too many sugary foods and carbonated beverages causes the blood to leach minerals from the brain—as well as from body tissues, including the bones and teeth.[50]

Obesity

One of the greatest impacts of nutrition on health relates to obesity, an excessive accumulation of body fat. Generally, body fat should constitute about 15 to 22 percent of body tissues in men, and 20 to 27 percent of body tissues in women. Obesity is generally determined by a measurement called body mass index (BMI); you are considered overweight if your BMI is greater than 25, and you are considered obese if your BMI is greater than 30. (To determine your BMI, multiply your weight in pounds by 705, then divide twice by your height in inches.) People normally gain weight as they age; both metabolism and physical activity decline as people get older. Those who do not want to gain weight need to take in fewer calories, increase physical activity, or do both to avoid weight gain.

Obesity has become so commonplace that it has begun to replace malnutrition as the most important dietary contributor to poor health worldwide. In the United States, it has reached epidemic proportions. An estimated 6 in 10 Americans is overweight, and almost one-third are obese; slightly more women than men are overweight or obese in the United States.

Obesity itself is a health risk, causing an estimated 300,000 deaths in the United States every year.[51] It can create conditions—such as high blood pressure and high cholesterol—that become their own risk factors for disease. Overweight and obesity have also been associated with diseases such as hypertension, heart disease, stroke, type 2 diabetes, gallbladder disease, chronic fatigue, asthma, sleep apnea, and some kinds of cancer.[52] Overweight and obesity can also cause potentially serious risks from childbearing, surgery, and the administration of anesthesia. Finally, many of the things that people attempt in the treatment of overweight and obesity—such as fasting, diet pills, and the use of other medications—can cause their own health risks.

Even mildly overweight women have an increased risk of heart disease and heart attack when compared to women of normal weight, studies show.[53] One study determined that women who are 30 percent overweight are more than three times as likely to develop heart disease as women who are of normal weight; that risk increased to five times if the women were also smokers.[54]

Interestingly, risks seem related to where the fat is deposited. Recent evidence suggests that the most dangerous is fat that is localized to the abdomen rather than the hips, buttocks, or thighs; localized abdominal fat is associated with a particular increase in high blood pressure, heart disease, diabetes, and some kinds of cancer. Also of interest is the apparent role of stress: people who carry their weight in the abdomen, rather than on the hips, tend to be more reactive to stress and show greater reaction of the cardiovascular,[55] nervous, and endocrine[56] systems to stress.

Recent research shows that one of the worst effects of obesity is actually mental: feeling bad about being fat may be even more harmful than actually being overweight, according to a study of 170,000 U. S. adults. The study, conducted by researchers at Columbia University, showed that the difference between actual weight and perceived ideal weight was a better indicator of physical and mental health than was a measurement of body mass index.[57]

The best solution for achieving and maintaining a healthy weight is one that is gradual and that involves permanent lifestyle changes. It's important to choose a realistic goal; most physicians advise losing no more than one to two pounds per week. The best approach is to eat a balanced diet with smaller portions consisting of plenty of whole grains, vegetables, fruits, and lean protein sources and reducing fats and refined sugars. Exercise is important; in addition to burning calories, it increases the body's metabolism, reduces body fat, and preserves lean tissue; the effects of exercise accumulate over time, so that the body's resting metabolism actually increases over time with exercise. Other approaches can include nutrition and exercise counseling, self-help or support groups, and various behavioral techniques (such as keeping a food diary, setting up a system of rewards, eating only while sitting down at the table, or putting the fork down after every bite). Reducing stress is essential; stress hormones help contribute to obesity. Social support is also important—losing weight is always easier with the support of friends, family, or caring members of a support group. Those who have a high degree of confidence and who get support from family members and important others generally do the best in achieving permanent weight loss.

Insulin Resistance

As stated in the *New England Journal of Medicine,* the "sweet death" associated with too much refined sugar "is a secret killer."[58] Too much refined sugar in the diet leads to insulin resistance, a situation in which the cell can't utilize insulin properly. Basically, the cell membrane becomes rigid and loses its ability to function normally. As mentioned earlier, cell membranes need to be flexible and fluid in order for molecules to move in and out of the cell successfully. Floating on the membrane layer are protein receptors, or "gates," where messengers of cell communication attach in a lock-and-key fashion. These protein receptors have undergone various modifications to maximize their structure and function through a process called glycosylation.[59]

In order for the protein receptors to work properly, the correct kind of carbohydrates need to be attached to them. Protein receptors that have too much processed sugar become resistant to other glycoproteins that come to the cell membrane as messengers. The most classic example is insulin: a cell inundated with too much sugar resists insulin—a condition known as insulin resistance, which causes diabetes. Other factors can cause insulin resistance as well; for example, too many transhydrogenated and saturated fats also cause the cell membranes to become rigid.

The correct glycosylation of proteins plays a major role in how both the body and the mind work. Studies have shown that improving glycosylation helps reduce the craving for tobacco and alcohol and can help in the treatment of Alzheimer's disease, attention deficit disorder, and dyslexia. According to research,[60] insulin resistance is also related to both depression and coronary artery disease.

The Connection Between Insulin Resistance, Depression, and Cardiovascular Disease Insulin resistance actually has a bidirectional relationship with depression. When cell membranes resist insulin, the pancreas starts to produce more insulin, creating a condition known as hyperinsulinemia. Insulin also has central effects on the brain: Some of those effects include, but are not limited to, glucose metabolism by brain cells, stability of the blood-brain barrier, control of blood flow, and regulation of the autonomic nervous system. Insulin resistance combined with cardiovascular disease decreases blood flow to the brain, which in turn leads to more depression; and, as discussed elsewhere in this book, depression increases the risk of cardiovascular disease. As one example, depression is associated with proinflammatory cytokines, which contribute to both cardiovascular disease and insulin resistance.

It has been shown that antidepressants reduce insulin resistance; 60 mg per day of fluoxetine (Prozac) decreases insulin resistance by 20 percent. Antidepressants have also been shown to increase the amount of L-tryptophan in the brain; too little L-tryptophan not only can cause carbohydrate craving, binge eating, and obesity but also has been associated with depression and insulin resistance. Finally, antidepressants help regulate serotonin—and we know that serotonin disturbances increase the platelet-binding sites associated with depression, which in turn may contribute to clotting and narrowed blood vessels and thereby increase the risk of cardiovascular events.[61]

Depression, insulin resistance, and cardiovascular disease have many risk factors in common. Stress, smoking, obesity, and alcohol lead the list. In other words, the same factors—mostly nutritional—that contribute to heart disease also contribute to depression.

The journal *Family Practice Recertification* says that the cause of depression "is still poorly understood, but it is probably not due to a simple deficiency of one neurotransmitter or another. Neuroscientists are coming to the realization that, although many patients improve with a drug that inhibits the reuptake of a neurotransmitter (like Prozac does), that doesn't necessarily mean those patients were depressed because of a neurotransmitter deficiency. It now appears such thinking is akin to saying that a skin rash that improves with a steroid cream is due to a steroid deficiency."[62]

Recent research suggests that depression, bipolar disorder, and many other mental illnesses might be related to cell membrane dysfunction—specifically inflammation of the cell membrane, particularly in the microglial cells, which are now recognized to be integral parts of the brain's "immune system."[63]

The Connection Between Insulin Resistance and Brain Function The same factors discussed above may well affect the brain in other ways. Researchers at the 2004 Annual Meeting of the American Neurology Association reported that the same factors that cause heart disease are at play in Alzheimer's disease, concluding that "what is good for the heart may also be good for the brain."

A diet low in refined sugars lowers the chance of cell membrane problems. According to research, hyperinsulinemia causes inflammatory plaques to form in the brain; MRIs of people with type I diabetes show accelerated aging.[64] Insulysin, a chemical that breaks down insulin, has also been shown to be lacking in people with Alzheimer's disease.[65] Even patients who have insulin resistance but not diabetes show brain changes years before they are diagnosed with Alzheimer's disease. In other words, a sugar-laden diet leading to a prediabetic condition can have deleterious effects on the brain.

Normal levels of insulin and the insulin growth factor IGF-1 clear inflammatory plaques from the brain. Both insulin and IGF-1 are secreted by the brain—and both hormones have a number of functions in protecting cells of the nervous system. When there is not enough insulin or IGF-1, the inflammatory plaques remain in the brain.[66] Because of that, researchers conclude that IGF-1 has promise in the treatment of degenerative nerve disorders, including multiple sclerosis. The connection underscores the importance of diet on brain function.

Diabetes has been clearly associated with an increase in degenerative nerve diseases of the brain, like Alzheimer's disease and Parkinson's disease, partly because of the formation of inflammatory plaques. These plaques play a role in diseases, that we know to be inflammatory conditions, such as Lou Gehrig's disease (also called amyotrophic lateral sclerosis, or ALS), multiple sclerosis, and Parkinson's disease.[67] However, high-sugar diets also affect the brain directly: the blood-brain barrier, which normally weakens with age, also becomes weak from loss of insulin sensitivity.[68] Research shows that hyperglycemia makes the blood-brain barrier more porous, which allows toxins to penetrate the brain,[69] and sugar at high levels is itself toxic to the central nervous system.

People with diabetes have reduced cognitive functioning because they do not get as much blood flow to the brain, which can also increase the risk of stroke. They also have more neurological problems everywhere—feet, stomach, intestines, and eyes, for example—because of poor blood flow to the nerves wiring those areas. Even in people without diabetes, transient ischemic attacks (TIAs, or "mini-strokes") and strokes often result in insulin resistance.[70] Research shows that the elderly people who have impaired glucose tolerance or a prediabetic condition have greater cognitive dysfunction. Even in healthy people, the reduction of blood sugar that occurs following an excessively large meal can cause emotional stress and hypersensitivity of the neurons.[71]

Insulin Resistance and Thyroid Dysfunction Hyperinsulinemia is the most common cause of thyroid dysfunction. Because the hormone produced by the thyroid gland is a powerful neurotransmitter, a poor diet high in sugar has yet another marked effect on the brain.

Treating thyroid dysfunction has been shown to be effective in the treatment of major depression.[72] Given the epidemic of depression in the United States and the fact that traditional treatment with antidepressants is effective only about 50 percent of the time, thyroid treatment might be considered as a treatment for depression, even when thyroid dysfunction isn't obvious. Treatment with low levels of thyroid hormone, even in those with normal thyroid functions, has been shown to cause significant improvement in cognitive functions.[73]

The "Second Brain": The Gastrointestinal Tract

A landmark symposium in Oxford, England,[74] reflects the increasing understanding that many nerve and psychiatric disorders actually begin in the gut—not surprising in light of the fact that 95 percent of the body's serotonin and other neurotransmitters are found in the gastrointestinal tract, not in the brain. After 40 years of rejection by the medical community, the physician who authored *The Second Brain*,[75] a book about the role of the gastrointestinal (GI) tract, is now being hailed as a pioneer in neuroscience. A recent symposium held in Paris[76] resurrected similar ideas advanced by the winner of the 1908 Nobel Prize in Medicine. Unfortunately, these concepts have not received the attention they deserve because we have developed a health care system that tends to deemphasize nutritional research. Fortunately, and thanks to these pioneers, this is slowly changing.

The Paris symposium—titled "The Intelligent Intestine"—also highlighted the concept that 60 percent of the immune system is in the GI tract, from which it exerts significant influence on the systemic immune system, where the other 40 percent is found. Thus, "The intestine is the primary immune organ of the body represented by the gut-associated lymphoid tissue . . . the microflora and the mucosal barrier." This is extremely important: when the mucosal barrier of the intestine is inflamed, toxic foods and food additives can leak through it, exerting significant influence on how our brains and minds work.

Several other significant ideas were discussed at the Paris symposium:[77]

- If the intestine is considered "intelligent," it must be able to send, receive, and understand messages.

- Carbohydrates line the membranes of the intestine and facilitate reception of messengers. Eating processed carbohydrates compromises this communication, resulting in problems such as adhesion of harmful bacteria, which slowly begin to gain power over the normal bacteria (flora) of the digestive tract.

- Loss of the gastric acid barrier results in altered intestinal bacteria.

- Mucosal cells produce antimicrobial peptides called defensins.

- An unhealthy balance of intestinal flora will disrupt the immune system, causing inflammation throughout the body and brain. According to the symposium report, antibiotic treatment has a considerable effect on the equilibrium of bacteria in the intestinal tract. Regular doses of probiotics can help, as will a diet high in fiber and low in refined sugar.

An editorial in the journal *Gut* says that "the fathers of gastroenterology clearly recognized the relationship between the brain and the gut." However, the attitude that "if you can't measure something you don't know that it exists" banished recognition of the link between the brain and the gut for a time. Fortunately, thanks to pioneers like those mentioned above and the laser Doppler flow-meters that measure brain-gut activity, this knowledge is now considered to be sound science.[78]

Brain-gut activity goes both ways. An article in the *American Journal of Gastroenterology* pointed out that while irritable bowel syndrome (IBS) is very much associated with psychological issues and significant stress, it would be a mistake to think that the relationship is only one way (from mind to guts). There is ample evidence that IBS also works from gut to brain. That theory was also spelled out in the journal *Gastroenterology*[79] by H. Tomblom and associates.

Furthermore, the vagus nerve, traditionally thought to be a nerve originating in the brain to send messages to the intestines and stomach, is composed of many neurons. One-third of those neurons do indeed travel from the brain to the stomach, but the other two-thirds originate in the stomach and travel to the brain. R. A. Floto and K. G. Smith explained that stimulation of the vagus nerve decreases inflammation, an effect generally attributed to the immune system.[80] Interestingly, vagus nerve stimulation has been used to treat problems such as seizures, schizophrenia, bipolar disorder, and depression.[81]

A landmark study by H. C. Lin and reported in the *Journal of the American Medical Association*[82] pointed out that the clinical criteria for IBS diagnosis don't include symptoms outside the intestine, such as fatigue or pain. Instead, it says, these complaints are viewed as symptoms of other problems that coexist with IBS and fibromyalgia. In reality, 78 percent of patients with IBS have an overgrowth of bacteria in the small intestine, which can disrupt normal brain-gut interaction and prevent immune activation. The overgrowth of the bacteria is also responsible for intolerance to sugar, altered neuro-transmitter levels, and disrupted brain responses—an effect that is made clear as a result of the two-way communication between the immune system and the autonomic nervous system of the intestines and the brain.[83]

N. E. Rosenstein and colleagues reported a very interesting case of a child with colitis who had psychological problems. When a flare-up of his colitis was treated with antibiotics, his psychosis disappeared! The researchers concluded that "maybe an opportunistic bacteria colonizing the colon produced a neurotoxin."[84] Intestinal flora can mutate and become toxic to the body. Why do intestinal flora mutate? Wouldn't you try to adapt if you were constantly subjected to antibiotics, toxic foods, water chlorination, and who knows what else?[85]

This same process is probably why antifungal medication is effective in treating "atypical" depression.[86] Perhaps it wasn't so atypical after all but was a misdiagnosed problem of the "second brain." This point of view is supported by research showing that 5-hydroxytryptophan (5-HTP) and L-tryptophan (dietary precursors of the neurotransmitter serotonin) have antifungal activity in the laboratory.[87] High-sugar diets encourage the growth of toxic organisms in the intestines, which taxes the brain-gut connection. This is compounded in carbohydrate-sensitive people, who lose serotonin more readily, especially when eating too much sugar.[88] Research shows that a diet too high in carbohydrates can cause depression[89] and that migraine headaches and depression not only are bidirectionally associated but also have gut connections.[90]

There may be other important ways that the intestinal tract impacts the brain. Half of all children with autism have gastrointestinal problems, such as bloating, diarrhea, and pain. Many are diagnosed after a course of antibiotics.[91] Most of them have enlarged lymph nodes in the intestines and a condition called "leaky gut."[92] Also, a significant proportion of children with developmental disorders have enterocolitis.[93]

An article by James A. Komer and Rudolf L. Leibel further emphasizes the hormonal connection between the gut and the brain. Hormones other than insulin, such as ghrelin, have been found to "talk" to the brain and subsequently alter behavior, including eating habits. The article concludes that "it is unlikely that any one molecule or derivative will provide a magic bullet to induce and maintain weight loss. Successful pharmacological treatment for obesity may be possible only by simultaneously targeting the interlocking, redundant systems that drive food intake and act to resist the loss of body fat."[94]

The same theory explains why Parkinson's disease is associated with constipation. People who have fewer than one bowel movement a day have three times the risk of developing Parkinson's disease when compared to people who have more than one movement a day, and are four and a half times more likely to develop Parkinson's disease than men who have more than two movements a day. The reason? They cannot detoxify the agents associated with Parkinson's disease—mostly pesticides—and they have disrupted the brain-gut connection.[95]

A story published in *Scientific American* drives the brain-gut connection home; Robert Sapolsky, one of the foremost neuroscientists of our age, specializes in the psychoneuroimmune-endocrine system and the mind-body-spirit concept. He describes a recent experience he had at the last Annual Meeting of the Society for Neuroscience,[96] where 28,000 scientists found themselves overwhelmed by how little they know about the workings of the human brain. Reflecting on this humble thought, he sat on the steps of the convention center, "bludgeoned by information and a general sense of ignorance."

He then noticed a murky stagnant puddle of water by the curb, which reminded him of a recent extraordinary paper he had read on how certain parasites control the brain of their host. He felt the bugs in the puddle knew more about the human brain than he did. He continues to cite many examples—perhaps the most remarkable being rabies and toxoplasmosis. The rabies virus affects exactly those neurons that guarantee that the rabies virus survives, that is, the virus makes its victims aggressive and prone to bite, which allows the infected saliva to be passed along to a hew host. *Toxoplasma gondii* is the parasite that pregnant women need to avoid in cat litter. Rats have developed a fear of cats to keep them alive, but this instinct is overridden in their brains by a chemical produced by *Toxoplasma*. Losing their fear of cats, they get eaten, thus assuring the parasites' survival. Sapolsky concludes,

> Many of us hold the deeply entrenched idea that primate mammals are the most evolved [organisms]. . . . If you [agree,] you are not just wrong but a step away from a philosophy that most evolved human beings are Northern Europeans. . . . So, remember, there are creatures out there that can control our brains . . . with even more power than Big Brother. . . . My reflection on a curbside puddle brought me to the opposite conclusion that Narcissus reached in his watery reflection. We need humility. We are not the most evolved species, nor the least vulnerable. Nor the cleverest.[97]

Changes in intestinal flora, caused mostly by poor nutrition, affect our minds. Is it possible that the new dominant flora are also affecting human behavior by promoting a switch to a diet that is higher in refined sugars?

Conclusion

At a workshop in the Netherlands, practitioners were told,

> It is essential that practicing physicians develop a working knowledge of herbs and stay abreast of these emerging findings in order to best advise their patients on the value of health promoting diets in disease and prevention. . . . These are heady days for nutritional scientists as newer understandings of food and health promise to bring clinical nutrition to the forefront of clinical medicine. Practitioners must become nutritionally educated and oriented if they are to maintain their patients' confidence and stay abreast of this aspect of continuously evolving modern medicine.[98]

These are indeed "heady days" when nutrition is coming to the "forefront of clinical medicine." It won't be long before we restore the principles that built the practice of medicine—that "food is the best medicine," as proposed by pioneers like Hippocrates, a founder of ancient medicine; Sir William Osler, one of the founders of modern medicine; Maimonides, a twelfth-century Arab-Spanish physician; and Hildegard of Bingen, a twelfth-century saint and health care worker.

Even though testimonials are not the mainstay of scientific validation, they are legitimate tools of expanding knowledge.[99] More than 90 percent of clinical problems can be corrected by empowering patients to live better lifestyles, including improvement in their nutrition, environment, and behavioral/spiritual well-being. Unfortunately, there are some physicians who may not agree, having not seen the research—possibly because of a "dumbing down" in clinical circles.[100]

A focus on nutrition and the mind-body connection is time consuming and is, as a result, deemphasized by busy health maintenance organizations (HMOs) that continue to offer a "disease-care system." There is also a pervasive attitude in our society to treat symptoms quickly and pharmaceutically. The drug companies have capitalized handsomely on that attitude, perpetuating the use of drugs for medical problems, especially mental disorders. How else could we explain the fact that nutrition is now categorized as an "alternative" mode of providing care? Plato states in *The Republic* that "doctors who treat slaves prescribe medications, while doctors who treat free men teach health lifestyles to prevent disease."

Despite the fact that 9 out of 10 independent studies never found antidepressants to be any better than placebos in the treatment of depression, antidepressant drugs are now the "standard of care" for behavioral issues.[101] This has created a deeply rooted belief that nutrition, environmental toxins, and mind-body issues are not worth pursuing. Fortunately, recent books published by Harvard-connected doctors (*Overdosed America*),[102] a former *New England of Journal of Medicine* editor (*The Truth About Drug Companies*),[103] Pulitzer Prize winners (*Critical Condition*),[104] and the Institute of Medicine (*Crossing the Quality Chasm*)[105] are addressing these vital concerns.

WHAT DID YOU LEARN?

1. What are the basic principles of nutrition?
2. How does nutrition affect the brain and physical health?
3. Why do we consider the gastrointestinal tract the "second brain"?
4. What seems to be the best way to control obesity?

ENDNOTES

1. Symposium on Nutrition for Physicians, "What is Nutrition?" *American Journal of Clinical Nutrition* 77 (2003): 149.
2. C. B. Pert, *Molecules of Emotion* (New York: Touchstone, 1999).
3. H. Hu and M. Wu, "Spin-mediated Consciousness Theory," *Medical Hypotheses* 63 (2004): 633–46.
4. M. A. Aller et al., "Neuro-Immune-Endocrine Functional System and Vascular Pathology," *Medical Hypotheses* 57 (2001): 561–9.
5. Shirley Vanderbilt, "Food: Your Body's Natural Healer," *Body Sense* (Spring/Summer 2007): 37.

6. M. L. Fitzgibbon, M. R. Stolley, and D. S. Kirschenbaum, "Obese People Who Seek Treatment Have Different Characteristics Than Those Who Do Not Seek Treatment," *Health Psychology* 12 (1993): 342–5.

7. Vanderbilt, "Food: Your Body's Natural Healer."

8. "Micronutrients for Older Adults," *Linus Pauling Institute,* Oregon State University, http://lpi.oregonstate.edu/infocenter/olderadultnut.html, accessed May 23, 2008.

9. "Body Image and Nutrition," *Teen Health and the Media,* http://depts.washington.edu/ themedia/view.cgi?section=body image, accessed May 28, 2008.

10. "USDA's Continuing Survey of Food Intakes by Individuals 1994–1996, 1999," from www.usda.gov.

11. Ibid.

12. T. Peregrin, "The New Frontier of Nutrition Science: Nutrigenomics," *Journal of the American Dietetic Association* 101 (2001): 1306.

13. D. Kritchevsky, "Diet and Cancer: What Is Next?" *Journal of Nutrition* 133 (2003): 386s.

14. J. Diamond, *Guns, Germs and Steel* (New York: W. W. Norton & Company, 1999).

15. L. Pauling and D. Hawkins, "Orthomolecular Psychiatry," *Science* 160 (1968): 265–71.

16. C. Boult et al., "The Validity of Nutritional Status as a Marker for Future Disability and Depressive Symptoms Among High Risk Older Adults," *Journal of the American Geriatrics Society* 47 (1999): 995–9.

17. D. S. Kays, G. J. Naylor and A. H. Smith, "The Therapeutic Effect of Ascorbic Acid and EDTA in Manic Depressive Psychosis, a Double Blind Trial," *British Journal of Psychiatry* 109 (1963): 294.

18. A. A. Shaheen, et al., "Effect of Pretreatment with Vitamin E or Diazepam on Brain Metabolism of Stressed Rats," *Journal of Biochemistry Pharmacology* 46 (1993): 194.

19. J. R. Davidson, K. Abraham and K. M. Connor, "Effectiveness of Chromium in Atypical Depression, a Placebo-Controlled Trial," *Biological Psychiatry* 53 (2003): 261.

20. R. C. Hall and J. R. Joffe, "Hypomagnesemia. Physical and Psychiatric Symptoms," *Journal of the American Medical Association* 224 (1973): 1749.

21. "Mediterranean-Style Diet Pattern Could Reduce Risk of Alzheimer's Disease," *Tufts University Health & Nutrition Letter* (April 2007).

22. A. Lapillonne and S. D. Clarke, "Polyunsaturated Fatty Acids and Gene Expression," *Current Opinion in Clinical Nutrition and Metabolic Care* 7 (2004): 151.

23. P. M. Kidd, "Bipolar Disorder and Cell Membrane Function," *Alternative Medicine Review* 9 (2004): 107–135.

24. B. M. Cohen and A. L. Miller, "Lecithin in Mania," *American Journal of Psychiatry* 137 (1980): 242; and S. Delion, S. Chalon, and D. Guilloteau, "Age-Related Changes in Phospholipid Fatty Acid Composition and Monoaminergic Neurotransmission in the Hippocampus of Rats Fed a Balanced or an N-3 Polyunsaturated Fatty Acid-deficient Diet," *Journal of Lipid Research* 38 (1997): 680.

25. A. C. Logan, "Neurobiological Aspects of Omega-3 Fatty Acids: Possible Mechanisms and Therapeutic Value in Major Depression," *Alternative Medicine Review* 8 (2004): 410.

26. M. Peet and D. F. Horrobin, "A Dose-Ranging Study of the Effects of -Ethyl-Eicosapentaenoate in Patients with Ongoing Depression Despite Apparently Adequate Therapy with Standard Drugs," *Archives General Psychiatry* 59 (2002): 913.

27. Russell L. Blaylock, "DHA Supports Brain Development and Protects Neurological Function," *Life Extension* (January 2008): 45–57.

28. R. A. Waterland and R. L. Jirtle, "Transposable Elements: Targets for Early Nutritional Effects on Epigenetic Gene Regulation," *Molecular Cell Biology* 23 (2003): 5293.

29. B. W. Penninx and J. M. Guralnik, "B-12 Deficiency and Depression in Physically Disabled Older Women: Epidemiologic Evidence from the Women's Health and Aging Study," *American Journal of Psychiatry* 157 (2000): 715.

30. S. E. Andres, E. Noel, and N. H. Loukili, "Vitamin B12 Deficiency in Older Adults," *Geriatrics* 58 (2003): 12.

31. Symposium in Santa Barbara on SAMe, *American Journal of Clinical Nutrition* 76 (2002): 1145S.

32. W. Poldinger, B. Calanchini and W. Schwartx, "A Functional-Dimensional Approach to Depression: Serotonin Deficiency as a Target Syndrome in a Comparison of 5-Hydroxytryptophan and Fluvoxamine," *Psychopathology* 24 (1991): 53–81.

33. J. Walinder and A. Skott, "Potentiation of the Antidepressant Action of Clomipramine by Tryptophan," *Archives of General Psychiatry* 33 (1976): 1384.

34. M. Eubanks, "Allergies A La Carte. Is There a Problem with Genetically Modified Food?" *Environmental Health Perspectives* 110 (2002): A130–3.

35. V. Heresco-Levy, D. C. Javitt, and M. Emilov, "Efficacy of High Dose Glycine in the Treatment of Enduring Negative Symptoms of Schizophrenia," *Archives General Psychiatry* 56 (1999): 29.

36. Z. Farfel and H. R. Bourne, "The Expanding Spectrum of G Protein diseases," *New England Journal of Medicine* 340 (1999): 1012.

37. G. W. Lambert, C. Reid, and D. M. Kaye, "Effect of Sunlight and Season on Serotonin Turnover in the Brain," *Lancet* 360 (2002): 1840.

38. J. S. Bland, "Vitamin D update," *Functional Medicine Update* 24, no. 8 (2004): 317.

39. Tim Batchelder, "Alpha-Lipoic Acid, Acetyl-L-Carnitine, and Carnosine: The Latest Significant Research on This Powerful Life Extension Tool," *Life Extension Magazine* (September 2003).

40. "Antioxidant Alpha Lipoic Acide (ALA) Significantly Improves Symptoms of Diabetic Neuropathy," Mayo Clinic, April 7, 2003 newsletter.

41. Ibid.

42. "Lipoic Acid," *Linus Pauling Institute,* Oregon State University, http://lpi.oregonstate.edu/infocenter/othernuts/la/, accessed May 23, 2008.

43. Bruce N. Ames, Proceedings of the National Academy of Sciences, USA, February 19, 2002, 99(4) 2356–61.

44. R. McManus and D. Kelleher, "Celiac Disease, the Villain Unmasked," *New England Journal of Medicine* 348 (2003): 2517.

45. J. A. Murray, "Effect of a Gluten-Free Diet on Gastrointestinal Symptoms," *The American Journal of Clinical Nutrition* 79, no. 44 (2004): 669–73.

46. A. De Rosa, A. Trocone, and M. Vacca, "Characteristics and Quality of Illness Behavior in Celiac Disease," *Psychosomatics* 45 (2004): 325, 336.

47. M. Hadjivassiliou, A. Gibson, and G. A. Davies-Jones, "Does Cryptic Gluten Sensitivity Play a Part in Neurological Illness?" *Lancet* 347(1996): 369; and M. Hadjivassiliou, R. A. Grunewald, and G. A. Davies-Jones, "Gluten Sensitivity: A Many Headed Hydra," *British Medical Journal* 318 (1999): 1710–11.

48. M. Gabrielli, F. Cremonini, and G. Fiore, "Association Between Migraine and Celiac Disease," *American Journal of Gastroenterology* 98 (2003): 625.

49. A. Hernanz and I. Polanco, "Plasma Precursor Amino Acids of Central Nervous System Monoamines in Children with Celiac Disease," *Gut* 32 (1991): 1478.

50. Fred Pulver, "Genius and Madness," *Macrobiotics Today* (January/February 2007): 24–5.

51. D. B. Allison et al., "Annual Deaths Attributable to Obesity in the United States," *Journal of the American Medical Association* 282 (1999): 1530–8.

52. "Mind/Body Health: Obesity," *American Psychological Association Help Center,* http://apahelpcenter.org/articles/article.php?id=106, accessed June 5, 2008.

53. J. E. Manson et al., "A Prospective Study of Obesity and Risk of Coronary Heart Disease in Women," *New England Journal of Medicine* 322 (1990): 882–8.

54. Ibid.

55. M. C. Davis, E. W. Twamley, N. A. Hamilton, and P. D. Swan, "Body Fat Distribution and Hemodynamic Stress Responses in Premenopausal Obese Women: A Preliminary Study," *Health Psychology* 18 (1999): 625–33.

56. E. S. Epel et al., "Stress and Body Shape: Stress-Induced Cortisol Secretion Is Consistently Greater Among Women with Central Fat," *Psychosomatic Medicine* 62 (2000): 623–32.

57. "Feeling Fat May Be Worse for You Than Being Fat," *Reuters,* from www.reuters.com/article/healthNews/idUSTON07916120080130 accessed January 30, 2008.

58. D. W. Foster, "Insulin Resistance: A Secret Killer?" *New England Journal of Medicine* 320 (1989): 733.

59. S. Hurtley, R. Service, and P. Szumori, "Carbohydrates and Glycobiology," *Science* 291 (2001): 237.

60. R. Ramasubbu, "Insulin Resistance, a Metabolic Link Between Depressive Disorder and Atherosclerotic Vascular Diseases," *Medical Hypotheses* 59 (2002): 537.

61. Ibid.

62. Michael W. O'Hara, "Depression: Causes and Consequences," *Family Practice Recertification* (Princeton, NJ), 1992.

63. D. Ongur and W. C. Drevets, "Glial Reduction in the Subgenual Prefrontal Cortex in Mood Disorders," *Proceedings of the National Academy of Science* 95 (1998): 13290.

64. Z. Arvanitakis et al., "Diabetes Mellitus and Risk of Alzheimer's Disease and Decline in Cognitive Function," *Archives of Neurology* 61 (2004): 661.

65. B. C. Miller, E. A. Eckman, and K. Sambamurti, "Amyloid-Beta Peptide in Brain Are Inversely Correlated with Insulysin Activity in Vivo," *Proceedings of the National Academy of Science* 100 (2003): 6221.

66. L. Gasparini and H. Xu, "Potential Roles of Insulin and IGF-1," *Trends in Neuroscience* 26 (2003): 404.

67. G. Cohen, "Is the Brain on Fire?" *Annals of Neurology* 36 (1994): 333.

68. R. N. Kalaria et al., "The -Glucose Transporter of the Human Brain and Blood Brain Barrier," *Annals of Neurology* 24 (1988): 757.

69. J. M. Starr, J. Wardlaw, and K. Ferguson, "Increased Blood Brain Barrier Permeability in Type II Diabetes Demonstrated by Gadolinium Magnetic Resonance Imaging," *Journal of Neurology, Neurosurgery & Psychiatry* 74 (2003): 70.

70. W. N. Kerman, S. E. Inzucchi, and C.M. Viscoli "Impaired Insulin Sensitivity Among -Non-Diabetic Patients with a Recent TIA or Ischemic Stroke," *Neurology* 59 (2002): 809–815.

71. I. Berlin, A. Grimaldi, and C. Landau, "Suspected Postprandial Hypoglycemia Is Associated with Beta Adrenergic Hypersensitivity and Emotional Stress," *Journal of Clinical Endocrinology and Metabolism* 79 (1994): 1428.

72. D. L. Ginsberg, "T4 Augmentation Effective in Partial Responders with Major Depression," *Primary Psychiatry* 9(7) (2002): 23.

73. S. Volpato and J. M. Guralnik, "Serum Thyroxine Levels and Cognitive Decline in Euthyroid Older Women," *Journal of Neurology* 58 (2002): 1055.

74. D. H. Raybould and F. Azpiroz, "2001: A Brain-Gut Odyssey," *Digestion* 63 (2001): 247–279.

75. M. D. Gershon, *The Second Brain* (New York: Harper Collins, 1998).

76. Pierre Bourlioux, Berthold Koletzko, Francisco Guarner, and Veronique Braesco, The Danone Symposium (Paris, France, 2002); and "The Intelligent Intestine," *American Journal of Clinical Nutrition* 78 (2003): 675.

77. Ibid.

78. D. G. Thompson, "Descartes and the Gut: I'm Pink, Therefore I am," *Gut* 49 (2001): 165.

79. H. Tomblom, G. Lindberg, B. Nyberg, and B. Veress, "Full Thickness Biopsy of the Jejunum Reveals Inflammation and Enteric Neuropathy in IBS," *Gastroenterology* 123 (2002): 1972.

80. R. A. Floto and K. G. Smith, "The Vagus Nerve, Macrophages and Nicotine," *Lancet* 361 (2003): 1069.

81. G. Elger, C. Gittopec and P. Falka, "Vagus Nerve Stimulation Is Associated with Mood Improvement in Epileptic Patients," *Epilepsy Research* 42 (2000): 203.

82. H. C. Lin, "Small Intestinal Bacterial Overgrowth," *Journal of the American Medical Association* 292 (2004): 852.

83. Ibid.

84. N. E. Rosenstein, S. A. Stocker, and T. Popovic, "Relief of Psychiatric Symptoms in a Patient with Crohn's Disease After Metronidazole Therapy," *Clinical Infectious Diseases* 30 (2000): 214.

85. E. Pennisi, "Close Encounters: Good, Bad, Ugly," *Science* 290 (2000): 1491.

86. R. Sovner and S. Fogelman, "Ketoconazole Therapy for Atypical Depression," *Journal of Clinical Psychiatry* 57 (1996): 227.

87. C. Lass-Flörl et al., "Antifungal Properties of -5-Hydroxytryptamine (Serotonin) Against *Candida* In Vitro," *Journal of Medical Microbiology* 52 (2003): 169–71.

88. J. S. Bland, "Functional Medicine Update," (2) 21 (2002): 199.

89. R. J. Wurtman and J. J. Wurtman, "Carbohydrates and Depression," *Scientific American* 260 (1989): 68.

90. N. Breslau, R. B. Lipton, and W. F. Stewart, "Comorbidity of Migraine and Depression: Investigating Potential Etiology and Therapy," *Journal of Neurology* 60 (2003): 1308.

91. A. J. Wakefield, "Ileal-Lymphoid-Nodular Hyperplasia and Nonspecific Colitis and Pervasive Development Disorder in Children," *Lancet* 351 (1998): 637.

92. P. D'Eufemia, M. Cell, and R. Finocchiaro, "Abnormal Intestinal Permeability in Children with Autism," *Acta Pædiatrica* 85 (1996): 1076.

93. A. J. Wakefield, A. Anthony, and S. H. Mursh, "Enterocolitis in Children with Developmental Disorders," *American Journal of Gastroenterology* 95 (2000): 2285.

94. J. Komer and R. L. Leibel, "To Eat or Not to Eat: How the Gut Talks to the Brain," *New England Journal of Medicine* 349 (2003): 9236.

95. R. D. Abbott, H. Petrovich, and L. R. White, "Frequency of Bowel Movement and the Future Risk of Parkinson's Disease," *Neurology* 57 (2001): 456.

96. R. Sapolsy, "Bugs in the Brain," *Scientific American* 288 (2003): 94.

97. Ibid., 95.

98. Proceedings of the Third Heelsum International Workshop (Netherlands, December 2001). "Nutrition Guidance of Family Doctors Towards Best Practice," *American Journal of Clinical Nutrition* 77 (2003): 1001S.

99. K. Malterud, "The Art and Science of Clinical Knowledge: Evidence Beyond Measures and Numbers," *Lancet* (2001): 397.

100. H. W. Horowitz, "A Piece of My Mind: Dumbing Down," Journal of the American Medical Association 289 (2003): 1349.

101. J. Abramson, *Overdosed America: The Broken Promise of American Medicine. How the Pharmaceutical Companies Distort Medical Knowledge, Mislead Doctors, and Compromise Your Health* (New York: Harper Collins, 2004).

102. Ibid.

103. M. Angell, *The Truth About Drug Companies: How They Deceive Us and What to Do About It* (New York: Random House, 2004).

104. D. L. Barlett and J. B. Steele, *Critical Condition: How Health Care in America Became Big Business and Bad Medicine* (New York: Doubleday, 2004).

105. Institute of Medicine, *Crossing the Quality Chasm: A New Health Care System for the 21st Century* (Washington, DC: National Academy Press, 2001).

CHAPTER 21

Behavioral Medicine Treatment: The Effects of Mind-Body Interventions on Health Outcomes

To a great extent, the very term psychosomatic has lost meaning. No longer can we talk about "psychosomatic illnesses," but we must acknowledge that most, if not all, disease is potentially influenced by psychosocial factors. Even dividing the body into systems—such as the immune system or the nervous system—has lost meaning as we observe the overlap and communication among systems.

—Stanford B. Friedman, 1988 Presidential Address
to the American Psychosomatic Society

LEARNING OBJECTIVES

- Understand how to best substantiate the mind-body connection; that is, the relationship between mental processes and physical illness.

- Examine medical outcome data when mental interventions are added in treating physical illness for high utilizers of medical care, for specific medical illnesses, or to reduce health costs.

- Explore the use of behavioral medicine (mind-body) interventions to fill the hole in current medical approaches.

Outcome research is a hot item these days. At the top of medical research priorities is demonstrating whether a treatment or preventive measure significantly changes the incidence, costs, morbidity, or mortality of a disease—or, for that matter, of health in general. When we do something to change morbidity (and impact of an illness), we should not only reduce symptoms and disability but also improve a person's quality of life.

What are Optimal Medical Outcomes?

In the past, a main focus of research has been mortality rates. We now know that a powerful treatment that reduces the severity of the disease or that prolongs life may not be the best treatment if it creates more misery for the patient or if it is tremendously expensive. A person who is ill may prefer a treatment program that improves quality of life even more than a treatment that merely prolongs life. Optimally, of course, we would hope for an approach that does both.

Medical research has often focused on intermediate effects that were easy to measure and that were presumed to lead to beneficial outcomes. For example, researchers knew that high blood pressure (hypertension) was a risk factor in heart disease and stroke. The goal, then, has been to reduce blood pressure, with the assumption that lower blood pressure will result in a lower incidence of death from heart disease and strokes. One type of drug that works fairly well to lower blood pressure is a diuretic (sometimes referred to as a "water pill"). Higher doses of these worked even better than lower doses to reduce pressure. As long as the focus was on intermediate steps, such as lowering blood pressure, everyone was happy with the diuretics. Once actual studies started looking at the outcome, however, researchers realized that high doses of diuretics were causing even more cardiac deaths than were caused by untreated hypertension. Why? Probably because they cause problems in the blood chemistry that subsequently lead to irregular heart rhythm. So even though the intermediate result was good, the overall outcome was not.

Studies that look at the larger desired result of a specific treatment are called *outcome studies*. Outcome studies that look at the bottom line are often eye-openers. They can readjust our focus from the intermediate goals to the result that really counts and can dispel mistaken myths that seem like common sense.

That's what we're starting to see with the outcome effects of several behavioral medicine interventions. These treatment programs are directed primarily at three things:

- Creating mental skills that are directed at reducing medical symptoms and disease processes
- Bringing behaviors and attitudes in congruence with those of optimal health and with the patient's own deepest values
- Achieving optimal well-being (health) and quality of life

These are best done as an adjunct to, but not in place of, other proven medical treatments.

Saying that mental stress is the cause of a disease is a great oversimplification. However, if mental factors really play a role in the evolution of an illness, then interventions that address mental factors should improve the outcome of treatment. It generally takes three things to document that a factor (such as mental distress) contributes to or helps cause a disease process:

1. You must show that when the factor is present, the disease is worse.

2. You must demonstrate that the factor worsens the pathophysiological processes that lead to the disease.

3. You must prove that interventions that reduce or remove the factor subsequently improve the disease incidence or the eventual outcome. Health outcomes are measured by fewer adverse disease effects, fewer deaths, and improved quality of life and function.

Of these three requirements, the third—showing that active intervention (to reduce the risk factor) actually changes the outcome of the disease—is usually the most convincing and is the most important from a practical point of view.

A well-known example is the role of a high-cholesterol diet in contributing to coronary artery disease. Let's look at the three requirements as they apply to high cholesterol:

1. **Correlations: If the factor is present, the disease is worse.** Early epidemiological studies, such as those in Finland,[1] showed that people who ate a high-fat diet had a higher incidence of heart attacks and strokes. This association did not prove that fatty diets were the cause because people who eat high-fat diets may also have other undetected factors that lead to heart disease. One tongue-in-cheek researcher responded by showing a correlation between wearing a pocket watch, as the elderly then did, and increased heart attacks; then, with a grin, he suggested outlawing pocket watches as a major public hazard. Another light hearted maxim called Mersky's second rule states, "More people die in bed than out of bed. So keep the patient out of bed!" While a high rate of an illness is associated with a certain factor, clearly more is needed to show cause and effect.

2. **Mechanisms: The suspected factor worsens pathophysiological processes.** High fat intake was then shown to increase the cholesterol that in turn formed plaques on the walls of the arteries. Those plaques narrowed the arteries that supplied blood to the heart and to the brain, leading to the occlusions that eventually caused heart attack and stroke. There are, however, other parts of the pathological processes (such as inflammation, blood vessel spasm, and clotting) that can reduce blood flow but that are not known to be prominently affected by fat intake.

3. **Treatment Outcomes: Interventions that reduce the suspected factor improve disease outcomes.** Active programs to lower dietary fat intake, with the subsequent lowering of blood cholesterol levels, were shown to reduce the incidence of cardiovascular events by about 12 percent. Medications that lowered cholesterol more brought about an even higher reduction in heart attacks—about 40 percent. Despite the somewhat modest benefits, this intervention effect was really the evidence needed, triggering major public education efforts to reduce cholesterol levels.

Demonstrating the role of mental factors in disease has followed a similar pattern. In the case of cardiovascular disease, improved mental states had even more profound effects on outcomes than did reducing dietary cholesterol alone. First came the studies correlating mental distress (or loneliness, or hopelessness, or depression) with higher incidences of various physical illnesses. For example:

- Half or more of general medical outpatients have physical ailments significantly related to psychosocial factors; about half of primary care patients have various diagnosable depressive and anxiety disorders, while the rate of these disorders in the general population is only about 15 percent. Others feel "stressed" without a diagnosable mental disorder, and many have high-risk behaviors.[2]

- Sixty percent of all medical visits are primarily for stress-related symptoms;[3] among high utilizers of health care services, this percentage increases substantially.

- One-third to one-half of hospitalized medical patients have a psychiatric diagnosis in addition to their medical problem. When mental illness or significant stress is present, health care costs substantially increase.[4]

Again, these are only associative correlations; if examined alone, they don't prove cause and effect. However, in previous chapters we have discussed the pathophysiological mechanisms of stress (see Chapter 2), anger (see Chapter 4), anxiety (see Chapter 5), and depression (see Chapter 6)—all conditions by which these correlations might be causally explained. The most substantial evidence, however, lies in showing medical improvement with conscious interventions to improve the mental factors.[5]

The Connection Between Mental Stress and Medical Symptoms

Correlations

In a classic study in primary care medical clinics, Kurt Kroenke and his colleagues evaluated the most common physical symptoms that patients presented. After three years of testing and follow-up, they found that, on average, fewer than 17 percent had a clear-cut organic diagnosis to explain those symptoms! That is, 84 percent were "unexplained" pathologically.

Certain bothersome medical symptoms, particularly if otherwise unexplained, are likely to have a high percentage of underlying mental anxiety or depression.[6] These include the following:[7]

- Insomnia (87 percent)
- Fainting (47 percent)
- Constipation (46 percent)
- Headaches (44 percent)
- Palpitations (40 percent)
- Shortness of breath (33 percent)
- Diarrhea (29 percent)
- Numbness (28 percent)
- Chest pain (28 percent)
- Persistent fatigue (55 to 58 percent)[8]
- Dizziness (48 percent)[9]
- Menstrual problems (56 percent) and premenstrual syndrome[10]
- Multiple allergies (62 percent)[11]
- Prolonged convalescence from viral infections (such as influenza)[12]
- Irritable bowel syndrome (91 percent)[13]

Patients with *combinations* of such symptoms, especially those that involve multiple body systems, are highly likely to have underlying anxiety, depression, or other mental distress. For example, one study showed that of those who have a combination of both dizziness and numbness/tingling, 93 percent have an anxiety disorder. Of those with both a pain symptom and an unrelated symptom of autonomic dysregulation (such as palpitations, nausea, bowel problems, or shortness of breath), more than 80 percent have an anxiety problem.[14] Recognizing these correlations can greatly help either patient or physician to explore the potential mental issues involved.

The above correlations still do not prove that mental distress causes physical illness, however, because numerous other risk factors could easily be present. For example, anxious and depressed people smoke at a much higher rate, often tend to eat a richer diet, and use more alcohol and illicit drugs. Also, since many of these correlation studies were retrospective (that is, they looked at the person after the illness had already appeared) some might argue that the mental distress was brought on by the illness, rather than the other way around. Understanding mind-body connections involved some new ways of viewing the world medically (new health paradigms), so skeptics about the importance of those connections were, of course, abundant.

Mechanisms

Next came many studies correlating mental distress, or mental conditioning, to the pathophysiological processes that lead to disease. Significant mental distress results in dysregulation of protective immune and hormone balance, as well as discoordinated autonomic nervous system control. The three systems most affected by mental factors—the hormonal, immune, and nervous systems—form the communication networks that provide the homeostatic balance that maintains good health. That is, when health is challenged, these systems allow for a response that is neither too much nor too little but just enough to keep the challenge in control and to maintain well-being. If emotional responses are too much (as with anxiety) or too little (as with severe depression), physiological responses tend to follow suit. Even the process of damage to the blood vessels that eventually causes heart attacks can be traced in part to disruptions in these three systems that are caused by mental factors such as hostility or depression.

Intervention Outcomes

Once again, however, the truly convincing evidence will come with intervention outcome studies. For example, does a treatment program that reduces hostility or depression also reduce heart attacks, cardiac death, or the costs and disability associated with them?

Much effort is now being directed at these mental intervention issues, with interesting and often impressive results. The treatment interventions have been behavioral, spiritual, psychological, psychoeducational, and even psychopharmacological in nature, with measurement of resulting medical and health outcomes. An example of such an intervention would be a program to create stress resilience.

What does participating in such a program do to subsequent health outcomes and costs? For example, how does treating depression impact the physical diseases shown to be associated with it—and the pathophysiological processes that cause those diseases?

Or what does a psychoeducational program that helps a person manage the full mental impact of a serious disease (such as breast cancer or rheumatoid arthritis) do to the activity and prognosis of the disease itself? Does it improve the quality of life of the person who has that illness?

Although behavioral medicine is still in its childhood, and such intervention studies are really just beginning, some highly interesting results are beginning to emerge. One fact is becoming increasingly clear: Particularly in chronic disease, using the old, strict disease model to treat the many people with stress-related medical illness (or psychosomatic dysfunction) is not only costly but also ineffective and frustrating to all involved. In this chapter, only a few of the better-known of many psychobehavioral intervention studies and those pertaining to some of the larger medical issues will be considered to create a perspective and give a flavor of future potentials.

Outcome Data from Behavioral Medicine (Mind-Body) Interventions

In the near future, a question like this might appear on a National Board Examination for physicians in training:

Which one of the following has *not* clearly been shown to have an improved medical outcome by adding stress management to the usual medical care?

1. Myocardial infarction

2. Metastatic breast cancer

3. Hip fracture repair in the elderly

4. Obstetrical delivery

5. Hypertension

6. High medical care utilization and costs

7. Psoriasis

While clearly relevant, such a question is not likely to appear for some time because most who take the exam are probably not familiar with the data. Curiously, the best answer right now is hypertension; treating mental stress has substantially and consistently improved the medical aspect of all of the above conditions *except* high blood pressure. Some stress interventions have been useful for hypertension and others have not, but when they are taken all together in a meta-analysis, no persistent clear-cut benefit for lowering blood pressure over the long term was found from treating mental stress. (These interventions reducing the dangerous *effects* of hypertension, such as heart attacks, has been another story, however.)

Some researchers who conducted the successful hypertension trials might, of course, argue that the type and style of the stress reduction program may be crucial. For example, was the intervention purely didactic—talking about better ways to deal with stress, as many older stress management programs have been—or was it predominantly experiential, which involves mentally living the changes and feeling them in the body? Experiential approaches are increasingly being shown to be far more effective than talk alone in improving both behavioral and medical outcomes.

Another question: Did the intervention simply elicit the relaxation response alone, or did it also couple relaxation with the reframing of upsetting thinking and the reprogramming of habitual, distressed responses? The answers to these questions appear to play an important role in the effectiveness of behavioral medicine interventions. Moving beyond the relaxation response alone to include changing behaviors provides better outcomes.

Behavioral medicine as a "specialty" probably began formally with the 1978 Yale conference called to form the Academy of Behavioral Medicine Research. "Specialty" is in quotes because, by its nature, behavioral medicine goes in the opposite direction of specialties. By delving progressively deeper into the function of a specific organ system, specialization in medicine has been of great value in creating special expertise. Behavioral medicine, on the other hand, goes upward to higher levels of integrating all systems in an interdisciplinary way, explicitly reuniting the body systems and mind—and even the spiritual issues—that make up the whole person. As you can see from the data provided in this book, the past few years have brought a flood of research following those beginnings; some is very solid, while others were uncontrolled or had too few patients to draw broad conclusions.

Behavioral medicine attempts to reliably create new clinical methods to diagnose, treat, and prevent many of our most perplexing health problems. While the field is still new, some very real possibilities for changing our approach to patient care and health prevention are surfacing. Some examples of treatment studies leading to these conclusions follow. Perhaps one bottom line that speaks loudest to the health system, and may most reflect overall benefits, is the effect on reducing both medical costs and the need to utilize health care services.

High-Volume Users of Medical Care and Resources

Overall, people who use more medical care and who have multiple medical maladies tend largely to have much more stress-related medical illness (and more depression and anxiety disorders.)[15] For example, half of specialty visits and hospitalizations come from the top 10 percent of health care utilizers.[16] (Utilization is measured by the number of medical visits, tests, and procedures and the associated costs.) Among this same top 10 percent, 68 percent have major depression and 32 percent have chronic low-grade depression; in other words, nearly all of them have depression to some degree. Many also have anxiety disorders.

Certain groups of medical problems are more likely to cluster in patients with mental or stress disorders; examples include gastrointestinal problems, atypical chest pain, chronic pain, or unexplained neurological symptoms. These are all very common problems seen in primary care medicine as well as in specialty clinics. For example, of all patients entering a gastroenterology clinic, one-third were depressed (33 percent), one-third had panic disorder (34 percent), and one-third had anxiety-related somatization disorder (38 percent)—obviously with some overlap. The most common diagnosis coming out of a gastroenterology clinic is irritable bowel syndrome (IBS). Over the lifetime of gastroenterology patients with IBS, 80 to 90 percent will have a diagnosed anxiety or depression disorder.[17] It is people with these types of disorders who tend to be high utilizers.

Another example is the high rate of multiple-system symptoms seen in patients with low back pain. Among those, anxious somatization is four to six times the usual rate in the population.[18]

Despite the fact that huge numbers of medical patients have stress and mental disorder problems, a large percentage go unrecognized and untreated. Only about one-fifth of that half of medical patients with diagnosable depression and anxiety disorders get help from mental health professionals. Despite considerable recent improvement, medical physicians, even those in primary care, usually only make such diagnoses about half the time.[19] The missed mental diagnosis is more understandable as we observe that most patients (and physicians) focus largely on the associated physical problems, and patients are often reluctant to bring up the mental issues, even if the mental issues are causing the most suffering. Even when diagnosed with a mental component, patients are reluctant to "see a shrink," and medical physicians typically are not taught the needed skills to deal well with such psychosomatic problems. All this adds up to the fact that there is a huge hole in our total health delivery system, leaving many medical patients untreated for the real underlying issues. These patients are likely to return repeatedly and chronically with more stress-related medical problems. Some new treatment options are, however, beginning to emerge.

Medical Outpatients

With the above realizations in mind, researchers in the Harvard Community Health Plan (a large health maintenance organization [HMO] managed care program in the Boston area) decided to see if stress-reduction programs, which patients do tend to accept, would benefit high utilizers and reduce health care needs and costs.[20] Patients who utilized health services more than twice as often as average were randomly assigned to one of three different stress-reduction programs available in the Harvard system:

1. An informational, "talk only" group discussing the role of stress in illness and methods for managing stress (much like many older stress-management classes).

2. An intervention centered on "mindfulness meditation," experiencing deep relaxation and focused attention in the present moment, with daily practice.

3. An intervention that combined cognitive and language restructuring (new ways of thinking about the stressor) with both relaxation and the mental experience of visualizing how to respond more effectively in areas of recurrent struggle.

Note that both the second and third methods are "experiential" interventions, in which participants used mental practice in the group; in the first method, participants only talked about how to manage stress without actually practicing stress reduction. The experiential programs were reasonably brief, with 90-minute sessions held once a week for six weeks.

Researchers measured changes in physical and mental symptoms as well as how frequently the patients utilized health care systems over the subsequent six months. The results, as shown in Table 21.1, are as follows:

1. The "talk only" group ("good ideas") did not experience any change in physical or mental symptoms, and their frequency of using health care systems did not change.

Table 21.1 Utilization of Health Care Systems

	Mental Distress (BI POMS Test Score, 0–36)	Physical Symptoms (25-Symptom List)	Utilization (In 6 Months)
Mindfulness meditation	−4.7	−6.2	−1.6 visits
Combining cognitive change with meditation and imagery	−4.0	−14.7	−3.9 visits

2. The two experiential groups significantly reduced both symptoms and utilization.

3. The third group, which combined experiential methods (relaxation and visualization) with "good ideas," was more effective than the group that focused primarily on meditation alone. One might use the analogy here of left-brain approaches (logical reasoning), right-brain approaches (experiential), and combining a whole-brain approach (both logical reasoning and experiential, which was the most effective).

A similar difference between experiential and cognitive interventions was found in chronic pain patients at the University of New Mexico. Again, meditative methods were more effective than only using cognitive reframing (new ways of thinking, or cognitive therapy).[21] Cognitive therapy is highly useful for anxiety and depression, but, for the physical outcomes, adding the experiential component seems important.

Does such an intervention just add more cost? This depends on how long the study goes. In general, short-term costs include adding those of the intervention; but, over the long term, the overall health costs decrease. For example, in the Seattle area, Wayne Katon showed that treating depressed diabetics improved greatly their medical care without adding additional cost.[22] Unfortunately, at times medical insurance companies look only at the short-term costs and attempt to avoid covering these interventions.

Most behavioral medicine intervention programs are very low in cost, particularly when done in groups. For the majority of participants (those without severe mental issues), group participation is usually even more effective than individual approaches. (Some of the reasons why will be addressed in Chapter 22.) Usually, people are much more ready to accept such psycho-educational programs—to learn how to become more stress resilient—than they are to start individual psychotherapy, as valuable as that would likely be for them.

For the Harvard treatment programs discussed above, overall cost savings were evident in addition to the health and life quality benefits to the patients. For the number of patients attending the two experiential programs, averaging their effects, the estimated net cost savings (after costs for the interventions were included) were $6,900 per year. With ten such programs offered per year, the Harvard Health Care Plan saw potential first-year savings of $69,000 (with compounding savings if the beneficial effects held in subsequent years).

Hospitalized Medical Inpatients

The Department of Behavioral Medicine at Hohf Clinic and Hospital in Victoria, Texas, studied 235 hospitalized patients referred for stress-related disorders.[23] Using a more intensive intervention averaging 11 full inpatient days, they analyzed the subsequent need for hospitalization compared to before the intervention. The intervention program was multimodal, was somewhat tailored to individual patient needs, and used modalities such as biofeedback training, self-management activities, and outpatient psychotherapy if needed.

Comparing the subsequent two years to the five years before the intervention, hospitalization days dropped dramatically: from 22.8 days per year to 7.3 (a 68 percent reduction). Also note that the 7.3-day average over two years included the 11 days of inpatient behavioral medicine treatment program. Total calculated savings were more than $3 for each $1 invested in the intervention. Additionally, the program improved the overall well-being and health risk of those participating.

Some Implications of Behavioral Medicine Interventions Effects

Behavioral medicine interventions such as those described in the previous section represent an effective but nontraditional approach to some of our most common and perplexing medical problems. Rather than simply attempting to control physical symptoms with medications (as helpful as that might be), patients are taught to quiet their overarousal and to become aware of their thinking and bodily responses to typical stressful situations. They are then taught how to consciously recreate new, healthier automatic responses that are in line with their reflective values about how they would most like to be in such situations. The processes involved are empowering to patients, giving them a sense of personal control to react to stress as they most deeply would want to respond. When the relationships between thoughts, values, and behaviors are thus experientially addressed, the physical health (and economic) benefits follow naturally. In addition, behavioral interventions have been shown to improve risky health behaviors such as poor nutrition, smoking, drug and alcohol abuse, and sedentary lifestyles.[24]

One significant problem with researching behavioral medicine interventions is that there are several potential variations in the way they are done; another is the need to tailor such interventions to the individual. One person does better with body or movement therapies (such as tai chi, yoga, or progressive muscle relaxation) and another with cognitive reframing and mentally practicing new responses. Men often need a different approach (directive) than women (supportive). The style of the therapist affects the results. Medical studies, by their very nature, need to be standardized, or uniform across locations where they are being conducted, which makes them less adaptable to the individual than would be optimal. People with multiple other medical problems are often excluded in medical studies, making the study somewhat artificial but more controllable. It should be noted that multiple problems are common in patients with stress-related illness, and it is often difficult to have a truly blinded control group (who don't know if they are getting the active or placebo treatment). Thus, the results of a behavioral intervention may be more difficult to interpret, and more complicated to replicate, than pharmacological treatments.

Nevertheless, a number of outcomes have been quite remarkable, and the American Board of Family Practice published a review of outcome studies that endorses the importance of these interventions in several disorders.[25] Outcome reviews have found "mind-body" interventions significantly helpful both for specific diseases and for symptoms such as pain (headaches, back pain, muscle pain, and surgical pain).[26] For example, a chronic back pain study published in the *Annals of Internal Medicine* compared outcomes of patients who used yoga, traditional back exercises, or a self-care book. Yoga improved function and bothersomeness better than either of the other two traditional treatments.[27] Back pain is commonly impacted greatly by stress. In 2007, the American College of Physicians conducted an exhaustive and scientifically meticulous review of every published treatment of back pain and created clinical guidelines for what works best.[28] Important in those guidelines for physicians was the use of cognitive behavioral therapy.

Overall the strength and quality of the evidence for mind-body treatment of medical disorders increased considerably between 2000 and 2005.[29] Some examples are given in the next section.

Outcomes for Specific Medical Illnesses

Coronary Artery Disease

After a heart attack, in order to prevent recurrent heart attacks or cardiac death, many approaches to reducing risk factors are undertaken. These include low-fat diets, treatment of high blood pressure, exercise, smoking cessation, aspirin (to reduce clotting), and other medications. These interventions reduce the risk of a second heart attack by 8 to 20 percent. Stopping smoking or taking aspirin can result in close to a 30 percent reduction, and using beta-blocker medication can result in a 25 percent reduction. It now appears, however, that some group behavioral programs are even better, particularly those designed to reduce stress and transform hostile and socially isolating behaviors into the protective behaviors described earlier in this book (see Chapters 4 and 8).

Among heart attack survivors, more than eight well-controlled studies have compared individuals who were provided this behavioral modification approach in addition to the above standard preventive measures to patients who received standard prevention without the behavioral program. These results are summarized in Table 21.2. Taken together, the studies reveal a 39 percent decrease in recurrent heart attacks and a one-third reduction in cardiac death. Some of the interventions were more effective than others. (The key elements are described in Chapter 22.) The large Friedman study showed a 46 percent reduction in heart attacks.

Adding treatment of depression when appropriate further improves on these outcomes (see Chapter 6). One trial demonstrated that treating depression after myocardial infarction reduced cardiac mortality by 61 percent compared to those who were depressed but not treated.[30] In a similar second study, medically treated depression after heart attacks resulted in a 41 percent reduction in coronary death (which was substantially better than using stress reduction alone in these clinically depressed patients).[31]

A later study at Duke University compared the effects of stress reduction versus a good exercise program in reducing second heart attacks. The results showed recurrent

Table 21.2 Secondary Coronary Prevention: Studies of Behavioral Medicine Interventions

	Number of Patients	Years of Follow-Up	% Risk Nonfatal MIs	Reduction in Cardiac Death
Friedman (1986–1987)	862	4.5	−46	−28
Frasure-Smith (1985)	453	1.0		−50
Frasure-Smith (1989)	355	7.0	−33	−15
Ibrahim (1974)	105	1.5		−3
Rahe (1979)	44	3.5	−100	−100
Patel (1985)	169	4.0	−54	−100
Fielding (1979)	45	1.0	−100	
Horlick (1984)	116	0.5		+60
Stern (1983)	64	1.0	+149	
Weighted risk reduction			**−39%**	**−33%**

attacks in 30 percent of those having the usual preventive care, 20 percent if exercise alone was added to usual care, but only 7 percent if stress reduction alone was added to usual care.[32]

On the other hand, for people with high-risk psychobehavioral styles (such as cynical hostility and social alienation, as described in Chapter 4), one might wonder if using a similar behavioral program would effectively prevent the *first* heart attack. One controlled European study, if reproducible, suggests the answer is clearly yes— and in spades. Of a group of middle-aged people with a high personality risk profile for coronary disease, half were treated with a behavioral modification program over several weeks and half were not. Thirteen years later, twice as many of the treated people were still alive.

Do such mental interventions actually affect the arterial wall pathology that leads to heart attacks and strokes? The answer appears to be yes. For example, meditation has been shown to reverse several of the processes by which mental stress and depression were shown to cause increased arterial plaque, spasm, and clot (detailed in Chapter 6). Excess peripheral norepinephrine, which contributes to vessel wall damage, and low central nervous system serotonin, which contributes to spasm and increased clotting, are both improved by meditative techniques and gaining a sense of personal control. Do those neurochemical changes actually reduce vascular lesions? A study of African Americans with high blood pressure looked at their carotid artery thickness in response to either practicing transcendental mediation or following good instruction for reducing the usual other cardiovascular risk factors.[33] Those meditating regularly had significant reduction in carotid artery thickness, while those in the education-only group had progression of the artery thickening. Carotid artery thickening also closely correlates with thickening of the coronary (heart) arteries as well. Thus, we see that these mental interventions provide documented benefits for both the disease mechanisms and the clinical outcomes as well.

It should be noted, however, that such intervention for coronary patients (after an infarction) may need to be done differently for women than for men. A stress reduction program that showed a striking benefit for men (50 percent reduction in cardiac mortality)[34] did not work at all well for women. The authors concluded that men prefer to have a task given that they can work on, while women do not like being told what to do and have much better outcomes when they are listened to and emotionally supported.

There is some evidence as well that such behavioral interventions may be the best chance we have for changing other risk factors (such as smoking or overeating). Is it possible that these kinds of behavioral interventions, coupled with the usual measures, could become our most important cardiac prevention?

Hypertension

Earlier chapters documented the associations of mental stress, depression, and lack of social support with:

- Persistent elevations of hormones that cause high blood pressure (catecholamines, aldosterone, vasopressin, and cortisol), and increased blood vessel spasm
- Observations of blood pressure elevations in anxious people being examined
- Later development of hypertension

These associations have logically led many health care professionals and researchers to conceive of treating the problem with stress management methods instead of with medication. Relaxation techniques, occasionally including biofeedback, have been the main methods used. A review of 25 controlled trials (including more than 1,400 patients total, though most trials were small in number) showed significant benefit in 12 of the 25 studies but not in the others.[35] The benefits, however, tended to be lost over time and were better at three months after the intervention than at one year. This emphasizes the fact that experiential stress reduction techniques need to be continued over the long term. These types of interventions do not represent a "quick fix."

One might wonder if adding substantially more than just relaxation or adding periodic refresher sessions would improve the results. However, a meta-analysis that also included some cognitive (thinking-change) methods also showed no benefit.[36]

Overall, state-of-the-art stress management methods alone cannot be fully endorsed for treatment of high blood pressure. At the same time, the reason for treating hypertension is the prevention of heart attacks, strokes, and kidney failure. So if cardiac outcomes are considered, rather than simply blood pressure reduction per se, adding hostility reduction and improved social connectedness to the relaxation methods that have been shown to prevent the heart attacks may be wise in people at high risk for hypertension anyway. So, once again, the mixed results may depend on the details of the intervention goals and methods. It may be difficult to interpret analyses that lump many different types of interventions together as "stress management."

Noncardiac Chest Pain

People who have chest pain but who have normal coronary arteries (as shown on arteriograms) are well-known to have high rates of associated depression, anxiety disorders, and stress[37] (as much as seven to nine times the normal incidence of depression and panic disorder.) Spasm of the esophagus, coronary arteries, and/or chest wall muscles may be involved in creating the pain, but usually it is best managed when seen as a complex interaction between mind and body. More than half of new patients referred to cardiac clinics for chest pain fall in this group, and often they are simply reassured and discharged rather than treated. Follow-up studies show that most continue to have the pain, have considerable anxiety about the pain, continue to use medical resources to reevaluate it, and usually limit their activities because of it.[38]

In a controlled study of 31 patients with resistant atypical chest pain, clinical psychologists at Oxford used a program (averaging seven sessions) that sensitively explained how "real" chest pain can be caused by stress factors. They then used progressive muscle relaxation, breathing control, distraction, thought checking, and skills for responding differently to triggering cues. The results were striking: Significant reductions were achieved not only for chest pain (one-third became pain free) but also for other physical symptoms—dizziness, breathlessness, nausea, and palpitations. Psychological benefits included reductions in diagnosable depression, anxiety, and functional limitations. The improvements continued to be fully maintained four to six months later.

The treatment program was effective for patients both with and without diagnosable anxiety disorders. Pain medication use was eliminated by all but one patient. Cost savings were not calculated; but, with these degrees of improvements in patients traditionally high in medical resource utilization, the savings were probably substantial. Whether the savings would exceed the cost of the intervention, as it usually does in such studies, is not known here, but the savings in patient suffering are considerable.

Arthritis

Kate Lorig at Stanford University studied arthritis patients who were taught self-management skills at very low cost by a trained layperson who also had arthritis.[39] Four hundred patients with both osteoarthritis and rheumatoid arthritis participated in the controlled study, holding six two-hour sessions to learn how to have more self-efficacy; that is, how to increase their sense of control and capability despite the arthritis. The results:

- Self-efficacy was improved.

- Pain was reduced by 20 percent.

- Inflammation was reduced, and there were fewer swollen joints (demonstrating an actual decrease in disease activity).

- Medical office visits were reduced by 43 percent.

- Costs were reduced an average of $648 for each rheumatoid arthritis patient and $189 for each osteoarthritis patient over a period of four years.

How could the inflammation and disease activity be reduced by a "mental" intervention? Inflammation is triggered by the immune system (and to some extent by the neurological system.) Remember the discussions in Chapters 1 and 2 about how the nervous system impacts pain and the immune system? Improved "control" in the nervous system is reflected in improved control over immunity as well.

Also, interventions that increase self-efficacy improve a patient's capacity for self-management of many types of medical illness, which improves outcomes substantially.[40]

Chronic Obstructive Pulmonary Disease

People who have asthma, chronic bronchitis, emphysema, and other problems in breathing are frequently anxious—and understandably so. Unfortunately, their anxiety usually compounds the airway spasm, making symptoms worse. In one study, only 39 percent of medical outpatients complaining of shortness of breath were able to get relief with medications.[41] And medications that relax the airway can occasionally be dangerous if the patient also has heart disease.

It would seem that mentally learning to relax, particularly to relax the airways (which it now appears possible to learn), could potentially provide great relief and perhaps improved breathing. Despite active breathing-education programs that are being conducted nationally, well-controlled treatment studies in this area have been few and usually involve small numbers of patients.

One very economical approach used four weekly sessions of learning progressive muscle relaxation from a recorded audiotape (measuring the relaxation effectiveness by Bensen's criteria)[42] then practicing at home daily with the tape. Compared to controls who just sat quietly for 20 minutes, this simple intervention achieved significant reductions in anxiety and in the subjective feeling of shortness of breath, as well as a mildly improved peak expiratory flow rate—a measure of ease of airflow (6 percent, compared to 7 percent worsening in the controls).[43] There was no long-term follow-up, but the taped intervention could presumably be continued at home indefinitely. Asthmatics would likely have better improvements in measurable airway flow from relaxation than those with structure lung damage such as emphysema.[44]

Other similar behavioral interventions in children showed reduction in medication and fewer lost school days. For asthmatics, however, the stress issues vary greatly, and the mental interventions may need to be individually tailored. Interventions that work well for one individual may not be as effective for another.

Menopausal Symptoms

The discomforts of going through menopause can be pervasive; and, while not always dangerous (unless depression sets in), they can be very uncomfortable and disruptive. Taking estrogen replacement therapy is often helpful in alleviating symptoms, but what about women who can't use these medications or who prefer not to do so?

One study described a program of simple relaxation methods using deep, quieting breathing and mindfulness training over eight one-hour training sessions.[45] The program significantly relieved symptoms of menopause, including:

- Hot flashes

- Night sweats

- Disturbed sleep

- Distressed emotions

This simple approach illustrates an interesting characteristic about behavioral medicine approaches that are different (and perhaps easier for physicians to understand) from many other psychological therapies. They involve specific techniques initiated by the patient that can, if desired, be directed at changing unwanted symptoms (such as insomnia), unwanted observable behaviors (such as anger outbursts or lighting a cigarette when stressed), or even physiological reactions (such as hot flashes) in much the same way a medication might be used. Results are often observable and measurable. In these regards, behavioral medicine is much closer to traditional biophysical medical approaches than are most other psychological interventions.

These techniques, however, can also often create a relaxed, disengaged state where the patient is able to see more clearly the real solution to his or her underlying distresses and to "reprogram" habitual responses to be those most desired.

Chronic Insomnia

One-third of the population has sleep problems. In addition to a significant increase in accidents and loss of social and performance function, sleep deprivation can produce some significant health problems. Longevity is reduced, pain worsens, insomniacs often gain weight, and depression or anxiety exacerbates. (People with chronic insomnia have 40 times the normal risk for developing depression and have an increased family history of depression, suggesting a common neurochemical link between the two.[46]) As with depression, immune function and autonomic nervous system regulation are decreased when a person is deprived of sleep. These effects of sleep loss were detailed in Chapter 7.

Treatment of insomnia with medication alone has in the past been somewhat suboptimal because of a tendency to lose effectiveness after a month or so. Older sleeping pills can also adversely affect the parts of sleep that are most restorative for the body, often leaving some fatigue the next day. Newer medications are much better; but, if used alone, insomnia tends to return when the patient stops taking them. Most persistent sleeplessness has a strong conditioned component to it; that is, the brain learns that what happens on going to bed—often feeling frustrated and anxious about the next day's events—causes one to struggle to try to sleep. Trying to do anything is arousing. After that has been practiced a while, then just approaching the bed automatically elicits that aroused response, resulting in a self-fulfilling prophecy. Such adverse conditioning needs to be behaviorally changed. This is done with "stimulus control," which means doing nothing in bed except practicing deep relaxation and sleeping (and occasionally having sex). Anything else is done outside the bedroom.

A number of other behavioral treatment approaches have been developed to specifically address the particular components of sleep that are disturbed. These were detailed in Chapter 7. For example, progressive relaxation before bedtime improves deep sleep, while stimulus control (reversing the conditioned part) can be more useful for initially getting to sleep. Medication used over the short term (particularly medications that don't interfere with deep or dreaming sleep) can be helpful to recondition the expectation of what happens when one climbs into bed—that relaxation and sleep will occur. The health improvement can be substantial.

A meta-analysis of 21 studies compared the effects of cognitive behavioral treatment (CBT) to medication for insomnia. Both were equally effective in the short term.[47] A recent trial in young to middle-aged people compared CBT for insomnia to medication over a period of eight weeks. The CBT was superior to medication and nearly as good as combining the two.[48] In general, however, combining behavioral techniques with at least short-term medication works over a longer period better than does either alone.[49] Treating these sleep problems early is much more helpful in preventing the associated medical problems than is treating sleep difficulty later.

Irritable Bowel Syndrome and Related Disorders

As discussed earlier, irritable bowel syndrome (IBS) is the most common problem seen in the gastroenterologist's office. It is diagnosed when a person has abdominal pain and dysregulated bowel movements, despite normal bowel tissue. In the medical setting, it is highly related to stress, depression, and anxiety. Usual methods of treatment involving antispasmodic medications and fiber are often unsatisfactory. Studies of the effects of stress reduction and behavioral methods on the physical symptoms are quite interesting.

A combination of relaxation techniques and mindfulness meditation exercises taught during four to six sessions produced a good response in two-thirds of the participants—considerably better than did antispasmodic medication.[50] Results were maintained one year later.

Another study using eight sessions of progressive muscle relaxation plus thermal biofeedback and cognitive coping training produced a 73 percent improvement in IBS symptoms with effectiveness maintained in the majority one year later.[51] The response was not as good if anxiety was chronic and severe.

Hypnosis was dramatically effective for IBS, and better than psychotherapy. With only 7 sessions, the results persisted, even one year later.[52] Nevertheless, two studies have shown that psychotherapy, particularly that focusing on interpersonal and forgiveness issues, has also been effective.[53] Eight sessions of such psychotherapy produced good results, particularly for pain and diarrhea, in patients resistant to medical treatment. The benefits were also maintained one year later.

Irritable bowel syndrome is a "hyperalgesic" or "hypersensitivity" disorder; that is, it has a neurochemical abnormality that causes excessive nervous system responsiveness to a bowel stimulus. Similar overresponsiveness to a stimulus is seen in other very common problems: nonulcer dyspepsia (stomach sensitivity), migraine (light and sound sensitivity), and fibromyalgia (muscle hypersensitivity). Half of fibromyalgia patients have IBS, as both conditions are related to this "twitchy nervous system." While these are not psychiatric problems per se, stress can clearly make them worse, and stress reduction approaches are highly beneficial. More than six studies have shown significant improvement in fibromyalgia using behavioral medicine (cognitive-behavioral) methods.[54]

Cancer

In considering the use of psychobehavioral interventions for medical diseases, few areas have been met with as much emotion and controversy as that of applications for cancer patients. Common sense suggests that helping with the stress of having cancer would be useful. Linda Carlson and colleagues in Canada showed that a meditation-based stress-reduction program for cancer patients significantly improved stress, sleep, and quality of life[55] and improved some physiological markers of stress and immunity.[56] These benefits persisted many months after the intervention itself was finished.[57] While few would argue with the need for psychological support for most people with a diagnosis of cancer, claims that psychological treatment might improve a patient's medical prognosis or survival have been met with skepticism.

David Spiegel at Stanford University was such a skeptic, but he believed that a group program to create an opportunity for personal expression, comfort, loving support, and finding meaning in and healing of one's life would be of value to women with metastatic breast cancer, regardless of the effects on the disease itself. He set out in a well-designed and controlled study to determine the outcome effects of such a humanistic program. He was surprised. The women receiving the support lived almost twice as long as those without the program.[58] Part of the reason why such improved outcome could happen in the "healing" and psychologically supported group might be explained by improved immunity.

Better immune responses were seen during a similar intervention involving malignant melanoma patients. After only six weeks in the behavioral program, patients showed increases in lymphocytes and natural killer–cell activity that help suppress cancer activity.[59] The intervention—which included stress management, relaxation techniques, enhancement of problem-solving skills, and psychological support—resulted in significantly lower levels of distress and greater use of positive coping skills in the treated group members as compared to the individuals in the control group. These benefits were even more pronounced six months later.

In addition to physical effects, psychological treatments for cancer patients can provide tremendous overall well-being even while they are going through the significant stress of such a disease. A review of 22 studies on the effects of such psychological and behavioral treatment programs for those with cancer showed that the programs resulted in less distress, better sense of control, less pain and anxiety, and less nausea.[60] Calming, peace-bringing interventions may be more effective[61] than some of the "battle" imaging (visualizing killing of cancer cells) that was previously tried and recommended. The components of stress resilience derived from cancer studies will be enumerated in Chapter 22.

Cost and Medical Care Utilization Issues

Surgical Patients

Having surgery can be a frightening prospect. Much research interest has developed around how best to deal with the fear and anxiety around impending surgery and what happens to surgical outcomes when you do. A meta-analysis of psychoeducational interventions for surgery patients combined the findings of 191 controlled studies designed to create a positive expectation.[62] The average training required thirty minutes, and most training was provided by a registered nurse using audiovisual aids.

Eighty percent of the studies showed significant benefit for the following:

- Faster recovery
- Reduced length of hospital stay (an average of 1.5 days shorter)
- Fewer surgical or medical complications
- Improved breathing
- Less pain and reduced need for pain and sedative medications
- Less psychological distress

An earlier 13-study review of even modest psychosocial interventions for surgery and coronary care patients showed similar results, including a two-day reduction in hospital time. Of note, however, is the fact that the move to outpatient, same-day surgery has limited the logistics of providing these kinds of mental preparations.

Other studies of semihypnotic suggestion during anesthetic induction, when the unconscious mind is more receptive, have shown similar beneficial results (suggesting, for example, that pain would be minimal, that bowel function would return fairly quickly, and that healing would proceed well).[63] Some of the studies appear to confirm that such suggestion can be subconsciously incorporated even during deep anesthesia, leading to a conditioned automatic response following surgery. (Inadvertent negative remarks made in passing while the person is anesthetized may also be internalized.)

Even the aesthetics of the setting (such as color, light, and nature scenes) after surgery can play an important role in outcome and recovery rates. One study compared surgery patients who recovered in a room with a nature view to those in a room viewing a brick wall.[64] The average patient with a nature view required less pain medication, had less postoperative distress, and left the hospital one day earlier than those with the brick wall. Sounds odd, perhaps, but try staring at a dull wall for a while, and then compare the feelings of savoring a look at trees and meadows. Perhaps the "healing" influence is not so odd after all.

Labor and Delivery

Like surgery, childbirth can be bewildering and frightening. In Latin American countries, this anxiety is sometimes dealt with quite well with the help of a *doula*—a gentle woman experienced in childbirth who is essentially a hand-holder, informing the mother-to-be about what to expect and providing caring reassurance. When Latin American physicians and patients anecdotally observed that mothers with a doula seemed to have better birth outcomes than women who did not have a doula's services, a group in Texas decided to run a controlled study.[65] They randomly assigned 600 first-time mothers in labor to one of three groups: one with a doula, one with an uninvolved observer in the room, and one with usual care (a nurse who periodically came in to check monitoring and respond to questions). The cost of having a doula in the room was less than $200. The results of this study are presented in Table 21.3.

Table 21.3 Reductions in Number of Events When Using Doula Support Compared with Usual Care (Control) in First Time Mothers

Outcome Reduced	Control	Supported	Percentage Reduction
Caesarean section rates	18%	8%	Reduced 56%
Duration of labor	9.4 hours	7.4 hours	Reduced 25%
Epidural anesthesia	55%	9%	Reduced 85%
Oxytocin to increase labor	44%	17%	Reduced 61%
Forceps delivery	26%	8%	Reduced 70%
Baby hospitalized more than 48 hours	24%	10%	Reduced 58%

Note: The group simply observed by a person in the room had about half the improvement.
Source: J. Kennel et al., "Continuous Emotional Support During Labor in a U.S. Hospital: A Randomized Controlled Trial," *Journal of the American Medical Association* 265 (1991): 2197–201.

Dr. David Sobel, an internist who analyzes such outcome studies for the Kaiser-Permanente health plans in California, has observed that if we had a perfectly safe pill or device that could result in those kinds of reductions in obstetrical complications, every delivering woman would likely use it. With the cost of the doula less than $200, large overall savings were also projected from reductions in operating room and hospital time, medications, and nursing staff time.

A review of other published mind-body approaches to labor and delivery came to the same conclusion.[66] In fact, new delivery guidelines are suggesting routine use of a doula for delivery.[67]

Hip Fracture in the Elderly

Hip fracture can have surprisingly devastating effects on an elderly person's life, and the costs of surgical repair are substantial. James J. Strain and his colleagues wondered what effect psychological consultation might have, not only on resulting disability but also on treatment outcomes and costs. They studied 452 patients admitted for surgical repair of fractured hips at two different hospitals in New York and Chicago.[68] They screened patients for their psychological needs and then, if clearly indicated, referred them for psychological care. Sixty percent had a significant psychological diagnosis, and psychological consultations increased from 5 percent before the screening to 70 percent after screening, suggesting that psychological need may be significantly overlooked in the usual care. Medical costs were affected by the psychological referral in the following ways:

- Hospital stays were reduced by 1.7 to 2.2 days per patient.

- Overall costs were cut by $270,000 (the psychological interventions cost $40,000).

- There was little difference in hip healing characteristics or location of placement after discharge.

These results confirm the findings of S. J. Levitan and D. S. Kornfeld: They found that general orthopedic patients who had psychiatric care reduced their hospital length of stay by 29 percent, saving five times the cost of the psychological interventions.[69]

Overall Medical Cost Reduction

As noted in some of the examples above, in addition to the quality-of-life (and often medical) benefits afforded by adding behavioral and psychological interventions to the usual medical care, the costs of those interventions are usually low compared to the often substantial savings in medical costs and use of resources. A number of other examples might be cited. For example, a Harvard study of 109 chronic pain patients, often a costly and frustrating group, found that adding behavioral medicine approaches reduced clinic visits by 36 percent and produced savings of $35,000 over two years, including the cost of the intervention.[70]

Emily Mumford and her colleagues provided a much more global summary of the cost issues in two large-scale analyses. The first was a meta-analysis of 58 controlled studies of medical and surgical patients comparing results when mental issues were addressed to when they were not. The studies also included some well-controlled, unpublished doctoral dissertations to eliminate any bias toward positive results that might occur by including only published reports. Those results were then compared to the insurance files of 32,450 federal employees' families, looking to see if there were any differences in the changes in medical costs of those who received outpatient (but not inpatient) mental health services compared to those who did not.[71]

Once again, the savings were quite remarkable. The major savings came with reduced hospitalization. The meta-analysis revealed that attention to mental health gave a 73.4 percent reduction in inpatient costs and a 22.6 percent reduction in outpatient costs—impressive particularly when noting that only one of the 58 studies was an exception to that pattern. They noted that, despite a higher need for psychological support in the elderly, they were not psychologically treated as often as younger people.

The four-year insurance data for federal employees calculated the change in medical utilization before mental health treatment to that after the treatment and compared the same trends in patients who did not receive mental interventions.[72] Before mental treatment, those later needing it had medical costs substantially (50 percent) higher than those not needing mental treatment, a finding consistent with what you might suspect from the evidence in this book. The costs after mental health treatment fell substantially below the inflation rate for those years, while costs for those not treated rose well above the inflation rate. After four years, the costs for the two groups nearly equalized—that is, the higher utilizers treated for their mental health were no longer higher utilizers. Again, the major savings came with less hospitalization, implying less severe medical illness after mental treatment. Older people showed greater savings after mental health treatment than younger people. The medical savings roughly equaled the cost of 20 mental health visits,[73] though seldom are that many visits used.

In the group behavioral medicine programs, the costs are usually considerably lower than with individual therapy and provide more interactive time and feeling of group support. And sometimes, for the person stressed out without severe psychological issues, the experiential nature of these group approaches can change behavioral responses even more quickly.

Another entire area with great potential for expanded treatment possibilities (but somewhat beyond the scope of this book) is that of use of the medications (such as antidepressants) in stress-related medical illnesses that do not meet the full criteria for depression. Much of the physiological dysregulation we have explored in this book is mediated by changes in the mesolimbic brain neurochemistry that also underlies depression and anxiety disorders. For example, pain systems share striking neurochemical similarities with mood and stress systems.[74] Many common medical problems, particularly those enumerated above, are related to a hypersensitized or "twitchy" central nervous system that over-responds to many different kinds of stimuli (e.g. bowel, pain, neurological, immune or stress stimuli). Thus, a little pain or gut signal becomes a big one, becoming very bothersome. Many of the techniques described above are designed to bring this over-responsive nervous system back into balance. Sometimes, however, the abnormal neurobiology needs to be treated directly with medicine before these methods can be fully effective. Medications that work to normalize the nervous system would include "anticonvulsants" and "antidepressants." By correcting underlying neural dysfunction they can be effective for many physical problems (particularly pain) well beyond their mood or convulsion benefits.

We might use the analogy of a computer. The behavioral and psychotherapeutic approaches we have been considering here are much like reprogramming the software of a computer to elicit a new response. However, if the computer hardware is not working well, the software changes don't work well either—or may not even be possible to create. Antidepressants are not just symptom-relieving pills that cover up the learned responses. They work by correcting the underlying brain dysfunction, which then allows for much more effective "software reprogramming" to get the results for which a person hopes or even just by enabling the possibility of the relaxed state that allows the needed healing. Once the now refunctioning brain has done well for a period of time (often with temporary medication), nonpharmacological approaches work to *keep* it that way much better than they could have done trying to attain that well-functioning state in the first place. When nonpharmacological treatment approaches are not enough, medical improvement of these overlapping neurochemical abnormalities can often be highly useful.

There are many examples of medical problems which improve with antidepressant medication whether or not depression is actually present. Some illustrations are captured by the many studies shown in Table 21.4, in which "antidepressant" medications are found highly effective in the treatment of many medical problems, even when depression is not present. For example, one study found an 80 percent reduction in noncardiac chest pain among patients treated with an antidepressant, even though no one in the study had been diagnosed with depression or anxiety disorders.[75] Many studies for chronic widespread muscle pain show great benefit of antidepressants in reducing pain even in the absence of depression.[76] Irritable bowel often responds well to antidepressants as well.[77] Almost surprisingly, they can even improve medical outcomes in cardiovascular disease and stroke,[78] and even for people with multiple allergies.[79] These medications, which often also work well for some kinds of pain, are usually called antidepressants because that was the disorder for which they were first studied, but in fact they work as well as stabilizers of the nervous system, which then stabilizes other systems also. The fact that both the mind *and* the body respond to these medications once again illustrates the tight interaction between the two.

Table 21.4 The Use of Antidepressant Medications for Medical Disorders Other than Pure Depression

Of Demonstrated Benefit

1. Chronic Pain Disorders[82]
   a. Myofascial pain disorder and fibromyalgia[83]
   b. Migraine and tension headaches[84]
   c. Some types of arthritis[85]
   d. Trigeminal neuralgia[86]
   e. Diabetic neuropathy[87]
   f. *Herpes zoster* neuralgia[88]
   g. Idiopathic pelvic pain[89]
   h. Temporomandibular joint syndrome[90]
   i. Chronic facial pain[91]
   j. Back pain[92]
   k. Fibromyalgia[93]
   l. Noncardiac chest pain[94]
2. Other psychiatric disorders
   a. Panic disorder[95]
   b. Eating disorders: anorexia nervosa and bulimia[96]
   c. Obsessive-compulsive disorder[97]
   d. Addiction and alcoholism control[98]
   e. Pseudodementia of the elderly[99]
   f. Appetite and weight loss in the elderly[100]
   g. Hypochondriasis[101]
   h. Posttraumatic stress disorder[102]
   i. Attention deficit disorder[103]
   j. Personality disorders[104]
3. Dementia[105]
4. Chronic fatigue syndrome[106]
5. Premenstrual syndrome[107]
6. Irritable bowel syndrome[108]
7. Sleep disorders (including sleep apnea)[109]
8. Urinary incontinence[110]
9. Peptic ulcer[111]
10. Recurrent hives, dermatitis, eczema, pruritus[112]
11. Preventing heart attacks[113]
12. Preventing strokes[114]
13. Functional bowel disorders[115]

Of Probable Benefit

1. Medical illnesses to which stress contributes substantially[116]
   a. Some asthma patients
   b. Multiple allergies[117]
2. Other endorphin deficiency states
3. Somaticization disorder (particularly in the aged)[118]
4. HIV dementia[119]

Curiously, when treatment is discussed, even among many interested in mind and body integration, there still tends to be the old divisions between the "mind people" and the "body people." Rather than being forced to choose either the "mind" approaches (such as psychotherapy or behavioral therapy) or the body chemistry (medication) approach, it is likely that well-timed integration of both will often provide the best solutions. This synergy has been proven, for example, with all both depression (with all its physical effects) and sleep disturbances.

The bottom line suggested by most of these studies is that some of our best possibilities for reducing health care costs while substantially improving health quality may lie in conscious and organized attention to the mental aspects of medical illness.[80]

Filling the Hole in the Health Care Delivery System?

Earlier in this chapter, we noted the large numbers of general medical patients (more than half) who have documented stress-related medical problems and the small percentage of those in which the mental component is being actually diagnosed and treated. A lot of people are not feeling well and are uncertain how to get help. Large numbers of patients with some of the most common problems of pain, fatigue, gastrointestinal disorders, and strange neurological symptoms fall into this category. This leaves a big hole in the health care delivery system: about 40 percent of primary care patients have stress-related medical illness that is not being addressed by mental health professionals, and most of the physicians they are seeing are not being trained in behavioral interventions. A major barrier in medical offices to using these methods is not enough time and a lack of reimbursement for that time.[81] Thus the medical system itself is a barrier, even though this integrated approach works and saves money. We are beginning to see, however, a move toward bringing multidisciplinary care, including behaviorists as part of the team, into the primary care setting, and if the system can accommodate this move, many physicians would welcome it.

One solution may be to provide low-cost group behavioral medicine and psychoeducational intervention programs—a solution that is patient-friendly, generally well received, and usually even enjoyable. Perhaps more practical in day-to-day clinical life (but with more cost), these methods can also be learned individually. And perhaps the treatment approaches that integrate mind and body will be even more effective—especially in the long run—than some of the traditional ways we have approached these perplexing, chronic problems.

WHAT DID YOU LEARN?

1. Describe the three types of research studies that demonstrate a cause-and-effect relationship between mental factors and physical illness. Which of these types is most convincing?
2. Give three reasons why mind-body medical research studies are more complicated than simple medication studies.

3. What is your overall impression of the outcome effectiveness of mind-body interventions? Give three specific examples of why you feel that way.

4. Explain the "huge hole" in the medical system regarding treatment of stress-related illness.

5. Describe at least two barriers that explain why the current medical system has difficulty implementing these methods, and propose a possible solution to those barriers.

ENDNOTES

1. J. T. Salonen et al., "Coronary Risk Factor Clustering Patterns in Eastern Finland," *International Journal of Epidemiology* l0(3) (1981): 203–10.

2. J. D. Stoeckle, I. K. Zola, and G. Davidson, "The Quantity and Significance of Psychological Distress in Medical Outpatients," *Journal of Chronic Disease* (1964): 959–70; R. A. Crum, L. Cooper-Patrick, and D. E. Ford, "Depressive Symptoms Among General Medical Patients: Prevalence and One-Year Outcome," *Psychosomatic Medicine* 56 (1994): 109–17; and H. C. Schulberg and B. J. Burns, "Mental Disorders in Primary Care: Epidemiologic, Diagnostic and Treatment Research Directions," *General Hospital Psychiatry* 10 (1985): 79–87.

3. N. A. Cummings and G. R. VandenBos, "The Twenty Year Kaiser-Permanente Experience with Psychotherapy and Medical Utilization: Implications for National Health Policy and National Health Insurance," *Health Policy Quarterly* 1 (1981): 159–75.

4. C. Shen, U. Sambamoorthi, and G. Rust, "Co-Occurring Mental Illness and Health Care Utilization and Expenditures in Adults with Obesity and Chronic Physical Illness," *Disease Management* 11, no. 3 (June 2008): 153–60.

5. R. E. Glasgow et al., "Practical Behavioral Trials to Advance Evidence-Based Behavioral Medicine," *Annals of Behavioral Medicine* 31, no. 1 (February 2006): 5–13. Also see the editorial comment in *Annals of Behavioral Medicine* 31, no. 1 (February 2006): 3–4.

6. K. Kroenke and A. D. Mangelsdorff, "Common Symptoms in Ambulatory Care: Incidence, Evaluation, Therapy, and Outcome," *American Journal of Medicine* 86 (1989): 266–6.

7. K. Kroenke and R. K. Price, "Symptoms in the Community: Prevalence, Classification and Psychiatric Comorbidity," *Archives of Internal Medicine* 153 (1993): 2474–80.

8. D. W. Bates et al., "Prevalence of Fatigue and Chronic Fatigue Syndrome in a Primary Care Practice," *Archives of Internal Medicine* 153 (1993): 2759–65.

9. M. Sullivan et al., "Psychiatric and Otologic Diagnosis in Patients Complaining of Dizziness," *Archives of Internal Medicine* 153 (1993): 1479–84.

10. J. Bancroft, D. Rennie, and P. Warner, "Vulnerability to Perimenstrual Mood Change: The Relevance of a Past History of Depressive Disorder," *Psychosomatic Medicine* 56 (1994): 225–31.

11. A. I. Terr, "Environmental Illness: A Clinical Review of 50 Cases," *Archives of Internal Medicine* 146 (1986): 145–9.

12. J. B. Imboden, A. Canter, L. E. Cluff, "Convalescence fron Influenza: Study of Psychological and Clinical Determinants, *Archives of Internal Medicine* 108 (1961): 393–9.

13. R. B. Lydiard, M. D. Fossey, W. Marsh, and J. C. Ballenger, "Prevalence of Psychiatric Disorders in Patients with Irritable Bowel Syndrome," *Psychosomatics* 34 (1993): 229–34.

14. N. L. Smith, "Physical Symptoms Predictive of Depression and Anxiety," American Psychosomatic Society Annual Meeting (May 8–10, 1996, Williamsburg, Virginia), *Psychosomatic Medicine* Abstracts 1996, and J. Shavers, "The Identification of Depression and Anxiety in a Medical Outpatient Setting and Their Correlation to Presenting Physical Complaints" (PhD dissertation, University of Utah, 1996).

15. W. Katan et al., "Distresses High Utilizers of Medical Care," *General Hospital Psychiatry* 12 (1990): 355–62.

16. P. Vedsted and M. B. Christensen, "Frequent Attenders in General Practice Care: A Literature Review with Special Reference to Methodological Considerations," *Public Health* 119, no. 2 (February 2005): 118–37.

17. R. B. Lydiard et al., "Prevalance of Psychiatric Disorder."

18. N. M. K. Bacon et al., "Somatization Symptoms in Chronic Low Back Pain Patients," *Psychosomatic Medicine* 56 (1994): 118–27.

19. P. Freeling et al., "Unrecognised Depression in General Practice," *British Medical Journal* 290 (1985): 1880–3; and S. M. Anderson and B. H. Harthorn, "The Recognition, Diagnosis and Treatment of Mental Disorders by Primary Care Physicians," *Medical Care* 27 (1989): 869–86.

20. C. J. C. Hellman et al., "A Study of the Effectiveness of Two Group Behavioral Medicine Interventions for Patients with Psychosomatic Complaints," *Behavioral Medicine* 16 (1990): 165–73.

21. B. W. Smith et al., "A Pilot Study Comparing the Effects of Mindfulness-Based and Cognitive-Behavioral Stress Reduction," *Journal of Alternative and Complementary Medicine* 14, no. 3 (April 2008): 251–8.

22. W. J. Katon et al., "Long-Term Effects on Medical Costs of Improving Depression Outcomes in Patients with Depression and Diabetes," *Diabetes Care* 31, no. 6 (June 2008): 1155–9. Also see W. Katon et al., "Cost-Effectiveness and Net Benefit of Enhanced Treatment of Depression for Older Adults with Diabetes and Depression," *Diabetes Care* 29, no. 2 (February 2006): 265–70.

23. U. L. Gonik et al., "Cost Effectiveness of Behavioral Medicine Procedures in the Treatment of Stress Related Disorders," *Journal of Clinical Biofeedback* 4 (1981): 16–24.

24. L. Gordon, N. Graves, A. Hawkes, and E. Eakin, "A Review of the Cost-Effectiveness of Face-to-Face Behavioural Interventions for Smoking, Physical Activity, Diet and Alcohol," *Chronic Illness* 3, no. 2 (June 2007): 101–29.

25. J. A. Astin, S. L. Shapiro, D. M. Eisenberg, and K. L. Forys, "Mind-Body Medicine: State of the Science, Implications for Practice," *Journal of the American Board of Family Practice* 16, no. 2 (March/April 2003): 131–47.

26. J. A. Astin, "Mind-Body Therapies for the Management of Pain," *Clinical Journal of Pain* 20, no. 1 (January/February 2004): 27–32.

27. K. J. Sherman et al., "Comparing Yoga, Exercise, and a Self-Care Book for Chronic Low Back Pain: A Randomized, Controlled Trial," *Annals of Internal Medicine* 143, no. 12 (December 20, 2005): 849–56. Also see comments in: "Yoga, Exercise, and Education for the Treatment of Chronic Low Back Pain," *ACP Journal Club* 145, no. 1 (2006): 16; "Summaries for Patients: Comparison of Yoga, Exercise, and Education for the Treatment of Chronic Low Back Pain," *Annals of Internal Medicine* 20; 143, no. 12 (2005): I–18; and C. J. Standaert, "Is Yoga an Effective Therapy for Chronic Low Back Pain?" *Clinical Journal of Sport Medicine* 17, no. 1 (January 2007): 83–4.

28. R. Chou, L. H. Huffman, American Pain Society, and American College of Physicians, "Nonpharmacologic Therapies for Acute and Chronic Low Back Pain: A Review of the Evidence for an American Pain Society/American College of Physicians Clinical Practice Guideline, *Annals of Internal Medicine* 147, no. 7 (October 2, 2007): 492–504.

29. E. Ernst, M. H. Pittler, B. Wider, and K. Boddy, "Mind-Body Therapies: Are the Trial Data Getting Stronger?" *Alternative Therapies in Health and Medicine* 13, no. 5 (September/October 2007): 62–4.

30. A. H. Glassman, "Sadhart Trial: Sertraline Treatment of Depression After Myocardial Infarction," *Journal of the American Medical Association* 289 (2002): 701–9.

31. S. M. Czajkowski, and the Writing Committee for the Enriched Investigators, "Effects of Treating Depression and Low Perceived Social Support on Clinical Events after Myocardial Infarction: The Enhancing Recovery in Coronary Heart Disease Patients (ENRICHD) Randomized Trial," *Journal of the American Medical Association* 289 (2003): 3106–16.

32. J. A. Blumenthal et al., "Stress Management and Exercise Training in Cardiac Patients with Myocardial Ischemia. Effects on Prognosis and Evaluation of Mechanisms," *Archives of Internal Medicine* 157 (1997): 2213–23.

33. Amparo Castillo-Richmond et al., "Effects of Stress Reduction on Carotid Atherosclerosis in Hypertensive African Americans," *Stroke* 31 (2000): 568–73.

34. N. Frasure-Smith and R. Prince, "The Ischemic Heart Disease Life Stress Monitoring Program: Impact on Mortality," *Psychosomatic Medicine* 47 (1985): 431–45; also N. Frasure-Smith and R. Prince "Long-term Follow-up of the Ischemic Heart Disease Life Stress Monitoring Program," *Psychosomatic Medicine* 51 (1989): 485–513.

35. D. W. Johnson, "The Behavioral Control of High Blood Pressure," *Current Psychological Research Review* 6 (1987): 99–114.

36. D. M. Eisenberg et al., "Cognitive Behavioral Techniques for Hypertension: Are They Effective?" *Annals of Internal Medicine* 118 (1993): 964–72.

37. L. J. Lantinga et al., "One Year Psychosocial Follow-up of Patients with Chest Pain and Angiographically Normal Coronary Arteries," *American Journal of Cardiology* 62 (1988): 209–13.

38. R. A. Mayou, "Invited Review: Atypical Chest Pain," *Journal of Psychosomatic Research* 33 (1989): 393–406; and R. C. Pasternak et al., "Chest Pain with Angiographically Insignificant Coronary Arterial Obstruction," *American Journal of Medicine* 68 (1980): 813–7.

39. K. Lorig, et al., "Outcomes of Self-Help Education for Patients with Arthritis," *Arthritis and Rheumatism* 28 (1985): 680–85.

40. R. B. Curtin et al., "Self-Efficacy and Self-Management Behaviors in Patients with Chronic Kidney Disease," *Advances in Chronic Kidney Disease* 15, no. 2 (April 2008): 191–205.

41. K. Kroenke, M. E. Arrington, and A. D. Manglesdorf, "The Prevalence of Symptoms in Medical Outpatients and the Adequacy of Treatment," *Archives of Internal Medicine* 150 (1990): 1685–9.

42. H. Bensen, J. F. Beary, and M. P. Carol, "The Relaxation Response," *Psychiatry* 37 (1974): 37–45.

43. A. G. Gift, T. Moore, and K. Soeken, "Relaxation to Reduce Dyspnea and Anxiety in COPD Patients," *Nursing Research* 41 (1992): 242–6.

44. P. D. Freedberg, L. A. Hoffman, W. C. Light, and M. K. Kreps, "Effect of Progressive Muscle Relaxation on the Objective Symptoms and Subjective Responses Associates with Asthma," *Heart and Lung* 16 (1987): 24–30.

45. R. R. Freedman, "Pathophysiology and Treatment of Menopausal Hot Flashes," *Seminars in Reproductive Medicine* 23(2) (2005): 117–25. Also R. R. Freedman and S. Woodward, "Behavioral Treatment of Menopausal Hot Flashes Evaluation by Ambulatory Monitoring," *American Journal of Obstetric Gynecology* 167 (1992): 436–9.

46. D. E. Ford and D. B. Kamerow, "Epidemiologic Study of Sleep Disturbances and Psychiatric Disorder: An Opportunity for Prevention?" *Journal of the American Medical Association* 263 (1989): 1479–84.

47. M. L. Perlis et al., "On the Comparability of Pharmacotherapy and Behavior Therapy for Chronic Insomnia," *Journal of Psychosomatic Research* 54 (2003): 51–9.

48. G. D. Jacobs, E. F. Pace-Schott, R. Stickgold, and M. W. Oho, "Cognitive Behavior Therapy and Pharmacotherapy for Insomnia," *Archives of Internal Medicine* 164(17) (2004): 1888–96.

49. C. M. Morin, "Combined Therapeutics for Insomnia: Should Our First Approach be Behavioral or Pharmacological?" *Sleep Medicine* 7 Suppl 1 (2006 Aug): S15–19; also C. M. Morin, R. R. Bootzin, D. J. Buysse, et al, "Psychological and Behavioral Treatment of Insomnia: Update of the Recent Evidence (1998–2004). *Sleep* 29(11) (2006): 1398–414.

50. G. Shaw, "Stress Management for Irritable Bowel Syndrome: A Controlled Trial," *Digestion* 50(1991): 36–42.

51. S. P. Schwarz, E. B. Blanchard, D. F. Neff, "Behavioral Treatment of Irritable Bowel Syndrome: A 1-year Follow-up Study," *Biofeedback and Self Regulation* 11(3) (1986): 189–98.

52. P. J. Whorwell, A. Prior, E. B. Faragher, "Controlled Trial of Hypnotherapy in the Treatment of Severe Refractory Irritable-Bowel Syndrome," *Lancet* 2 (1984): 1232–4.

53. E. Guthrie, et al, "A Controlled Trial of Psychological Treatment for the Irritable Bowel Syndrome," *Gastroenterology* 100 (1991): 450–457; and J. Svedlund, et al, "Controlled Study of Psychotherapy in Irritable Bowel Syndrome," *Lancet* 2 (1983): 589–91; and J. Svedlund and I. Sjdin, "A Psychosomatic Approach to Treatment in the Irritable Bowel Syndrome and Peptic Ulcer Disease with Aspects of the Design of Clinical Trials," *Scandinavian Journal of Gastroenterology* 20, Issue S109(1985): 147–151.

54. R. Bennett and D. Nelson, "Cognitive Behavioral Therapy for Fibromyalgia." *Nature Clinical Practice in Rheumatology* 2(8) (2006): 416–24. Also D. L. Goldenberg, "Multidisciplinary Modalities in the Treatment of Fibromyalgia." *Arthritis and Rheumatism* 57(5) (2007): 830–6.

55. L. E. Carlson and S. N. Garland, "Impact of Mindfulness-Based Stress Reduction (MBSR) on Sleep, Mood, Stress and Fatigue Symptoms in Cancer Outpatients," *International Journal of Behavioral Medicine* 12, no. 4 (2005): 278–85.

56. L. E. Carlson, M. Speca, P. Faris, and K. D. Patel, "One Year Pre-Post Intervention Follow-Up of Psychological, Immune, Endocrine and Blood Pressure Outcomes of Mindfulness-Based Stress Reduction (MBSR) in Breast and Prostate Cancer Outpatients," *Brain, Behavior and Immunity* 21, no. 8 (November 2007): 1038–49 (E-published May 22, 2007).

57. L. E. Carlson et al., "The Effects of a Mindfulness Meditation-Based Stress Reduction Program on Mood and Symptoms of Stress in Cancer Outpatients: 6-Month Follow-Up," *Support Care Cancer* 9, no. 2 (March 2001): 112–23.

58. D. Spiegel, H. C. Kraemer, J. R. Bloom, and E. Gottheil, "Effect of Psychosocial Treatment on Survival of Patients with Metastatic Breast Cancer," *Lancet* 2 (October 14, 1989): 888–91.

59. I. F. Fawzy, "A Structured Psychiatric Intervention for Cancer Patients: Changes over Time with Methods of Coping and Affective Disturbance and in Immunological Parameters," *General Hospital Psychiatry* 13 (1991): 361–2.

60. R. W. Trijsburg, F. C. E. van Knippenberg, and S. E. Rijpma, "Effects of Psychological Treatment on Cancer Patients: A Critical Review," *Psychosomatic Medicine* 54 (1992): 489–517.

61. L. Freeman et al., "Imagery Intervention for Recovering Breast Cancer Patients: Clinical Trial of Safety and Efficacy," *Journal of the Society for Integrative Oncology* 6, no. 2 (Spring 2008): 67–75.

62. E. C. Devine, "Effects of Psychoeducational Care for Adult Surgical Patients: A Meta-Analysis of 191 Studies," *Patient Education and Counseling* 19 (1992): 129–42.

63. R. P. Blankfield, "Suggestion, Relaxation and Hypnosis as Adjuncts in the Care of Surgery Patients: A Review of the Literature," *American Journal of Hypnosis* 33 (1991): 172–86.

64. R. Ulrich, "View Through a Window May Influence Recovery from Surgery," *Science* 224 (1984): 420–1.

65. J. Kennel et al., "Continuous Emotional Support During Labor in a U.S. Hospital: A Randomized Controlled Trial," *Journal of the American Medical Association* 265 (1991): 2197–201.

66. A. E. Beddoe and K. A. Lee, "Mind-Body Interventions During Pregnancy," *Journal of Obstetric, Gynecologic and Neonatal Nursing* 37, no. 2 (March/April 2008): 165–75.

67. J. Green, D. Amis, B. A. Hotelling. "Care Practice #3: Continuous Labor Support." *Journal of Perinatal Education* 16(3) (2007): 25–8.

68. James J. Strain et al., "Cost Offset from a Psychiatric Consultation Liaison Intervention with Elderly Hip Fracture Patients," *American Journal of Psychiatry* 148 (1991): 1044–9.

69. S. J. Levitan and D. S. Kornfeld, "Clinical and Cost Benefits from Liaison Psychiatry," *American Journal of Psychiatry* 138 (1981): 790–3.

70. M. Caudill et al., "Decreased Clinic Use by Chronic Pain Patients: Response to a Behavioral Medicine Intervention," *Clinical Journal of Pain* 7 (1991): 305–10.

71. E. Mumford et al., "A New Look at Evidence About Reduced Cost of Medical Utilization Following Mental Health Treatment," *American Journal of Psychiatry* 141 (1984): 1145–58.

72. E. Mumford, H. J. Schlesinger, and G. V. Glass, "The Effect of Psychological Intervention on Recovery from Surgery and Heart Attacks: An Analysis of the Literature," *American Journal of Public Health* 72 (1982): 141–151.

73. H. J. Schlesinger et al., "Mental Health Treatment and Medical Care Utilization in a Fee-for-Service System: Outpatient Mental Health Treatment Following the Onset of a Chronic Disease," *American Journal of Public Health* 73 (1983): 422–9.

74. P. L. Delgado, "Common Pathways of Depression and Pain," *Journal of Clinical Psychiatry* 65, suppl 12: (2004) 16–9; M. Briley, "Clinical Experience with Dual Action Antidepressants in Different Chronic Pain Syndromes," *Human Psychopharmacology* 19, suppl. 1 (October 2004): S21–5; and S. K. Brannan et al., "Duloxetine 60 mg Once-Daily in the Treatment of Painful Physical Symptoms in Patients with Major Depressive Disorder," *Journal of Psychiatric Research* 39, no. 1 (January/February 2005): 43–53.

75. I. Varia, "Sertraline Treatment of Noncardiac Chest Pain," *American Heart Journal* 140 (2000): 367–72.

76. L. M. Arnold et al., "A Double-Blind, Multicenter Trial Comparing Duloxetine with Placebo in the Treatment of Fibromyalgia Patients With or Without Major Depressive Disorder," *Arthritis and Rheumatism* 50, no. 9 (September 2004): 2974–84; and Vitton et al., "A Double-Blind Placebo-Controlled Trial of Milnacipran in the Treatment of Fibromyalgia," *Human Psychopharmacology* 19, suppl 1 (October 2004): S27–35.

77. M. D. Crowell et al., "Antidepressants in the Treatment of Irritable Bowel Syndrome and Visceral Pain Syndromes," *Current Opinion in Investigational Drugs* 5, no. 7 (July 2004): 736–42.

78. A. Rasmussen et al., "A Double-Blind, Placebo-Controlled Study of Sertraline in the Prevention of Depression in Stroke Patients," *Psychosomatics* 44, no. 3 (May/June 2003): 216–21; and K. R. Krishnan, "Depression as a Contributing Factor in Cerebrovascular Disease," *American Heart Journal* 140, 4 suppl. (October 2000): 70–6.

79. J. S. Seggev and R. C. Eckert, "Psychopathology Masquerading as Food Allergy," *Journal of Family Practice* 26, no. 2 (February 1988): 161–4.

80. We are indebted to David S. Sobel, MD, MPH, editor of *Mental Medicine Update* (special report, 1993), for bringing several of these studies to our attention.

81. V. Sierpina, R. Levine, J. Astin, and A. Tan, "Use of Mind-Body Therapies in Psychiatry and Family Medicine Faculty and Residents: Attitudes, Barriers, and Gender Differences," *Explore (NY)* 3, no. 2 (March/April 2007): 129–35.

82. Briley, "Clinical Experience"; I. G. Egbunike and B. J. Chaffee, "Antidepressants in the Management of Chronic Pain Syndromes," *Pharmacotherapy* 10, no. 4 (1990): 262–70; K. R. Krishman and R. D. France, "Antidepressants in Chronic Pain Syndromes," *American Family Physician* 39, no. 4 (April 1989): 233–7; M. Valdes et al., "Psychogenic Pain and Depressive Disorders: An Empirical Study," *Journal of Affective Disorders* 16, no. 1(1989): 21–5; R. D. France, "The Future for Antidepressants: Treatment of Pain," *Psychopathology* 20, suppl. 1 (1987): 99–113; and Z. Herman, "Enkephalins and the Action of Psychotropic Drugs," *Polish Journal of Pharmacology and Pharmacy* 39, no. 5 (1987): 633–9

83. D. H. Finestone and S. K. Ober, "Fluoxetine and Fibromyalgia," *Journal of the American Medical Association* 264, no. 22 (1990): 2869–70; and D. L. Goldenberg, "Diagnostic and Therapeutic Challenges of Fibromyalgia," *Hospital Practice* 24, no. 9A (1989): 39–52.

84. A. Bonazzi, "Fluoxetine vs. Amitriptyline in the Prophylaxis of Tension Type Headache," *Cephalalgia* 11 suppl. 11 (1991): 341–2; S. Diamond and F. G. Freitag, "The Use of Fluoxetine in the Treatment of Headache," *Clinical Journal of Pain* 5 no. 2 (1989): 200–1; H. G. Markley et al., "Fluoxetine in Prophylaxis of Headache: Clinical Experience," *Cephalalgia* 11, suppl. 11 (1991): 164–5; G. Sandrini et al., "Antalgic and Antidepressant Activities of Fluoxetine in Daily Chronic Headache," *Cephalalgia* 11 suppl. 11, (1991): 280–1; and P. J. Orsulak and D. Waller, "Antidepressant Drugs: Additional Clinical Uses," *Journal of Family Practice* 28, no. 2 (February 1989): 209–16.

85. M. Gringas, *Journal of International Medical Research* 4, suppl. 2: 41; M. Scott, *Practitioner* 202: 802; Krishman and France, "Antidepressants in Chronic Pain Syndrome"; and France, "The Future for Antidepressants."

86. M. B. Max et al., "Efficacy of Desipramine in Painful Diabetic Neuropathy: A Placebo-Controlled Trial," *Pain* 45, no. 1 (April 1991): 69, discussion 1–3; K. A. Theesen and W. R. Marsh, "Relief of Diabetic Neuropathy with Fluoxetine," *DICP* 23, nos. 7–8 (July/August 1989): 572–4; Krishman and France, "Antidepressants in Chronic Pain Syndrome"; and France, "The Future for Antidepressants."

87. F. A. Bucci, Jr., and R. A. Schwartz, "Neurologic Complications of Herpes Zoster," *American Family Physician* 37, no. 3 (March 1988): 185–92; and C. E. Argoff, N. Katz, and M. Backonja, "Treatment of Postherpetic Neuralgia: A Review of Therapeutic Options," *Journal of Pain and Symptom Management* 28, no. 4 (October 2004): 396–411.

88. M. B. Hahn et al., "Idiopathic Pelvic Pain," *Postgraduate Medicine* 85, no. 4 (March 1989): 263–6, 268, 270.

89. M. Harris, "Medical Versus Surgical Treatment of Temporomandibular Joint Pain and Dysfunction," *British Journal of Oral and Maxillofacial Surgery* 25, no. 2 (April 1987): 113–20.

90. Krishman and France, "Antidepressants in Chronic Pain Syndrome."

91. France, "The Future for Antidepressants."

92. L. M. Arnold et al., "A Double-Blind, Multicenter Trial Comparing Duloxetine with Placebo in the Treatment of Fibromyalgia Patients With or Without Major Depressive Disorder," *Arthritis and Rheumatism* 50, no. 9 (September 2004): 2974–84; and O. Vitton et al., "A Double-Blind Placebo-Controlled Trial of Milnacipran in the Treatment of Fibromyalgia," *Human Psychopharmacology* 19, suppl 1 (October 2004): S27–35.

93. W. M. Wong and R. Fass, "Noncardiac Chest Pain," *Current Treatment Options in Gastroenterology* 7, no. 4 (August 2004): 273–8; and I. Varia, "Sertraline Treatment of Noncardiac Chest Pain," *American Heart Journal* 140 (2000): 367–72.

94. R. J. Baldasserini, "Current Status of Antidepressants: Clinical Pharmacology," *Journal of Clinical Psychiatry* 50, no. 4 (April 1989): 117–26.

95. J. M. Gorman et al., "An Open Trial of Fluoxetine in the Treatment of Panic Attacks," *Journal of Clinical Psychopharmacology* 7, no. 5 (1987): 329–32; K. Brady, M. Zarzar, and R. B. Lydiard, "Fluoxetine in Panic Disorder Patients with Imipramine-Associated Weight Gain," *Journal of Clinical Psychopharmacology* 9, no. 1 (1989): 66–7; F. R. Schneier et al., "Fluoxetine in Panic Disorder," *Journal of Clinical Psychopharmacology* 10, no. 2 (1990): 119–21; Orsulak and Waller, "Antidepressant Drugs,"; and L. Solyom, C. Solyom, and B. Ledwidge, "Fluoxetine in Panic Disorder," *Canadian Journal of Psychiatry* 36, no. 5 (June 1991): 378–80.

96. H. G. Pope, Jr., et al., "Bulimia Treated with Imipramine," *American Journal of Psychiatry* 140 (1983): 554–8; R. G. Granet, "Fluoxetine Treatment of Obsessive Compulsive Disorder," *Journal of Clinical Psychiatry* 50, no. 11 (1989): 436; H. E. Gwirtsman, B. H. Guze, J. Yager, and B. Gainsley, "Fluoxetine Treatment of Anorexia Nervosa: An Open Clinical Trial," *Journal of Clinical Psychiatry* 51, no. 9 (1990): 378–82; D. B. Herzog, A. W. Brotman, and I. S. Bradburn, "Treating Eating Disorders with Antidepressants," *Australian Paediatric Journal* 24, no. 3 (1988): 169–70; S. H. Kennedy and D. S. Goldbloom, "Current Perspectives on Drug Therapies for Anorexia Nervosa and Bulimia Nervosa," *Drugs* 41, no. 3 (1991): 367–77; M. R. Trimble, "Worldwide Use of Clomipramine," *Journal of Clinical Psychiatry* 51 suppl. 8 (1990): 51–4; P. L. Hughs et al., Treating Bulimia with Desipramine," *Archives of General Psychiatry* 43 (1986): 182–6; C. P. L. Freeman and M. Hampson, "Fluoxetine as a Treatment for Bulimia Nervosa," *International Journal of Obesity* 11, suppl 3 (1987): 171–7; M. Fava et al., "Long-Term Use of Fluoxetine in Bulimia Nervosa: A Retrospective Study," *Annals of Clinical Psychiatry* 2, no. 1 (1990): 53–6; and L. Solyom, C. Solyom, B. Ledwidge. "The Fluoxetine Treatment of Low-weight, Chronic Bulimia Nervosa," *Journal of Clinical Psychopharmacology* 10 (1990): 421–5.

97. Orsulak and Waller, "Antidepressant Drugs."

98. C. A. Naranjo et al., "Fluoxetine Differentially Alters Alcohol Intake and Other Consummatory Behaviors in Problem Drinkers," *Clinical Pharmacology and Therapeutics* 47, no. 4 (1990): 490–8; D. A. Gorelick, "Serotonin Uptake Blockers and the Treatment of Alcoholism," *Recent Developments in Alcoholism* 7 (1989): 267–81; and J. Rosecan: World Congress of Psychiatry, 1983.

99. J. T. Moore, "The New Antidepressants,"pp. 3–23 in R. Ham, ed., *Geriatric Medicine Annual* (1986).

100. J. Talley, "Geriatric Depression: Avoiding the Pitfalls of Primary Care," *Geriatrics* 42, no. 4 (1987): 53–60, 65–6.

101. D. V. Sheehan, J. Ballenger, and G. Jacobsen, "Treatment of Endogenous Anxiety with Phobic, Hysterical and Hypochondriacal Symptoms," *Archives of General Psychiatry* 37 (1980): 51–9; and N. Fernando, "Monosymptomatic Hypochondriasis Treated with a Tricyclic Antidepressant," *British Journal of Psychiatry* 152 (June 1988): 851–2.

102. C. J. McDougle, S. M. Southwick, D. S. Charney, and R. L. St. James, "An Open Trial of Fluoxetine in the Treatment of Posttraumatic Stress Disorder," *Journal of Clinical Psychopharmacology* 11, no. 5 (1991): 325–7; and J. Davidson, S. Roth, and E. Newman, "Fluoxetine in Post-Traumatic Stress Disorder," *Journal of Traumatic Stress* 4, no. 3 (1991): 419–23.

103. Orsulak and Waller, "Antidepressant Drugs."

104. M. J. Norden, "Fluoxetine in Borderline Personality Disorder," *Progress in Neuro-Psychopharmacology & Biological Psychiatry* 13, no. 6 (1989): 885–93; and J. R. Cornelius, P. H. Soloff, J. M. Prel, and R. F. Ulrich, "A Preliminary Trial of Fluoxetine in Refractory Borderline Patients," *Journal of Clinical Psychopharmacology* 11, no. 2 (1991): 116–20.

105. W. M. McDonald et al. "Pharmacological Management of the Symptoms Dementia," *American Family Physician* 42, no. 1 (1990 Jul): 123–32.

106. M. Sharpe, "Psychiatric Management of Post Viral Fatigue Syndrome," *British Medical Bulletin* 47, no. 4 (1991): 989–1005; D. A. Matthews, P. Manu, and T. J. Lane, "Evaluation and Management of Patients with Chronic Fatigue," *American Journal of the Medical Sciences* 302, no. 5 (1991): 269–77; P. J. Goodnick, "Bupropion in Chronic Fatigue Syndrome," *American Journal of Psychiatry* 147, no. 8 (1990 Aug): 1091.

107. R. Rickles et al., "Fluoxetine in the Treatment of Premenstrual Syndrome," *Current Therapeutic Research* 48, no. 1 (1990): 161–6; and A. B. Stone, T. B. Pearlstein, and W. A. Brown, "Fluoxetine in the Treatment of Late Luteal Phase Dysphoric Disorder," *Journal of Clinical Psychiatry* 52, no. 7 (1991): 290–3.

108. D. S. Greenbaum et al., "Effects of Desipramine on Irritable Bowel Syndrome Compared with Atropine and Placebo," *Digestive Diseases and Sciences* 32, no. 3 (March 1987): 257–66; J. I. Hudson and H. G. Pope Jr., "Affective Spectrum Disorder: Does Antidepressant Response Identify a Family of Disorders with a Common Pathophysiology?" *American Journal of Psychiatry* 148, no. 2 (February 1991): 280; also 148, no. 4 (April 1991): 548–49.

109. J. C. Ware and J. T. Pittard, "Increased Deep Sleep after Trazodone Use: A Double Blind, Placebo Controlled Study in Healthy Young Adults," *Journal of Clinical Psychiatry* 51, suppl. (1990 Sep): 18–22; R. L. Manfrede and A. Kales, "Clinical Neuropharmacology of Sleep Disorders," *Seminars in Neurology* 7, no. 3 (1987): 286–95.

110. Orsulak and Waller, "Antidepressant Drugs."

111. Orsulak and Waller, "Antidepressant Drugs"; and D. S. Singh, S. Sunder, and K. K. Tripathi, "Tricyclic Antidepressant Therapy in Duodenal Ulcer," *Journal of the Indian Medical Association* 85, no. 9 (September 1987): 265–7.

112. M. A. Gupta, A. K. Gupta, and C. N. Ellis, "Antidepressant Drugs in Dermatology: An Update," *Archives of Dermatology* 133, no. 5 (May 1987): 647–52; and B. A. Harris, E. F. Sherertz, and F. P. Flowers, "Improvement in Neurotic Excoriations with Oral Doxepin Therapy," *International Journal of Dermatology* 26, no. 8 (October 1987): 541–3.

113. Glassman, "Sadhart Trial"; and S. M. Czajkowski,"Effects of Treating Depression and Low Perceived Social Support on Clinical Events after Myocardial Infarction: The Enhancing Recovery in Coronary Heart Disease Patients (ENRICHD) Randomized Trial," *Journal of the American Medical Association.*

114. A. Rasmussen et al., "A Double-Blind, Placebo-Controlled Study of Sertraline in the Prevention of Depression in Stroke Patients," *Psychosomatics* 44, no. 3 (May/June 2003): 216–21; and K. R. Krishnan, "Depression as a Contributing Factor in Cerebrovascular Disease," *American Heart Journal* 140, 4 suppl. (October 2000): 70–6.

115. M. D. Crowell et al., "Antidepressants in the Treatment of Irritable Bowel Syndrome and Visceral Pain Syndromes," *Current Opinion in Investigational Drugs* 5, no. 7 (July 2004): 736–42.

116. Hudson and Pope, "Affective Spectrum Disorder."

117. J. S. Seggev and R. C. Eckert, "Psychopathology Masquerading as Food Allergy," *Journal of Family Practice* 26, no. 2 (February 1988): 161–4.

118. R. G. Ruegg, S. Zisook, and N. R. Swerdlow, "Depression in the Aged: An Overview," *Psychiatric Clinics of North America* 11, no. 1 (March 1988): 83–99; and R. H. Gerner, "Geriatric Depression and Treatment with Trazodone," *Psychopathology* 20, suppl. 1 (1987): 82–91.

119. J. K. Levy and F. Fernandez, "Neuoropsychiatric Care for Critically Ill AIDS Patients," *Journal of Critical Illness* 4, no. 3 (1989): 33–42.

Principles of Resilience and Methods of Implementing Them

He who cannot change the very fabric of his thought will never be able to change reality.

—Anwar Sadat

- Explain the principles of stress resilience.
- Describe the central core of what mental, physical, and even spiritual well-being are about.
- Examine a synthesis of the research and thought described in previous chapters.

Life is stress . . . in fact, it's one stressor after another. Finding life meaningful involves finding the stress meaningful. Having fun with life requires having some "fun" with the challenge of solving problems—or at least seeing the personal opportunity that comes along with them. That holds true even for depression; noting that all episodes of depression are not bad, Scott Peck speaks of the "healthiness of depression."[1]

Much of the effect of stress depends on how you choose to respond to it. One response is, "I want to get back to where I was before." Quite another is a response of humility: "I need to change. I think I'm wiser now."

Times of great stress or crisis provide a catalyst for change and, at times, quantum leaps in growth. We joke about smaller trials being for our growth, but the fact is that problems do indeed provide the opportunity to become wiser, stronger, and more resilient. For millennia the Chinese have recognized that fact in their language: The pictogram character for crisis combines those for danger and opportunity.

Three simple factors define whether stress is productive or destructive:

- The way you see and regard stress: is it an opportunity or an intolerable burden?
- Whether you can see both the pros and the cons—and whether you can create solutions (simply stated, whether you have a healthy brain)

- Whether you have mental or behavioral tools and principles that enable you to deal well with stress

The first of these factors, the way you choose to look at the stressful situation, is the basis of cognitive therapy. It may be the most rapidly effective of today's traditional psychotherapy approaches. The way you think about stress is heavily influenced by your propensity to see the world either in rational and even positive (optimistic) terms or in pessimistic ways.

The second factor, a healthy brain, requires normally functioning tissues and neurochemistry. Reversible neurochemical abnormalities, such as depression and anxiety disorders, are actually far more common barriers than is organic brain tissue disease. Both the pleasure and pain centers in the midbrain need to be adequately functioning if you're to deal well with stress; for example, neurochemically depressed people have trouble seeing the pros because the brain pleasure centers don't work well. Everything begins to look negative, so positive solutions become difficult to imagine. For that reason, medication may occasionally be needed, at least temporarily, to get the brain working well so that you can see both the pros and the cons. Good nutrition, exercise, and sleep are also highly important in preserving the brain's health.

The third requirement, the tools and principles, form the central focus of this final chapter. With this perspective, we'll describe some tools for transforming thought, behavior, and physiology into a condition congruent with the principles of total health.

Lessons from Cancer Studies

As mentioned in the previous chapter, few areas of behavioral medicine have been as emotionally charged and controversial as the treatment of cancer patients. In *The Type C Connection: The Mind-Body Links to Cancer and Your Health*, Lydia Temoshok and Henry Dreher originally best summarized the studies in this field.[2] An enormous paradigm shift is required to see behavioral and mental interventions as a form of "adjuvant" cancer therapy that improves prognosis (in this context, "adjuvant" refers to something that enhances how the primary therapy works in the body); such new concepts will likely be met with resistance. Less controversial is the attempt to use behavioral interventions as "supportive measures" to help a person emotionally deal optimally with the immense stress of confronting cancer and all its specters.

As discussed, the following associations exist between mental factors and cancer risk, morbidity, and mortality:

Good Prognosis

- Feeling a sense of personal control
- Hope of survival
- Trust in one's ability to deal with crisis
- Determination to live and a sense of purpose
- Connectedness
- Good coping ability
- Ability to express distressed feelings

Worse Prognosis

- Helplessness/hopelessness
- Lack of assertiveness
- Lack of meaning in life; apathy
- Unsatisfactory personal relationships
- Ineffectiveness at solving problems
- Clinical depression or anxiety
- Stoicism; inability to discuss problems

We bring these qualities and characteristics up here because, as you have seen throughout the pages of this book, these same issues are related to many other kinds of health outcomes as well.

Temoshok and Dreher concluded that, for cancer, the most important of the mental risk factors listed above—and the pathological core of their risky "type C behavior"—were the suppression of anger and other negative feelings in an attempt to be "nice." This suppression involves passively giving up important parts of your own values so you'll be acceptable to others, which is a violation of personal integrity. Such a behavior pattern may be more associated with the progression of and mortality from some existing cancers than it is with getting cancer in the first place. It should also be noted that certain mental factors have been associated with certain kinds of cancers, such as melanoma, lymphoma, or breast cancer, and it's not certain whether they apply to cancer in general. For the most part, the cancers that are more affected by hormones and immunity (such as cancers of the reproductive system and breast lymphomas, and skin cancers) seem to be impacted more by the central nervous system issues that modulate those hormones and immunity.

Even with these caveats in mind, would clinical programs that help cancer patients develop "better-prognosis" mental states also improve outcomes—at least in those cancer types we know to be associated with such psychological factors? We believe that the immune factors of protective cancer surveillance (such as natural killer–cell activity) may be involved because they are improved by some of the same mental factors that benefit cancer patients (see Chapter 1).

Dr. Sandra Levy at the Pittsburgh Cancer Institute has shown that prognosis in breast cancer can be improved with an optimistic rather than a pessimistic expectational style; she extended that knowledge to a therapeutic program designed to boost optimism in colon cancer patients. It worked—and it helps confirm hope as one of the principles we are looking for. (You may recall the central role of hope in the placebo effect described in Chapter 14, where we discussed that hope was able to even change cellular responses.)

This same principle was confirmed by Steven Greer's 15-year follow-up on British breast cancer patients. Those with a sense of hope and personal control had four times the survival rate of those who felt hopeless and helpless (80 percent versus 20 percent).[3] Leonard R. Derogatis similarly documented what physicians have sensed for hundreds of years: that an increased will to live, and having a purpose for that living, increased breast cancer survival.[4]

You must, however, tread lightly when creating hope in a therapeutic setting. Why? Although large numbers who have positive expectation may survive longer, a particular individual with a great deal of hope may die early. To have a sense of control, you need to accept responsibility, but it can be devastating to imply that a person is to blame for either developing cancer or failing to survive longer. Exactly what are we "responsible" for? The answer is simple: We're not so much responsible for the cancer as for how we choose to respond to the cancer. David Spiegel's support intervention that doubled life expectancy in breast cancer patients (see Chapter 21 was based not so much on expectations but rather on providing a sense of personal control in dealing with caregivers, a sense of meaning and purpose, a sense of connectedness to others struggling with the same crisis, the ability to deal wisely with the stress, and an opportunity to express and explore distressed feelings. (It also involved a longer period of time—a full year—than the usual psychobehavioral group intervention.)

Caroline Bedell Thomas's landmark study of physicians over a period of 25 years confirmed the importance of close, meaningful relationships as a protection from cancer. She found a four times greater incidence of cancer in those who lacked that connectedness.[5] She also found optimistic expectations to be important to overall health.

Again, the lessons we've discussed about healing and protective principles as they relate to cancer apply to many other diseases as well.

Four Core Principles Underlying Stress Resilience and Well-Being

If we pull together the healing principles outlined in the previous chapters, we might construct the following "stress-resilient" qualities around which behavioral interventions might best be directed:

1. **A sense of empowerment and personal control** (Chapters 2, 8, and 18)

   - Control over one's responses, not necessarily over the environment
   - The ability to live by one's deepest values (personal integrity) regardless of external pressures (authenticity)
   - A sense of feeling heard and valued

2. **A sense of connectedness and acceptance** (Chapters in Part III)

   - To one's deepest self
   - To other people
   - To the earth and the cosmos
   - To all regarded as good and to the sources of one's spiritual strength—an attitude that involves kindness, forgiveness, and humor

3. **A sense of meaning and purpose** (Chapters 14 and 15)

   - Giving of self for a purpose of value; a caring sense of mission
   - Finding meaning and wisdom in here-and-now difficulties
   - Enjoying the process of growth and creativity
   - Having a vision of one's potential

4. **Hope** (Chapters 14, 16, and 17)

   - Positive, optimistic expectations
   - A sense of being able to deal well with whatever situation arises
   - The ability to envision what one wants before it happens

This group of core principles arises not only from the multitude of medical and health studies reviewed in this book but also from careful studies of highly healthy and effective people. The key characteristics of such people include:

- The seventeen common characteristics of Maslow's self-actualizers (see Appendix A)[6]

- The three components of Kobasa's and Maddi's "stress-hardy" people (see Chapter 8)

- The seven habits of Covey's highly effective people (see Appendix B)[7]

- The characteristics of Garfield's peak performers [8]

- The characteristics of Friedman's "cardio-protected" Type B individuals (see Appendix C)

- The characteristics of Seligman's optimistic expectational style (see Chapters 16 and 17) and those characteristics exhibited in studies of human happiness[9] (see Table 8.1)

If you synthesize the underlying "ways of being in the world" by which these people function, you find that the four core principles listed above tie all of them together. (Even Maslow's 17 self-actualizing principles are largely variations on these four principles.) That's not all: the studies discussed throughout this book show that they underlie optimal physical health as well.

Also common to all these groups of healthy people are the values that led them to the above ends. When people in a relaxed, introspective state in a clinical setting are asked to reflect on who they really are—on the values they most deeply cherish—a small set of what seems to be nearly universal core values keeps appearing. Interestingly, they're the same core values by which well-functioning, healthy people actually operate, the core values that motivate them to do what they do.

What are some of those deeper, more universal values?

- **Caring love:** the kind that lifts and empowers both the person who is loved and the one who loves

- **Responsible free will:** feeling in charge of your own experience and responses to what happens in life

- **Integrity:** being the way you want to be; acting out of your clearly defined core values and wisdom

- **Growth:** enjoying a challenge, the love of continually getting wiser and more capable

From the studies cited earlier, we know that well-functioning people seem to operate through variants of these four "universal" values, which are in turn closely linked with the four core principles listed above that have been proven to bring better health. Interestingly, these principles hold true in a corporate environment as well: the most "healthy" companies (those whose success lasts longest) also tend to operate through these same principles.[10] These principles seem to be basic qualities of well-being, and they seem to be the deeper longings of most people who don't have them. How, then, do these stress-resilient principles work? Table 22.1 gives a handful of examples.

Keep in mind that the brain needs to be working well to implement these principles. If depression or anxiety disorders are present, a person may also need to treat the neurochemical abnormalities that accompany those disorders—even, at times, in the absence

Table 22.1 Stress-Resilient Principles

Major Issues Causing Distress	Core Values and Principles That Can Resolve the Distress
Issues of personal worth: low self-esteem, uncertain identity	Integrity to unconditional love, acceptance
Aloneness	Connectedness
Blaming, victimization, and feeling "forced"	Responsible free will, bringing choice and a sense of control
Demanding that things be different than they are	Acceptance of self and others; understanding cause and effect, and working with it (wisdom)
Threat, worry, and negative expectation	Hope, optimism, caring love
Perfectionism or giving up	Enjoying continued growth; a sense of purpose and meaning

of significant situational stress. It can be almost impossible to make the kind of mental change required with these four principles if the mental instrument needed to do it isn't working properly. When that's the case, medication—even on a temporary basis—can be of immense benefit (see Chapters 5, 6, and 21).

A Sense of Empowerment and Personal Control

Creating a personal sense of control in the face of stress is no trivial matter. This sense appears to lie at the heart of stress resilience because the bottom line about feeling distressed is that the stressful situation feels beyond control. In fact, all four core principles of stress resilience contribute to a natural sense of personal control—of how to be in the world. Many medical and mental disorders arise from an over-aroused nervous system with the loss of good homeostatic control. Treatment methods that calm the over-arousal can move the body toward the reestablishing of that homeostasis. Feeling a mental sense of control brings better physiological control. Table 22.1 contains further observations about a sense of personal control that will help demonstrate why some of the behavioral treatment approaches work.

Stressed Animals and Control

A mental state of being "out of control" is accompanied by physiology that's "out of control"—a dysregulation of autonomic, hormonal, and immunological balance that protects from disease. An example comes from the work of Madelon Visintainer, Martin Seligman, and his colleagues.

In their studies,[11] animals were placed in a classical stress setup: They were confined in a box, and an electrode that delivered intermittent shocks was attached to their tails. Each shock was preceded by a warning bell. Each animal was assigned to one of three groups:

1. The first group was given a wheel that, when turned, aborted the shock, as the animals quickly learned. The bell rang, the animals spun the wheel, and no shock occurred. They were captains of their destiny. They were in control, despite the stressor.

2. The second group had no wheel. They were truly victims, cowering at the bell that signaled the imminent misery.

3. The third group acted as controls; they were not given shocks.

The animals were then injected with cancer cells to see which were most likely to develop cancer and which were best able to immunologically reject the cancer and stay healthy. Those in the group who had control over the stress were able to reject sarcoma cells 70 percent of the time compared with only 27 percent of the victims. Interestingly, the group that had control over stress did even better than the group that had no stress at all: Only 50 percent of the unstressed animals rejected the cancer cells. When researchers measured the immune responses in the different groups, those with control over stress had the best immune response; the victims had the worst.

The same pattern holds up across many types of studies dealing with stress: It's not the stressor that matters as much as the ability to control the response to stress. Like the animals, those who are stressed but have a sense of control, in fact, are often even healthier than those who are not stressed at all. Out of control, stress becomes distress; under control, it becomes eustress. And, as noted in Chapter 2, the neurochemical and physiological responses differ between the two.

It should be noted that a fascinating paradox exists about how to achieve a sense of control. The more you attempt to control the external situation (such as what others do), the more out of control things feel, simply because the external world can seldom be reliably controlled. On the other hand, the more you let go—the less you try to control the external world and the more you respond with wisdom and maturity—the greater the sense of *personal* control. When you accept that things exist as they are for a reason (whether good or bad), you can respond with creative, persuasive wisdom to draw others in a different direction.

Brain Neurochemistry and the Sense of Control

Finding a sense of control also seems to improve the neurochemical abnormalities associated with extreme stress, depression, and anxiety. Raleigh and McGuire at the University of California–Los Angeles studied how gaining and losing social control affect serotonin levels.[12] (Serotonin is a key player, not only in depression and anxiety but also in keeping physical and emotional responses "in balance" and under control.) They studied the difference in serotonin levels in dominant versus submissive males in vervet monkeys.

The results were fascinating. Serotonin levels were twice as high in the alpha male, the dominant ("in control") monkeys, as in the submissive ones. Then researchers "dethroned" the dominant monkey by placing him behind a one-way mirror where he could watch the submissive males eating his special food, getting their needs met, and cozying up to his harem of females, but none of the others could see or hear him. He ranted and raved, as he always did to maintain power, but—unheard and unseen—to no avail. As he began to give up, feeling helpless and hopeless, his serotonin levels dropped. Some dropped to the level of the formerly submissive males; some dropped even lower. Interestingly, as the previously submissive monkeys started to gain some control, their serotonin levels rose toward those of the previously dominant male. Thus, it was demonstrated that a sense of control has an antidepressant-like effect on serotonin.

In the second part of the study, Raleigh and McGuire used drugs to change the serotonin levels then watched the resulting behaviors.[13] When drugs were given to raise serotonin levels in passive males, they acted dominant. When drugs were given to inhibit serotonin in dominant males, they acted subordinate—and were anxious over tests they had previously done with confidence. Another fascinating observation was that researchers could predict which monkey would soon dominate by watching which monkey the females were cozying up to, regardless of which monkey was winning all the battles. The brain serotonin levels in the male being sought by the females increased, and within two weeks, he dominated the others.

Social dominance also affects the immunity of animals. In response to stress, dominant animals show a more optimal antibody response; that of submissive animals is decreased.[14] Dominance increases not only brain serotonin levels but also natural painkillers (opioids), such as endorphins. These opioids, in turn, affect immunity; animals with high endorphin levels have increased resistance to cancer. On the other hand, higher cortisol levels—seen with chronic submission and "helplessness"—are correlated with decreased immune competence. It all plays into why people who feel depressed or helpless have more difficulty clearing infections and a worse prognosis for certain treated cancers (see Chapters 1 and 6).

Boston University researcher David McClelland showed that, when frustrated, students with a need to exercise power over others had significantly increased blood adrenaline levels and decreased salivary immunoglobulin A (Ig-A) antibody levels. The effect? More upper respiratory infections when under academic stress.[15] Students under the same stress but not under the same need for control didn't have the same rate of infections or the same drop in antibodies. Interestingly, the brain tends to elicit behavior to help get the chemicals it needs.

McClelland's study illustrates another paradox about a sense of control: Those people lower in brain serotonin function are often driven to seek control—maybe in an attempt to get levels back up. That is, a strong need for control can be a symptom of deficient brain serotonin. Examples are seen in people with compulsive behaviors, perfectionism, or hostility toward competitors. Seeking power and control is often a symptom of the underlying insecurity that accompanies diminished serotonin function (as may also be seen in some type A behavior). Treatment that improves serotonin function often helps these behaviors.

So, if you find yourself with an excessive need to control, consider doing other things to increase serotonin function: get good sleep, meditate mindfully, and eat high-tryptophan foods[16] (tryptophan converts into serotonin) (and maybe get some female monkeys interested in you!). Best of all, recognize the paradox of control: Stop trying to control the external world, and take back your power to be the way you want to be, regardless of external forces. Refuse to blame others for making you feel or behave in ways you don't want to. With those resolves, a personal kind of control begins to settle in, and serotonin function naturally improves.

Cognitive Structuring and Therapy

Many intervention approaches are built around giving a greater sense of integrity and personal control. One of the most rapidly effective forms of psychotherapy for converting distressed responses into healthier responses is cognitive (thinking) therapy. Cognitive restructuring underlies both cognitive therapy and some of its spinoffs (such as rational behavioral therapy or rational emotive therapy).[17] These therapies are based on the realization that stressful situations do not really cause our feelings and physiological responses nearly as much as does the way we choose to think about those situations.

The sequence creating feelings and behavior is sometimes called the ABCs of creating feelings and behavior:

A. The perceived situation
B. Our thinking about the situation
C. Our responses: feelings, physical responses, and behavior

The situation is the event around which our thinking forms. We choose how to think about the situation—how we regard the situation and its meaning for us. The way we think about the situation leads to our response: feelings, physiological responses, and behavioral responses. Each time this process occurs for a specific situation, it becomes more automatic.

Note that feelings and behavioral responses are not caused directly by the situation at all but rather by the way we choose or learn to think about the situation. As soon as the thinking changes, the response changes. The situation is only the event around which the thinking forms. It is the thinking, rather than the event, that creates the reality for that person. That's why one person feels "blown away" by the same situation that another person sees as a creative challenge. When you blame the situation for your feelings and behaviors, you become a victim—you give up your sense of control. On the other hand, if you recognize that most situations aren't as distressing as the way you've chosen to think about them, you open up many possibilities for regarding the situation in more mature and wise ways. If the response is destructive and distressful, almost invariably a more rational way of thinking can be found that fits much better with one's deeper values and wisdom. This new thinking will create a more productive response, will result in less distress, and will bring back a sense of control, even though the situation is the same.

The following is an example. If a father felt upset and angry when his teenaged daughter rebelled with provocative remarks, he might think, "She makes me so angry!" Remember, however, it's not her that makes him angry. The way he chooses to think about her does make him angry. (It may seem there's only one way to think and feel about her behavior, but that's not the case.) Instead of trying to control her, he could regain personal control by refusing to blame the teen's behavior (the situation) for "making" him feel bad or for "causing" him to react in destructive ways toward his daughter. By realizing that he himself created the way he thought about his daughter, which in turn caused the disturbing reaction, he can—in a more reflective, disengaged moment—create new ways of thinking and dealing with a struggling teenager, ways of thinking congruent with his deeper, wiser hopes as her dad, to lift and encourage his daughter instead of putting her down. As he does so, his anger begins to disappear. Identifying this deeper wisdom, he could then mentally practice his new, more compassionate response repetitively, helping his new reaction become more automatic. Instead of being extremely distressful and alienating, his new reaction could be creatively empowering—and even bonding.

At first, the way you think about a situation may seem like the only way to regard it. At that point, it's easy to be misled about what the most rational thoughts are. But there's a key guideline as to whether thinking is maturely rational: Look at the feelings and behavior it engenders. If the feelings or behavior are destructive, then the thinking that caused it has two characteristics:

- It is in some way irrational (that is, it's not totally reliable; if you examine it closely, you'll find you don't totally believe it).

- It in some way violates your deepest values.

By destructive feelings and behavior, we mean those feelings and behaviors that make you miserable, hurt relationships or other people, or keep you from doing or becoming what you more deeply want.

Let's look again at the example of the father struggling with his teenaged daughter. What's so irrational about getting angry over his daughter's rude remarks? It's irrational to think that the father *has* to be angry and upset. He can choose to respond with anger and putdowns, or he can choose instead to react in some wiser way. Instead of judgmental anger, the father may try to understand his daughter's struggle with identity and independence, which is what is really causing her behavior, and he may respond with gentle wisdom that encourages his daughter instead of trying to put her down. In the long run, that kind of reaction is probably more in harmony with his deepest values, anyway: He wants to lift and encourage his daughter rather than make her feel diminished. Just being aware that it is not her that is causing the anger, but rather his old ways of thinking about her that causes the anger, gives him some new choices. There's an important caveat here, too: In responding differently, the father isn't suppressing his anger. Instead, when he thinks about his daughter differently, his anger simply dissipates. His new feelings toward her may even be compassionate for her struggle to find independence.

Remember: If feelings are destructive, there is always a wiser, more rational way of thinking that is more in harmony with your deeper values—and that will result in a very different response to the same situation. The first step to gaining control of your responses is giving up blame, fully realizing that you create your own thinking and responses (or have simply learned them from somewhere). Accepting that responsible free choice to respond with wisdom is the first step to control.

Typical ways of thinking that cause distress have to do with:

- The "shoulds" (How does the situation fit with what "should" be true?)

- Issues of worth (What does this situation mean about my worth and value?)

- Threat (Am I likely to lose something of value because of this situation?)

- Force (Am I feeling forced to do something I don't want to do?)[18]

What is the most effective way of dealing with a recurrently distressful situation? First (after getting calm) clarify your thoughts about the situation. You might want to write them down in the ABC format, and ask yourself whether there is anything a bit irrational about the thought. (In his classic book on self-applications of cognitive therapy, *Feeling Good: The New Mood Therapy,* David Burns describes ways to recognize and reframe these thought distortions.[19] You might, for example, ask yourself, "If a panel of wise, uninvolved people were evaluating my thoughts here, would they all agree, or might some have a more mature way of seeing it?" Just thinking about your irrational thoughts takes the emotional power out of them and starts the formation of wiser ones.

Second, discover a more rational way of regarding the situation (something more in line with your deeper values and wisdom). Perhaps ask yourself, "If a person of great wisdom, strength, and goodness were handling this, how would he or she think and respond?" Doing this taps into your own deeper, wise mind, where many solutions reside.

And, finally, use an experiential technique like visualization or other forms of imagery to help your new way of thinking and responding become automatic. (Visualizing and imagery are discussed below.) The result? A sense of personal control that is in harmony with your values. With repeated practice, your new response will become as automatic as the way you tie your shoes: you've done it so many times that you do it without any conscious thought. What is involved here is replacing old automatic, habitual responses (based on practiced unconscious pictures in the brain) with a new practiced picture of responding more rationally. If your old practiced way of tying your shoes wasn't working for you because your shoes weren't staying tied, what would you do? You would probably go back to the drawing board to figure out a new way of tying the shoes (thinking and responding differently), and then you would practice the new way of tying over and over again until it becomes automatic. At first, the new way of thinking may seem awkward or artificial just as tying your shoes a new way would seem awkward at first. That's because it doesn't fit with your old habit. It's awkward at first, but it's not artificial; in fact, it's more real.

Notice also how this process begins to create hope. You'll notice an expectation that you can deal well with both this situation and others like it.

Basic Elements of Behavior Change

To change distressed behaviors, whether emotional or physiological:

1. Clarify the present state—awareness (including awareness of automatic thoughts).

2. Clearly determine in explicit, specific terms what you wholly desire your new thinking and behavior to be.

3. Experientially practice your new behavioral response (for example, by relaxing and visualizing it or experiencing it with other types of imagery).

Research has shown that it's very difficult to mentally "reprogram" yourself if you're overly aroused—which is likely if you're also distressed. The key is to become deeply relaxed and receptive through "meditative methods," behaviors that help you relax, become calm, disengage from destructive thinking, and create and practice new mental models. This usually involves becoming centered in the present moment (which is the only moment in which you can feel a personal sense of control).

There are some meditative methods that elicit the relaxation response, helping you to become calm and mentally disengage from old ways of thinking. Other meditative methods help you experience transformation, thus bringing change to a new, better behavior. You'll need to use both.

Methods of Eliciting the Relaxation Response

Meditative Breathing   Using your breathing can be a very effective method for calming the mind. This is a body-to-mind technique because the mind automatically associates certain patterns of breathing with either anxiety or calm. For example, if you right now breathe in very, very deeply and hold it. Don't let it out—in fact, breathe in even more air and hold it, and then, without letting much air out, breathe shallowly high in your lungs (with nearly a full breath still held in, using your chest muscles rather than those of your abdomen). Breathing like this, you're likely to start feeling anxious. That's because this is the way you breathe when you're anxious. Check it out next time you are very stressed: notice how you are breathing—it's likely to be shallow and high in the chest.

Now, shift gears and breathe slowly in such a way that a hand on your abdomen rises and falls, as though you were breathing gently down into your belly (a technique known as diaphragmatic breathing). You will probably find your mind calming and becoming more focused. This type of breathing is how you breathe when you're relaxed. Sometimes adding three counts—1, 2, 3—on each in-breath and each out-breath makes this even more calming. Putting your hand on your abdomen to feel it rising and falling eventually creates a conditioned cue, such that, after practice, when you place your hand there, over-aroused becomes automatically calmed. Such breathing can then be used even during an anxious moment to bring back focus and calm.

Practice relaxed breathing for a few minutes. Sense that you are breathing in energy and life (which, after all, is exactly what you are doing) and that you are breathing out the unnecessary things (which is also physiologically true). Sense the metaphor in this: as you breathe, feel energy (and even insight) flowing into your mind and out to your extremities, and feel letting go of that which no longer needs to be held. Perhaps you will even find yourself being grateful for this remarkable, automatic process that has kept you alive for so long. As you focus on the bodily feelings of letting go with the breath, you will find an interesting paradox: as your body and mind calm, you become more keenly aware of what is going on. In some cultures, this simple breathing practice has been used for millennia to facilitate spiritual insight.

After getting good at this by practicing it repeatedly, when you notice anxious breathing during the day, simply change it to relaxed breathing, and your mind and body will follow.

Progressive Muscle Relaxation   With this method, you tense specific muscles as you inhale, become aware of the feeling of tension, then totally "let go" to relax those same muscles as you exhale, closely noticing the difference between tension and relaxation. To try it, breathe in as you tightly tense one arm and fist; make sure to notice how tension feels. Hold the breath and the associated tension for a moment. Then, as you breathe out, let your arm and hand flop into your lap, and notice the feeling that flows through your arm into your hand. Give it great attention. As you do this, figure out exactly how muscle relaxation feels. (Does it cause some warmth or tingling?) Notice how that hand feels different from the other one. Next, sequentially involve all the muscles in your body in a systematic way, starting with your foot and leg, for example, and then moving up the body step by step to the buttocks, trunk, chest, shoulders, arms, hands, neck, and face. Once you know the difference between feeling tense and relaxed, you can recognize situations ("cues") that make you feel tense. You can then practice relaxing, using an "anchor"—a certain kind of breath, body position, or touch—to signify that deep relaxation is present. After regular practice, the anchor becomes a conditioned trigger of relaxation, and then it becomes your cue to quickly elicit deep relaxation when needed.

Autogenic Training   This technique has been used for more than a century, particularly among European athletes to enhance performance. It creates a trance much like self-hypnosis. You simply sense different parts of your body, such as your hands and feet, getting heavy and warm (and tell yourself so), and then the stomach and gut getting relaxed and calm, and the heartbeat slowing and becoming more regular. When this semi-hypnotic state is reached, gentle suggestions or visualizations about optimal performance can be more fully realized.

Mindfulness Meditation   This method involves living fully in the present moment, giving complete, caring attention to whatever you choose.[20] You focus attention on one thing at a time, allowing intruding or distracting thoughts to pass; as a result, you feel a quiet sense of control instead of a frazzled attempt to concentrate on several thoughts at once. To practice, you can devote complete concentration and attention to simple things like breathing or eating, the sensations of these, and the increased awareness that accompanies such attention. You give full, caring attention to whatever single task is at hand, rather than multitasking. The brain seems to love mindfulness, and gets distressed when multitasking. This calm, focused attention and awareness in the present moment has been used very effectively in a number of stress-reduction programs, including those at the University of Massachusetts, Harvard, and the University of Utah. Deeper states of mindfulness meditation go well beyond simple relaxation to facilitate self-transformation (discussed below).

Imagery   Imagery involves mentally going to a safe, beautiful place—a place that you then totally experience with all your senses: the visual beauty, the smells, the sounds, the touch, the feelings of being there. With practice, you can take a "mental trip" every day to the mountains or the seashore—and not only experience the sensations but also the mental detachment, perspective, and rejuvenation that come from actually traveling to a similar place for a few days.

"Body Work"   Techniques like yoga usually involve "relaxed stretching," putting the body under stress while you relax your mind. This can become a type of experiential metaphor for life: calmness under stress or while in pain. Other useful relaxing body work methods include tai chi, qi gong, and Feldenkrais, or even massage (you can find directions for many of these online[21]).

Which of all the techniques described above is best? It really doesn't matter so much which you use, as long as it best matches your preferred way of mental processing. Those who are auditory (liking words and dialogue) may prefer to mindfully meditate on a meaningful word or phrase, letting the sound and its meaning resonate within. A visual processor may prefer imaging a beautiful place or meditating on an image. Someone who likes physical feelings and touch may do best with breathing and muscle relaxation methods. Someone geared spiritually may enjoy a deeper experience like transcendental meditation.

Some (especially men) like to do the breathing and muscle relaxation first because it feels more tangible, feeling the level of tension or relaxation (similar to a built-in biofeedback gauge). Once they have those techniques mastered, other methods become more attractive.

Meditative Methods of Changing Behavior

Several meditative methods help to clarify your core values and solutions from your inner, wise mind. As a result, they help you change your behavior to that which you desire.

Quiet Contemplation   In a peaceful, quiet environment free of distraction, think about and record those things that have the deepest meaning in your life. This exercise is a key way of clarifying your values. The more sensory detail you put into your written record, the more effective it will be for change. Imagine that what you want most is happening right now. Record what you would be seeing, feeling, hearing, and sensing as your desired outcome is in place. This will make it easier to visualize. Record what having this outcome does for you beyond the outcome itself (at even higher levels of meaning). This will motivate you to accomplish your most desired outcome.

Guided Imagery   Dr. Martin Rossman effectively pioneered the use of guided imagery for self-healing.[22] Two kinds of guided imagery particularly may help you reprogram your thoughts and change your behavior.[23] The first, imagery to the "inner child,"[24] helps you mentally visit yourself as a child who is going through a disturbing event. You then reprogram the meaning of that event through mature eyes—you nurture and heal by giving the child new ways of dealing well with the event. This creates a new memory for the meaning of the old event.

In the second kind of guided imagery, imagery to the "inner advisor," you personify your inner wisdom and values into an "inner advisor." While picturing the interaction, that imagined wise advisor then provides you rapid access to solutions congruent with your own values.

More recently, other methods of such imagery have developed. Some of which are very useful for medical problems such as headaches, sleep or fatigue, and appear to be the most effective for healing past trauma.[25]

Visualization   Through visualization,[26] you actually practice "seeing" yourself performing or functioning in the way you want. It's a highly effective way of rapidly changing your behavior, and it hinges on four techniques:

- You need to define your desired goal or outcome in clear detail. The brain doesn't process "don'ts" very well; to be effective, you need to define the outcome only in terms of what you *do* want. Your outcome, of course, needs to be compatible with your deepest values—and all parts of you must intensely want that outcome.

- You must be totally relaxed.

- You must see and feel yourself achieving the desired result in great detail. In essence, you need to "experience" it completely—including the place, cues, who is there, your style of behavior, and your physical sensations. This goes beyond fantasizing; instead, you see yourself with enough feeling and trust that you generate the energy to actually carry out the vision. You may find it easier to first visualize this happening by observing yourself as if in a movie. Then, when you are comfortable with that, shift to visualizing what's going on from within the event (seeing through your eyes, sensing the feelings of being actually in the event). This needs to be repeated at least three or four times for each specific event.

- You need to practice regularly. Soon the capacity to respond wisely and well to many kinds of events begins to generalize.

Other Ways to Change Behavior

There are other keys to changing behavior—ways of achieving a personal sense of control. Although they've been discussed in greater detail earlier in this book, they deserve to be mentioned here.

Increasing the Internal Locus of Control   Training in self-assertion helps you become aware of your own needs and values; use the combined principles of honesty and kindness to express them. An internal locus of control engenders a proactive spirit; you refuse to choose helplessness or being hopeless as a response. Key to this self assertion is coupling respectful kindness with authentically communicating your position.

Practicing Forgiveness   Entire treatment approaches have been built around the practice of forgiveness (see Chapter 14).[27] To some, forgiving someone who has been offensive or who has caused pain seems like giving a gift to an undeserving person. In reality, genuine forgiveness is giving a gift to yourself. It involves regaining personal control by refusing to blame someone else's actions for your feelings and behavior. Forgiveness involves choosing to act in ways that are wise and mature, regardless of how someone else has acted. Experiencing real forgiveness is at the heart of gaining personal control.

Keeping a Journal   When you write about your feelings, you become aware of how you think and behave in response to stressful situations. The troublesome thoughts become more objectified—something to observe and analyze—and thus lose their destructive emotional power. When you capture the experience on paper, you "get a handle on it" and achieve some sense of how to deal with it. Keeping a journal has the added benefit of creating a sense of who you really are and the values for which you stand. Include a description of how you would have wanted to respond to a recorded situation. Also record what you hope to become. Your written words create newness.

Building Social Support   To create social support:

- Identify a type of relationship that would be deeply satisfying for you.

- Write down in detail the words that describe what makes the relationship so great: ways you would treat and regard each other in such a meaningful relationship.

- Choose to be that way no matter how the other is currently acting: experiment with this, even if only for one day.

- Practice being that way (both during visualization and in reality).

- Anticipate others responding in like manner, but don't get unduly disturbed if they fail to respond as you would hope. Be patient; as you keep doing this others will gradually be drawn in.

Social support not only increases your quality of life but also increases overall health and longevity (and even reduces your risk of coronary disease).[28] For detailed information on the benefits of creating social support, see the chapters in Part III.

Summarizing the Process for Rapid Change to Healthier, More Resilient Behavior

At times, we seem to have two minds. One is the mind by which we operate in the world, creating thoughts by which we function. Some of those thoughts cause us trouble. Then we also seem to have a deep, wise mind that knows the solutions and the values by which we want to live. The key in this process is getting the operating mind to become one with the wise mind, resulting in behaviors that follow our own deep wisdom.

Using the above elements, changing old destructive habits and stress reactions might go something like this:

1. **Practice conscious awareness:** "I can respond as I choose." Half the solution is won with this realization: "I am no longer a victim."

2. **Develop and practice relaxation skills.** Let go of old thoughts and get mindfully centered.

3. **Clarify deep values and wisdom.** Ask yourself how you want to be—then write your answer in great detail and in positive, not negative, terms.

4. **Visualize (experience with imagery) being the new way.** You'll need several repetitions for each situation you want to change. The new style then becomes easier, almost like a habit.

It's very important that you visualize what *to* do instead of what *not* to do. For example, don't try to not be Type A hostile and cynical. Instead, define what you want to be: the healthy Type B described in Appendix C. Behaviors are created by mental pictures. The visualizing brain cannot visualize not doing something; it needs to know what to do instead. You might, for example, explore whether some of the characteristics of Maslow's self-actualizers in Appendix A resonate with your values as solutions; if they do, then picture yourself responding in similar ways that suit you. If you can't create visual images (and even if you can), bring in all the other senses and feelings at to what would be going on when you are being and doing as you desire.

The Spiritual Connection

Professionals who do the hands-on work with patients struggling over mind-body issues often comment that stress finally resolves when "the spiritual issues resolve." They sense, in other words, that spiritual well-being underlies much of both mental and physical well-being (see Chapter 14).

In Chapter 14, we described some of the polls of Americans in pain. People who were questioned claimed that their pain was relieved as much by spiritual counseling and practices as by medical methods. How could this be? Perhaps the answer lies in what good spiritual practices bring about in an individual. Solid spiritual practices are designed to:

- Help people identify and live by their deepest values and wisdom (providing personal control)

- Empower people to live with integrity and to forgive (again, providing personal control)

- Provide support, caring, and a greater capacity to love (creating connectedness)

- Give purpose and structure to life, transforming the meaning of life's events

- Foster hope

The World Health Organization defines health as "a state of complete physical, mental, and social well-being and not merely the absence of disease or infirmity."[29] In Chapter 14 we found strong evidence that these dimensions of health are also often linked to spiritual well-being as well.

What is meant by "spiritual well-being"? The answers are varied, and the condition is difficult to measure in a study. We can measure with considerable precision optimal physical health and function. We can even measure with fair accuracy the condition of mental well-being. Yet, even though spiritual well-being escapes the precise measurement of these others, practitioners claim that it may be possible to demonstrate the essence of spiritual well-being.

How? In essence, the four core principles listed near the beginning of this chapter make up the components of overall wellness. They are also the ends toward which many spiritual traditions are working: empowerment, deep integrity, connectedness, a sense of purpose and meaning, and hope (see Chapter 14). It is no coincidence that these principles are also what many in the world are hungering for. Based on the science of creating physical and mental well-being, the four principles and the four "universal values" above may well be the essence of spiritual well-being, and practices that foster these principles are likely to be valuable for one's mental and spiritual life.

It's important to note that what undermines these principles in the name of "spirituality" is likely to be a misconception. For example, being angrily judgmental of "imperfect" people doesn't empower; it puts down. It doesn't foster connectedness; instead, it causes alienation. It doesn't promote hope but instead promotes discouragement. With this in mind, are such misguided attempts to be spiritual more likely to advance physical health or to cause physical illness?

Simply stated, the essence of genuine spiritual growth is expanding the sense of control, connectedness, meaning, and hope that have been proven to bring about healing.

When health interventions or spiritual practices are directed toward these four ends, the evidence suggests that total well-being (health) is a likely result. Markers of spiritual well-being would likely include a sense of gratitude for life, oneness, recognition of beauty, and wholeness. Healing, after all, is about making separated things whole.

Mind-Body Treatment: Can It Change the Course of Disease?

With all of our knowledge about behavioral techniques, we come to a sobering question: If someone starts practicing the techniques described in this chapter at an early age, will it actually prevent or alter the course of disease?

The answer lies in results of pioneering studies in the field of mind-body treatment. For example, Jon Kabat-Zinn at the University of Massachusetts Medical Center Stress Reduction Clinic takes on patients with difficult medical problems that other physicians have given up on. In turn, he uses methods based on mindfulness meditation. Among more than 4,000 patients he treated over a period of 10 years, that simple but also profound technique reduced medical illness in these difficult cases by 35 percent.[30] Even diseases as specific and resistant as psoriasis have responded positively.[31] Among the elderly, other forms of meditation have had even greater health benefits.[32] Chapter 21 describes the medical outcome effects of many such interventions.

As noted in Chapter 1, distressed thinking can adversely affect the immune system—with an obvious link to disease. Behavioral interventions that have been shown to improve immune response include:

- Clinical biofeedback
- Meditation
- Autogenic training
- Progressive relaxation
- Visualization
- Hypnosis
- Behavior modification[33]

Although the results of such studies have been encouraging, they have also been somewhat inconsistent; the field of achieving stress resilience is filled with paradox. A good example is the controversial use of imagery for "healing" cancer.[34] Many years ago, Ainsley Mears used two different types of imagery with cancer patients. The first created a state of relaxed peacefulness and acceptance; patients used the crisis to focus on their deepest values and heal their lives. The result? Cancer progression slowed; more patients actually went into remission.

For the second part of his study, Meares instructed patients to use imagery to imagine the active destruction of the cancer cells by white blood cells and macrophages. His aim was rejection of the tumor by the immune system. That didn't happen, though; for a majority of the patients, tumor recurrences began to increase. What went wrong? Maybe it was just a function of time; because the second part of the study took longer, there was time for recurrences to happen. But a greater issue involves whether creating an aroused, hostile state aimed at destroying the tumor may actually be counterproductive; instead of creating a sense of inner peace, it involves a threat to one's sense of control.

The first approach—creating a state of relaxed peacefulness—allowed patients to accept things as they are and to respond with wisdom, maturity, and love to the situation. It let patients use the crisis to get focused on healing the parts of their lives that had been neglected or had gone unresolved. That kind of approach, argue researchers, creates a greater sense of personal control even if the tumor goes uncured.

Other methods of mental control, such as biofeedback to change body temperature, have been beneficial in the treatment of autoimmune diseases, such as rheumatoid arthritis.[35] Treatments that have included social support, guided imagery, and progressive relaxation have also helped rheumatoid arthritis patients; the psychological interventions have been more effective than social support alone.[36] In one study, 81 percent said that relaxation training was a major factor in reducing pain, reducing inflammation, and decreasing levels of serum rheumatoid factor. In another study,[37] patients were given a cognitive-behavioral treatment designed to boost self-efficacy in managing the disease; patients were taught self-relaxation, cognitive pain management, and goal setting. The more the patients enhanced self-efficacy (a measure of their sense of control), the more their pain and inflammation were reduced.

Ohio State University researcher Janice Kiecolt-Glaser has extensively studied the effects of mental distress on immune function. One such study involved 45 nursing home residents who were taught progressive relaxation and guided imagery as a way to gain control over their world. This simple step resulted in significantly less mental distress, as well as better prognosis and greater longevity. Furthermore, those who used progressive relaxation and guided imagery had significantly improved cellular immune response, including an increase in natural killer cell–activity.

We know that mental conditioning can affect immune response (see Chapter 1). A classic example occurred when University of Rochester researcher Robert Ader mentally conditioned a group of mice to suppress their immune response.[38] Here's how he did it: He gave the mice a mixture of the drug cyclophosphamide, which suppresses the immune response, and saccharine (a sweetener). Later, he gave the mice saccharine but no cyclophosphamide. What happened? The taste of the saccharine triggered the memory of the cyclophosphamide, causing the immune response of the mice to be suppressed by that memory alone (a conditioned mind-body response).

Ader then extended his experiment to a group of New Zealand mice that genetically get lupus erythematosus, an autoimmune disease in which an overactive immune system destroys the kidneys and causes death at a predictable age.[39] The drug cyclophosphamide diminishes the extra immune function and, as a result, delays kidney failure and prolongs life. Ader gave the mice saccharine with the first few doses of cyclophosphamide their immune suppression was linked in the brain to the saccharine taste. Later, giving them saccharine alone suppressed the immune response with this mind-body conditioned effect. The result? Saccharine alone (the conditioned expectation) delayed kidney failure and prolonged life. In the animals who received saccharine without conditioning with the drug, nothing happened.

Perhaps as we learn more precisely to understand the fascinating interactions between the mind and the body and how to effectively work with them, we can embark on new and safe therapies in the future that we haven't even considered today.

Changing Directions

An interesting point is that the behavioral interventions described in this book are going in the opposite direction of the growing medical trend toward superspecialization. That specialization—reaching now to the molecular level—has reaped great benefits but has also tended to separate the parts of a person and his or her overall care. The studies cited in this book call for a focused and concerted effort to treat the whole person and integrate each part of an individual's care. Combining both approaches will provide the most optimal outcome.

That integration requires the targeted use of not only behavioral and psychological interventions but strong educational efforts as well—all preferably in both the medical and health prevention settings. In fact, these principles and methods could be taught effectively in school health classes and, based on the data you have seen in this book, could quite possibly become the most effective preventive medicine. Perhaps the most potent mind-body intervention of all is a deeply trusting and caring relationship with the medical caregiver who is sensitive to these issues and who truly understands how these interventions work.

We have seen some major medical revolutions in the past:

1. The surgical revolution (which began with ether anesthesia, about 1846)

2. The scientific revolution (the ability to clearly demonstrate repeatable results, which began in earnest about 1870)

3. The chemical revolution (which began with penicillin, about 1936)

4. And now: the behavioral revolution (since about 1979)

   This phase is seeing shifts from

- Organ-based medicine toward a person-based emphasis

- Technological approaches toward humanely based approaches

- Treatment of symptoms toward prevention

- Paternalistic approaches toward cooperative care

Revolutions do not come easily, but each of the revolutions above has been very valuable. We seem to be in a moment in time where new ways of thinking in mind-body terms are being proven to be very fruitful.

As we move into that future, we discover the truth of what mathematician Charles Muses proclaimed when he said, "The potentials of consciousness remain well nigh the last reachable domain for man not yet explored—the Undiscovered Country." We anticipate a time and system in which we will, as French neurologist Frederic Tilney challenged us, "We will by conscious command evolve cerebral centers which will permit us to use powers that we now are not even capable of imagining."[40]

WHAT DID YOU LEARN?

1. Describe four core principles of mental resilience that are highly associated with better health, happiness, and fulfillment. Give a brief explanation of each of these.

2. Describe two mechanisms by which an internal locus of control might improve health, and describe the paradox of control.

3. Decribe the ABCs of creating feelings and behavior. Why is it important to understand that situations are not the real cause of feelings?

4. Describe six methods of eliciting the relaxation response.

5. Describe three experiential methods for rapidly changing behavior.

6. Summarize a process for fairly rapid change.

ENDNOTES

1. Scott Peck, *The Road Less Traveled: A New Psychology of Love, Traditional Values and Spiritual Growth* (New York: Simon & Schuster, 1978), 69.

2. Lydia Temoshok and Henry Dreher, *The Type C Connection: The Mind-Body Links to Cancer and Your Health* (Random House, 1992. Paperback: Plume, 1993).

3. S. Greer et al., "Psychological Response to Breast Cancer and 15-Year Outcome," *Lancet* 1 (1990): 49–50.

4. Cited in Constance Holden, "Cancer and the Mind: How are They Connected?", *Science*, 200: 1363–9.

5. C. B. Thomas et al., "Cancer in Families of Former Medical Students Followed to Midlife: Prevalence of Subjects with and without Major Cancer." *Johns Hopkins Medical Journal* 151 (1982): 193–202.

6. Abraham Maslow, *Personality and Motivation* (HarperCollins Publishers; 3 Sub. edition 1987), ch. 11.

7. Stephen R. Covey, *The Seven Habits of Highly Effective People* (New York: Fireside–Simon & Schuster, 1989).

8. Charles Garfield. *Peak Performers* (New York: Harper Paperbacks: 1987).

9. Martin Seligman, Christopher Peterson, Tracy Sheen, and Nansook Park, "Positive Psychology Progress: Empirical Validation of Interventions," *American Psychologist* 60 (2005): 410–21. Also see these websites: www.positivepsychology.org and www.apa.org/science/postivepsy/html.

10. Thomas J. Peters and Robert H. Waterman, Jr., *In Search of Excellence: Lessons from America's Best-Run Companies* (New York: Harper & Row, 1982).

11. M. Visintainer, J. Voipicelli, M. Seligman "Tumor Rejection in Rats after Inescapable or Escapable Shock." *Science* 216 (1982): 437–439. Also see story behind this in Martin E. P. Seligman, *Learned Optimism* (New York: Pocket Books: 1990) 169–171.

12. M. J. Raleigh, M. T. McGuire, "Social and Environmental Influences on Blood Serotonin Concentrations in Monkeys," *Archives of General Psychiatry* 41(4) (1984): 405–10; Also M. J. Raleigh, M. T. McGuire, et al., "Serotonergic Mechanisms Promote Dominance Acquisition in Adult Male Vervet Monkeys," *Brain Research* 559(2) (1991): 181–90.

13. M. J. Raleigh, M. T. McGuire, G. L. Brammer, et al., "Serotonergic Mechanisms Promote Dominance Acquisition in Adult Male Vervet Monkeys," *Brain Research* 559(2) (1991): 181–90.

14. Bessel A. van der Kolk, *Psychological Trauma* (Washington, DC: American Psychiatric Press, 1987), 47.

15. D. C. McClelland, G. Ross, V. Patel, "The Effects of an Academic Examination on Salivary Norepineprine and Immunoglobulin Level, "*Journal of Human Stress* 11(2) (1985): 52–9.

16. Foods which supply the amino acid tryptophan include: dairy products, turkey, nuts (walnuts and peanuts are good sources), egg white, soy, fish (cod, halibut, shrimp, crab) and the seaweed spirulina.

17. Some useful guides to cognitive therapy principles include Maxie C. Maultsby, *Rational Behavior Therapy* (Englewood Cliffs, NJ: Prentice-Hall, 1984); Donald Meichenbaum, *Cognitive Behavior Modification: An Integrative Approach* (New York: Plenum Publishing, 1977); and Donald Meichenbaum, *Stress Inoculation Training: A Clinical Guidebook* (Boston: Allyn & Bacon, 1985).

18. Maultsby, *Rational Behavior Therapy.*

19. David Burns, *Feeling Good: The New Mood Therapy* (New York: HarperCollins; 1980 and 1999); see also see http://www.feelinggood.com.

20. Early books describing the clinical use of mindfulness meditation include Jon Kabat-Zinn, *Full Catastrophe Living* (New York: Delacorte Press, 1990); Joan Borysenko, *Minding the Body, Mending the Mind* (New York: Bantam Books, 1988); Herbert Benson, *The Relaxation Response* (New York: Morrow, 1975); Thich Nhat Hanh, *The Miracle of Mindfulness: A Manual of Meditation* (Boston: Beacon Press, 1976); and H. Benson and E. Stuart, *The Wellness Book* (New York: Carol Publishing Group, 1993).

21. Some useful websites for tai chi and yoga include those at the Mayo Clinic: http://www.mayoclinic.com/health/tai-chi/SA00087 http://www.mayoclinic.com/health/yoga/MM00650 http://www.mayoclinic.com/health/yoga/CM00004

22. Martin L. Rossman, *Guided Imagery for Self Healing* (Tiburon, CA: Starseed Press, 2000). This excellent book is viewable online at http://books.google.com/books?id=a9nsXVNGyI0C.

23. William Fezler, *Creative Imagery: How to Visualize in All Senses* (New York: Fireside–Simon & Schuster, 1989).

24. Joan Borysenko, *Guilt Is the Teacher, Love Is the Lesson* (New York: Warner Books, 1990), Chapters 3 and 4.

25. Bellruth Naparstek, *Staying Well with Guided Imagery,* (New York: Wellness Central: 1995) (Headache pp.169–175; Sleep pp. 187–191; Fatigue pp. 192–197). Other websites discussing guided imagery include: http://www.helpstartshere.org/mind_and_spirit/stress_management/current_trends/stress_management_-_current_trends.html http://www.guidedimageryinc.com/guided.html.

26. Adelaide Bry, *Visualization: Directing the Movies of Your Mind* (New York: Harper & Row, 1978).

27. Robin Casarjian, *Forgiveness: A Bold Choice for a Peaceful Heart* (New York: Bantam Books, 1992).

28. W. Ruberman, "Psychosocial Influences on Mortality of Patients with Coronary Artery Disease," *Journal of the American Medical Association* 267 (1992): 559–60.

29. Preamble to the Constitution of the World Health Organization as adopted by the International Health Conference, New York, 19–22, June, 1946; signed on 22 of July 1946 by the representatives of 61 states (Official Records of the World Health Organization, no. 2, p. 100) and entered into force on 7 April 1948.

30. Kabat-Zinn, *Full Catastrophe Living.*

31. J. Bernhard, J. Kirsteller, and J. Kabat-Zinn, "Effectiveness of Relaxation and Visualization Techniques as an Adjunct to Phototherapy and Photo-chemotherapy of Psoriasis," *Journal of the American Academy of Dermatology* 19 (1988): 572–3.

32. C. N. Alexander, et al., "Transcendental Meditation, Mindfulness, and Longevity: An Experimental Study with the Elderly," *Journal of Personality and Social Psychology* 57(6) (1989): 950–964.

33. J. K. Kiecolt-Glaser, et al., "Psychoneuroimmunology and Psychosomatic Medicine: Back to the Future," *Psychosomatic Medicine* 64(1) (2002): 15–28. Also J. K. Kiecolt-Glaser and R. Glaser, "Psychoneuroimmunology: Can Psychological Interventions Modulate Immunity? *Journal of Consulting and Clinical Psychology* 60(4) (1992): 569–75; K. R. Pelletier and D. L. Herzing, *Advances in Mind-Body Medicine* 5, no. 1 (1988): 27–56.

34. A. Meares, "Regression of Cancer after Intensive Meditation," *Medical Journal of Australia* 2(5) (1976): 184.

35. J. Achterberg, P. McGraw, and G. F. Lawis, "Rheumatoid Arthritis: A Study of Relaxation and Temperature Biofeedback as an Adjunctive Therapy," *Biofeedback and Self-Regulation* 6 (1981): 207–23; and K. A. Applebaum, E. B. Blanchard, and E. J. Hickling, "Psychological and Functional Measurement in Severe Rheumatoid Arthritis Before and After Psychological Intervention: A Controlled Evaluation [Summary]," in *Proceedings of the 17th Annual Meeting of the Biofeedback Society of America* (1986), 5–7.

36. L. A. Bradley et al., "Effects of Psychological Therapy on Pain Behavior of Rheumatoid Arthritis Patients," *Arthritis and Rheumatism* 30 (1987): 1105–14.

37. A. O'Leary, S. Shoor, K. Lorig, and H. R. Holman, "A Cognitive-Behavioral Treatment for Rheumatoid Arthritis," *Health Psychology* 7 (1988): 527–44.

38. R. Ader and N. Cohen, "Behaviorally Conditioned Immunosuppression and Murine Systemic Lupur Erythematosus," *Science* 215 (#4539) (1982): 1534–6.

39. R. Ader, "Conditioned Immune Responses and Pharmacotherapy," *Arthritis Care Research* 2(3) (1989): S58–64.

40. Frederick Tilney. *The Brain in Relation to Behavior.* American Museum of Natural History James Arthur Lecture Series, Washington DC, March 15, 1932.

The Elements of Human Fulfillment

According to famed researcher Abraham Maslow, human fulfillment is based on the following characteristics, which describe his studies of self-actualized people:

Growth-motivated rather than deficiency-motivated. As Maslow stated, "The motivation of ordinary men is a striving for the basic need gratifications they lack. But for self-actualizing people, motivation is just character growth, character expression, and maturation." Simply stated, fulfillment rests in the ability to distinguish between living and preparing to live.

Good sense of reality. Self-actualized people, says Maslow, have "an unusual ability to detect the spurious, the fake, and the dishonest in personality. . . . They are far more apt to perceive what is there rather than their own wishes, hopes, fears, anxieties, their own theories (prejudices) and beliefs or those of their cultural group . . . unfrightened by the unknown. . . . Doubt, tentativeness, and uncertainty, which are for most a torture, can be for some a pleasantly stimulating challenge, a high spot in life rather than a low."

Acceptance of self and others. Human fulfillment is characterized by a relative lack of crippling guilt, though self-actualized people do feel bad about the discrepancy between what is and what ought to be; the ability to see through unnecessary guilt and anxiety; the ability to accept the frailties and imperfections of human beings (in other words, the ability to see human nature as it is instead of as they would prefer it to be); a relative lack of disgust and aversion toward average people; a lack of defensiveness, and distaste for such artificiality in others; and an unusual lack of hypocrisy, game-playing, and attempts to impress others.

Honest authenticity and naturalness. Self-actualized people have a tendency toward unconventional thinking, though not necessarily unconventional behavior; an internalized code of high ethics (not necessarily the same as those around them); and a superior awareness of who they are, what they want, and what they believe.

Commitment and problem centering. Self-actualized people have a strong sense of purpose outside themselves—a "task they must do." They are concerned with the good of mankind, and work for that which they love; they have a great sense of care for others. They see problems as a stimulating challenge rather than an intolerable dilemma.

Autonomy. The self-actualized have a greater sense of "free will"; they are less dependent on or determined by their circumstances or other people. Self-movers, they are self-disciplined and have a sense of determining their own destiny through their personal choices.

Independence and resistance to enculturalization. Human fulfillment is characterized by relative independence from the need for approval, respect, and even love; the tendency to act conventionally in affairs regarded as important or unchangeable; and patient entrepreneurialism in wanting to change the status quo for the better.

An element of detachment and privacy. Self-actualized people practice objectivity; they are able to withstand personal misfortunes without reacting as violently as most would.

Continued freshness of appreciation. The self-actualized have, as Maslow states it, "the wonderful capacity to appreciate again and again (with newness), freshly and naively, the basic goods of life, with awe, pleasure, wonder, even ecstasy, however stale these experiences have become to others." They avoid taking things for granted; instead, they "retain a constant sense of good fortune and gratitude for it."

High energy levels, peak experiences. "Their energy is not supernatural," Maslow says of the self-actualized; "it is simply the result of loving life and all the activities in it. They don't know how to be bored. . . . They are aggressively curious. They never know enough. They search for more and want to learn each and every present moment of their lives. . . . They are mystic, with peak experiences of transcendence of self; they have a sense of limitless horizons opening up to vision, coupled with ecstasy and a transforming feeling of strength."

Deep interpersonal relations. Human fulfillment is characterized by the capability of more fusion, intimacy, and obliteration of ego boundaries than seen in most people. The self-actualized tend to be kind to—or at least patient with—almost everyone, particularly children, yet they often have few profoundly close relationships because of the time required to maintain them. When they express hostility, it is not toward someone's character but to achieve some good end.

Democratic character structure. The self-actualized are oblivious to barriers of class, education, politics, or race; they possess a certain sense of humility that allows them to learn from anyone and to be aware of how little they know when compared with what could be known.

Discrimination between ends and means. Ethically, the self-actualized believe that means are subordinated to ends, but means are usually enjoyed as ends in themselves. Simply, the self-actualized appreciate the process of doing for its own sake.

Philosophical, unhostile sense of humor. Humor for the self-actualized is usually directed at self or at people who are trying to be big when they are small; humor extends to work—which, though taken seriously, is approached with a sense of play. They find that humor often has an educational function beyond the simple value of laughter.

Creativity. The self-actualized are often not creative in the usual artistic forms; their creativity is more a process and attitude than a product. Their creativity extends to a way of approaching all of life; they find fresh, direct solutions with naive newness.

Guiltless acceptance of sexuality. For the self-actualized, sex is fused with love and full of underlying intimacy; they do not usually seek sex for its own sake. Theirs is a paradox: They seem to enjoy their sexuality far more than average, yet consider it much less important.

Resolution of complementary opposites. Finally, the self-actualized seem to enjoy—even thrive on—differences rather than fear them. They creatively seek overarching principles that make seeming opposites synergic (complementary) rather than antagonistic; peak experiences often occur during the resolution.

Source: Abraham Maslow, *Motivation and Personality* (New York: Harper & Row, 1954).

The Seven Habits of Highly Effective People

According to Steven R. Covey, the seven habits of highly effective people are as follows:

1. **Be proactive.** Use the responsible free will to act as you desire, with integrity.

2. **Begin with the end in mind.** Have clearly defined values; cultivate a sense of purpose and mission; and visualize the results ahead of time.

3. **Put first things first.** Be able to distinguish core values from lesser values and act with integrity toward the deeper ones (with discipline and sacrifice as necessary).

4. **Think win/win.** Aim for mutual acceptance and empowerment; strive for connectedness; and build on integrity, maturity, and an abundance mentality.

5. **Seek first to understand, then to be understood.** Use caring love and acceptance and a sense of connectedness when dealing with others.

6. **Synergize.** Accept, and even appreciate, differences; try creative cooperation and connectedness; work from a common sense of mission and purpose; and have a positive expectation.

7. **Renew yourself.** Experience a sense of purpose and mission (commitment); continued growth; and meditative reflection and visualization.

Source: Stephen R. Covey, *The Seven Habits of Highly Effective People* (New York: Fireside–Simon & Schuster, 1989).

The Misunderstood Alternative: Effective Type B Personality Characteristics of Those Proven to Be Protected from Heart Disease

People with type B personality characteristics are often peak performers and hold many top positions. Below are protective traits that need fostering:

No time urgency

- More mindful in giving attention to the central task at hand
- Not easily bored or eager to move on to something else
- Usually keeps on schedule but without frenzy or rage
- Patient (no habitual haste)
- Contemplative: enjoys beauty and metaphor, tends to see the whole more than the parts
- Able to value and enjoy the things already done, or being now done, as much as those things to be done in the future

Able to relinquish control

- Good at delegation; team players—comfortable with this
- Tolerant of differences—even enjoys them
- Often good at inspiring creative involvement with others—good leaders

An internal locus of high self-value

- Appreciates self for what he or she *is* as much as what he or she *does*
- Accepts and values self as is
- Understands that self-identity and worth are far more important than numbers
- Feels valued and of worth regardless of achievement (often derived from parents)
- Often works as hard at something as type A's, but failure does not collapse self-esteem
- Loves growth, getting better (often through mistakes)
- Competes with self rather than with others

No free-floating hostility

- No need to find fault to bolster own ego
- Can accept with equanimity the trivial errors of subordinates ("They practice the art of being wise by knowing what to disregard.")
- Enjoys empowering and lifting others
- Uncommonly feels tense or induces tension in others
- Their self-confidence allows objectivity and ability to see through another's eyes
- Capable of both feeling and expressing affection—enjoys intimate Relationships

Source: See the discussion of the characteristics of noncoronary prone individuals in M. Friedman and D. Ulmer: *Treating Type A Behavior and Your Heart* (New York: Fawcett, 1984), chap 3.

Name Index

Subject Index